Temporal Bone Cancer

Paul W. Gidley · Franco DeMonte
Editors

Temporal Bone Cancer

Springer

Editors
Paul W. Gidley
Department of Head and Neck Surgery,
Otology-Neurotology
The University of Texas M.D. Anderson
Cancer Center
Houston, TX
USA

Franco DeMonte
Department of Neurosurgery
The University of Texas M.D. Anderson
Cancer Center
Houston, TX
USA

ISBN 978-3-030-09015-9 ISBN 978-3-319-74539-8 (eBook)
https://doi.org/10.1007/978-3-319-74539-8

Printed on acid-free paper

This Springer imprint is published by the registered company Springer International Publishing AG part of Springer Nature
The registered company address is: Gewerbestrasse 11, 6330 Cham, Switzerland

To my wife, Milvia. Thanks for your support and sacrifice over the years.

Paul W. Gidley, M.D.

To my wife, Paula. After more than 30 years together it would fill another book with all the reasons why!

Franco DeMonte, M.D.

Preface

This book comprehensively discusses temporal bone cancer. A book dedicated to this rare disease has been sorely needed. Primary squamous cell carcinoma of the temporal bone is rare, occurring in perhaps 1 person/million population/year. However, given the superficial nature of the external ear and ear canal and its proximity to the parotid gland and nearby lymph nodes, the temporal bone is frequently invaded by tumors from external ear, parotid or periauricular skin cancers.

The rarity of this disease has made it difficult to study and understand. Large, single institution studies generally include less than 100 patients. This book gathers the accumulated literature on temporal bone cancer into one volume and synthesizes this information into a usable reference.

Historically, primary temporal bone tumors had a dismal prognosis. Surgical resection of these large tumors could only rarely achieve negative margins and usually with significant morbidity. Newer techniques of radiotherapy and newer chemotherapeutic agents have offered patients with advanced disease an improved survival. Understanding the role of surgery and the place for adjuvant therapy is an important theme throughout this book.

This book is organized into four sections: (1) evaluation, (2) tumor types and behavior, (3) treatment options, and (4) rehabilitation and quality of life. The chapters on evaluation highlight the important aspects of the physical examination, radiologic evaluation, and pathologic diagnosis. Staging is critical for proper treatment and is discussed in detail. Next, several chapters are dedicated to the different tumor types that affect the ear canal and temporal bone. These chapters begin with the most common tumor type, squamous cell carcinoma, and proceed to cover many minor, rare, or unusual tumors. A chapter is devoted to the evaluation and management of hematologic malignancies and another to metastatic cancers to the temporal bone. Treatment options include surgery, radiotherapy, and chemotherapy. The many different surgical procedures are divided into separate chapters to highlight the indications, preoperative considerations, operative details and decisions, and the proper postoperative management. Radiotherapy and chemotherapy each have their own chapters outlining the newest techniques and protocols for temporal bone cancer. Temporal bone cancer and its treatment are often associated with facial paralysis, hearing loss, and changes to physical appearance. Chapters are dedicated to the rehabilitation of the paralyzed face, management of the eye, osseointegrated implants for hearing loss, and prosthetic rehabilitation for loss of the outer ear. The book culminates in a chapter devoted to quality of life, which has not been well studied in temporal bone cancer patients.

The experience presented in this book has been gained by a team of physicians who have seen more than 400 patients with tumors that affect the ear canal and temporal bone. The photographs, diagnostic imaging, and photomicrographs come from our patient population. We are indebted to our patients for giving us the privilege of serving them, and we are awed by the courage they demonstrate as they confront temporal bone cancer. Improving survival and treatment outcomes drives research on temporal bone cancer. The editors hope that readers will use the accumulated knowledge about temporal bone cancer to avoid the mistakes of the past and strive for greater advances in understanding, preventing, and treating this form of cancer.

Houston, TX, USA

Paul W. Gidley
Franco DeMonte

Contents

Contributors

Richard C. Allen, M.D., Ph.D., F.A.C.S. Section of Ophthalmology, Department of Head and Neck Surgery, The University of Texas M.D. Anderson Cancer Center, Houston, TX, USA

John R. de Almeida, M.D., M.Sc. Department of Otolaryngology — Head and Neck Surgery, University Health Network, Toronto, ON, Canada

Department of Otolaryngology — Head and Neck Surgery, Princess Margaret Cancer Centre, University of Toronto, Toronto, ON, Canada

Blair Barton, M.D. Department of Otorhinolaryngology — Head and Neck Surgery, Ochsner Health System, New Orleans, LA, USA

Beth M. Beadle, M.D., Ph.D. Department of Radiation Oncology, Stanford University, Palo Alto, CA, USA

Diana Bell, M.D. Departments of Pathology and Head and Neck Surgery, The University of Texas M.D. Anderson Cancer Center, Houston, TX, USA

G. Brandon Gunn, M.D. Department of Radiation Oncology, The University of Texas M.D. Anderson Cancer Center, Houston, TX, USA

Joseph T. Breen, M.D. Cincinnati, OH, USA

Matthew L. Bush, M.D., Ph.D. Department of Otolaryngology — Head and Neck Surgery, University of Kentucky Medical Center, Lexington, KY, USA

Mark S. Chambers, D.M.D., M.S. Section of Oral Oncology and Maxillofacial Prosthodontics, Department of Head and Neck Surgery, The University of Texas M.D. Anderson Cancer Center, Houston, TX, USA

Albert H. Chao, M.D. The Ohio State University Plastic Surgery, Columbus, OH, USA

Steven B. Chinn, M.D., M.P.H. Department of Otolaryngology — Head and Neck Surgery, University of Michigan Health System, Ann Arbor, MI, USA

J. Matthew Debnam, M.D. Section of Neuroradiology, The University of Texas M.D. Anderson Cancer Center, Houston, TX, USA

Franco DeMonte, M.D. Department of Neurosurgery, The University of Texas M.D. Anderson Cancer Center, Houston, TX, USA

Orlando M. Diaz, M.D. Department of Radiology, Houston Neurovascular Center, Houston, TX, USA

Renata Ferrarotto, M.D. Thoracic-Head and Neck Medical Oncology, Houston, TX, USA

Nathan Fowler, M.D. Department of Head and Neck Surgery, The University of Texas M.D. Anderson Cancer Center, Houston, TX, USA

Christopher D. Frisch, M.D. Department of Otolaryngology, Olmsted Medical Center, Rochester, MN, USA

Paul W. Gidley, M.D., F.A.C.S. Department of Head and Neck Surgery, The University of Texas M.D. Anderson Cancer Center, Houston, TX, USA

Matthew M. Hanasono, M.D. Department of Plastic Surgery, The University of Texas M.D. Anderson Cancer Center, Houston, TX, USA

Theresa M. Hofstede, D.D.S., F.A.C.P. Section of Oral Oncology and Maxillofacial Prosthodontics, Department of Head and Neck Surgery, The University of Texas M.D. Anderson Cancer Center, Houston, TX, USA

Badr Ibrahim, M.D. Division of Otolaryngology — Head and Neck Surgery, Université de Montréal, Centre Hospitalier de l'Université de Montréal (CHUM), Montreal, QC, Canada

Merrill S. Kies, M.D. Thoracic-Head and Neck Medical Oncology, Houston, TX, USA

Jamie A. Ku, M.D. Cleveland Clinic Head and Neck Institute, Cleveland, OH, USA

Elton Lambert, M.D. Pediatric Otolaryngology, Texas Children's Hospital/Baylor College of Medicine, Houston, TX, USA

Brandon D. Liebelt, M.D. Department of Neurosurgery, Methodist Hospital, Houston, TX, USA

Patricia C. Montgomery Section of Oral Oncology and Maxillofacial Prosthodontics, Department of Head and Neck Surgery, The University of Texas M.D. Anderson Cancer Center, Houston, TX, USA

Brian Moore, M.D. Department of Otorhinolaryngology — Head and Neck Surgery, Ochsner Health System, New Orleans, LA, USA

Jeffrey N. Myers, M.D., Ph.D. Department of Head and Neck Surgery, The University of Texas M.D. Anderson Cancer Center, Houston, TX, USA

Marc-Elie Nader, M.D., M.Sc., F.R.C.S.C. Division of Otolaryngology — Head and Neck Surgery, Université de Montréal, Centre Hospitalier de l'Université de Montréal (CHUM), Montreal, QC, Canada

Department of Head and Neck Surgery, The University of Texas M.D. Anderson Cancer Center, Houston, TX, USA

Sweet Ping Ng, M.B.B.S., B.Med.Sci. Department of Radiation Oncology, The University of Texas M.D. Anderson Cancer Center, Houston, TX, USA

Issam Saliba, M.D., F.R.C.S.C. Division of Otolaryngology — Head and Neck Surgery, Université de Montréal, Centre Hospitalier de l'Université de Montréal (CHUM), Montreal, QC, Canada

Robert A. Scranton, M.D. Department of Radiology, Houston Neurovascular Center, Houston, TX, USA

Natalie L. Silver, M.D., M.S. Department of Otolaryngology, University of Florida, Gainesville, FL, USA

Erich M. Sturgis, M.D., M.P.H. Department of Head and Neck Surgery, The University of Texas M.D. Anderson Cancer Center, Houston, TX, USA

Department of Epidemiology, The University of Texas M.D. Anderson Cancer Center, Houston, TX, USA

Christopher and Susan Damico Chair in Viral Associated Malignancies, The University of Texas M.D. Anderson Cancer Center, Houston, TX, USA

Randal S. Weber, M.D. Department of Head and Neck Surgery, The University of Texas M.D. Anderson Cancer Center, Houston, TX, USA

Owen Woods, M.D., M.Sc. Division of Otolaryngology — Head and Neck Surgery, Université de Montréal, Hôpital Maisonneuve-Rosemont, Montreal, QC, Canada

Overview and Historical Developments

1

Paul W. Gidley

Overview

The time has come for a book dedicated to the evaluation and management of temporal bone cancer. A rich literature on temporal bone cancer has accumulated over the years. A simple PubMed search using "temporal bone cancer" reveals more than 5000 articles, with more than 2700 published in the last 20 years. The outstanding articles in this body of literature are cited throughout the chapters in this book.

The main impetus to writing this book has been to encapsulate the learning and experience gained on managing temporal bone cancer. While cancers that involve the temporal bone are very rare, many of the recommendations in this textbook are based on the experience gained from managing over 400 patients with temporal bone cancer. These patients present with a wide array of tumor burden, from very small to prodigious primary tumors. Our approach to management utilizes a comprehensive, multidisciplinary team that includes otology-neurotology, head and neck surgery, neurosurgery, plastic and reconstructive surgery, oculoplastic surgery, anaplastology, audiology, medical oncology, and radiotherapy. These patients are evaluated by team members, and a comprehensive treatment plan is discussed and agreed upon at our weekly Tumor Board.

It is important to recognize that temporal bone cancer covers a wide range of tumor types and tumor locations. While squamous cell carcinoma (SCC) is the most common tumor to involve the temporal bone, many different primary tumor types can occur within the temporal bone. Squamous cell carcinoma is remarkable since it can be found as a primary tumor in the external auditory canal, middle ear, and mastoid. Other tumor types tend to have a more specific site of origin. For instance, adenoid cystic carcinoma occurs primarily in the ear canal since it arises from cerumen glands. Carcinoid tumors usually arise within the middle ear. Endolymphatic sac tumors (ELSTs) arise from the endolymphatic sac; and, as such, they destroy the posterior portion of the temporal bone.

These tumor types have vastly different behaviors. SCC has a propensity toward aggressive invasion and the potential for metastatic spread to parotid and cervical lymph nodes. Recurrence can occur within 2 years, and death quickly follows. In comparison, adenoid cystic carcinoma of the ear canal has proclivity for perineural spread and a tendency for delayed, distant metastasis. Recurrences can occur 10–15 years after primary tumor resection and are usually in the lungs. Both carcinoid tumors and ELSTs tend to recur locally if not completely excised, and their metastatic potential is very low. Clearly these tumor types have very different natural histories and behaviors should not be lumped together. Many chapters are dedicated to separate tumor pathologies in order to explore the natural histories of various histologic types.

Primary tumors of the temporal bone are rare. The incidence is perhaps one to two cases/million population/year. Skin cancer is very common, with an incidence of about 2800 cases/million population/year, with 75% of these occurring within the head and neck. The position and outstanding nature of the external ear makes it vulnerable to damaging rays from the sun. The temporal bone, especially the ear canal, is more likely to be involved secondarily by primary tumors of the periauricular skin and parotid gland (Fig. 1.1) [1].

The disease under the moniker "temporal bone cancer" seems to be changing. In the twentieth century, many case reports and case series showed high numbers of patients with chronic otitis media or chronic otorrhea as a precursor to squamous cell carcinoma of the ear canal, middle ear, or mastoid. In the setting of chronic infection, previous mastoidectomy patients developed large, fungating tumors that quickly spread throughout the temporal bone without the restriction of the ear canal wall. These patients seem to be less frequently encountered today in the USA than was previously reported.

P. W. Gidley, M.D., F.A.C.S.
Department of Head and Neck Surgery, The University of Texas M.D. Anderson Cancer Center, Houston, TX, USA
e-mail: pwgidley@mdanderson.org

P. W. Gidley, F. DeMonte (eds.), *Temporal Bone Cancer*, https://doi.org/10.1007/978-3-319-74539-8_1

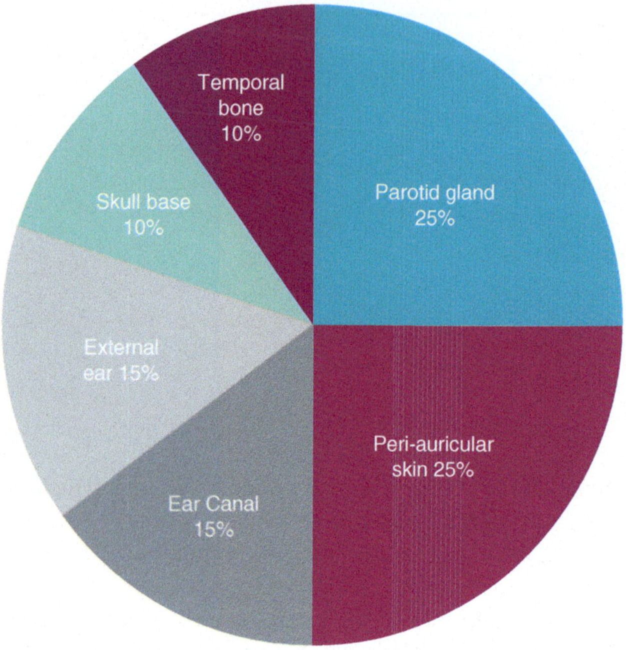

Fig. 1.1 Location of temporal bone primary tumors from the Department of Head and Neck Surgery at MD Anderson Cancer Center (used with permission from Gidley PW, DeMonte F. Temporal bone malignancies. Neurosurgery clinics of North America. 2013;24(1):97–110)

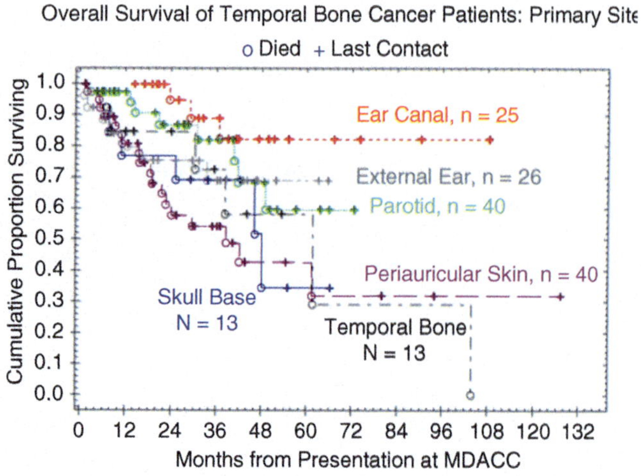

Fig. 1.2 Overall survival (used with permission from Gidley PW, Thompson CR, Roberts DB, et al. The oncology of otology Laryngoscope 2012;122(2):393–400) [2]

The reasons for this change are unclear. Perhaps the management of chronic otitis media has improved, and the persistent draining ear is much less common. Alternatively, as skin cancer rates have risen, more skin cancers occur which grow to involve the ear canal or temporal bone. Nonetheless, the percentage of temporal bone cancer patients with a history of chronic otitis media is decreasing.

The ear canal, external ear, mastoid and middle ear, parotid, periauricular skin, and skull base are all potential sites of primary tumors that involve the temporal bone. Some very large tumors involve the temporal bone, making it difficult to determine the site of origin. Establishing the site of origin is important since the overall survival varies widely based on tumor location (Fig. 1.2) [2].

Furthermore, staging systems are based on primary tumor location and extent. The staging of temporal bone cancer is discussed in Chap. 2. The staging system for skin cancer differs from the Pittsburgh staging system for temporal bone cancer in multiple ways (Chap. 6). An external ear cancer is properly staged using the AJCC system for skin cancer, while an external auditory canal cancer is properly staged using the Pittsburgh staging system. Melanoma and sarcoma have vastly different staging systems. Proper staging helps in treatment selection, allows appropriate comparisons on disease burden, and permits projections about prognosis.

As outlined in the History section of this chapter, many different surgical approaches have been developed to manage temporal bone cancer. The salient feature of surgical management is obtaining tumor-free margins. The very definition of "unresectable" is a final positive margin. Many factors contribute to unresectability in temporal bone cancer surgery. First, bone cannot be examined using frozen section technique. Second, resecting an important structure, such as the internal carotid artery, to obtain a negative margin might result in significant disability. Third, disease may have spread outside the temporal bone, such as to the lower cranial nerves or paraspinal muscles. Lastly, the anatomy of the temporal bone can make surgery within it difficult.

Management strategies and survival outcomes have greatly improved over the last century. For SCC and other tumors confined to the ear canal, the lateral temporal bone resection accomplishes an en bloc, no-touch, tumor-free margin and is associated with high rates of overall survival. The reason seems to be obvious, in that the tumor is confined by the bony canal. Santorini and Hyrtl's fissures are preformed pathways that facilitate spread to the parotid gland, the temporomandibular joint, or infratemporal fossa. These anatomic pathways permit spread of disease outside of the ear canal, and they contribute to shorter overall survival.

Much lower overall survival rates are reported for tumors that involve the middle ear or mastoid. In analogous terms, the eardrum can be considered the Ohngren's line for temporal bone cancer. In maxillary sinus cancers, Ohngren's line divides the sinus into an inferior-anterior compartment that has a favorable prognosis and a posterior-superior compartment that has a poor prognosis [3]. For the temporal bone, tumors that are contained within the ear canal have a more favorable prognosis than tumors that have spread from the ear canal to involve the middle ear.

Once tumors have invaded the middle ear, the air cell system allows unimpeded spread of malignant disease. The mastoid air cell system, the Eustachian tube, the jugular foramen, the carotid canal, and natural dehiscences in the tegmen each allow the spread of tumor to sites outside of the temporal bone. For this reason, tumors of the middle ear, mastoid, and other parts of the temporal bone are much harder to control surgically than tumors confined to the ear canal.

Several chapters in this book are dedicated to the surgical approaches to tumors in various parts of the temporal bone. Each surgical approach has unique challenges; however, the basic tenet remains the same: achieving a negative margin. The pursuit of a negative margin has led to wider and more extensive surgical resections, often entailing large soft tissue and bony defects.

Large soft tissue defects require proper reconstruction. Perhaps one of the greatest advances for the management of head and neck cancer has been the development and refinement of microvascular free tissue transfer. The role of free flaps is explored in the chapter on reconstruction of temporal bone defects. Facial paralysis is common in temporal bone cancer, and rehabilitation of the paralyzed face and care for the paralyzed eyelids are discussed in detail.

History has shown that surgery alone is not sufficient management for most temporal bone cancers beyond T2 stage tumors. Radiotherapy has been used as a definitive treatment and adjuvant treatment for temporal bone cancers since the birth of this medical field. The subsequent history section outlines some of the early pioneers of this modality. The efficacy of radiotherapy for primary temporal bone cancers has been established in its role as adjuvant, postoperative therapy. Multidrug chemotherapy protocols have been developed for the management of advanced head and neck cancer. A role for chemotherapy is emerging in the treatment of temporal bone cancer.

As part of the primary treatment plan, consideration must be given to hearing and cosmetic rehabilitation. Prosthetic rehabilitation of hearing can be through the use of osseointegrated implants and cochlear stimulators. These implants and speech processors replace the sound conducting mechanism of the ear canal and ossicular chain and help to restore hearing in those patients with an intact cochlea. Anaplastologists create extremely life-like prosthetic external ears which can be attached with either osseointegrated implants or adhesives to give patients an improved body image.

History of Temporal Bone Cancer

It has been 100 years since the first case series of temporal bone cancer was assembled by Newhart in 1907 [4]. Over these years, a significant body of literature has developed regarding cancers that affect the temporal bone. Observations have been made regarding the clinical presentation, natural history, histopathology, treatment, and outcomes for these tumors. Many different diagnostic techniques, staging systems, and treatment strategies have been proposed along the way. The authors who contributed to this body of knowledge were leaders in the field of otolaryngology, plastic surgery, radiotherapy, and neurosurgery. This section strives to provide the first comprehensive review on the subject of the history of temporal bone cancer treatment.

Developing the Diagnosis

In the nineteenth century, the field of otology was full of incompetents and charlatans [5]. Many treatments, elixirs, salves, and surgical procedures were proposed to treat hearing loss, tinnitus, and chronic ear infections. Few of these treatments produced beneficial results. Perhaps the only ear complaint that could be alleviated at the time was cerumen impaction.

In the middle of the nineteenth century, several individuals in Ireland, England, Austria-Hungary, France, and Germany began to dedicate themselves to the study of ear maladies. The first description of squamous cell carcinoma of the temporal bone was independently described by Drs. William Wilde and Hermann Schwartze in 1875 [6]. This date is erroneously cited as 1775 by Furstenberg [7] and repeated by subsequent authors [8, 9].

William Wilde (1815–1876) was the son of a physician and grew up in Roscommon in Ireland (Fig. 1.3). He learned medicine and surgery as an apprentice to Abraham Colles (1773–1843; known for Colles' fracture) in 1832. He also studied at Park Street Medical School of Trinity College under Robert James Graves (1796–1853; known for Graves' disease) and William Stokes (1804–1878; known for Stokes-Adams syndrome and Cheyne-Stokes respirations). As a young medical student, he saved a child's life by performing a tracheostomy [10].

During his last year of medical school, he contracted a severe fever; and Graves arranged for him to convalesce as a private physician to a wealthy patient aboard his private yacht, sailing to the Holy Lands. Upon return to Ireland, Wilde published his account of this adventure and the archeologic findings in a two-volume set, which brought him

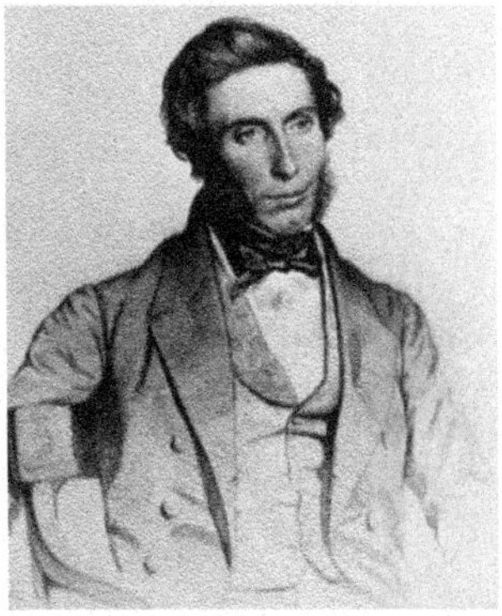

Fig. 1.3 William Wilde (public domain, https://commons.wikimedia.org/wiki/File%3AWilliam_Wilde_young.jpg)

financial success and fame throughout Ireland [11]. Shortly after this, the first of his three illegitimate children, Henry Wilson (1838–1877), was born. Wilson went on to become a famous Irish ophthalmologist in his own right. This book's success allowed Wilde to study ear and eye disorders in Vienna.

Wilde returned to Ireland and dedicated his early career to tending to the lower classes; news of his talent spread to the upper classes through their servants and maids [12]. Wilde's work elevated otology to clinical and scientific respectability [5]. He founded St. Mark's Hospital in 1844, which was the forerunner to the Royal Victoria Eye and Ear Hospital. He edited the *Dublin Quarterly Journal of Medical Science*, now called *The Irish Journal of Medical Science*. He wrote an early textbook on ear surgery in 1853 [13].

During the potato famine of 1845–1849, Wilde was appointed the census commissioner and recorded the progress of the famine in minute detail. He showed great ability in organizing and presenting statistical data, and he added questions about the "deaf and dumb," which led him to be the first to identify inherited forms of hearing loss. He was later knighted for this statistical and census work in 1864 [14].

He is known for Wilde's reflex (the light reflex) and Wilde's incision (the postauricular incision) for mastoid suppuration. However, his son, Oscar Wilde, the playwright and poet, probably has greater name recognition in today's era. Ironically, Oscar Wilde died of meningoencephalitis secondary to chronic otitis media [15].

Hermann Schwartze (1837–1910) was born in Neuhof, Germany, the son of a gentleman farmer (Fig. 1.4). He studied medicine in Wurzburg and Berlin, receiving his medical degree in 1853 from the University of Berlin. He studied ear disease under Anton von Tröltsch (1829–1890), known for the pouches of von Tröltsch in the middle ear. Schwartze settled in Halle and was professor of otology at the University of Halle. He published several textbooks on ear anatomy and pathology [16–18]. He described simple mastoidectomy using hammer and gouge (Schwartze mastoidectomy) in 1873, and his technique spread throughout the world as a treatment for chronic otitis media [19]. He is best remembered for his eponymous sign, a reddish discoloration behind the tympanic membrane seen in otosclerosis. In 1864, Schwartze, von Tröltsch, and Adam Politzer founded the *Archiv für Ohrenheilkunde*, the first journal dedicated to ear disorders. In the last years of his life, Schwartze suffered from a "nervous condition of restlessness, vertigo, and delusions." He died of heart failure at age 73. The Hermann-Schwartze medal at the University of Halle is named in his honor.

The first description of cancer involving the temporal bone with pathologic confirmation is attributed to Adam Politzer in 1883 [20]. Politzer (1835–1920) was a world famous Viennese physician and surgeon and is considered the founder of otology (Fig. 1.5). He developed many techniques and instruments for otologic examination and surgery. His book, *A Textbook of Diseases of the Ear*, became a standard treatise on otologic conditions and was translated into many languages. In his textbook, he gave an accurate description of cancer in the ear and temporal bone. He reported three cases; the first began in the outer ear and spread to include the ear canal and middle ear and progressed to the dura until death ensued. He reported a second tumor that began within the ear canal and spread to include the frontal bone, sphenoid wing, and inner ear and produced ipsilateral blindness, facial paralysis, and palate weakness. The third case began on the outer ear and extended to the ear canal. Histologically, this tumor invaded the bony spaces of the temporal bone and led him to conclude that surgery is not successful for treating this late-stage disease.

The great otologist and audiologist, Friedrich Bezold (1842–1908), at the University of Munich, only encountered four cases of ear carcinoma in his 24 years [21]. Bezold is

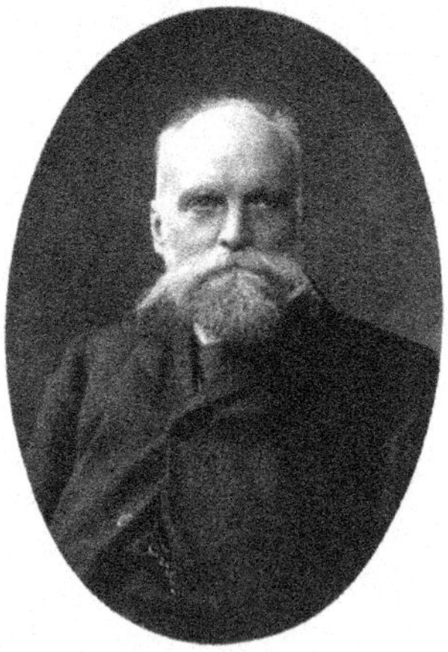

Fig. 1.4 Hermann Schwartze (public domain, https://commons.wikimedia.org/wiki/File%3AHermann_Schwartze.jpg)

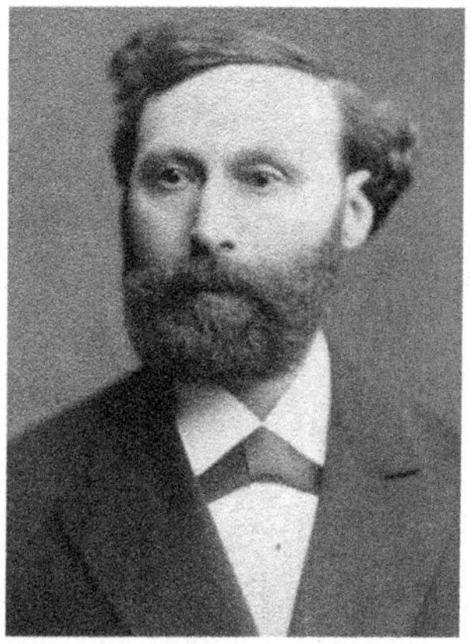

Fig. 1.5 Adam Politzer (public domain, https://commons.wikimedia.org/wiki/File%3ARudolf_Krziwanek_-_Adam_Politzer.jpg)

best remembered for his eponymous abscess caused by suppurative breakdown of the digastric ridge leading to neck abscess. Kretschmann complied 4 of his own cases of temporal bone cancer from private practice with 12 cases from the literature in 1887 [22]. Zeroni produced an exhaustive review of the literature from 1804 to 1899 and found 121 ear and temporal bone tumors, including 2 of his own cases [23]; however, the primary source could not be found.

The first large literature review published in the American literature was by Dr. Horace Newhart (1872–1945) of Minneapolis, Minnesota (Fig. 1.6). He cataloged and described 34 cases in the literature, and he noted that 85% had chronically discharging ears [4]. Newhart obtained his medical degree at the University of Michigan (1898) and performed postgraduate training in Vienna. He took three trips to Vienna, spending about 3 years in total there. It is unclear if he studied with Politzer. He became Director of the Division of Otolaryngology at University of Minnesota [24]. He wrote several articles on the ear and hearing, especially on testing hearing in children and the use of hearing aids. His article on carcinoma of the middle ear is his most highly cited paper. He served as president of the American Otological Society in 1939–1940.

Ceruminoma was first described by Rud Haug, from the Universitäts-Ohrenpoliklinik, Munich, Germany, in 1894 [25]. Haug wrote 11 papers, and this one on ceruminoma was his most highly cited paper. Unfortunately many tumors were classified under this moniker, thus creating confusion for years about the natural history and behavior of ear canal tumors [25]. Given the confusion attached to this term, it was later rendered obsolete by the World Health Organization in 1991.

In 1898, Leopold Treitel of Berlin described the first case of adenocarcinoma of the middle ear [26]. In his paper he describes a 77-year-old woman with a history of lightheadedness and dizziness. She had a tumor involving the middle ear and mastoid. The hand-drawn depiction of the microscopic findings shows a clear papillary pattern to this tumor. Nearly, 100 years later, in 1989, Dennis K. Heffner, Armed Forces Institute of Pathology, proposed that papillary adenocarcinoma of the petrous bone is derived from the endolymphatic sac [27]. His paper on lower-grade papillary adenocarcinoma of the endolymphatic sac is his most highly cited paper.

Piecemeal resection of temporal bone cancers was first reported by Hermann Heyer of Worms, Germany, in 1899 [28]. His paper describes how he excised this tumor under chloroform anesthesia. A wide resection involving the zygoma, parotid, sigmoid sinus, and temporal bone down to the cochlea was accomplished. The dura remained intact. This procedure was performed without the use of an operating microscope, high-speed drill, or electrocautery. Hemostasis was achieved with an iodoform-soaked gauze. The resulting wound was allowed to heal by secondary intention with granulation tissue, and the patient was discharged from hospital 1 month later. The patient apparently returned back to work until his tumor recurred on the dura at the margin of the excision; and he died about 1 year after the operation. Heyer advocated such an operation as palliation since the only alternative was morphine.

Furstenberg (1924) from the University of Michigan reported on two cases of temporal bone cancer out of 40,000 patients seen at the University of Michigan [7]. He recommended radical excision by radical mastoidectomy, "employment of a technique that will allow inspection of the cavity for the remainder of the patient's life" for future cauterizations in the event of recurrence. Albert Carl Furstenberg (1890–1969) was born in Saginaw, Michigan, and graduated from the University of Michigan with a BS degree in 1913 and from the medical school in 1915 (Fig. 1.7). He remained there for residency training under Dr. Roy Bishop Canfield and for his entire professional career [29]. He was promoted to professor and chairman of Otolaryngology at the University of Michigan in 1932. In 1934, he initiated a 4-year residency program in otolaryngology, preceding by 30 years this requirement in the USA. In 1935, he was named

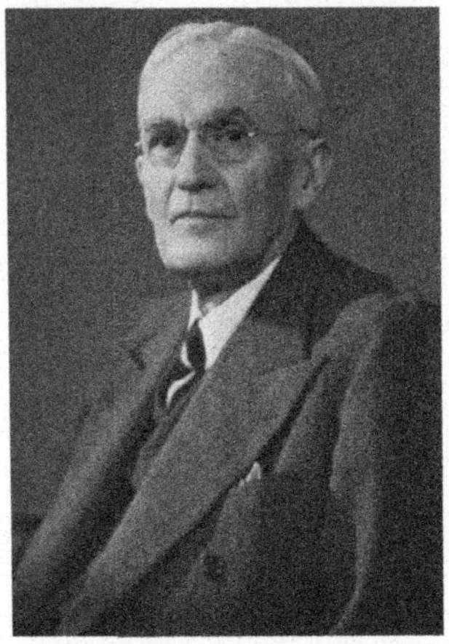

Fig. 1.6 Horace Newhart (photo reprinted with permission) [24]

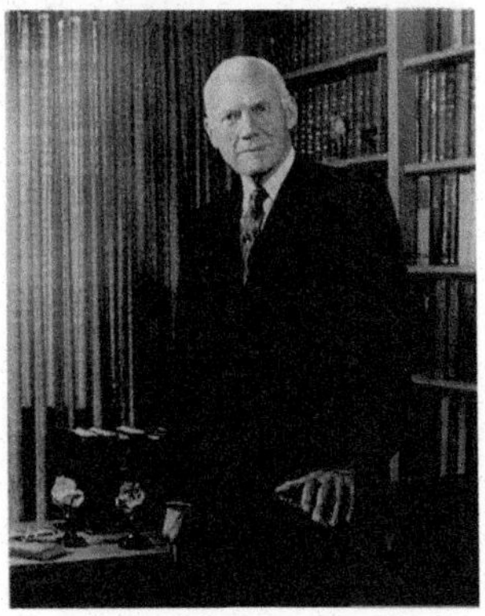

Fig. 1.7 A.C. Furstenberg (reprinted with permission) [29]

dean of the medical school and remained in that position for 28 years [30]. Under his direction the University of Michigan Medical School grew remarkably, adding eight new buildings to the medical center and founding the Kresge Hearing Research Institute. He was a tremendous promoter of medical education and research in otolaryngology [31, 32]. His greatest contribution to otology is recognizing the amelioration of Meniere's disease with sodium restriction [33]. He served two terms as president of the Triological Society and a term as president of the American Association of Medical Colleges (1946) and president of the American Otological Society (1953) [29]. He died in 1969 after suffering a subarachnoid hemorrhage.

Development of Radical Mastoidectomy and Radiotherapy

In 1930 Fraser recommended radical surgery followed by radium or radiation [34]. J.S. Fraser (1874–1936) was a Scottish otologist who studied in London and Vienna (Fig. 1.8). In 1905 he became a fellow in the Royal College of Surgeons of Edinburgh. He was recognized as a world expert on temporal bone pathology, and he later became president of the Otological Section of the Royal Society of Medicine in 1927–1928 [35, 36].

In 1935, Thorell in Stockholm reported on 13 patients with temporal bone cancer treated with radium [37]. Dr. Ivan Thorell wrote many papers on the therapeutic use of radium. A biography or obituary of him could not be located.

In 1943, Figi and Hempstead from the Mayo Clinic were first to report a large series of patients with middle ear and mastoid cancer including radical mastoidectomy, electrodessication, and implantation of radium [38]. Their report covers 48 patients with cancers in the middle ear and mastoid of whom 10 cases were beyond treatment, and they quote an incidence at the Mayo Clinic of 0.003% of all patients registered. This paper set the treatment for the next decade and was highly cited by contemporary authors [39]. This form of treatment always meant radiating an open mastoid cavity.

Frederick A Figi (1892–1970) was an alumnus of the University of Nebraska and was a fellow at the Mayo Clinic in 1918 and served that institution for 39 years (Fig. 1.9). He received his American Board of Otolaryngology certification in 1926. He specialized in head and neck cancer, especially laryngeal cancer, and he earned the nickname "fearless Fred." He was unusually short and required specially made surgical gowns and operating room steps. During his time at the Mayo Clinic, the medical specialties were not sorted out in their current form, and he served in the section of Plastic Surgery and Laryngology. Later in life, Figi dedicated himself to plastic and reconstructive surgery. He served as the president of the American Society of Plastic and Reconstructive Surgeons and as chair of the American Board of Plastic Surgery in 1957–1958.

In a second paper, Figi writes, "If it is true that here 'fools rush in where angels fear to tread,' it is no less true that a defeatist attitude and a halfhearted attempt at eradication on the part of the surgeon is tantamount to the death sentence for most patients" [40]. In this report he recommended radical mastoidectomy, occasionally preceded by ligation of the carotid artery and electrocoagulation of tumor, followed by implantation of radium and subsequent external beam radiation. The wound was packed with iodoform gauze impregnated with petrolatum and allowed to heal by secondary intention. Unfortunately, despite these extreme and heroic efforts, he could not show a survival benefit.

Adams and Morrison in 1955 described a case series of 27 patients from the UK [41]. It must be borne in mind that these patients with middle ear and mastoid cancers were examined only with plain radiographs and that mastoidectomy was not only therapeutic but also diagnostic. They cite the method of Figi and Hempstead as the usual course of treatment. Radiotherapy was given postoperatively in all cases and consisted either of radium inserted into the operative cavity or

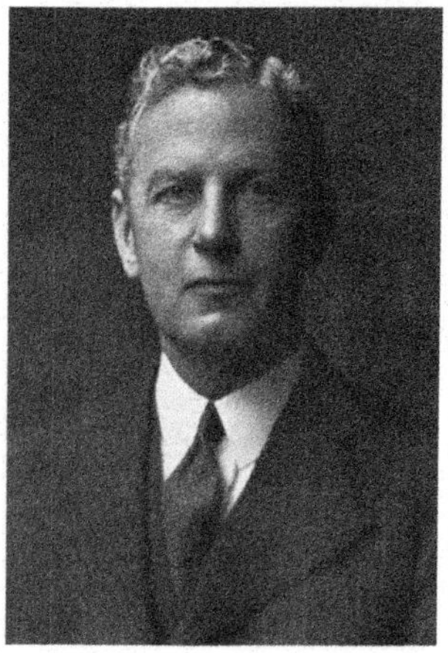

Fig. 1.8 J.S. Fraser (reprinted with permission) [35]

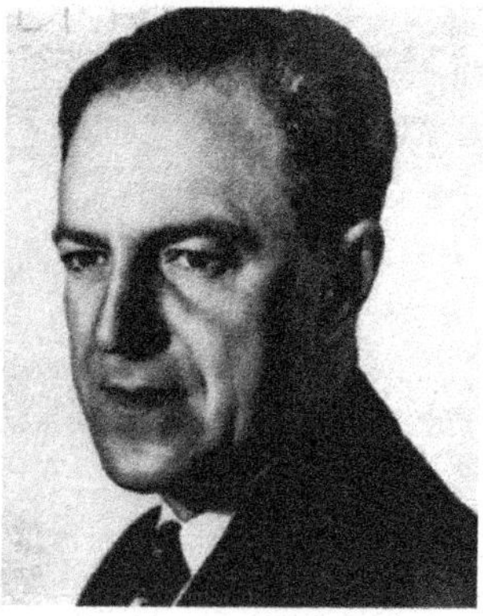

Fig. 1.9 Frederick A. Figi (reprinted with permission) [88]

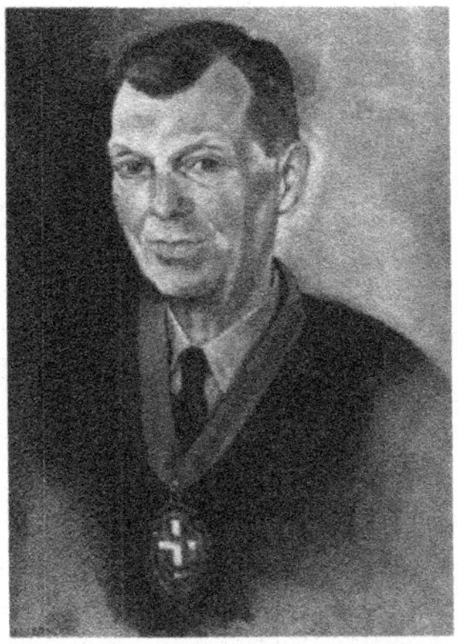

Fig. 1.10 William Stirk Adams (reprinted with permission) [89]

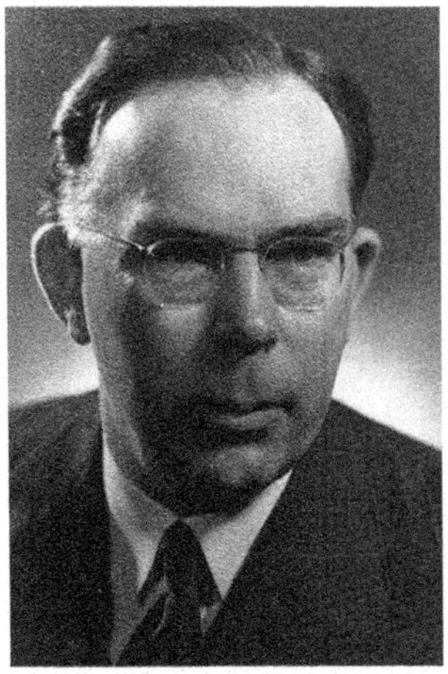

Fig. 1.11 Ralston Paterson (https://commons.wikimedia.org/wiki/File:Ralston_Paterson_(1897–1981).png)

external "radium beam" [41]. Their paper highlights the fact that these patients died of local disease and not regional or distant metastasis.

William Stirk Adams (1896–1976) was born in Acocks Green, Worcestershire, England, and attended Birmingham University (Fig. 1.10). His studies were interrupted by World War I, and he served as a "surgeon probationer" and as a boat spotter, perched high up in a balloon. Given the shortage of surgeons during the war, surgeon probationers were third- and fourth-year medical students enrolled into the navy with some basic medical training. He received his MB from Birmingham University in 1921. He began his surgical residency in obstetrics, but he switched to otolaryngology. He obtained his FRCS in 1924, and he was appointed assistant surgeon at General Hospital Birmingham in 1926. He spent his entire career in Birmingham until his retirement from the National Health Service in 1961. He was a Hunterian Professor at the Royal College of Surgeons in 1944. Although a general otolaryngologist, he demonstrated interest in otology and the Eustachian tube. He was part of a research council charged with studying the effects of radiation to the nasopharynx in cases of otitis media with effusion. In 1947, he founded the Midland Institute of Otology (MIO) for the sole purpose of postgraduate training in otolaryngology. He had many hobbies and was an accomplished gardener, bee keeper, and sailor. He drove a 1933 Rolls-Royce 20/25 four-door saloon until his death in 1971. He remained a bachelor, and upon his death, his library and the proceeds from his estate helped to fund the MIO.

His colleague Robert B.I. Morrison (1913–1992) graduated from Edinburgh University in 1935. He went on to obtain his FRCP, FRCS, and MD from Edinburgh. He earned his Diploma in Radiology followed by Fellowship in FCR in 1951. In 1953, he joined the Radiotherapeutic Research Unit at Hammersmith Hospital and was responsible for the first linear accelerator for clinical use [42]. Over his long career, he saw many changes in radiotherapy. He wrote 44 papers, principally on radiotherapy techniques. He was a president of the Royal College of Physicians, Radiology section, 1977–1978. His presidential address was entitled "Progress of radiotherapy and oncology from radium to platinum." [43]

Boland and Paterson described their radiotherapy technique in 1955 [44]. They reported results of radiotherapy in 14 patients with carcinoma limited to the ear canal. The overall survival rate was 23%, but the end point was not clearly defined. They described the complications of osteoradionecrosis and brainstem damage with radiation in this location. Boland published just this one paper. Ralston L. Paterson (1897–1981) published 28 papers (Fig. 1.11). He served in World War I with the Argyll and Sutherland Highlanders and received the Military Cross. He completed his medical training at the Royal Infirmary of Edinburgh in 1923. He received his training in radiotherapy at the Mayo Clinic. Along with Herbert Park, he pioneered the development of the Paterson-Parker rules for the Radium Dosage system, also called the Manchester system.

The earliest reported case series of sarcoma of the temporal bone is from Eggston and Wolff (1947), where they reported five cases all presenting with facial paralysis [45]. In 1952, Aub described the first case of epidermoid carcinoma of the middle ear in a radium dial painter [46]. The first case of temporal bone carcinoma from therapeutic radiation was described by Ruben et al. in 1977 [47].

Development of Surgical Techniques

Radiotherapy was the mainstay of temporal bone cancer treatment until 1951 when Ward et al. [48] described piecemeal excision of the temporal bone and surrounding structures, even if this required a radical operation, with the goal of trying to achieve negative margins. Grant Eben Ward (1896–1958) was born in Lorain, Ohio (Fig. 1.12). He graduated

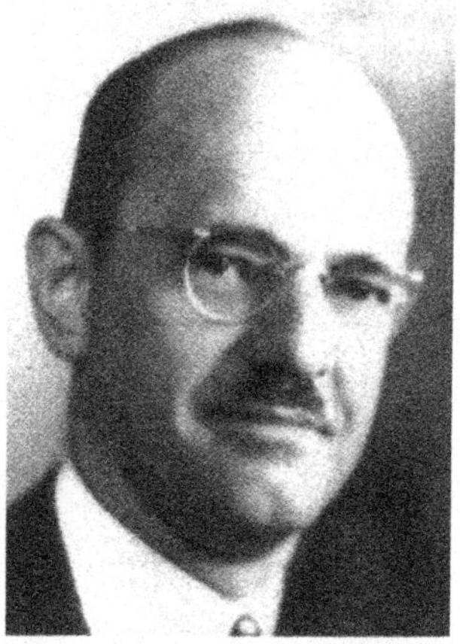

Fig. 1.12 Grant Ward (reprinted with permission) [49]

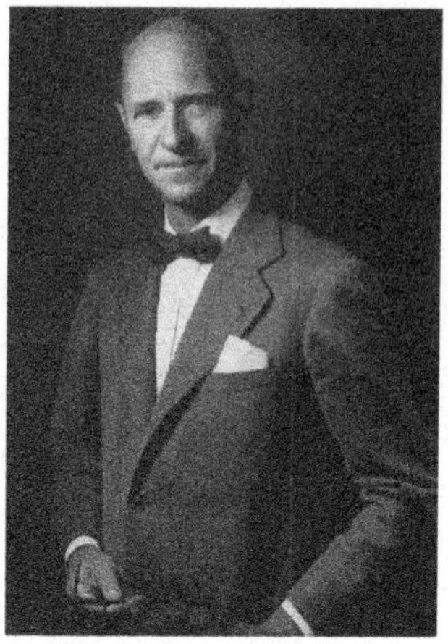

Fig. 1.13 Eldridge Houston Campbell (reprinted with permission) [90]

from Johns Hopkins Medical School in 1921. He became a fellow in the American College of Surgeons in 1928 and certified by the American Board of Surgery in 1939.

Dr. Ward overcame significant personal medical hurdles in his career. He had ulcerative colitis and required an ileostomy in 1940. He developed a benign spinal cord tumor in 1942; and following resection, he developed severe weakness of his dominant right arm. Through perseverance and ingenuity, he worked with engineers to develop an orthotic device to support his right hand and to continue to perform surgery, developing significant dexterity with his left hand [49].

He developed an interest in electrosurgery and authored a book on the subject with Dr. Howard Kelly in 1932. He performed the first composite resection for oral cavity cancer in 1932. He wrote papers on the composite resection of oral cavity cancers and neck dissection along with radical operation of middle ear and temporal bone cancers. In 1950 he co-wrote with James Hendrick the first comprehensive textbook of head and neck surgery, *Tumors of the Head and Neck*. The foundation of the Society of Head and Neck Surgeons (SHNS) has its start with Drs. Hayes Martin and Grant Ward in 1953 [50]. Ward was elected to the presidency of the SHNS in 1957, but his death from rectal cancer in 1958 prevented him from serving his term [49]. Forty year later, The SHNS merged with the American Head and Neck Society in 1998 [51].

In 1951, Campbell et al. [52] suggested that *en bloc* resection of the temporal bone would be possible. Eldridge Houston Campbell (1901–1956) did his undergraduate work at the University of Virginia and graduated from medical school at Johns Hopkins University in 1927 (Fig. 1.13). His undergraduate honors include Phi Beta Kappa and 2 years as a Rhodes scholar. He spent his entire residency training with the eminent neurosurgeon, Dr. Walter Dandy. He joined the faculty of Albany Medical College in 1934 and served as professor and chairman of the department of surgery from 1946 until his death in 1956. During World War II, he served as chief of Surgery in the 33rd General Hospital and as consultant in Neurosurgery in the Mediterranean Theater of Operation. Given his war experiences, he wrote many papers regarding penetrating trauma to the head. He wrote the obituary of Dr. Dandy for the American Association of Neurological Surgeons [53].

However, it was not until 1954 that Parsons and Lewis actually performed the first one-stage subtotal temporal bone resection in 1954 [54]. This marked a major departure from the previous treatment paradigm of radical mastoidectomy followed by radiotherapy and fostered the trend toward *en bloc* resection of temporal bone tumors [55]. After soft tissue surgery in the neck controls the major vessels, posterior and middle fossa craniotomy allows osteotomy across the petrous portion of the temporal bone just lateral to the internal auditory canal and removal of an intact specimen. Reconstruction was with local flaps, fascia lata, and abdominal fat grafts. The operative mortality rate was around 10% [56].

Herbert Lynn Parsons (1909–1995) was born in New York City and attended Yale University and Harvard Medical School. He did his training at St. Luke's Hospital in New York and served during World War II in the European Theatre of Operations (ETO) as a neurosurgeon. He was an attending physician at many NYC hospitals including New York Presbyterian Hospital, Department of Neurosurgery.

John S. Lewis (1919–2005) was born in Medicine Hat, Alberta and graduated from medical school at the University of Alberta, Edmonton, in 1943 (Fig. 1.14). He served in the Royal Canadian Army Medical Corps ETO in 1943–1946 [57]. He did graduate training in surgery and pathology before completing his otolaryngology training at the University of Pennsylvania (1948–1950) and fellowship in head and neck surgery at Memorial Sloan-Kettering in 1951. He spent his entire medical career at the Memorial Sloan-Kettering Cancer Center, New York. He received numerous awards including the Newburn Medal for Surgery from the

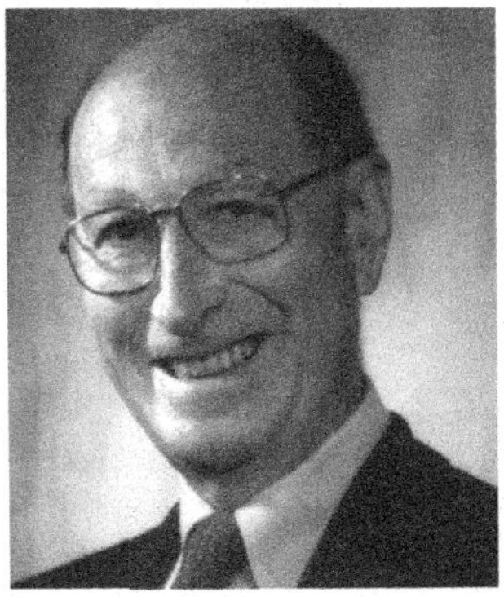

Fig. 1.14 John S. Lewis (reprinted with permission) [57]

University of Alberta and the Newcomb Award from the American Laryngological Society. He served as president of the American Society of Head and Neck Surgery (1970–71) and American Otolaryngological Society (1983–84).

Lewis ultimately published 10 papers dedicated to cancers of the ear and temporal bone. In 1975, Lewis reported his 20-year experience with 100 cases of temporal bone cancer, 86% of which were squamous cell carcinoma. His 5-year survival rate was 25%, and the operative mortality dropped from around 10% to 5% [56]. He attributed improved results to the use of hypotensive anesthesia, high-speed drills, and adequate soft tissue coverage of the defect. His most widely cited paper, "Temporal Bone Resection: Review of 100 cases" [56], has lasting relevance today.

In 1960 Conley and Novak describe *en bloc* resection of the bony ear canal lateral to the facial nerve [58]. This description is the earliest for today's lateral temporal bone resection (LTBR). In their series, 66% of the cases were SCC; and their 5-year survival rate was 18%. They observed that tumors that extended beyond the Eustachian tube had a very poor prognosis and that the goal of surgery should be palliation [58].

In 1965, Conley described his experience with middle ear cancers [59]. He pointed out the difficulty in curing patients when the tumor involves the Eustachian tube, petrous portion of the temporal bone, the dura, the base of skull, or extension into the neck. In the same article, he utilizes the hypoglossal-facial graft for facial paralysis. In these first articles, Conley used a chisel for lateral temporal bone resection. It was not until later that the use of high-speed drill and microsurgical dissection was described for LTBR [60].

John J. Conley (1912–1999) was born in Carnegie, PA, a small steel mill town outside of Pittsburgh (Fig. 1.15). He received his medical degree from the University of Pittsburgh. He interned at Mercy Hospital in Pittsburgh, and the nuns there advised him to study cardiology. He left Pittsburgh to do cardiology training at Kings County Hospital in Brooklyn. Ironically, during that training, he developed an arrhythmia, paroxysmal atrial tachycardia. He was counseled that cardiology was too stressful, and he should go into a field with better working hours, like ENT. Following otolaryngology training at Kings County, he served in the US Army for 4 years during World War II. The experience of treating war wounds was invaluable for his future as a head and neck surgeon [61]. After the war, he returned to NYC to work with Dr. George Pack at Memorial Hospital. He trained many residents and fellows during his long tenure at the College of Physician and Surgeons at Columbia University. He authored more than 300 papers and published 13 books in otolaryngology. He developed many innovative techniques in otolaryngology and reconstructive surgery. In addition to his scientific works, he wrote many papers on medical ethics and 11 volumes of poetry. He was fond of classical music and proficient on the flute.

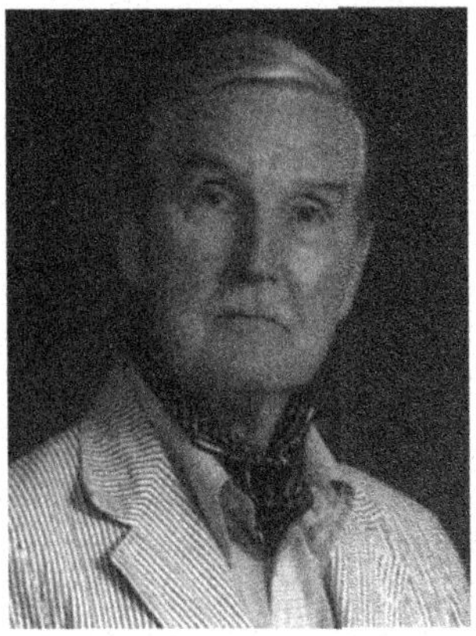

Fig. 1.15 John Conley (reprinted with permission) [61]

He is perhaps the most famous American head and neck surgeon since Dr. Hayes Martin. He was the president of the American Academy of Ophthalmology and Otolaryngology (1974) at a time when it was being restructured to separate these two surgical specialties. He also served as president of the American Academy of Facial Plastic and Reconstructive Surgery. As the first president of the American Society of Head and Neck Surgery, he calmed the inter-specialty tension among general surgeons, plastic surgeons, and otolaryngologists. He established the John Conley Foundation for Ethics and Philosophy in Medicine. He stopped performing surgery at age 80 and retired from Columbia University's College of Physicians and Surgeons, Columbia-Presbyterian Medical Center, and St. Vincent's Hospital in Manhattan. As a lasting tribute, he is remembered through the John Conley lecture of the AHSN.

In another ironic twist of fate, he died from a primary tumor at the skull base, involving the facial nerve, and another malignant growth in the parotid region [61].

Hilding and Selker [62] in 1969 described a total temporal bone resection utilizing an approach first described by Julius Lempert in 1937 [63]. Lempert described an approach to the anterior petrous apex for petrous apicitis by exposing and following the carotid artery. The key step in this procedure is exposure of the carotid artery through the glenoid fossa after removal of the mandibular condyle, thus avoiding any surgery within the middle ear or temporal bone. In Hilding and Selker's procedure, the carotid artery, jugular bulb, sigmoid sinus, and middle fossa dura are separated from the temporal bone. A curved osteotome is inserted through the posterior fossa, and sharp blows are used until the bone fractures free. The advantage of this procedure, over that from Parsons and Lewis, is the removal of the anterior portion of the temporal bone.

David A Hilding (1930–2016) was born in Duluth, Minnesota. He received his MD degree from the University of Minnesota in 1951. He was a resident at Columbia Presbyterian Hospital in New York before serving as a medical army officer during the Korean War. He spent a year conducting research at the Karolinska Institute in Stockholm before joining the faculty at Yale Medical School. His main research interest was hearing loss, and he helped to develop technology to test newborn hearing [64]. He published more than 60 articles; his most highly cited papers deal with the development of the organ of Corti and the anatomy and physiology of the onset of auditory function.

Robert G. Selker (1930–2010) grew up in Squirrel Hill neighborhood of Pittsburgh, Pa, and attended University of Pittsburgh [65]. His college career was interrupted by military service during the Korean War. After the war, he completed his undergraduate training and later his medical school at the University of Pittsburgh. He did his neurosurgical residency training at the University of Pennsylvania. He served a number of academic centers including Yale, Emery, University of Chicago, the NIH, and then Pittsburgh. He held the position of chief of neurosurgery at UPMC Montefiore. He wrote more than 100 papers, with the majority dedicated to gliomas. He developed a pioneering shunt, the "Selker reservoir." He is the lead author on the influential paper regarding the Brain Tumor Cooperative Group NIH trial 87-01 [66].

In 1984, Graham et al. described the first successful, single-stage total temporal bone resection with carotid artery sacrifice [67]. This procedure built on the experience of prior surgeons. A key preliminary step to this procedure is application of a Kindt clamp to the internal carotid artery, with gradual occlusion over 4 days if tolerated by the patient. Total temporal bone resection is then performed, using fascia lata grafts for the dura and packed with abdominal fat graft. This procedure invariably produced deficits of cranial nerves VII through XII and was used successfully in a few reported cases. In 1987, Sataloff et al. reported the extended temporal bone resection, which includes the lower cranial nerves, petrous apex, carotid artery, jugular vein, sigmoid sinus, and most of the middle fossa floor [68]. However, the operative morbidity is significant without significant survival benefit, and current chemotherapy and radiotherapy techniques have largely rendered this procedure obsolete.

Malcolm D. Graham graduated medical school from McGill University in Montreal, Quebec, in 1957. He did an internship at University of Colorado Hospital in Denver, Colorado, and then returned to Canada for residency in General Surgery at Veteran's Hospital in Victoria, BC, before completing his otolaryngology training at the University of Iowa under Dr. Dean Lierle. He did fellowship training at House Ear Clinic in Los Angeles. He became board certified in otolaryngology in 1962. He served as professor at the University of Michigan in Ann Arbor from 1978 to 2004, followed by a short time at the University of North Carolina, then Mercer University, and is currently emeritus professor at Emory University in Atlanta, Georgia. He published more than 120 papers on all areas of otology-neurotology. His most highly cited paper deals with residual and recurrent cholesteatoma. He did pioneering work on the use of homograft tympanic membranes in cases of chronic otitis media. He has served as president of the American Neurotology Society and received a Presidential Citation (2006) and Award of Merit (2008) from the American Otological Society.

Lateral temporal bone resection has undergone refinements since its first description. Crabtree et al. described several modifications such as using an endaural incision with a preauricular incision to preserve the external ear. They describe a method for dissecting and preserving the facial nerve when parotidectomy is indicated [69]. In 1990, Medina et al. proposed a classification of the types of temporal bone resection, describing four different variations of lateral temporal bone resection [70]. In 1997, Moffat et al. described an extended temporal bone resection with preservation of the internal carotid artery and piecemeal resection of the petrous apex [71].

The Impact of Diagnostic Imaging and the Development of Staging Systems

Contemporary surgeons cannot fathom operating on temporal bone cancer without the benefit of cross-sectional imaging. In the first half of the twentieth century, clinical examination and plain films (AP, Stenver's, Laws and Owen Mayer, and Poschl views) were the main guides for otologic surgeons [72]. Polytomography became the primary radiographic diagnostic test in the 1960s [73, 74]. Polytomographs could be made at 2 mm intervals and gave some definition to the middle and inner ear structures; however, the images are blurry and rather difficult to interpret. Polytomography led to both overestimation and underestimation of disease; Goodwin and Jesse found that this modality was accurate in only 1 of 13 cases [75]. This modality was quickly replaced by computerized axial tomography in the late 1970s, which was further supplanted by magnetic resonance imaging in the 1990s.

The development of cross-sectional imaging fostered the birth of rational staging systems for temporal bone cancer. In 1980, Goodwin and Jesse divided their cases into three groups based on the location of the primary: group 1 in the cartilaginous ear canal, group 2 in the bony canal, and group 3 in the middle ear and deeper structures [75]. Absolute 5-year survival rates were 57%, 45%, and 29% in groups 1–3, respectively.

In the late 1980s, Kinney and Wood [76] and Kinney [77] were unable to develop an accurate staging system based on examination and radiographic imaging. Instead, they relied on a stepwise approach to resection of ear canal and temporal bone cancers. They categorized tumors as (1) limited to the external ear canal, (2) extension to the middle ear and TM, (3) extensive disease into the mastoid, stylomastoid foramen, skull base, and dura. They reported survival rates of 85%, 83%, and 40%, respectively, and they used radiotherapy only for those cases with positive margins on final pathology.

In 1990, Shih and Crabtree converted from polytomography to CT scan imaging. They improved on the staging system proposed by Kinney and Wood by adding preoperative CT findings and devising a three-stage system: (1) localized disease, (2) extension into the temporal bone but not beyond, and (3) tumor beyond the temporal bone into surrounding structures such as parotid, neck, skull base, and dura [73]. They identified involvement of the facial nerve as a poor prognostic factor since all patients with facial nerve involvement died of disease. They recognized that early CT had limitations with soft tissue extension. They stated that disease localized to the canal can be adequately treated with *en bloc* lateral temporal bone resection.

In that same year (1990), Arriaga et al. describe a staging system based on preoperative clinical findings and CT findings [78]. This paper describes the earliest version of the Pittsburgh temporal bone staging system. This system used a TNM format and has been verified as a predictor of survival outcomes, and it has become a standard for reporting results in temporal bone cancer.

Contemporary Approaches to Temporal Bone Cancer

The landmark paper by Prasad and Janecka marks a clear delineation between antecedent studies and contemporary studies [79]. They evaluated 96 publications on SCC of the temporal bone and analyzed the results of 26 papers covering 144 patients. Their findings can be distilled into five major points: (1) patients with tumors confined to the ear canal fared equally with mastoidectomy, lateral temporal bone resection (LTBR), or subtotal temporal bone resection; (2) patients with tumors that involve the middle ear fared better with subtotal temporal bone resection than with LTBR or mastoidectomy; (3) the value of surgical resection for tumors that involve the petrous apex remains unclear; (4) resection of dura does not improve survival; and (5) there is insufficient data regarding resection of brain or carotid artery. As an early form of meta-analysis, this paper advanced the study of temporal bone SCC by combining and analyzing results of prior work and decanting the salient features while pointing out the gaps in knowledge about SCC of the temporal bone. The importance of this paper is underscored by the frequency in which it has been cited by other papers (89 citations identified by www.scopus.com). However, as explained in many of the following chapters, ear canal tumors have much higher survival with lateral temporal bone resection than with mastoidectomy alone. The other observations continue to hold true.

Intra-arterial chemotherapy was first reported by Tucker [80] in 1965 as part of treatment for middle ear cancers. He stated that five out of six patients had good results with this type of treatment. The use of intra-arterial chemotherapy has fallen out of favor in the USA, but it is still used with success in Japan and Europe [81–86].

The Japanese have led the way in the use of chemotherapy and radiotherapy for treatment of temporal bone cancer [87]. Nakagawa et al. described a group of temporal bone cancer patients treated with combination chemotherapy and radiotherapy. The encouraging results in this paper have led others to try similar protocols for large, advanced T3 and T4 tumors. This paper marks the beginning of the modern era of temporal bone cancer.

Conclusions

A rich literature regarding temporal bone cancer has evolved over the last century. While squamous cell carcinoma is the most common tumor to involve the temporal bone, many different primary tumor types can occur within the temporal bone. These different tumor types have very different biologic behaviors, and it is important to understand the natural history of each of these tumors. Equally, many different primary locations, such as periauricular skin and parotid, can involve the temporal bone. Recognizing the similarities and differences of these primary sites from the ear canal, middle ear, and mastoid is essential.

The history of temporal bone cancer treatment reveals a refinement in understanding and techniques for management. Temporal bone cancer has been recognized from the origin of otology as a field of study. As the field of otology developed, surgical techniques to treat chronic infection were applied to temporal bone cancer. The contemporaneous development of diagnostic and therapeutic uses of radiation helped to improve on the outcomes gained by surgery alone. The improvements in temporal bone resection and the reliable use of microvascular free flaps denote the current state-of-the-art for temporal bone surgery. The development of a cogent staging system has allowed physicians to compare results and to apply appropriate treatment to disease burden. The development of multidrug chemotherapy protocols marks the dawn of a new age in temporal bone cancer.

References

1. Gidley PW, DeMonte F. Temporal bone malignancies. Neurosurg Clin N Am. 2013;24(1):97–110.
2. Gidley PW, Thompson CR, Roberts DB, DeMonte F, Hanna EY. The oncology of otology. Laryngoscope. 2012;122(2):393–400.
3. Öhngren G. Malignant disease of the upper jaw: (Section of laryngology and section of otology). Proc R Soc Med. 1936;29(11):1497.
4. Newhart H. Primary carcinoma of the middle ear: report of a case. Laryngoscope. 1917;27:543–55.
5. Walsh M. William Wilde: his contribution to otology. Ir J Med Sci. 2016;185(2):291–2.
6. Weinberger HL. Carcinom am ohr1908.
7. Furstenberg AC. XLII. Primary adenocarcinoma of the middle ear and mastoid. Ann Otol Rhinol Laryngol. 1924;33(3):677–89.
8. Peele J, Hauser GH. Primary carcinoma of the external auditory canal and middle ear: review of the literature; Report of a case of cystic adenoid epithelioma (Brooke's tumor) of the external auditory canal. Arch Otolaryngol. 1941;34(2):254–66.
9. Moffat DA, Wagstaff SA, Hardy DG. The outcome of radical surgery and postoperative radiotherapy for squamous carcinoma of the temporal bone. Laryngoscope. 2005;115(2):341–7.
10. Wilson TG. Historical Vignette: William Wilde. Arch Otolaryngol. 1965;81(6):626–9.
11. Wilde WR. The narrative of a voyage to madeira, teneriffe, and along the shores of the mediterranean. Dublin: William Curry, Jun. and Co.; London: Longman, Orme, Browne and Co.; 1840.
12. Sunder S, Jackler RK, Blevins NH. Virtuosity with the mallet and gouge: the brilliant triumph of the "modern" mastoid operation. Otolaryngol Clin N Am. 2006;39(6):1191–210.
13. Wilde WR. Practical observations on aural surgery and the nature and treatment of diseases of the ear: Blanchard & Lea; 1853.
14. Seaton A. Wilde thoughts. QJM. 2012;105(11):1137–8.
15. Robins AH, Sellars SL. Oscar Wilde's terminal illness: reappraisal after a century. Lancet. 2000;356(9244):1841–3.
16. Schwartze H. Die Chirurgischen Krankheiten des Ohres. Leipzig; 1873.
17. Schwartze H. Pathologische anatomie des ohres: Verlag von August Hirschwald; 1878.
18. Schwartze H. Lehrbuch der chirurgischen Krankheiten des Ohres: Enke; 1885.
19. Schwartze H, Eysell C. Uber die kunstliche eroffnung des warzenfortsatzes. Arch Ohrenheilkd. 1873;7:157–62.
20. Politzer A. Textbook of diseases of the ear, translated and edited by HC Cassells. Philadelphia: Lea & Son; 1883.
21. Bezold F. Übersicht über den gegenwärtigen stand der ohrenheilkunde [Overview of the present state of ear medicine]. Wiesbaden; 1895.
22. Kretschmann F. Ueber Carcinome des Schläfenbeines. Archiv für Ohrenheilkunde. 1887;24(4):231–62.
23. Zeroni. Uber das Carcinom des Gehoerorgans. Archiv f Ohrenhlk. 1899;8:141.
24. Boies LR. Horace Newhart, MD. SAGE Publications Sage CA: Los Angeles, CA; 1945.
25. Haug R. Beiträge zur Klinik und mikroskopischen Anatomie der Neubildungen des äusseren und mittleren Ohres. Eur Arch Otorhinolaryngol. 1894;36(3):170–206.
26. Treitel L. Ueber des carcinom des ohres. Z Ohrenheilkunde. 1898;33:152–64.
27. Heffner DK. Low-grade adenocarcinoma of probable endolymphatic sac origin A clinicopathologic study of 20 cases. Cancer. 1989;64(11):2292–302.
28. Heyer H. Ueber einen Fall von Ohrcarcinom, behandelt mit Resection des Felsenbeines. Deutsche Zeitschrift für Chirurgie. 1899;50(5):522–33.
29. Shambaugh GE Jr. Albert c. furstenburg, md. Arch Otolaryngol. 1965;82(1):38–41.
30. Work WP. Albert c. furstenberg, md: In memoriam. Arch Otolaryngol. 1970;91(3):215.
31. Furstenberg A. A chronicle of 100 years of otolaryngology. Laryngoscope. 1947;57(9):596–615.
32. Furstenberg AC. LXIII address of president. Ann Otol Rhinol Laryngol. 1953;62(3):712–9.
33. Furstenberg AC, Lashmet FH, Lathrop F. LXXXIV. Meniere's symptom complex: medical treatment. Ann Otol Rhinol Laryngol. 1934;43(4):1035–46.
34. Fraser J. Malignant disease of the external acoustic meatus and middle ear. SAGE Publications; 1930.
35. Mollison W, Fraser JS. SAGE Publications Sage CA: Los Angeles, CA; 1936.
36. Rankin MNM. I Wimpole Street, London, W. i. Section of Laryngology.—The Opening Meeting of the Session 1927–28 will be held on Friday, 4th November, at 5 PM President, Mr Harold S. Barwell, FRCS; Hon. Secretaries, Mr WM Mollison, M. Ch., 23 Devonshire Place, London, W. 1, and Mr Lionel Colledge, FRCS.
37. Thorell I. Treatment of malignant tumours of the middle ear at Radiumhemmet, Stockholm. Acta Radiol. 1935;16(2):242–53.
38. Figi FA, Hempstead BE. Malignant tumors of the middle ear and the mastoid process. Arch Otolaryngol. 1943;37(2):149–68.
39. Mattick WL, Mattick JW. Some experiences in management of cancer of middle ear and mastoid. AMA Arch Otolaryngol. 1951;53(6):610–21.
40. Figi FA, Weisman PA. Cancer and chemodectoma in the middle ear and mastoid. J Am Med Assoc. 1954;156(12):1157–62.
41. Adams WS, Morrison R. On primary carcinoma of the middle ear and mastoid; its incidence, etiological factors and clinical course, with the results of treatment by surgery and radiotherapy. J Laryngol Otol. 1955;69(2):115–31.
42. Deeley TJ. Robert Morrison 1913–1992. Clin Oncol. 1992;4(4):271.
43. Society Notices. J R Soc Med. 1978;71.
44. Boland J, Paterson R. Cancer of the middle ear and external auditory meatus. J Laryngol Otol. 1955;69(7):468–78.
45. Eggston AAW. Histopatology of the ear, nose and throat; 1947.
46. Aub JC, Evans RD, Hempelmann LH, Martland HS. The late effects of internally-deposited radioactive materials in man. Medicine. 1952;31(3):221–329.
47. Ruben RJ, Thaler SU, Holzer N. Radiation induced carcinoma of the temporal bone. Laryngoscope. 1977;87(10 Pt 1):1613–21.
48. Ward GE, Loch WE, Lawrence W Jr. Radical operation for carcinoma of the external auditory canal and middle ear. Am J Surg. 1951;82(1):169–78.
49. Shedd DP. Historical landmarks in head and neck cancer surgery: The American Head and Neck Society; 1999.
50. Jaques DA. The fraternity of strangers. Am J Surg. 1984;148(4):426–7.

51. Francis HW, Papel I. Otolaryngology–head and neck surgery at Johns Hopkins: The first 100 years (1914–2014). Laryngoscope. 2015;125(09):S1.
52. Campbell E, Volk BM, Burklund CW. Total resection of temporal bone for malignancy of the middle ear. Ann Surg. 1951;134(3): 397–404.
53. Campbell E. Walter E. Dandy—Surgeon 1886–1946. J Neurosurg. 1951;8(3):249–62.
54. Parsons H, Lewis JS. Subtotal resection of the temporal bone for cancer of the ear. Cancer. 1954;7(5):995–1001.
55. Tabb HG, Komet H, McLaurin JW. Cancer of the external auditory canal: treatment with radical mastoidectomy and irradiation. Laryngoscope. 1964;74:634–43.
56. Lewis JS. Temporal bone resection. Review of 100 cases. Arch Otolaryngol. 1975;101(1):23–5.
57. Obituary: John S. Lewis 2005. Available from: http://www.legacy.com/obituaries/nytimes/obituary.aspx?n=john-s-lewis&pid=14203127.
58. Conley JJ, Novack AJ. Surgical treatment of cancer of the ear and temporal bone. Trans Am Acad Ophthalmol Otolaryngol. 1960;64:83–92.
59. Conley J. Cancer of the middle ear. Ann Otol Rhinol Laryngol. 1965;74:555–72.
60. Shotton JC, Sergeant RJ, Tanner NS, Allen JP. Lateral temporal bone resection for extensive pinnal malignancy. Has anything changed in forty years? J Laryngol Otol. 1993;107(8):697–702.
61. Mccabe BF. John J. Conley, MD, 1912–1999—In celebration of a life—A meeting of fellows and friends. Ann Otol Rhinol Laryngol. 2000;109(1):1–8.
62. Hilding DA, Selker R. Total resection of the temporal bone for carcinoma. Arch Otolaryngol. 1969;89(4):636–45.
63. Lempert J. Complete apicectomy (mastoidotympano-apicectomy). Arch Otolaryngol Head Neck Surg. 1937;25(2):144–77.
64. Obituary: David Hilding. Salt Lake Tribune. 2016 Nov. 13, 2016.
65. Obituary: Robert Selker 2010. Available from: http://www.post-gazette.com/news/obituaries/2010/11/04/Obituary-Robert-G-Selker-Renowned-neurosurgeon-who-advanced-treatment-for-brain-tumors/stories/201011040521.
66. Selker RG, Shapiro WR, Burger P, Blackwood MS, Deutsch M, Arena VC, et al. The Brain Tumor Cooperative Group NIH Trial 87-01: a randomized comparison of surgery, external radiotherapy, and carmustine versus surgery, interstitial radiotherapy boost, external radiation therapy, and carmustine. Neurosurgery. 2002;51(2):343–57.
67. Graham MD, Sataloff RT, Kemink JL, Wolf GT, McGillicuddy JE. Total en bloc resection of the temporal bone and carotid artery for malignant tumors of the ear and temporal bone. Laryngoscope. 1984;94(4):528–33.
68. Sataloff RT, Myers DL, Lowry LD, Spiegel JR. Total temporal bone resection for squamous cell carcinoma. Otolaryngol Head Neck Surg. 1987;96(1):4–14.
69. Crabtree JA, Britton BH, Pierce MK. Carcinoma of the external auditory canal. Laryngoscope. 1976;86(3):405–15.
70. Medina JE, Park AO, Neely JG, Britton BH. Lateral temporal bone resections. Am J Surg. 1990;160(4):427–33.
71. Moffat DA, Grey P, Ballagh RH, Hardy DG. Extended temporal bone resection for squamous cell carcinoma. Otolaryngol Head Neck Surg. 1997;116(6 Pt 1):617–23.
72. Olsen KD, DeSanto LW, Forbes GS. Radiographic assessment of squamous cell carcinoma of the temporal bone. Laryngoscope. 1983;93(9):1162–7.
73. Shih L, Crabtree JA. Carcinoma of the external auditory canal: an update. Laryngoscope. 1990;100(11):1215–8.
74. Ross F. Polytomography of the Temporal Bone (Abridged). J Laryngol Otol. 1963;77(9):737–48.
75. Goodwin WJ, Jesse RH. Malignant neoplasms of the external auditory canal and temporal bone. Arch Otolaryngol. 1980;106(11):675–9.
76. Kinney SE, Wood BG. Malignancies of the external ear canal and temporal bone: surgical techniques and results. Laryngoscope. 1987;97(2):158–64.
77. Kinney SE. Squamous cell carcinoma of the external auditory canal. Am J Otol. 1989;10(2):111–6.
78. Arriaga M, Curtin H, Takahashi H, Hirsch BE, Kamerer DB. Staging proposal for external auditory meatus carcinoma based on preoperative clinical examination and computed tomography findings. Ann Otol Rhinol Laryngol. 1990;99(9 Pt 1): 714–21.
79. Prasad S, Janecka IP. Efficacy of surgical treatments for squamous cell carcinoma of the temporal bone: a literature review. Otolaryngol Head Neck Surg. 1994;110(3):270–80.
80. Tucker WN. Cancer of the middle ear; a review of 89 cases. Cancer. 1965;18:642–50.
81. van Es RJ, Nijsen JF, van het Schip AD, Dullens HF, Slootweg PJ, Koole R. Intra-arterial embolization of head-and-neck cancer with radioactive holmium-166 poly(L-lactic acid) microspheres: an experimental study in rabbits. Int J Oral Maxillofac Surg. 2001;30(5):407–13.
82. Balm AJ, Rasch CR, Schornagel JH, Hilgers FJ, Keus RB, Schultze-Kool L, et al. High-dose superselective intra-arterial cisplatin and concomitant radiation (RADPLAT) for advanced head and neck cancer. Head Neck. 2004;26(6):485–93.
83. Zuur CL, Simis YJ, Lansdaal PE, Hart AA, Rasch CR, Schornagel JH, et al. Risk factors of ototoxicity after cisplatin-based chemo-irradiation in patients with locally advanced head-and-neck cancer: a multivariate analysis. Int J Radiat Oncol Biol Phys. 2007;68(5):1320–5.
84. Ueda Y, Kurita T, Matsuda Y, Ito S, Nakashima T. Superselective, intra-arterial, rapid infusion chemotherapy for external auditory canal carcinoma. J Laryngol Otol Suppl. 2009;31:75–80.
85. Sugimoto H, Ito M, Yoshida S, Hatano M, Yoshizaki T. Concurrent superselective intra-arterial chemotherapy and radiotherapy for late-stage squamous cell carcinoma of the temporal bone. Ann Otol Rhinol Laryngol. 2011;120(6):372–6.
86. Sugimoto H, Hatano M, Yoshida S, Sakumoto M, Kato H, Ito M, et al. Efficacy of concurrent superselective intra-arterial chemotherapy and radiotherapy for late-stage squamous cell carcinoma of the temporal bone. Clin Otolaryngol. 2015;40(5): 500–4.
87. Nakagawa T, Kumamoto Y, Natori Y, Shiratsuchi H, Toh S, Kakazu Y, et al. Squamous cell carcinoma of the external auditory canal and middle ear: an operation combined with preoperative chemoradiotherapy and a free surgical margin. Otol Neurotol. 2006;27(2):242–8; discussion 9.
88. Johnson H. Obituary: Frederick A. Figi. Plast Reconstr Surg. 1970;46(6):618–9.
89. Pahor A, Stansbie J. The Midland Institute of Otology and its Founder: William Stirk Adams (1896–1978). J Laryngol Otol. 1997;111(12):1122–5.
90. Meirowsky A. Eldridge Campbell 1901–1956. J Neurosurg. 1957;14(1):114–6.

Evaluation and Staging of Temporal Bone Tumors

2

Joseph T. Breen and Paul W. Gidley

Abbreviations

AJCC	American Joint Committee on Cancer
BPPV	benign paroxysmal positional vertigo
CT	computed tomography
cVEMP	cervical vestibular-evoked myogenic potentials
EAC	external auditory canal
ENG	electronystagmography
ENoG	electroneuronography
MRI	magnetic resonance imaging
oVEMP	ocular vestibular-evoked myogenic potentials
PSS	Pittsburgh staging system
SCC	squamous cell carcinoma
TM	tympanic membrane
TNM	tumor node metastasis
VEMP	vestibular-evoked myogenic potentials
VNG	videonystagmography
VOR	vestibular-ocular reflex

Introduction

The comprehensive office evaluation is the foundation of optimal care for patients with any complaint. Patients with malignancies of the temporal bone are no exception to this rule, but there are elements of their clinical evaluation that are of particular importance in developing an appropriate treatment plan. Herein, the elements of a complete clinical assessment will be described in detail. While radiographic and histopathologic evaluations are additional crucial elements in the staging and decision-making process, they will be treated separately in this text.

J. T. Breen, M.D. (✉)
Cincinnati, OH, USA

P. W. Gidley, M.D., F.A.C.S.
Department of Head and Neck Surgery, The University of Texas M.D. Anderson Cancer Center, Houston, TX, USA

Patient Narrative

Hearing loss, otalgia, and otorrhea are the most common symptoms of temporal bone cancer [1–3]. Given the destructive nature of most temporal bone cancers, dysfunction of structures in contact with tumor is expected. As such, the examining physician should suspect symptoms related to structures of the temporal bone to be tumor-related until proven otherwise. Temporal bone malignancies are rarely found incidentally on imaging studies used to evaluate unrelated complaints.

Patients with temporal bone cancer commonly report hearing loss [4]. Hearing loss is a common symptom of otologic disease, and a long list of diagnoses are associated with hearing loss. Careful history and physical examination usually narrow the differential diagnosis. Objective evaluation with pure tone audiometry and speech discrimination testing to define the type and severity of this hearing loss is critical prior to embarking on any treatment, but the tests should be interpreted in light of the patient's history. The timing, symmetry, and functional impact of the hearing loss should be assessed. Associated aural fullness, autophony, or pulsatile tinnitus might suggest an effect of ear canal occlusion or middle ear pathology, while coincident vertigo or sudden complete hearing loss would be more consistent with tumor damaging the inner ear or central hearing pathway.

Otorrhea and otalgia are common complaints of otologic disease. These symptoms are most commonly associated with infectious processes—typically otitis externa or otitis media. Given the frequency of these symptoms and rarity of temporal bone cancer, pain or drainage will typically be initially attributed to infection. Symptoms of patients with otitis media or externa usually improve rapidly with conventional therapy: ear cleaning and ear drops. However, when these symptoms do not improve as expected, the treating physician should consider the presence of ear canal cancer.

Facial weakness or asymmetry should be evaluated with a high index of suspicion [5]. Gradual onset, sudden, or even transient episodes of paralysis can be associated with

P. W. Gidley, F. DeMonte (eds.), *Temporal Bone Cancer*, https://doi.org/10.1007/978-3-319-74539-8_2

tumor invasion. Associated hyperacusis (stapedius dysfunction), dysgeusia (chorda tympani involvement), or changes in lacrimation (involvement at or proximal to the geniculate ganglion) may provide clues as to the extent of facial nerve involvement by tumor. Any of these findings should prompt careful inspection of a high-resolution computed tomography (CT) or gadolinium-enhanced magnetic resonance imaging (MRI) scan for abnormal signal along the course of the nerve.

Dizziness is a common symptom in the general population, but is an unusual symptom in temporal bone cancer. Taking the required history to differentiate between its many causes can be laborious, but this history is often more useful than the vestibular laboratory evaluation. The acute onset of disequilibrium or true vertigo, a subjective sense of motion discordant with the patient's actual movement, would be expected with an insult to the inner ear. If there is radiographic evidence of tumor involving structures relevant to the peripheral vestibular apparatus, the patient should be asked about the presence and quality of these symptoms.

Headache, similarly, is an extremely common symptom that may have little to do with the tumor. However, significant changes in the patient's headache pattern or distribution should be viewed as potentially related to the malignancy, particularly when the pain is ipsilateral or worsening in tandem with tumor progression.

Dysphagia, dysphonia, or dysarthria warrants further evaluation in the context of temporal bone cancer. All patients should undergo a careful examination of all cranial nerves. Patients presenting with any of these complaints should be strongly considered for an in-depth examination of vocal fold and swallowing function. This may include flexible laryngoscopy with or without stroboscopy as well as video fluoroscopic swallowing studies. Even in the setting of preoperative dysfunction, treatment may further worsen lower cranial nerve function, and obtaining these baseline examinations may help counsel the patient on expected functional outcomes and need for supportive care.

Physical Examination

Mastery of the neuro-otologic physical examination is obtained over many repetitions and exposure to many kinds of pathology. However, physicians of all levels of experience benefit by performing the physical examination in a consistent, organized, and efficient manner. Being systematic, whether that means moving through the examination in a superior-to-inferior direction or always working with the same sequence of examinations, is recommended. There is a natural tendency to first examine the obviously relevant abnormalities that may lead to important exam components being omitted. Having an organized, comprehensive, and consistent approach will maximize the probability of detecting all relevant abnormalities.

Head, Scalp, and Skin

Careful examination of all skin-covered surfaces of the head and neck may reveal synchronous cutaneous malignancies. The significant sun exposure of this region of the body imparts a high risk of skin cancer relative to other sites. Primary squamous cell carcinoma (SCC) of the ear canal and temporal bone arises from the skin not directly exposed to the sun, but these patients, particularly those who are immunosuppressed, may be at higher risk of harboring additional skin cancers than the general population [6].

Patients reporting a history of previous surgery for skin cancer should be asked about pathology results, and the surgical sites should be identified. Delayed metastasis to the parotid or neck with subsequent temporal bone invasion and perineural spread tracking into the temporal bone are both diagnostic possibilities in this group.

Eye, Orbit, and Eye Movements

The eyes and eyelids should be examined for gross abnormalities or asymmetry. While temporal bone tumors will uncommonly involve the eye or orbit itself, careful inspection for downstream effects of cranial neuropathies is crucial. In particular, ectropion, epiphora, lagophthalmos, or corneal inflammation may be associated with facial paralysis. Documentation of these problems and providing appropriate eye care for the patient with weakness are of the utmost importance.

Eye Movements

Observing eye movements from the action of muscles within the orbit provides information regarding cranial nerves III, IV, and VI. The muscles supplied by these nerves, as well as their actions on the globe, are outlined in Table 2.1. Dysfunction of these cranial nerves may be incomplete and not isolated to a single nerve. This can lead to a constellation of abnormal eye movements that cannot be attributed to a classic mononeuropathy.

The patient should be asked to focus on the tip of the examiner's finger as it is moved through a field that examines all directions of gaze. The dysconjugate gaze that is associated with a unilateral abnormality in eye movements can often be detected on close inspection of the eyes. Additional clues to more subtle dysfunction can be gathered by asking the patient which directions of gaze produce diplopia.

Table 2.1 Innervation and actions of orbital musculature

Cranial nerve	Muscle(s)	Action	Secondary action	Deficit
III—oculomotor	Superior rectus	Elevation	In-cyclotorsion	When complete, "down and out" position of the eye
	Inferior rectus	Depression	Ex-cyclotorsion	
	Medial rectus	Adduction		
	Inferior oblique	Ex-cyclotorsion	Elevation	
IV—trochlear	Superior oblique	In-cyclotorsion	Depression	Relative elevation of the affected eye at rest Abnormal alternate cover testing
VI—abducens	Lateral rectus	Abduction		Weakness of abduction

Adapted from Kung et al. [47]

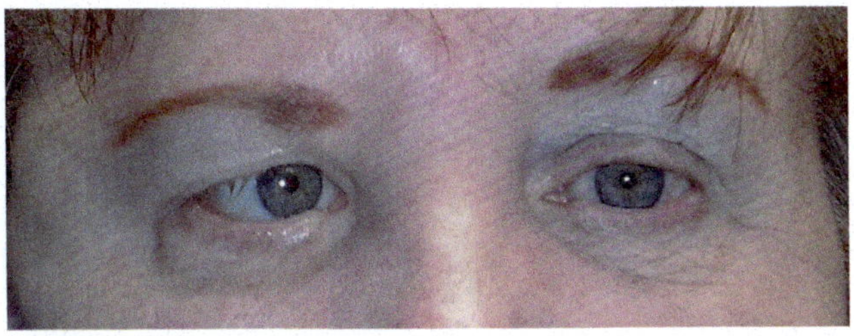

Fig. 2.1 Right abducens nerve palsy from recurrent adenoid cystic carcinoma of the right temporal bone and parotid gland

Diplopia only with gaze directed to the left, for example, would suggest a left-sided abducens nerve palsy or lateral rectus abnormality (Fig. 2.1).

The alternate cover test is performed by having the patient focus on an object, such as the examiner's nose, while the examiner first covers one eye and then moves the cover to the opposite eye. A corrective movement of the recently uncovered eye, usually seen in a vertical direction, may be associated with a 4th nerve palsy or an otolith organ abnormality.

Nystagmus

Nystagmus is an involuntary and rhythmic movement of the eyes that is typically produced by abnormalities along the vestibular-ocular reflex (VOR) pathway or elsewhere in the nervous system. Jerk nystagmus, which is comprised of alternating slow and fast components, is the more common and relevant form in the context of peripheral vestibular lesions, which can include temporal bone malignancies. Nystagmus is typically also described by the direction of the eye movements and can be horizontal, vertical, or torsional. In the case of jerk nystagmus, the direction of the fast eye movement component (the direction of the "beating") is reported.

Nystagmus that occurs without provocations of head movement, changes in gaze, or caloric stimuli is termed spontaneous nystagmus. Frenzel lenses or infrared camera systems reduce visual fixation while allowing the examiner to view eye movements. These may be helpful in uncovering subtler spontaneous nystagmus [7].

In the setting of an acute peripheral vestibular injury, a spontaneous horizontal and torsional jerk nystagmus is expected, beating away from the affected ear, with a torsional component rotating the superior pole of the globe away from the affected ear. Classically, the rotational velocity of the slow-phase component increases when the gaze is in the direction of the fast component. This phenomenon is known as Alexander's law, and several mechanisms of its action have been proposed [8].

Direction-changing, gaze-evoked nystagmus occurs with abnormalities of the mechanisms that keep the eye in an eccentric position. It is most commonly associated with central nervous system lesions or use of medications (such as sedatives or anticonvulsants) rather than peripheral vestibular insults. Bruns' nystagmus is associated with large cerebellopontine angle tumors. It is a form of gaze-evoked nystagmus with low-frequency high-amplitude fast phases when looking toward the side of the lesion and high-frequency low-amplitude fast phases when looking away from the lesion.

Ear

Auricle and External Auditory Canal

The majority of cancers involving the temporal bone arise from tissues of the auricle, external auditory meatus, external auditory canal, tympanic membrane, and middle ear [4]. Accurate identification and localization of tumor involving these structures are of great importance in making treatment decisions.

The lateral most external ear structure is the auricle, which is comprised of skin-covered elastic cartilage. Given the prominent location of the auricle on the head, it receives a relatively large amount of sunlight and ultraviolet (UV) radiation. This skin is at increased risk for the development of cutaneous malignancies and should be examined carefully for suspicious lesions. Malignancy may spread from the skin of the auricle medially into the EAC and temporal bone, or tumors originating medially may grow outward onto the auricle (Fig. 2.2).

The auricle should be both inspected and palpated. The elastic cartilage of the external ear is flexible and somewhat mobile in the majority of patients; the cartilage may become

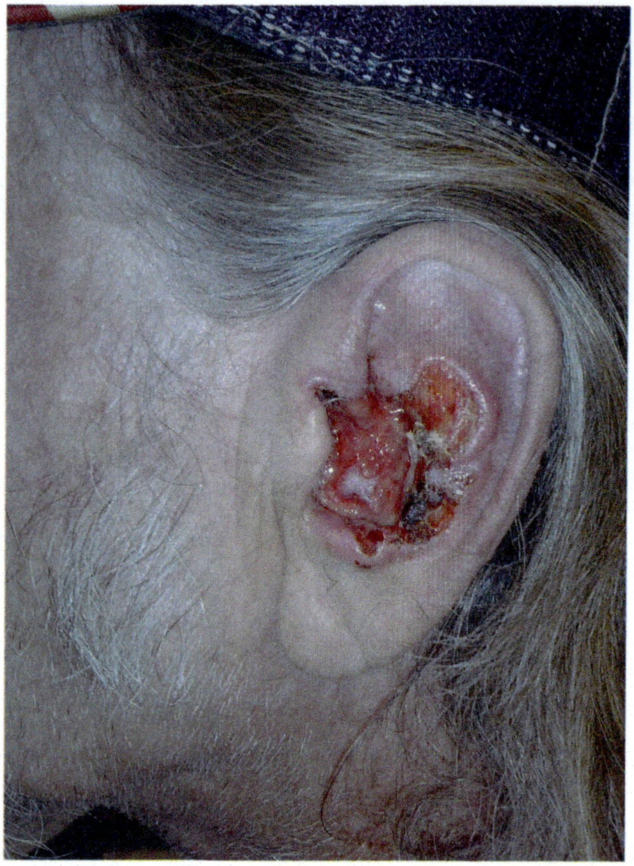

Fig. 2.2 Squamous cell carcinoma of the left outer ear invading the ear canal

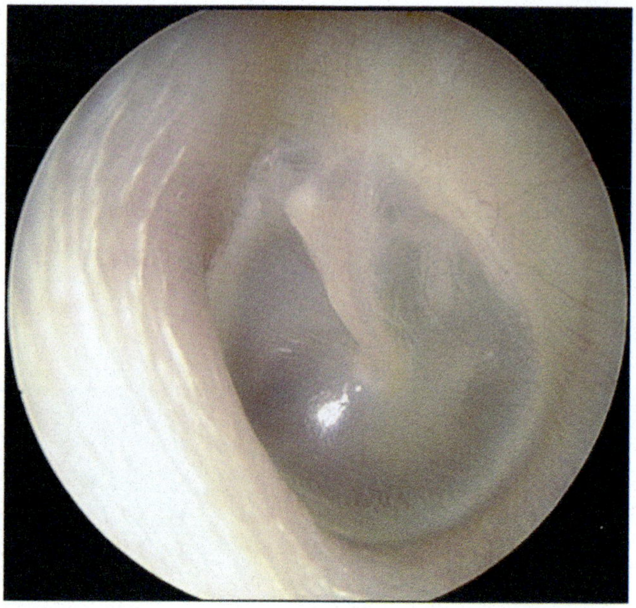

Fig. 2.3 Oto-endoscopic view of normal ear canal and eardrum

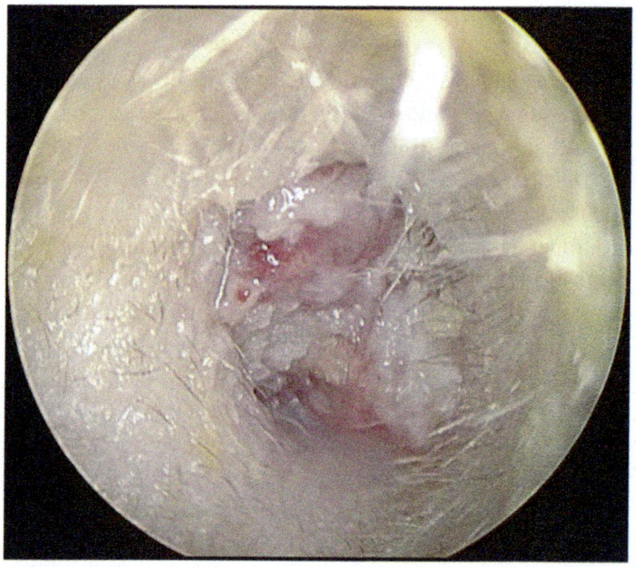

Fig. 2.4 Oto-endoscopic view of the external auditory meatus and canal, with squamous cell carcinoma involving the bony portion of the canal

stiff and calcified in older patients. In the setting of periauricular cutaneous malignancies, immobility of a portion of the cartilage may suggest invasion by tumor.

The entire ear canal can be examined by either a handheld otoscope, binocular microscopy, or a rigid oto-endoscope. Microscopy provides the advantage of binocular vision and the ability to remove debris or cerumen, obtain biopsies, and manipulate/palpate tumor within the EAC under direct vision. Endoscopy with straight or angled telescopes affords excellent visualization and the ability to obtain high-resolution photo-documentation (Fig. 2.3).

Working medially, the external auditory meatus and cartilaginous EAC are first encountered. These structures are covered in the skin that bears hair follicles, sebaceous glands, and ceruminous glands. The presence of abnormal skin, exophytic masses, drainage, granulation tissue, debris, and scarring should be noted.

The bony external auditory canal is lined by thinner skin, devoid of glandular elements or hair follicles. This creates visual contrast between the skin of the bony and cartilaginous parts of the EAC, helping the clinician accurately identify the extent of tumor (Fig. 2.4).

Recognizing the location of an ear canal tumor relative to the bony-cartilaginous junction is important. Tumors that are limited to the cartilaginous canal can usually be excised with the underlying cartilage. However, tumors that involve the bone canal require lateral temporal bone resection for complete excision.

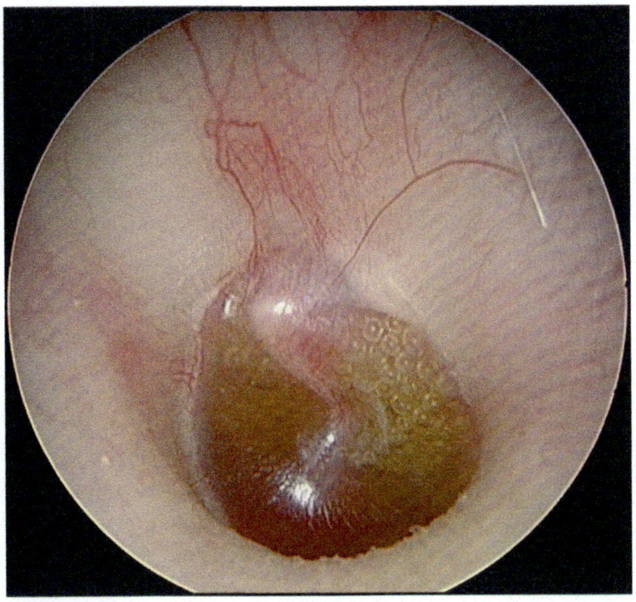

Fig. 2.5 Serous otitis media. Air bubbles can be seen in the posterior-superior quadrant

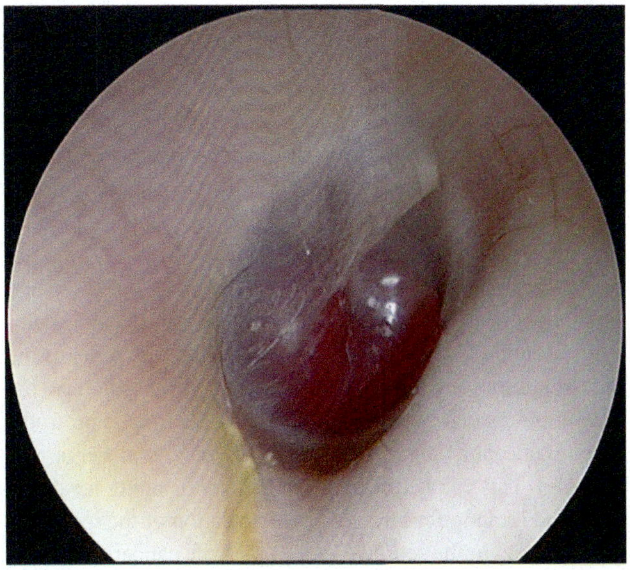

Fig. 2.6 Reddish and pulsatile mass in contact with the tympanic membrane consistent with tympanic paraganglioma

Tympanic Membrane and Middle Ear

The normal tympanic membrane (TM) will often be translucent, allowing for partial visualization of the middle ear contents. The aeration status of the middle ear should be noted. An effusion may be identified by seeing colored/opaque fluid through the TM, air fluid levels, or reduced mobility of the TM on pneumatic otoscopy (Fig. 2.5). There are many potential causes for a middle ear effusion, including Eustachian tube obstruction, inflammatory processes within the middle ear and mastoid, or cerebrospinal fluid leakage into the temporal bone. The examiner should consider all of these possibilities in the context of the patient's history.

A translucent TM can also reveal middle ear or retrotympanic masses. Vascular tumors can present as a retrotympanic, reddish mass (Fig. 2.6). If this tumor touches the TM, then pulsations can be seen in the tumor. Nonpulsatile reddish middle ear masses can be an indicator of neuroendocrine carcinoma. Pale or pinkish retrotympanic masses can be seen in meningioma.

Tuning Fork Examination

The audiogram is the gold standard for evaluation of hearing status, but tuning fork examinations serve as useful confirmatory and adjunctive data. The fork should be struck on a solid but partially dampened surface (such as the heel of a shoe, the knee, or the olecranon process) to produce a tone at the calibrated fundamental frequency and minimal overtones. The tuning fork can be held a short distance in front of either ear, asking the patient to report in which ear the tone is heard more loudly. This can grossly compare air-conduction thresholds between ears at the fork's frequency. The Weber test, typically performed with a 512 Hz fork, is performed by applying a struck tuning fork to a bony midline prominence on the head. Assuming roughly symmetric bone-conduction thresholds, the ear with the larger conductive hearing loss will tend to hear the sound more loudly. The Rinne test involves applying the base of the 512 Hz fork to the mastoid, then holding it in front of the ipsilateral ear with the tines in the coronal plane, asking the patient to compare the relative volume of the two sounds. If the bone-conducted sound is louder (the Rinne test is negative), this suggests a significant conductive loss in that ear at 512 Hz. Fair (up to approximately 50%) sensitivity for detection by the Rinne test of air-bone gaps as low as 10–19 dB has been demonstrated, with sensitivity of 88% for conductive losses between 20 and 29 dB [9].

Nose and Nasopharynx

The quality of the nasal mucosa can be assessed with a nasal speculum and light source or an endoscope. For patients with unilateral middle ear effusion or known lesions extending medially to involve the Eustachian tube, petrous apex, or clivus, rigid or flexible nasopharyngoscopy is used to assess the mucosa and rule out exophytic nasopharyngeal masses.

Oral Cavity and Oropharynx

The oral and oropharyngeal mucosa and teeth are carefully inspected and palpated when necessary. Infectious or neoplastic lesions of the oral cavity and oropharynx may generate referred otalgia and should be excluded in patients with this complaint. Cranial nerves IX (glossopharyngeal), X (vagus), and XII (hypoglossal) can be evaluated by assessing the gag reflex and looking for symmetry in movements of the palate and tongue. Sensory deficits (absent gag) suggest a glossopharyngeal nerve abnormality. Palatal elevation that pulls to one side suggests weakness of the contralateral musculature, primarily innervated by the vagus nerve. If the tongue protrudes to one side, this suggests ipsilateral hypoglossal nerve dysfunction. This can be further evaluated by listening for dysarthria and looking for atrophy or fasciculation of the ipsilateral hemitongue. In the setting of temporal bone cancer, deficits of the lower cranial nerves are indicators of far-advanced disease.

Larynx

The patient's voice should be listened to carefully for a breathy, coarse, or weak quality. The intrinsic muscles of the larynx are innervated by the vagus nerve and can be assessed by visualizing the larynx during respiration and phonation. Mirror examination of the larynx is possible in a subset of patients with favorable anatomy and a permissive gag reflex. If there are complaints of dysphonia and dysarthria, or if a temporal bone lesion approaches the jugular foramen, a finer examination of the larynx should be considered. Flexible laryngoscopy with topical nasal anesthesia can evaluate the laryngeal mucosa and vocal fold mobility in greater detail, as well as allow for photo-documentation.

Neck

The neck is carefully palpated for evidence of metastatic disease. The number, location, and size of palpable nodes should be carefully noted for staging purposes. The consistency, mobility, and presence of tenderness or inflammation for palpable neck nodes should also be assessed, as these characteristics may influence the likelihood that they harbor metastatic cancer. In cases where the clinical evaluation is indeterminate and results would influence treatment planning, fine needle aspiration (FNA) of palpable neck masses can be pursued. In the setting of temporal bone cancer, cervical lymphadenopathy is an ominous finding of late-stage disease.

The parotid glands should be palpated, as well, especially in patients with facial paralysis. If there is regional paralysis of the face, suggesting dysfunction of a branch of the facial nerve rather than the main trunk, parotid metastasis should be suspected.

The spinal accessory nerve (CN XI) is assessed during the neck examination by examining and palpating the trapezius and sternocleidomastoid muscles, assessing their bulk and strength. The patient can be asked to shrug their shoulders against resistance to assess trapezius strength. Turning the head into the examiner's hand when it is applied to one side of the patient's face assesses the contralateral sternocleidomastoid strength.

Cranial Nerves and the Neurologic Examination

Functional evaluation of the cranial nerves generally progresses in tandem with examination of the structures of the head and neck. As such, the proper evaluation of cranial nerves II, III, IV, VI, XI, XII, IX, X, XI, and XII has already been discussed. Olfaction (CN I) is not commonly relevant to the evaluation or treatment of patients with lateral skull base malignancies. However, patients who perceive changes in this sense should be further evaluated by nasal endoscopy, with particular attention to the cribriform area mucosa. Functional evaluation of olfaction can be performed by subjecting the patients to tests with standardized odorants [10].

Trigeminal Nerve: CN V

The trigeminal nerve originates at the brainstem and passes anteriorly through the posterior fossa. At the trigeminal depression, a surface landmark of the petrous apex where the nerve enters the middle cranial fossa, the trigeminal (Gasserian) ganglion resides. From this point, the nerve divides into three divisions, eventually passing through three distinct neural foramina of the sphenoid bone.

The ophthalmic nerve (V1) travels through the superior orbital fissure and eventually transmits sensation for the skin of the forehead, part of the scalp, and upper eyelid as well as the conjunctiva of the eye.

The maxillary nerve (V2) travels through foramen rotundum into the pterygopalatine fossa. From there, it innervates the skin of the nose, cheek, and upper lip, as well as the mucosa of the nose, maxillary teeth, and roof of the mouth.

The mandibular nerve (V3) travels through foramen ovale into the infratemporal fossa. It provides sensation to the skin of the lower lip, chin, and lower one-third of the face, as well as the mucosa of the cheeks, lower lip, and floor of mouth. It also carries general somatic afferents from the anterior two-thirds of the tongue.

Direct testing of light touch, pinprick, and temperature sensation can be performed for the skin supplied by all trigeminal divisions. Corneal reflexes can be tested by gently applying a wisp of cotton to the cornea and observing bilateral orbicularis oculi contraction, requiring integrity of the entire reflex pathway (including the facial nerves) to produce the normal response. When corneal anesthesia occurs in the setting of ipsilateral facial paralysis, significant problems with corneal abrasion or ulceration can result.

Integrity of the trigeminal nerve can be further assessed by examining its associated motor functions. The masticatory muscles, including the temporalis, masseter, and pterygoids, are innervated by V3. The masseter and temporalis can be palpated while asking the patient to clench their teeth to grossly assess bulk and strength. Asymmetric temporal hollowing can also be seen in the setting of V3 dysfunction.

Facial numbness can occur with perineural spread of squamous cell carcinoma of the face and periauricular skin. In the setting of temporal bone cancer, facial numbness indicates late-stage disease that may be unresectable.

Facial Nerve: CN VII

The facial nerve follows a complex course, beginning in the brainstem at the facial nucleus and traversing the posterior fossa to the internal auditory canal. From there, it follows a long and circuitous intraosseous route in the temporal bone. Branches within the temporal bone carry parasympathetic fibers to the sphenopalatine ganglion (greater superficial petrosal nerve), parasympathetic and special sensory fibers to the submandibular ganglion (chorda tympani nerve), and motor fibers to the stapedius muscle. Outside of the temporal bone, the nerve arborizes in a complex network of branches that supply the muscles of facial expression, as well as the posterior belly of the digastric. General sensory afferents from a small patch of periauricular skin are carried by the posterior auricular branch of the facial nerve, as well.

Complete examination of facial nerve function begins with assessment of resting facial symmetry. Lack of muscular tone and muscular atrophy from chronic denervation can lead to asymmetry at rest. Previous episodes of complete paralysis, with subsequent recovery, may lead to the development of midfacial contracture that is apparent at rest, as well.

The function of the muscles of facial expression can be assessed by asking the patient to proceed through a series of movements: "raise your eyebrows," "close your eyes tightly," "wrinkle your nose," "puff out your cheeks," "pucker your lips," and "show me your teeth." The examiner should press his or her thumbs in the midline in order to minimize distortion or pulling by the intact contralateral facial musculature. Synkinesis may occur after recovery from an episode of facial paralysis. This should be evaluated for by asking the patient to blink rapidly, looking for synchronous movement of other facial muscles.

Standardized scales for reporting facial nerve function have been proposed. The most widely adopted of these is certainly the House-Brackmann facial nerve grading scale [11]. The criteria used to assign a functional grade of 1 (normal) to 6 (complete paralysis) are outlined in Table 2.2. The House-Brackmann scale has been criticized, however, for having high interobserver variability and an inability to

Table 2.2 House-Brackmann facial paralysis grading scale [11]

Grade	Description	Characteristics
I	Normal	Normal facial function
II	Slight dysfunction	*Gross*: slight weakness noticeable on close inspection; may have very slight synkinesis *At rest*: normal symmetry and tone *Motion* Forehead: moderate to good function Eye: complete closure with minimum effort Mouth: slight asymmetry
III	Moderate dysfunction	*Gross*: obvious but not disfiguring difference between two sides; noticeable but not severe synkinesis, contracture, and/or hemifacial spasm *At rest*: normal symmetry and tone *Motion* Forehead: slight to moderate function Eye: complete closure with effort Mouth: slightly weak with maximum effort
IV	Moderately severe dysfunction	*Gross*: obvious weakness and/or disfiguring asymmetry *At rest*: normal symmetry and tone *Motion* Forehead: none Eye: incomplete closure Mouth: asymmetric with maximum effort
V	Severe dysfunction	*Gross*: only barely perceptible motion *At rest*: asymmetry *Motion* Forehead: none Eye: incomplete closure Mouth: slight movement
VI	Total paralysis	No movement

account for variability in function between different regions of the face [12, 13]. The Facial Nerve Grading System 2.0 was created by the Facial Nerve Disorders Committee of the American Academy of Otolaryngology—Head and Neck Surgery to address these concerns [14]. The criteria of this scale are presented in Table 2.3. Consistent adherence to a published functional grading system is recommended for communication of clinical findings as well as for scientific publications.

Table 2.3 Facial Nerve Grading System 2.0 [14]

	Region			
Score	Brow	Eye	Nasolabial fold	Oral
1	Normal	Normal	Normal	Normal
2	Slight weakness >75% of normal	Slight weakness >75% of normal Complete closure with mild effort	Slight weakness >75% of normal	Slight weakness >75% of normal
3	Obvious weakness >50% of normal	Obvious weakness >50% of normal Complete closure with maximal effort	Obvious weakness >50% of normal	Obvious weakness >50% of normal
4	Asymmetry at rest <50% of normal	Asymmetry at rest <50% of normal Cannot close completely	Asymmetry at rest <50% of normal	Asymmetry at rest <50% of normal
5	Trace movement	Trace movement	Trace movement	Trace movement
6	No movement	No movement	No movement	No movement
Secondary movement (global assessment)				
Score	Degree of movement			
0	None			
1	Slight synkinesis, minimal contracture			
2	Obvious synkinesis, mild to moderate contracture			
3	Disfiguring synkinesis, severe contracture			
Reporting: sum score for each region and secondary movement				
Grade	Total score			
I	4			
II	5–9			
III	10–14			
IV	15–19			
V	20–23			
VI	24			

Clinical Assessment of Vestibular Function, Balance, and Gait

The peripheral vestibular system can be grossly assessed by several clinical examinations, most of which assess the integrity of the vestibular-ocular reflex (VOR) pathway. The head thrust (or head impulse) test isolates the function of the lateral semicircular canal. The patient's head is gently grasped, and they are asked to keep their eyes focused on the tip of the examiner's nose. Small amplitude (5–10 degree), high acceleration (3000–4000 degrees/s^2) head thrusts are applied. If the lateral canal and remainder of the VOR pathway are intact, the patient's gaze appears to remain fixed at the examiner. If the thrust moves the gaze away from the examiner temporarily, followed by a corrective saccade, a lesion is indicated on the side toward which the head was thrust [15].

Positional testing is used to diagnose benign paroxysmal positional vertigo (BPPV), which most commonly affects the posterior semicircular canal. This very common disorder should not necessarily be assumed to be tumor-related. The Dix-Hallpike test involves rapidly moving the patient from a sitting to a head-hanging supine position, with the head rotated 45 degrees toward the side to be tested. Fatiguing episodes of nystagmus, typically starting within seconds of reaching the head-hanging position, suggests posterior canal BPPV [16].

Adjunctive Testing

Audiometry

Objective measurement of hearing status is of great importance in the evaluation of patients with any otologic complaint or disease process. Pure tone audiometry, speech discrimination testing, tympanometry, and acoustic (stapes) reflex testing comprise the basic audiogram. Understanding the hearing abilities of the patient via these tests can provide information regarding disease extent as well as guide treatment and rehabilitation options.

Pure tone audiometry is the measurement of thresholds at which the patient can hear tones of specific frequencies. These tones are presented via an over-the-ear headphone or ear insert for measurement of air-conduction sensitivity or via a bone oscillator for measurement of bone-conduction sensitivity. Each ear is measured independently, using masking noise as appropriate in the non-test ear to overcome the effect of partial routing of sound through the skull to the contralateral cochlea.

When tumor involves the external auditory canal, tympanic membrane, or ossicles, a conductive hearing loss may result. This is reflected on the audiogram by an increase in air-conduction thresholds relative to the bone-conduction threshold levels at the same frequencies. While there are many potential etiologies for conductive hearing loss, the relative accessibility of the conductive hearing apparatus to physical examination on microscopy usually allows the differential to be narrowed significantly. Typically, a significant proportion of the ear canal will need to be occluded for hearing to be impacted. However, a small amount of tumor contact with the tympanic membrane or ossicles may cause a clinically detectable conductive loss (Fig. 2.7).

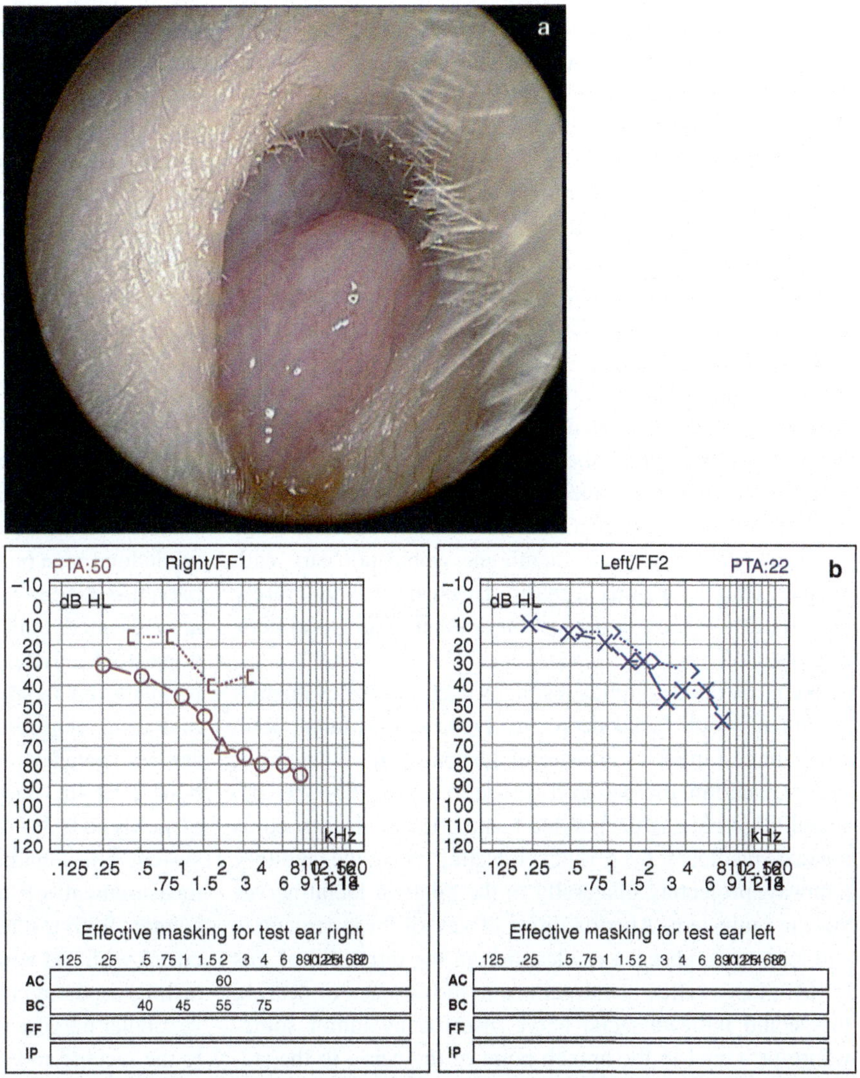

SRT PTA Right: 50.0 PTA Left: 21.7					
Transducer	Test type	Intensity	Masking	Aided I Binaural	ISF440 List
Right	HL	45	--		Spondee B
Left	HL	20	--		Spondee A

WR PTA Right: 50.0 PTA Left: 21.7						
Transducer	WR	Intensity	Masking	Score	Aided I Binaural	ISF440 List
Right	WR1	85	45	88		NU-6 LIST 1A
Left	WR1	60		100		NU-6 LIST 2A

Fig. 2.7 Squamous cell carcinoma filling right ear canal. (**a**) Oto-endoscopic view. (**b**) Audiogram

The bone-conduction thresholds should be carefully compared between the ears. Small (5–10 dB) threshold differences between ears, particularly when only at isolated frequencies, are commonly encountered and can be either attributed to test-retest variability or are considered clinically insignificant. Several definitions of asymmetric sensorineural hearing loss exist, typically for purposes of defining the unilateral hearing loss that is a part of a clinical syndrome (e.g., Meniere's disease). Erosion of tumor into the inner ear or auditory nerve may induce an asymmetric sensorineural loss, raising bone-conduction thresholds and worsening speech discrimination scores. The determination of inner ear involvement by temporal bone cancer cannot be made by audiometry alone, however.

Immittance audiometry is typically comprised of two components: tympanometry and acoustic reflex testing. Tympanometry involves the presentation of a tone via a sealed ear insert, while the pressure within the closed ear canal system is varied. The tympanic membrane vibrates most efficiently when the middle ear and ear canal pressures are equal. The immittance audiometer can detect this peak of movement efficiency (compliance) and can report an estimated pressure in the middle ear. If there is a perforation, or any pathology impedes the vibration of the tympanic membrane, the tympanogram will be flat (type B), since vibration of the tympanic membrane would not vary with pressure change in either scenario. This test rarely will rarely have much clinical significance in evaluating temporal bone cancers.

Acoustic (stapes) reflex testing is useful in the evaluation of patients with facial nerve involvement by tumor, however. The test involves measuring the compliance changes of the tympanic membrane in response to a loud (85–110 dB) sound. This change occurs due contraction of the stapedius muscle, mediated by a reflex traveling from the auditory pathway, projecting bilaterally to the bilateral facial nerves via the brainstem. Abnormalities of any of these structures can lead to an absence or elevation in the threshold of this reflex. Stapes reflex abnormalities in the absence of hearing loss could indicate facial nerve invasion by tumor somewhere proximal to the branch point of the nerve to the stapedius muscle. This would be most useful for patients with tumors that began extratemporally and subsequently invaded the skull base.

Electronystagmography/Videonystagmography (ENG/VNG)

ENG or VNG does not usually have a role in the evaluation of patients with skull base malignancies. It is a battery of tests that evaluate the peripheral vestibular system and vestibular-ocular reflex (VOR). Adequate vision and normal oculomotor function must be present for the test to be normal. Surface electrodes (ENG) or infrared video goggles (VNG) are used to measure eye movements in response to a variety of stimuli to the peripheral vestibular system.

Caloric testing assesses the functional integrity of the lateral semicircular canal, vestibular nerve, and the remainder of the vestibular-ocular reflex pathway. Air or water that is warmer or cooler than body temperature is introduced into the ear canal, and the resultant temperature change induces movement of endolymph in the lateral semicircular canal. This activates the VOR and produces nystagmus, the angular velocity of which is recorded. These velocities are compared between ears to assess for a relative weakness of one of the peripheral vestibular systems. Tumor which may be occluding the external or middle ear, however, might influence the caloric effect and invalidate the test results. Tumor invasion of the inner ear will often be evident by audiometry (sensorineural hearing loss) or imaging, and rarely would an abnormal ENG result be used to localize tumor. The test may be useful, however, to evaluate balance complaints in patients where the cancer would not be expected to induce these symptoms.

Vestibular-evoked myogenic potential (VEMP) testing analyzes EMG activity in response to auditory stimuli. In cervical VEMP (cVEMP) testing, the patient is laid supine, while loud tone bursts or clicks are presented to one ear. The patient is asked to lift their neck off the table while sounds are presented, tonically contracting the ipsilateral sternocleidomastoid muscle. Results are typically reported as a sound intensity threshold at which muscular activity response was first seen. Abnormally low thresholds (e.g., 70 dB or lower) are associated with 3rd window lesions, where defects in bone over the otic capsule allow for abnormal movement of perilymph and inappropriate activation of the vestibular system with sound. Ocular VEMP (oVEMP) testing involves measurement of orbital muscular EMG in response to sounds. With this test, abnormally high amplitudes are associated with 3rd window pathologies. Responses on oVEMP testing are thought to correlate with utricular and/or superior vestibular nerve activity, while cVEMP responses are related to the saccule and/or inferior vestibular nerve [17, 18].

Facial Nerve Testing

Standardized protocols for the electrical assessment of facial nerve function are widely used in neuro-otologic diagnosis, typically in the setting of acute injuries, such as Bell's palsy. Electroneuronography (ENoG) is used in cases of complete paralysis to assess the degree of Wallerian degeneration that occurs distal to an injury of unknown extent. The test is used to counsel the patient on prognosis or treatment options, such as decompressive surgery [19]. However, the usefulness of such tests in the assessment of tumor-related facial nerve complaints is limited. Spontaneous EMG activity of the facial musculature can be recorded and compared between sides to assess for subtle asymmetries when the weakness is not clinically obvious. The amplitude of EMG response can be subject to electrode placement and variable patient effort, and this information is not typically used to make treatment decisions.

Staging

The goal of staging is to group patients with equivalent disease burden to allow a fair comparison with respect to treatment outcomes. Staging is essential for patient counseling, treatment planning, and prediction of survival. In the case of temporal bone cancer, however, the relative rarity of the disease has precluded the creation of a universally accepted staging system. No system has been adopted by the American Joint Committee on Cancer. (AJCC) or the International Union for Cancer Control. Out of a desire to more specifically evaluate and risk-stratify patients with this rare and unique disease process, several staging systems for temporal bone cancer have been proposed.

Accurate staging improves external validity and allows for quality analysis of the effects of specific disease characteristics, comorbidities, and treatment [20]. Staging must account for local disease extension, since this is the main determinant of survival [21]. Regional and distant disease must also be included. The complex anatomy of the temporal bone and limitations of the physical examination in determining tumor extent have led to the integration of imaging and final pathologic findings in some staging systems [22, 23].

Several smaller single institution case series have been published, each with their own somewhat similar 2–4 level staging system. None of these have seen widespread use in the literature or have been subject to any prospective validation at other institutions. In general, increasing stage would be defined by involvement of more medial or functionally important structures, including the middle ear, facial nerve, mastoid, or structures beyond the temporal bone, such as dura. These are outlined in Tables 2.4, 2.5, and 2.6.

A few larger series are worth commenting on in further detail. Based on their series of 136 patients, Goodwin and Jesse proposed a classification system for temporal bone cancers in 1980, summarized in Table 2.7 [24]. Patients in groups 1 and 2 had similar 5-year overall survival rates, at 57% and 45%, respectively. Those in group 3 saw a lower survival rate of 29%. While the majority of tumors were squamous cell carcinoma, nearly 24% of the tumors in group 3 were of salivary gland origin.

Stell and McCormack (1985) [25] described a staging system based on their experience with 33 external ear canal tumors and 44 tumors of the middle ear (Table 2.8). Their system has 3T-stages. T1 tumors are limited to the site of origin. Interestingly, facial paralysis denotes a T2 tumor. Larger tumors with clinical or radiographic evidence of extension are listed as T3 tumors. This staging system has not been widely adopted but is still used in contemporary studies [26–34]. A modification was suggested by Clark et al. (1991), suggesting redefinition of T3 to include tumors with parotid, TMJ, and skin involvement, i.e., extracranial disease, and to make a T4 category for tumors with involvement of dura/base of skull, i.e., intracranial disease [35].

Table 2.4 Staging system proposed by Kinney and Wood (1987) [48]

Stage 1	Limited to the EAC
Stage 2	Erosion of bone or extension into the middle ear
Stage 3	Extension to dura, stylomastoid foramen, or skull base

Table 2.5 Staging system proposed by Shih and Crabtree (1990) [49]

Stage 1	Localized to the EAC
Stage 2	Extending into the temporal bone
Stage 3	Extending beyond the temporal bone into the parotid, neck, skull base, dura

Table 2.6 Staging system proposed by Spector (1991) [50]

Stage 1	Limited to the EAC
Stage 2	Superficial invasion
Stage 3	Deep invasion
Stage 4	Extension beyond the temporal bone

Table 2.7 Staging system proposed by Goodwin and Jesse (1980) [24]

Group 1	Tumors that involve the pinna and/or cartilaginous canal
Group 2	Tumors within the bony ear canal or mastoid cortex
Group 3	Tumors involving the deep structures of the temporal bone (middle ear, facial canal, skull base, or mastoid air cells)

Table 2.8 Staging system proposed by Stell and McCormack (1985) [25]

T1	Tumor limited to the site of origin, that is, with no facial nerve paralysis and no bone destruction
T2	Tumor extending beyond the site of origin indicated by facial paralysis or radiological evidence of bone destruction, but no extension beyond the organ of origin
T3	Clinical or radiological evidence of extension to surrounding structures (dura, base of the skull, parotid gland, temporomandibular joint, etc.)
TX	Patients with insufficient data for classification, including patients previously seen and treated elsewhere

Table 2.9 University of Cincinnati grading system for temporal bone tumors [2]

Grade I	Tumor in single site, <1 cm
Grade II	Tumor in a single site, but >1 cm
Grade III	Transannular tumor extension (i.e., ear canal and middle ear involvement)
Grade IV	Mastoid or petrous air-cell invasion
Grade V	Periauricular or contiguous extension (extratemporal)
Grade VI	Neck adenopathy, distant site, or infratemporal fossa

While this staging system might be accurate in predicting survival, it is less helpful in selecting treatment approach based on staging.

Pensak et al. (1996) published a staging system (Table 2.9) to describe a series of 46 patients with temporal bone cancer of differing histologic types [2]. A shortcoming of this scheme is that the use of "grade" to describe stage is potentially confused with histologic grading. Additionally, the lumping of distant disease with disease in the infratemporal fossa or neck would be obviated by using a TNM formulation.

This Manolidis staging system (Table 2.10) has been used by a few papers in reporting results of ear canal and temporal bone tumors [36, 37]. The advantage of this system is that it takes into account the spread of cancer from the auricle to the ear canal. It also considers progressively deeper sites as higher levels of staging. Furthermore, this staging system does not require measurement of tissue depth for adequate staging. One shortcoming is that infratemporal fossa and temporomandibular joint involvement are considered as an early-stage finding, which is not in keeping with the current understanding of temporal bone cancer invasion.

In 1990 Arriaga et al. [21] published a landmark study in which CT radiographic findings were correlated with pathologic findings for squamous cell carcinoma of the external auditory meatus. The authors excluded from consideration patients that had the ear canal involved secondarily by tumors of the auricle or surrounding skin. They identified 12 anatomic areas to be assessed: external osseous meatus erosion anteriorly, posteriorly, inferiorly, and superiorly; infratemporal extension; middle ear involvement; otic capsule erosion; mastoid involvement; jugular fossa erosion; carotid canal erosion; tegmen erosion with middle fossa involvement; and posterior fossa involvement. They identified a 98% concurrence between CT and pathologic extent of disease. This study highlights the fact that review of CT scans is required for accurate prediction of disease extent. Their staging system ranks tumors by extent of local destruction (e.g., canal wall or soft tissue extension) and by involvement of medial structures (e.g., ear canal, middle ear/mastoid, inner ear involvement) and uses a TNM format for squamous cell carcinoma of the external auditory meatus. In their schema, any lymph node involvement was automatically considered a sign of advanced stage disease.

Table 2.10 Staging system as proposed by Manolidis et al. (1998) [36]

Stage 1	Disease confined to external auditory canal including spread from auricular cancer to canal and confined to it
Stage 2	Disease spread from external auditory canal to one or more of the following: 1. Temporomandibular joint 2. Parotid 3. Infratemporal fossa
Stage 3	Spread of disease from external auditory canal to one or more of the following: 1. Middle ear 2. Mastoid 3. Facial nerve and Fallopian canal
Stage 4	Spread of disease to any one of the following: 1. Dura 2. Jugular bulb, sigmoid sinus 3. Carotid artery 4. Petrous apex extension

Table 2.11 Pittsburgh staging system for squamous cell carcinoma of the temporal bone (2000) [23]

Stage	Description
T classification	
T1	Limited to the EAC without bony erosion or evidence of soft tissue involvement
T2	Limited to the EAC with bon erosion (not full thickness) or limited soft tissue involvement (<0.5 cm)
T3	Erosion through the osseous EAC (full thickness) with limited soft tissue involvement (<0.5 cm) or tumor involvement in the middle ear and/or mastoid
T4	Erosion of the cochlea, petrous apex, medial wall of the middle ear, carotid canal, jugular foramen, or dura; with extensive soft tissue involvement (>0.5 cm, such as involvement of the TMJ or styloid process); or evidence of facial paresis
N classification	
N0	No regional nodes involved
N1	Single metastatic regional node <3 cm in size
N2	
N2a	Single ipsilateral node 3–6 cm in size
N2b	Multiple ipsilateral metastatic lymph nodes
N2c	Contralateral metastatic lymph node
N3	Metastatic lymph node >6 cm in size
Overall stage	
I	T1N0
II	T2N0
III	T3N0
IV	T4N0 and T1-4N1-3

EAC external auditory canal, *TMJ* temporomandibular joint

This system has become known as the Pittsburgh staging system (PSS) and has undergone several amendments (Table 2.11). The most notable of these amendments came in 2000, when Moody et al. modified the original PSS to classify patients with facial paresis or paralysis as having T4 disease [23].

The PSS has come to be the most widely used and externally validated staging system for temporal bone carcinoma, with several studies confirming the correlation between Pittsburgh T stage and prognosis [1, 22, 38–44]. Higgins and Moody-Antonio performed a systematic review of the literature regarding outcomes for patients with or without facial paralysis in the setting of SCC of the ear canal and temporal bone [20]. Their study encompassed 21 studies covering 348 patients. They demonstrated that patient with facial paralysis had a significantly worse disease-specific survival and overall survival when compared to patients without facial paralysis. Furthermore, they showed that overall survival was worse for patients with facial paralysis than those staged as Pittsburgh (2000) T3. There was no significant difference in overall survival between patients staged as Pittsburgh (2000) T4 and those with facial paralysis. From this analysis they concluded that facial paralysis rightfully should be staged as T4. They also showed that the Pittsburgh (2000) staging was superior to both the 1990 version and the Stell staging system by being able to discriminate overall survival in Stell T2 versus T3 disease and Pittsburgh T3 versus T4 disease.

Several criticisms and proposed amendments to the PSS have arisen. Breau et al. proposed a modification to the Pittsburgh system for early-stage lesions based on the site of disease in the canal with less emphasis on the size of the primary tumor or degree of bony invasion [45]. They argue that tumors on the anterior wall of the EAC have less impediment to spread beyond the temporal bone, finding that anterior canal wall tumors had a higher rate of local recurrence and decreased survival in their series.

However, even if anterior EAC tumors have a stronger tendency to spread beyond the temporal bone, Mazzoni et al. raise the point that tumor extension into the more anterior or lateral tissues (of the TMJ, parotid, or auricle) is more accessible and potentially resectable than tumor that invades in a posterior or medial direction [46]. They propose modifications to the PSS to account for this (Table 2.12).

Table 2.12 Proposed modification to the Pittsburgh staging system [39]

T1	Tumor in skin without bone involvement
T2	Tumor in skin with bone/cartilage involvement, but not full thickness
T3a	Tumor extending <5 mm from cartilage to periauricular soft tissues or tumor strictly limited to the anterior bone wall and growing <5 mm into the parotid space
T3b	Same as for T3a, but extending >5 mm
T4a	Tumor growing into mastoid, without 7th paresis
T4b	Tumor growing into mastoid with facial paresis, or infratemporal space, or medial wall of tympanum, labyrinth, petrous bone (jugular foramen, internal carotid canal, petrous apex)

Conclusion

Elements from all components of the clinical evaluation—including history, physical examination, imaging, and adjunctive testing—are important in the staging of temporal bone cancer. Important treatment decisions that significantly impact functional outcomes and survival rates stem from this evaluation. An accurate and precise characterization of tumor extent and the patient's functional status is therefore the cornerstone of care for patients with temporal bone cancer.

References

1. Gidley PW, Roberts DB, Sturgis EM. Squamous cell carcinoma of the temporal bone. Laryngoscope. 2010;120(6):1144–51.
2. Pensak ML, Gleich LL, Gluckman JL, Shumrick KA. Temporal bone carcinoma: contemporary perspectives in the skull base surgical era. Laryngoscope. 1996;106(10):1234–7.
3. Nyrop M, Grøntved A. Cancer of the external auditory canal. Arch Otolaryngol Head Neck Surg. 2002;128(7):834–7.
4. Barrs DM. Temporal bone carcinoma. Otolaryngol Clin N Am. 2001;34(6):1197–1218-x.
5. Jackson CG, Glasscock ME, Hughes G, Sismanis A. Facial paralysis of neoplastic origin: diagnosis and management. Laryngoscope. 1980;90(10 Pt 1):1581–95.
6. Manyam BV, Gastman B, Zhang AY, Reddy CA, Burkey BB, Scharpf J, et al. Inferior outcomes in immunosuppressed patients with high-risk cutaneous squamous cell carcinoma of the head and neck treated with surgery and radiation therapy. J Am Acad Dermatol. 2015;73(2):221–7.
7. Traccis S, Zoroddu GF, Zecca MT, Cau T, Solinas MA, Masuri R. Evaluating patients with vertigo: bedside examination. Neurol Sci. 2004, 25 Suppl 1:S16–9.
8. Jeffcoat B, Shelukhin A, Fong A, Mustain W, Zhou W. Alexander's Law revisited. J Neurophysiol. 2008;100(1):154–9.
9. Burkey JM, Lippy WH, Schuring AG, Rizer FM. Clinical utility of the 512-Hz Rinne tuning fork test. Am J Otol. 1998;19(1):59–62.
10. Doty RL, Shaman P, Dann M. Development of the University of Pennsylvania Smell Identification Test: a standardized microencapsulated test of olfactory function. Physiol Behav. 1984;32(3):489–502.
11. House JW, Brackmann DE. Facial nerve grading system. Otolaryngol Head Neck Surg. 1985;93(2):146–7.
12. Rickenmann J, Jaquenod C, Cerenko D, Fisch U. Comparative value of facial nerve grading systems. Otolaryngol Head Neck Surg. 1997;117(4):322–5.
13. Coulson SE, Croxson GR, Adams RD, O'Dwyer NJ. Reliability of the "Sydney," "Sunnybrook," and "House Brackmann" facial grading systems to assess voluntary movement and synkinesis after facial nerve paralysis. Otolaryngol Head Neck Surg. 2005;132(4):543–9.
14. Vrabec JT, Backous DD, Djalilian HR, Gidley PW, Leonetti JP, Marzo SJ, et al. Facial Nerve Grading System 2.0. Otolaryngol Head Neck Surg. 2009;140(4):445–50.
15. Schubert MC, Tusa RJ, Grine LE, Herdman SJ. Optimizing the sensitivity of the head thrust test for identifying vestibular hypofunction. Phys Ther. 2004;84(2):151–8.
16. Dix MR, Hallpike CS. The pathology, symptomatology and diagnosis of certain common disorders of the vestibular system. Ann Otol Rhinol Laryngol. 1952;61(4):987–1016.
17. Zuniga MG, Janky KL, Nguyen KD, Welgampola MS, Carey JP. Ocular versus cervical VEMPs in the diagnosis of superior

semicircular canal dehiscence syndrome. Otol Neurotol. 2013;34(1): 121–6.
18. Kantner C, Gürkov R. Characteristics and clinical applications of ocular vestibular evoked myogenic potentials. Hear Res. 2012;294(1–2):55–63.
19. Gantz BJ, Rubinstein JT, Gidley P, Woodworth GG. Surgical management of Bell's palsy. Laryngoscope. 1999;109(8):1177–88.
20. Higgins TS, Antonio SAM. The role of facial palsy in staging squamous cell carcinoma of the temporal bone and external auditory canal: a comparative survival analysis. Otol Neurotol. 2010; 31(9):1473–9.
21. Arriaga M, Curtin H, Takahashi H, Hirsch BE, Kamerer DB. Staging proposal for external auditory meatus carcinoma based on preoperative clinical examination and computed tomography findings. Ann Otol Rhinol Laryngol. 1990;99(9 Pt 1):714–21.
22. Essig GF, Kitipornchai L, Adams F, Zarate D, Gandhi M, Porceddu S, et al. Lateral temporal bone resection in advanced cutaneous squamous cell carcinoma: report of 35 patients. J Neurol Surg B Skull Base. 2013;74(1):54–9.
23. Moody SA, Hirsch BE, Myers EN. Squamous cell carcinoma of the external auditory canal: an evaluation of a staging system. Am J Otol. 2000;21(4):582–8.
24. Goodwin WJ, Jesse RH. Malignant neoplasms of the external auditory canal and temporal bone. Arch Otolaryngol. 1980;106(11): 675–9.
25. Stell PM, McCormick MS. Carcinoma of the external auditory meatus and middle ear. Prognostic factors and a suggested staging system. J Laryngol Otol. 1985;99(9):847–50.
26. Jia X, Liang Q, Chi F. Treatment and outcome of middle ear cancer. Eur Arch Otorhinolaryngol. 2014;271(10):2675–80.
27. Prabhu R, Hinerman RW, Indelicato DJ, Morris CG, Werning JW, Vaysberg M, et al. Squamous cell carcinoma of the external auditory canal: long-term clinical outcomes using surgery and external-beam radiotherapy. Am J Clin Oncol. 2009;32(4):401–4.
28. Cristalli G, Manciocco V, Pichi B, Marucci L, Arcangeli G, Telera S, et al. Treatment and outcome of advanced external auditory canal and middle ear squamous cell carcinoma. J Craniofac Surg. 2009;20(3):816–21.
29. Ogawa K, Nakamura K, Hatano K, Uno T, Fuwa N, Itami J, et al. Treatment and prognosis of squamous cell carcinoma of the external auditory canal and middle ear: a multi-institutional retrospective review of 87 patients. Int J Radiat Oncol Biol Phys. 2007;68(5):1326–34.
30. Bibas AG, Ward V, Gleeson MJ. Squamous cell carcinoma of the temporal bone. J Laryngol Otol. 2008;122(11):1156–61.
31. Lo W-C, Ting L-L, Ko J-Y, Lou P-J, Yang T-L, Chang Y-L, et al. Malignancies of the ear in irradiated patients of nasopharyngeal carcinoma. Laryngoscope. 2008;118(12):2151–5.
32. Pemberton LS, Swindell R, Sykes AJ. Primary radical radiotherapy for squamous cell carcinoma of the middle ear and external auditory canal – an historical series. Clin Oncol (R Coll Radiol). 2006;18(5):390–4.
33. Lim LH, Goh YH, Chan YM, Chong VF, Low WK. Malignancy of the temporal bone and external auditory canal. Otolaryngol Head Neck Surg. 2000;122(6):882–6.
34. Hashi N, Shirato H, Omatsu T, Kagei K, Nishioka T, Hashimoto S, et al. The role of radiotherapy in treating squamous cell carcinoma of the external auditory canal, especially in early stages of disease. Radiother Oncol. 2000;56(2):221–5.
35. Clark LJ, Narula AA, Morgan DA, Bradley PJ. Squamous carcinoma of the temporal bone: a revised staging. J Laryngol Otol. 1991;105(5):346–8.
36. Manolidis S, Pappas D, Doersten Von P, Jackson CG, Glasscock ME. Temporal bone and lateral skull base malignancy: experience and results with 81 patients. Am J Otol. 1998;19(6 Suppl): S1–15.
37. Testa JR, Fukuda Y, Kowalski LP. Prognostic factors in carcinoma of the external auditory canal. Arch Otolaryngol Head Neck Surg. 1997;123(7):720–4.
38. Madsen AR, Gundgaard MG, Hoff CM, Maare C, Holmboe P, Knap M, et al. Cancer of the external auditory canal and middle ear in Denmark from 1992 to 2001. Head Neck. 2008;30(10): 1332–8.
39. Prasad SC, D'Orazio F, Medina M, Bacciu A, Sanna M. State of the art in temporal bone malignancies. Curr Opin Otolaryngol Head Neck Surg. 2014;22(2):154–65.
40. Bacciu A, Clemente IA, Piccirillo E, Ferrari S, Sanna M. Guidelines for treating temporal bone carcinoma based on long-term outcomes. Otol Neurotol. 2013;34(5):898–907.
41. Zanoletti E, Marioni G, Stritoni P, Lionello M, Giacomelli L, Martini A, et al. Temporal bone squamous cell carcinoma: analyzing prognosis with univariate and multivariate models. Laryngoscope. 2014;124(5):1192–8.
42. Ito M, Hatano M, Yoshizaki T. Prognostic factors for squamous cell carcinoma of the temporal bone: extensive bone involvement or extensive soft tissue involvement? Acta Otolaryngol. 2009;129(11):1313–9.
43. Moffat DA, Wagstaff SA, Hardy DG. The outcome of radical surgery and postoperative radiotherapy for squamous carcinoma of the temporal bone. Laryngoscope. 2005;115(2):341–7.
44. Austin JR, Stewart KL, Fawzi N. Squamous cell carcinoma of the external auditory canal. Therapeutic prognosis based on a proposed staging system. Arch Otolaryngol Head Neck Surg. 1994;120(11):1228–32.
45. Breau RL, Gardner EK, Dornhoffer JL. Cancer of the external auditory canal and temporal bone. Curr Oncol Rep. 2002;4(1):76–80.
46. Mazzoni A, Danesi G, Zanoletti E. Primary squamous cell carcinoma of the external auditory canal: surgical treatment and long-term outcomes. Acta Otorhinolaryngol Ital. 2014;34(2): 129–37.
47. Kung NH, Van Stavern GP. Isolated ocular motor nerve palsies. Semin Neurol. 2015;35(5):539–48.
48. Kinney SE, Wood BG. Malignancies of the external ear canal and temporal bone: surgical techniques and results. Laryngoscope. 1987;97(2):158–64.
49. Shih L, Crabtree JA. Carcinoma of the external auditory canal: an update. Laryngoscope. 1990;100(11):1215–8.
50. Spector JG. Management of temporal bone carcinomas: a therapeutic analysis of two groups of patients and long-term followup. Otolaryngol Head Neck Surg. 1991;104(1):58–66.

Diagnostic Imaging of Temporal Bone Cancer

3

J. Matthew Debnam

Image Techniques

Multidetector computed tomography (MDCT) plays an important role in imaging tumors of the skull base and neck. A major advantage of MDCT is its short acquisition time, particularly in a patient population that may have difficulty tolerating the longer time required for magnetic resonance imaging (MRI) examinations. With MDCT, imaging is performed in the axial plane, and reformatted images can be provided in any plane deemed necessary. MDCT is superior to MRI in evaluating bony structures for conditions such as tumor-related bone destruction and osteoradionecrosis following radiation therapy. MDCT can also be used in the evaluation of patients who are incompatible with MRI, such as patients with claustrophobia and those with pacemakers, indwelling metallic devices, or foreign bodies in close proximity to the orbits.

Our CT protocol for imaging of the temporal bone and parotid tumors includes contrast-enhanced imaging in the axial plane at 1.25 mm slice thickness with reconstructed images in the coronal and sagittal planes. Both soft tissue and bone windows are provided for interpretation.

CT angiography (CTA) and CT venography (CTV) use a timed contrasted bolus to visualize the arterial or venous systems about the neck. CTA or CTV can be used, respectively, to assess tumors' arterial supply or venous drainage, to determine tumors' relation to the adjacent arterial or venous systems, and to rule out arterial or venous thrombosis.

MRI provides detailed imaging of soft tissue tumors about the skull base and neck. Patients are placed in a magnetic field, and a radio-frequency pulse is used to stimulate hydrogen protons and elevate them to a higher energy state. The protons then return to their normal lower resting energy state, releasing electromagnetic energy. A coil receives this electromagnetic energy, and computer manipulation converts it into an image. The time for the hydrogen protons to return to their normal resting state is called the relaxation time. Depending on their chemical composition, tissues have different relaxation times and thus create different signals for the image formation.

Our MRI protocol for temporal bone and parotid tumors includes an axial T1-weighted pre-contrast sequence, T1-weighted post-contrast images in three orthogonal planes, and an axial T2-weighted sequence. To highlight the enhancing characteristics and aid in tumor mapping, a fat suppression technique can be employed on both T1-weighted post-contrast and T2-weighted sequences. However, imaging without fat suppression may be necessary because the fat suppression technique increases magnetic susceptibility related to the patient's braces, makeup, and dental fillings. We use a 3 mm slice thickness with a 0.5 to 1.0 mm gap between the slices for all MRI sequences. Also, an axial T1-weighted post-gadolinium sequence of the brain can assess for intracranial spread of tumors and brain metastases. An axial T2-weighted sequence of the neck with fat suppression can evaluate for cervical lymphadenopathy.

The most common use of positron emission tomography (PET/CT) involves the administration of ^{18}F-fluorodeoxyglucose (FDG), a cyclotron-produced radionuclide. FDG is taken up by cells in the same manner as serum glucose. Tumors have a high metabolic demand with increased glucose uptake. When FDG is taken up by tumor cells, the FDG will decay and emit two photons that are detected by a coincidence scanner. The resulting images reflect the concentration of FDG within the tumor. An important clinical use of PET/CT is the detection of recurrent disease and distant metastasis. It should be noted that tumors of small size, low-grade, or containing significant necrosis may not be FDG-avid.

Ultrasonography (US) is a practical imaging modality for the assessment of the parotid gland and neck lymph nodes. US can reliably distinguish between simple cysts and solid tumors and demonstrate areas of vascular flow in a tumor;

J. Matthew Debnam, M.D.
Section of Neuroradiology, The University of Texas
M.D. Anderson Cancer Center, Houston, TX, USA
e-mail: matthew.debnam@mdanderson.org

P. W. Gidley, F. DeMonte (eds.), *Temporal Bone Cancer*, https://doi.org/10.1007/978-3-319-74539-8_3

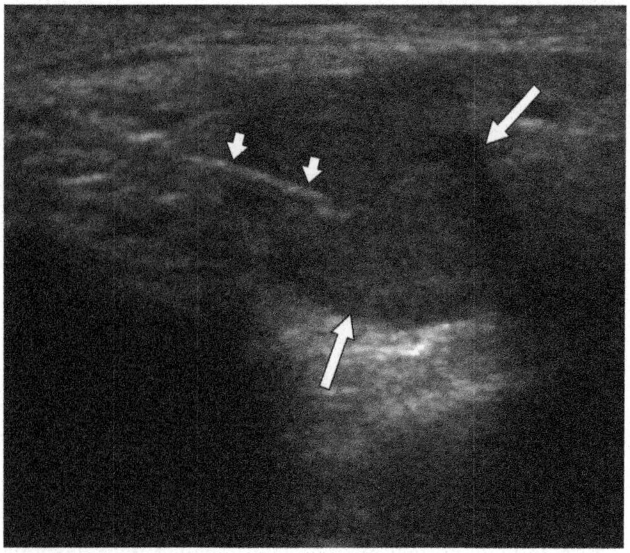

Fig. 3.1 Ultrasound-guided fine-needle aspiration: under ultrasonographic guidance, a needle (small arrows) is placed within a parotid mass (large arrows) for aspiration

however, differentiating benign from malignant disease has proved challenging because of similarities between the clinical presentation and sonographic appearance. US can be used to guide fine-needle aspiration (Fig. 3.1).

Skin Cancer (Ear and Preauricular)

Basal cell carcinoma (BCC) and squamous cell carcinoma (SCC) are the most common non-melanomatous cancers of the skin [1, 2]. BCCs are slow-growing neoplasms that invade locally, while SCCs are more aggressive [1–3]. Depending on the size of the lesion, BCCs and SCCs vary in appearance. Smaller lesions often appear as a soft tissue mass on the skin surface. When larger, the lesions invade the underlying soft tissues. Both the horizontal diameter and the thickness of skin cancers can be measured on imaging, and a large size is associated with an increased rate of metastasis [4–7]. The full extent of the tumor must be accurately mapped for treatment planning (Fig. 3.2a). This mapping includes the recognition of adjacent bony involvement (Fig. 3.2b) because such involvement will require lateral temporal bone resection. On T1-weighted MRI, these lesions are hypointense and demonstrate enhancement; on T2-weighted MRI, they are heterogeneously hyperintense [1]. BCCs and SCCs are FDG-avid on PET/CT [8]. While BCC rarely metastasizes (<0.1% incidence) [1, 9], the incidence of SCC metastasis varies from 5% to 30%; in approximately 55% of these cases, metastatic SCC is detected by imaging [10]. A higher rate of regional and distant metastasis occurs when there is perineural disease spread [11].

Tumors of the Ear Canal

The most common tumor of the ear canal is SCC [12, 13]. These tumors may arise in the external auditory canal (Fig. 3.3) and spread to the middle ear or originate in the middle ear. When patients present with large, destructive lesions, the site of origin may be obscured. SCC spreads by direct extension destroying the adjacent bony walls, commonly through the floor of the external auditory canal into the infratemporal fossa [14–16]. There may be further involvement of the mastoid temporal bone, periauricular soft tissues, parotid gland, or temporomandibular joint. In advanced stages, invasion of the middle and posterior cranial fossae, the carotid canal, and jugular foramen occurs [12, 17–19]. Often times, the otic capsule is spared [18, 20]. Metastatic adenopathy is uncommon and when present usually involves the preauricular region, parotid, upper cervical, or retropharyngeal nodes [21]. Extensive tumor spread, facial nerve paralysis, and adenopathy are poor predictors of patient outcomes [22].

Primary Bone Tumors

While osteosarcoma is the most common primary bone malignancy, involvement of the craniofacial bony structures is very rare, accounting for fewer than 2% of all osteosarcomas [23, 24]. Most osteosarcomas that occur in the skull bones are secondary malignancies. Predisposing factors for osteosarcoma include hereditary retinoblastoma, Paget disease, fibrous dysplasia, and trauma [25]. Osteosarcoma is a known complication of radiation therapy, usually occurring after a long latency period. Focal bone destruction is common, although dense sclerotic bone may also be present. On CT, there is often a "sunburst" periosteal reaction (Fig. 3.4a). Signal intensity on MRI depends on the tumor's bone content, usually demonstrating a hypointense T1-weighted signal and an intermediate T2-weighted signal intensity (Fig. 3.4b). Contrast enhancement is present on MRI, although generally not to the same degree as chondrosarcoma (Fig. 3.4c).

Chondrosarcomas occur at the cartilaginous junction of bones. On CT, a chondroid matrix mineralization is characterized by intraosseous calcification in the soft tissue mass (Fig. 3.5a). Bony erosion may also be present. The MRI signal is defined by the chondroid matrix and shows T1-weighted signal hypointensity, T2-weighted signal hyperintensity (Fig. 3.5b), and punctate hypointense foci on T1- and T2-weighted sequences suggestive of medullary calcifications. These tumors may demonstrate heterogeneous or homogeneous enhancement (Fig. 3.5c) [26].

Giant cell tumors are uncommon benign but potentially aggressive tumors. Approximately 2% occur in the head and neck, usually involving sites that develop from endochondral ossification such as the sphenoid, ethmoid, or temporal

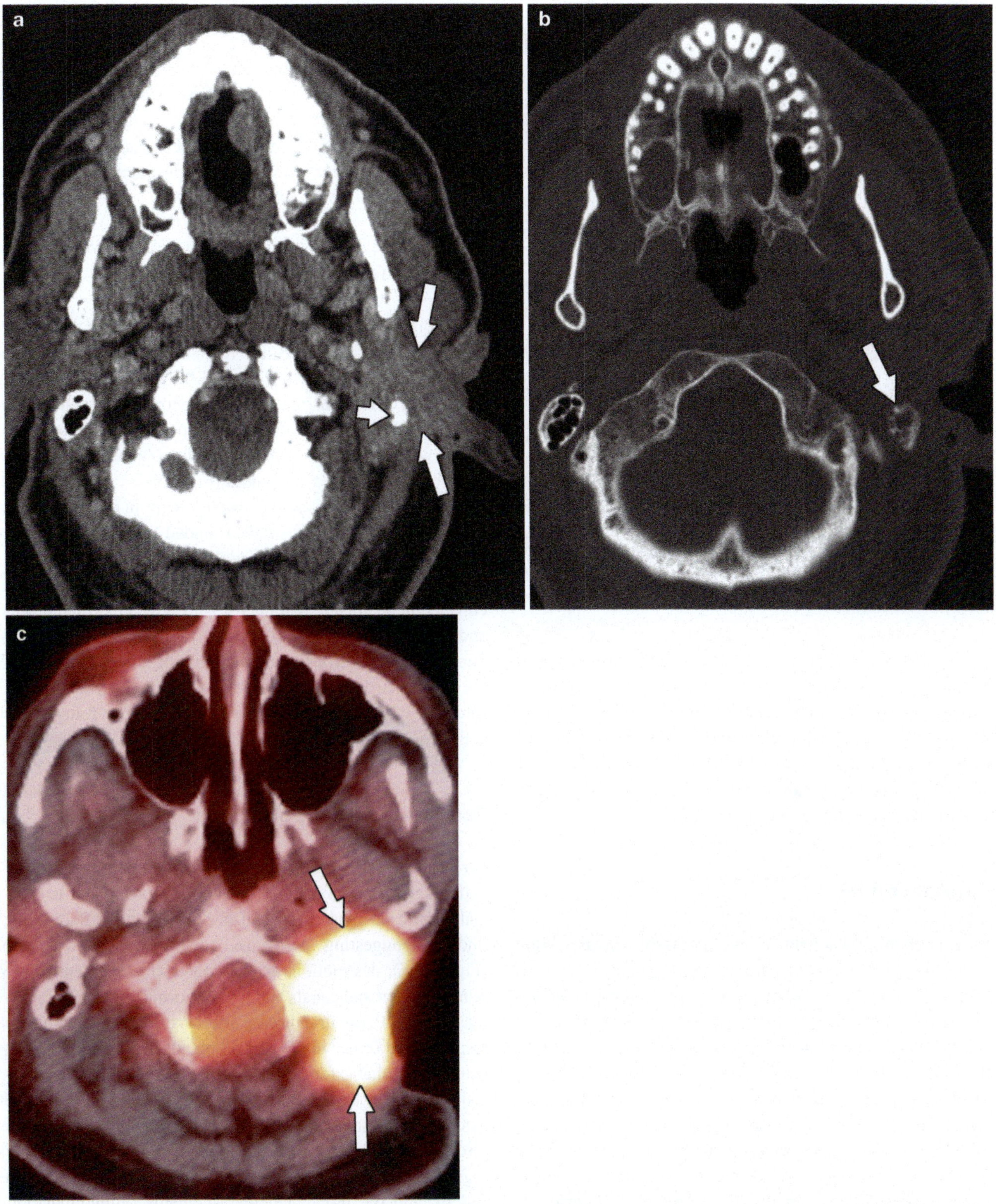

Fig. 3.2 A 60-year-old man with invasive SCC of the left post-auricular skin. (**a**) Axial CT with contrast, soft tissue window. Enhancing mass in the left parotid gland (arrows). Tumor can be seen engulfing the mastoid tip (small arrow). (**b**) Axial CT with contrast, bone window. Destruction of the left mastoid tip (arrow). (**c**) PET/CT, 5 years later. FDG-avid recurrent tumor in the superior left neck (arrows)

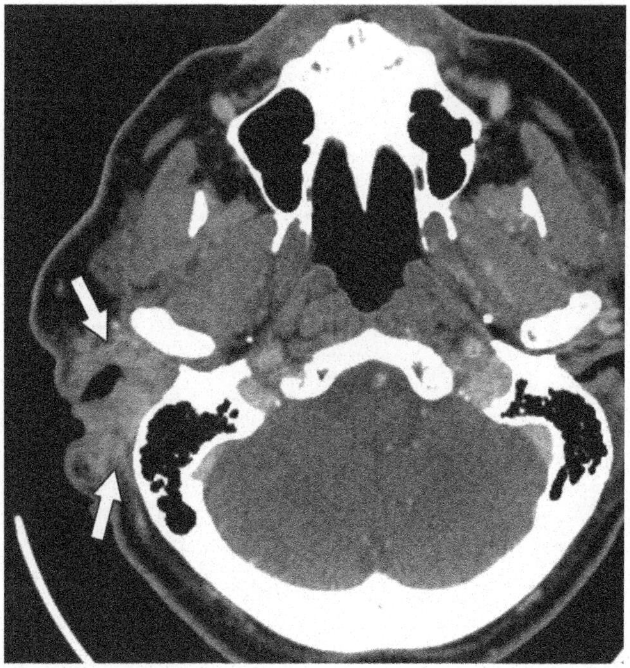

Fig. 3.3 A 73-year-old man with SCC of the right external auditory canal. Axial CT with contrast, soft tissue window. Homogeneously enhancing tumor about the right external auditory canal (arrows)

bones [27]. On CT, giant cell tumors show a tendency to destroy bone or to remodel bone with expansion and/or extend through bone with areas of loculation (Fig. 3.6a and b) [28] and demonstrate moderate enhancement [29, 30]. Calcifications are unusual. On MRI, giant cell tumors show signal hypointensity on all sequences (Fig. 3.6c) and demonstrate enhancement (Fig. 3.6d) [28–31].

Parotid Lesions

Mucoepidermoid carcinomas are tumors of salivary tissue, occurring most commonly in the parotid gland. Low-grade mucoepidermoid tumors have larger cystic components and few solid components, while higher-grade lesions have a solid appearance with poorly circumscribed margins. On CT the solid components demonstrate heterogeneous enhancement (Fig. 3.7a); calcifications are rare. Bone changes range from remodeling to destruction of the bony cortex. On MRI, lesions demonstrate low to intermediate signal on T1-weighted sequences, and there is heterogeneous enhancement of the solid components (Fig. 3.7b). T2-weighted signal intensity varies depending on the degree of cellularity, with signal hyperintensity in low-grade tumors (Fig. 3.7c) and signal hypointensity in high-grade tumors [32].

Adenoid cystic carcinomas of the salivary glands are slow-growing malignant tumors. Low-grade adenoid cystic carcinomas tend to have well-defined borders, while high-grade lesions are infiltrative (Fig. 3.8a). Adenoid cystic carcinomas are hypointense to isointense on T1-weighted MRI sequences and hyperintense on T2-weighted sequences; higher-grade lesions are markedly hyperintense on T2-weighted sequences. Both grades demonstrate homogeneous enhancement (Fig. 3.8a) [33]. Local recurrence, perineural spread, and late distant metastasis (Fig. 3.8b) can occur.

Pediatric Temporal Bone Cancers

Rhabdomyosarcoma is the most common middle ear tumor in children [34, 35]. Bone remodeling and destruction occur with rapid extension beyond the middle ear [35–37]. Rhabdomyosarcomas show homogeneous enhancement on CT and MRI, and the tumors are hypointense to isointense on T1-weighted MRI sequences and hypointense to hyperintense on T2-weighted sequences (Fig. 3.9).

Langerhans cell histiocytosis may occur in multiple bones and appear as multiple small, rounded radiolucent lesions with well-defined borders. Irregular lucent patches that have no reactive sclerosis occur. On MRI, lesions demonstrate enhancement and are hypointense on T1-weighted sequences and isointense to hyperintense on T2-weighted sequences. Temporal bone lesions involving only the anterior aspects of the bone (petrous apex and middle ear) suggest rhabdomyosarcoma, whereas lesions in the mastoid suggest Langerhans cell histiocytosis (Fig. 3.10) [38].

Perineural Tumor Spread

Perineural spread of SCC occurs in approximately 5–10% of patients, is often an incidental finding [39, 40], and is associated with decreased survival in SCC [41–43]. Radiologic findings suggesting perineural spread include widening (Fig. 3.11a), destruction, and extensive enhancement of the bony foramen and canals and loss of normal fat in the foramina [44–46]. Perineural disease affecting the facial nerve may result from a tumor in the parotid gland itself, from adjacent skin cancers that extend to involve the parotid, or from metastasis to the parotid. From the intraparotid facial nerve, there is retrograde disease spread of the facial nerve with extension through the stylomastoid foramen to involve the descending segment, posterior genu, geniculate ganglion (Fig. 3.11b and c), and the intracanalicular segments. Tumors involving the parotid can also spread along the auriculotemporal nerve [44]. Perineural spread along this nerve, which courses medially from the parotid gland through the stylomandibular tunnel, accesses the main trunk of the third division of the trigeminal nerve (Fig. 3.12b and c).

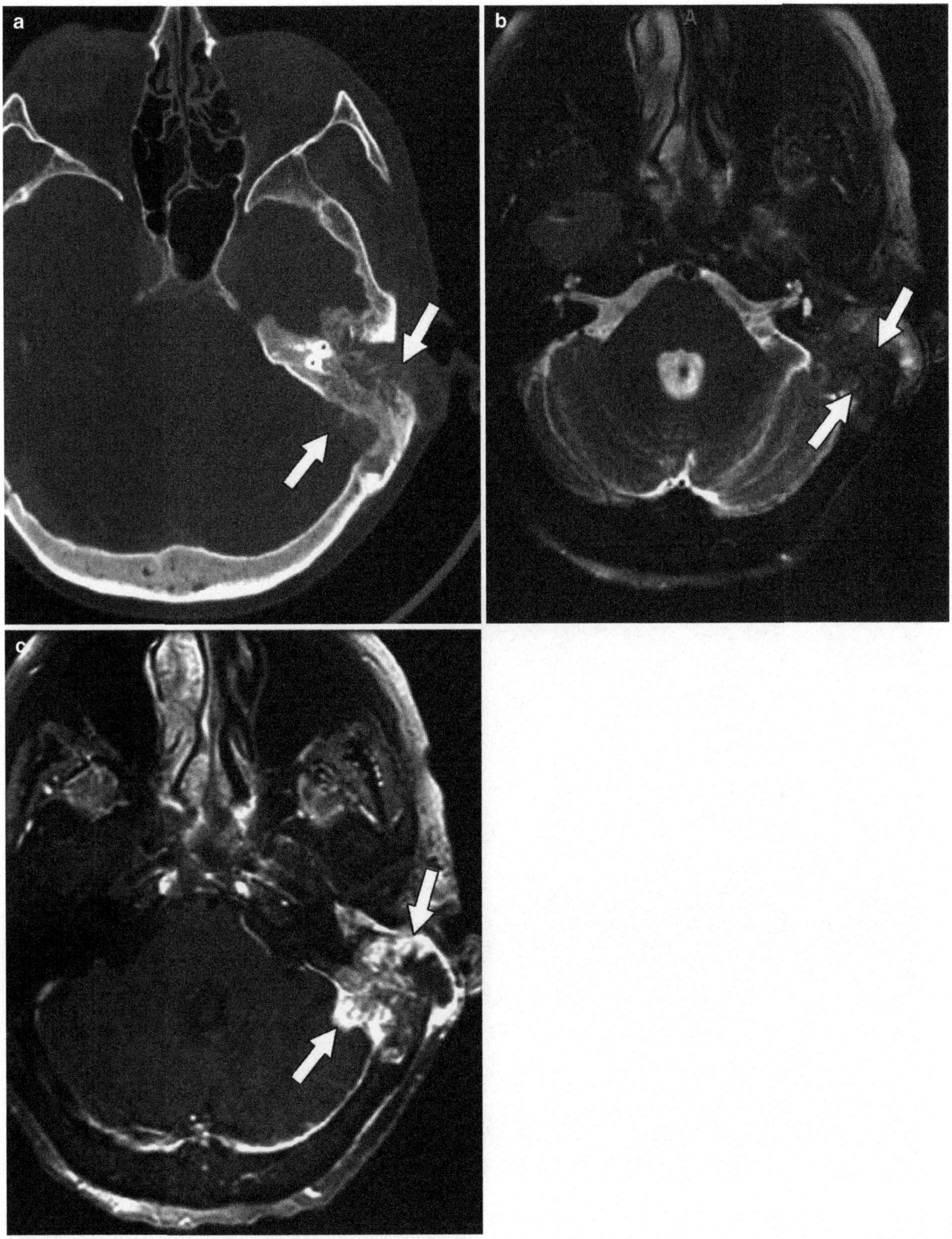

Fig. 3.4 A 69-year-old woman with a radiation-associated osteosarcoma of the left temporal bone 13 years after treatment for a mucoepidermoid tumor. (**a**) Axial CT with contrast, bone window. Destructive left temporal bone mass with a "sunburst" pattern of periosteal reaction (arrows). (**b**) Axial T2-weighted MRI sequence. Hypointense appearance of the mass (arrows). (**c**) Axial T1-weighted post-contrast MRI sequence. Heterogeneously enhancing mass (arrows)

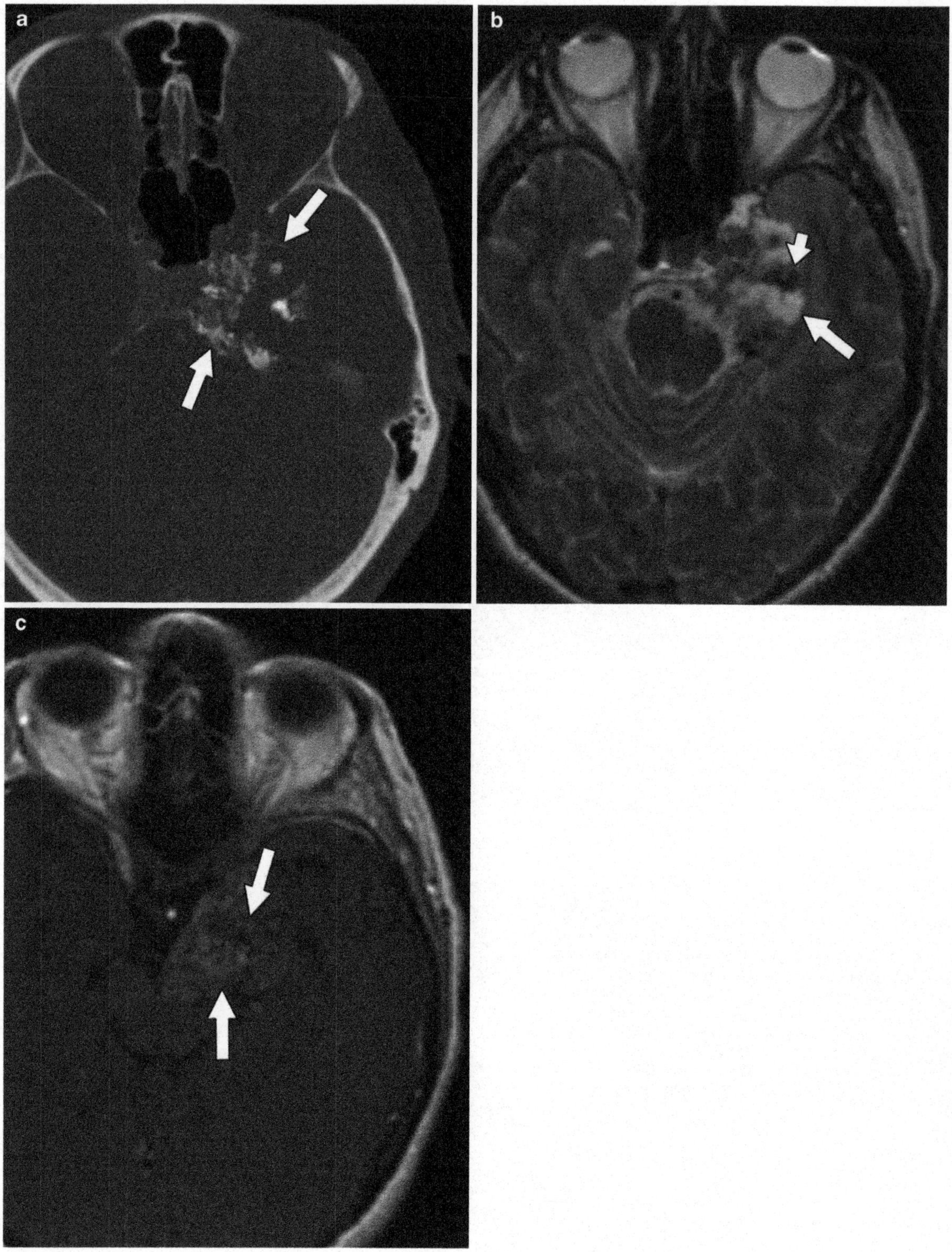

Fig. 3.5 A 57-year-old woman palatal mass from a chondrosarcoma involving from the left temporal bone. (**a**) Axial CT with contrast, bone window. Destructive left temporal bone mass with mineralization of the chondroid matrix (arrows). (**b**) Axial T2-weighted MRI sequence. Hyperintense appearance of the mass (arrow) with hypointense signal at sites of mineralization (small arrow). (**c**) Axial T1-weighted post-contrast MRI sequence. Mild, heterogeneous enhancement of the mass (arrows)

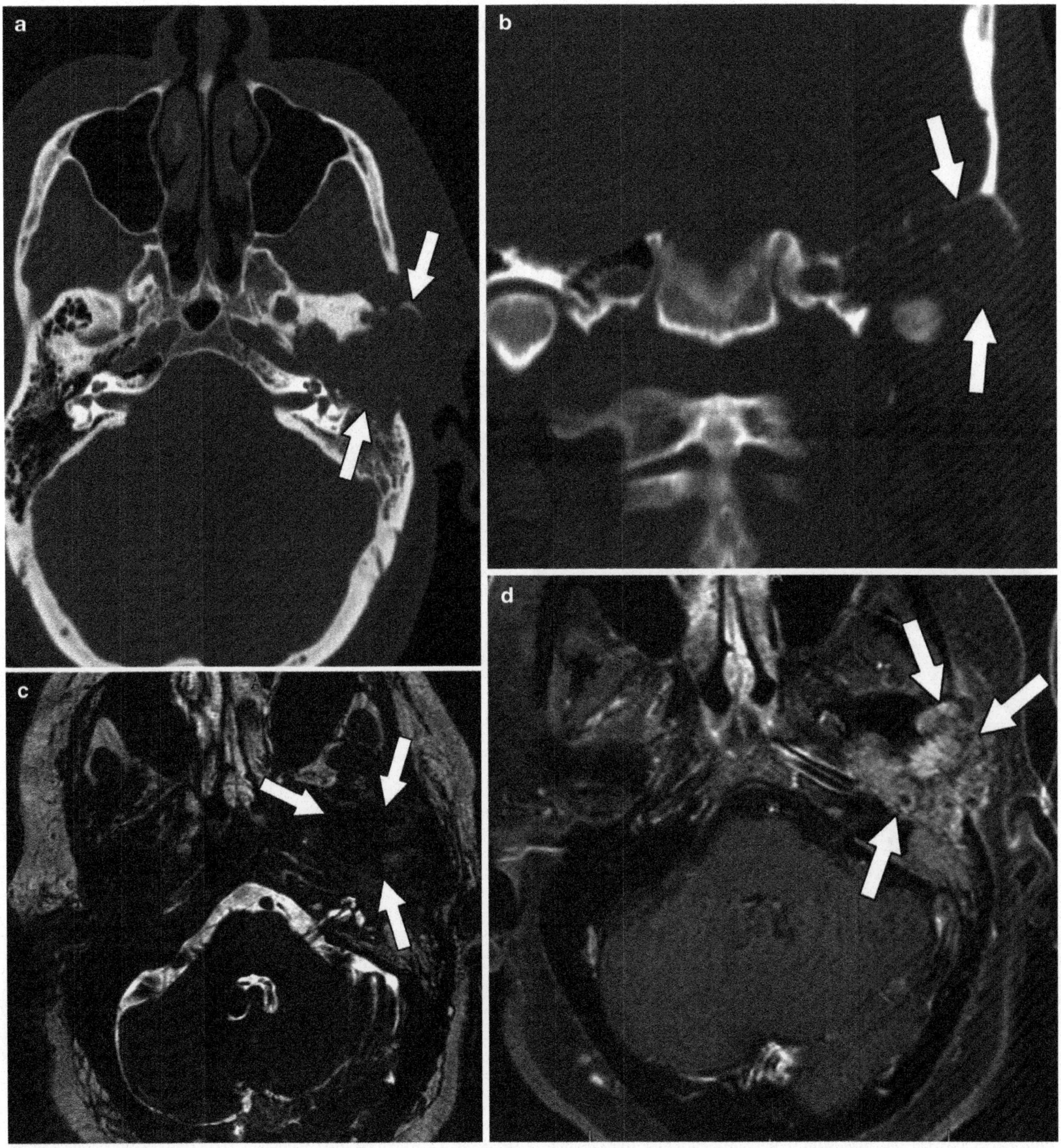

Fig. 3.6 A 49-year-old woman with left jaw pain caused by a left temporal bone giant cell tumor. (**a**, **b**) Axial and coronal CT with contrast, bone window. Expansile left temporal bone mass with bone loculation (arrows). (**c**) Axial T2-weighted MRI sequence. Hypointense appearance of the lobulated mass (arrows). (**d**) Axial T1-weighted post-contrast MRI sequence. Heterogeneous enhancement of the mass (arrows)

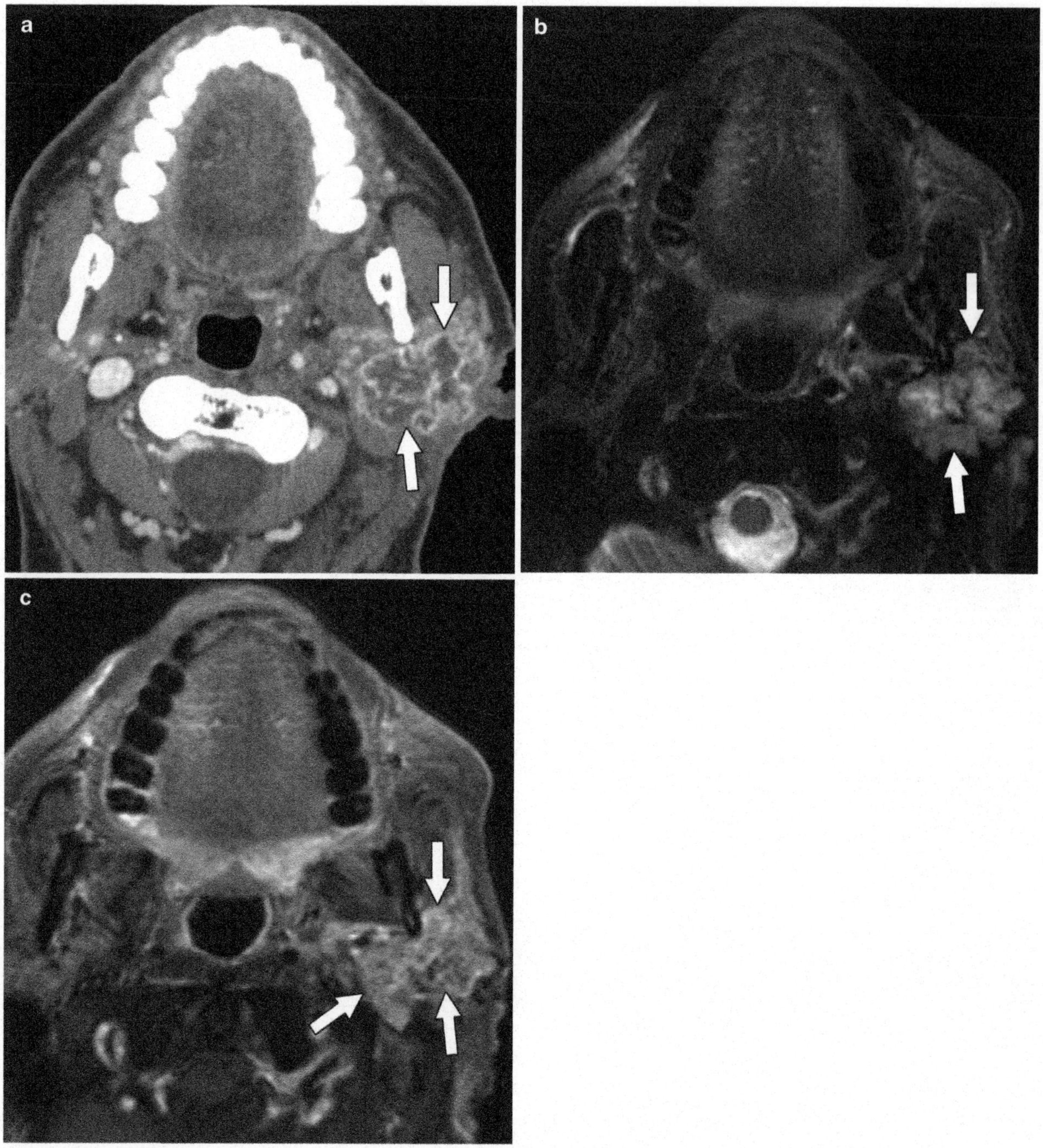

Fig. 3.7 A 63-year-old man with a left infra-auricular mucoepidermoid carcinoma. (**a**) Axial CT with contrast, soft tissue window. Peripherally enhancing left parotid mass with defined margins (arrows). (**b**) Axial T2-weighted MRI sequence. Hyperintense appearance of the mass (arrows). (**c**) Axial T1-weighted post-contrast MRI sequence. Heterogeneous enhancement of the circumscribed mass (arrows)

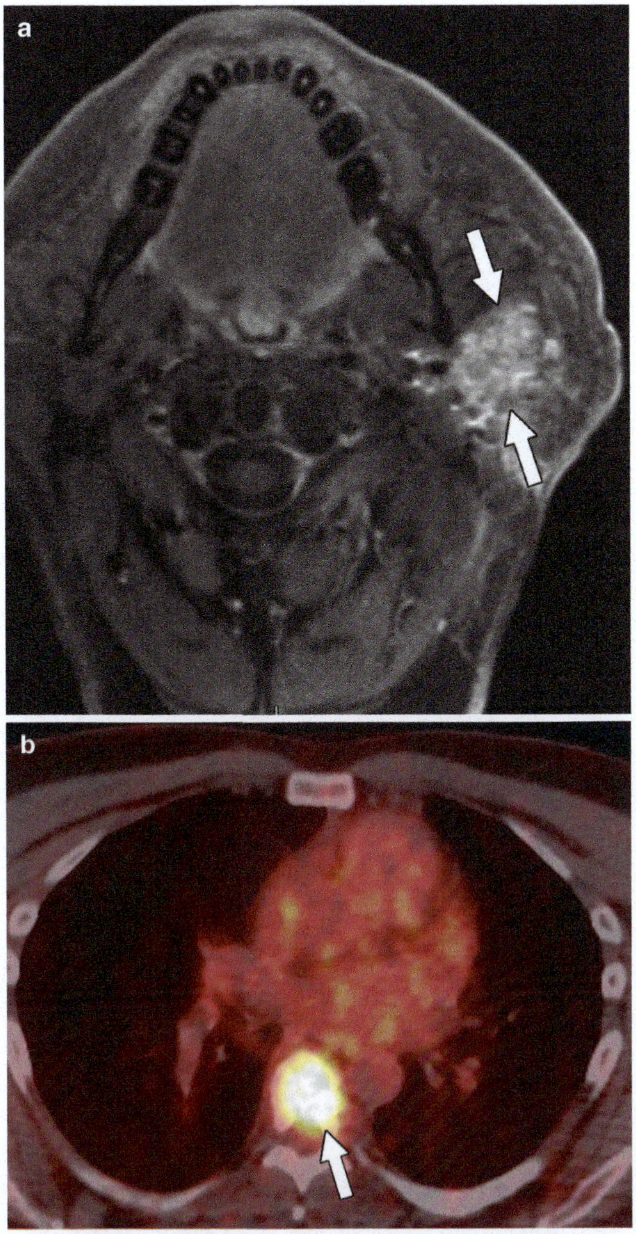

Fig. 3.8 A 43-year-old man presenting with facial nerve paralysis caused by adenoid cystic carcinoma left parotid. (**a**) Axial T1-weighted post-contrast MRI sequence. Left parotid enhancing mass (arrows). (**b**) PET/CT, 8 years later. FDG-avid recurrent tumor in the T6 vertebral body (arrow)

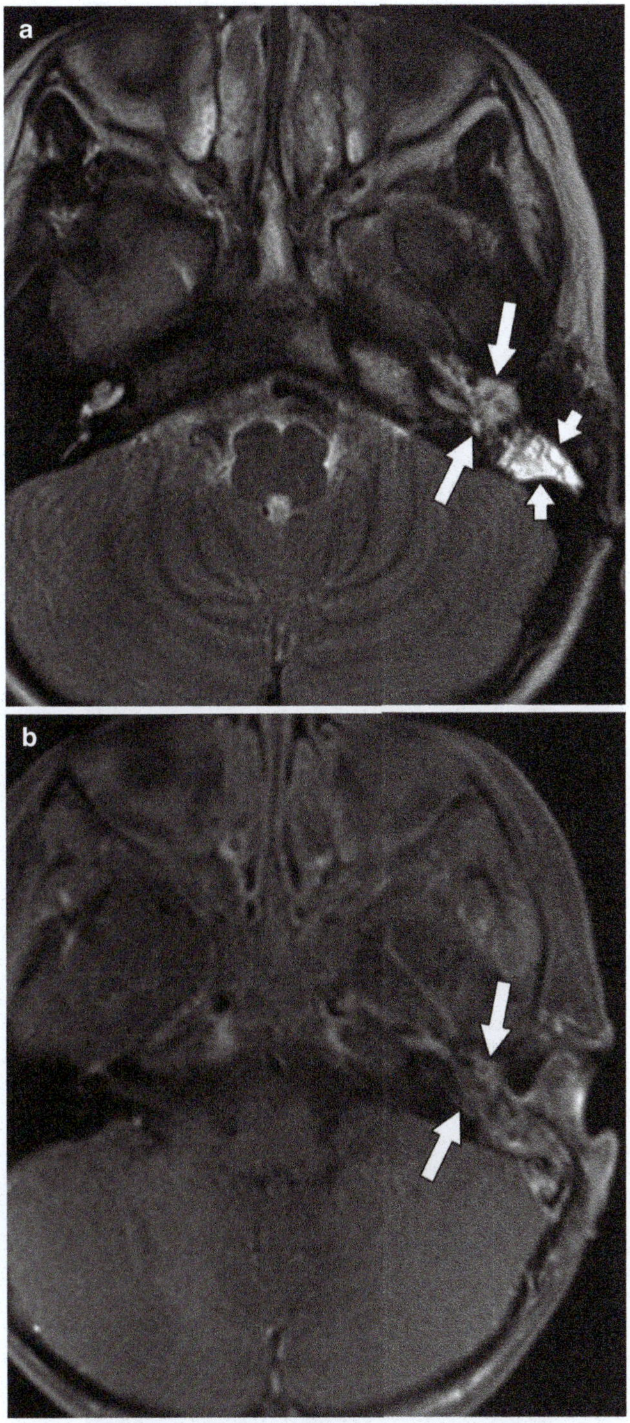

Fig. 3.9 A 4-year-old boy with left temporal bone rhabdomyosarcoma with extension in the infratemporal fossa. (**a**) Axial T2-weighted MRI sequence. Hyperintense mass involving the left middle ear (arrows). Note blocked secretions in the left mastoid are more hyperintense than the tumor (small arrows). (**b**) Axial T1-weighted post-contrast MRI sequence. Heterogeneous enhancement of the mass

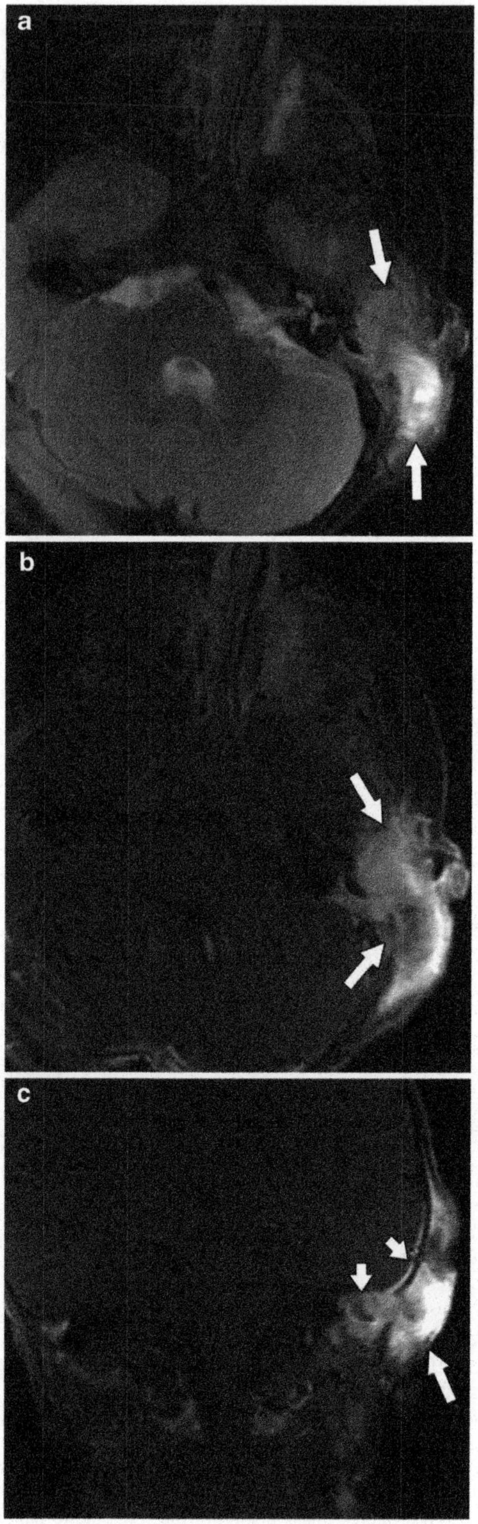

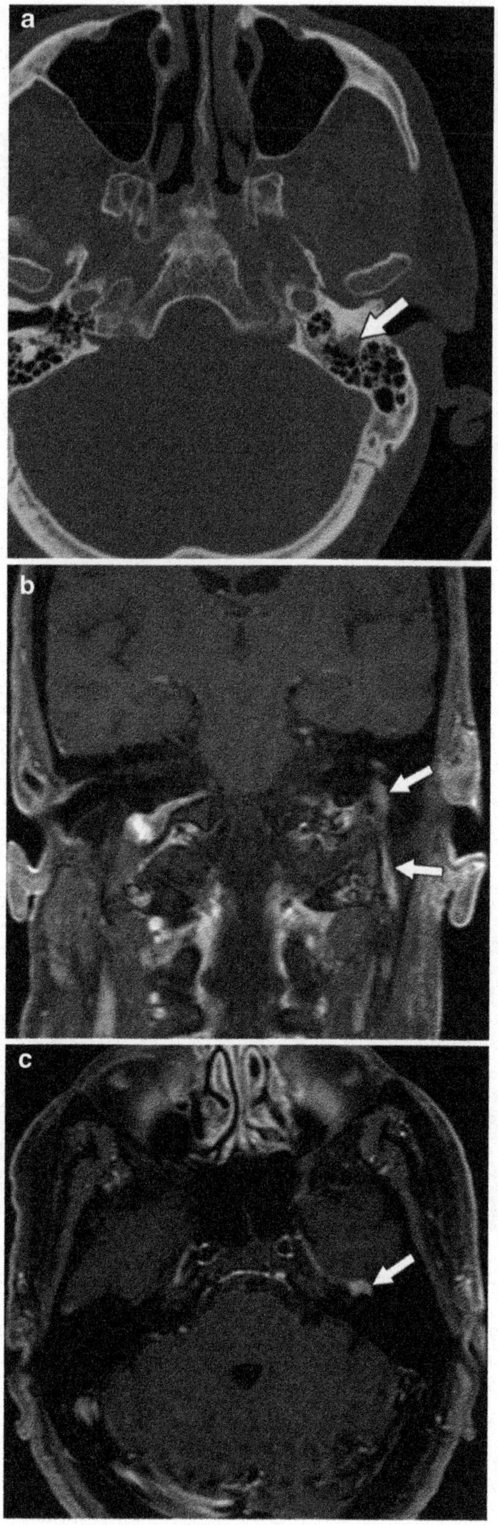

Fig. 3.10 A 2-year-old girl with left retro-auricular mass involving the mastoid temporal bone consistent with Langerhans cell histiocytosis. (**a**) Axial T2-weighted MRI sequence. A hyperintense mass is present in the left mastoid temporal bone and retro-auricular soft tissues (arrows). (**b**, **c**) Axial and coronal T1-weighted MRI sequences with contrast (arrows). Homogeneous enhancement of the mass. (**c**) Note the extension into the middle cranial fossa with dural reaction (small arrows)

Fig. 3.11 A 44-year-old man with left facial weakness caused by a left parotid adenoid cystic carcinoma with perineural spread to the seventh cranial nerve. (**a**) Axial CT with contrast, bone window. Enlargement of the facial nerve canal in the left temporal bone (arrow). (**b**) Coronal T1-weighted MRI sequence with contrast. Enhancement of the descending mastoid segment of the left facial nerve and in the parotid gland (arrows). (**c**) Axial T1-weighted MRI sequence with contrast. Perineural spread to the left geniculate ganglion (arrow)

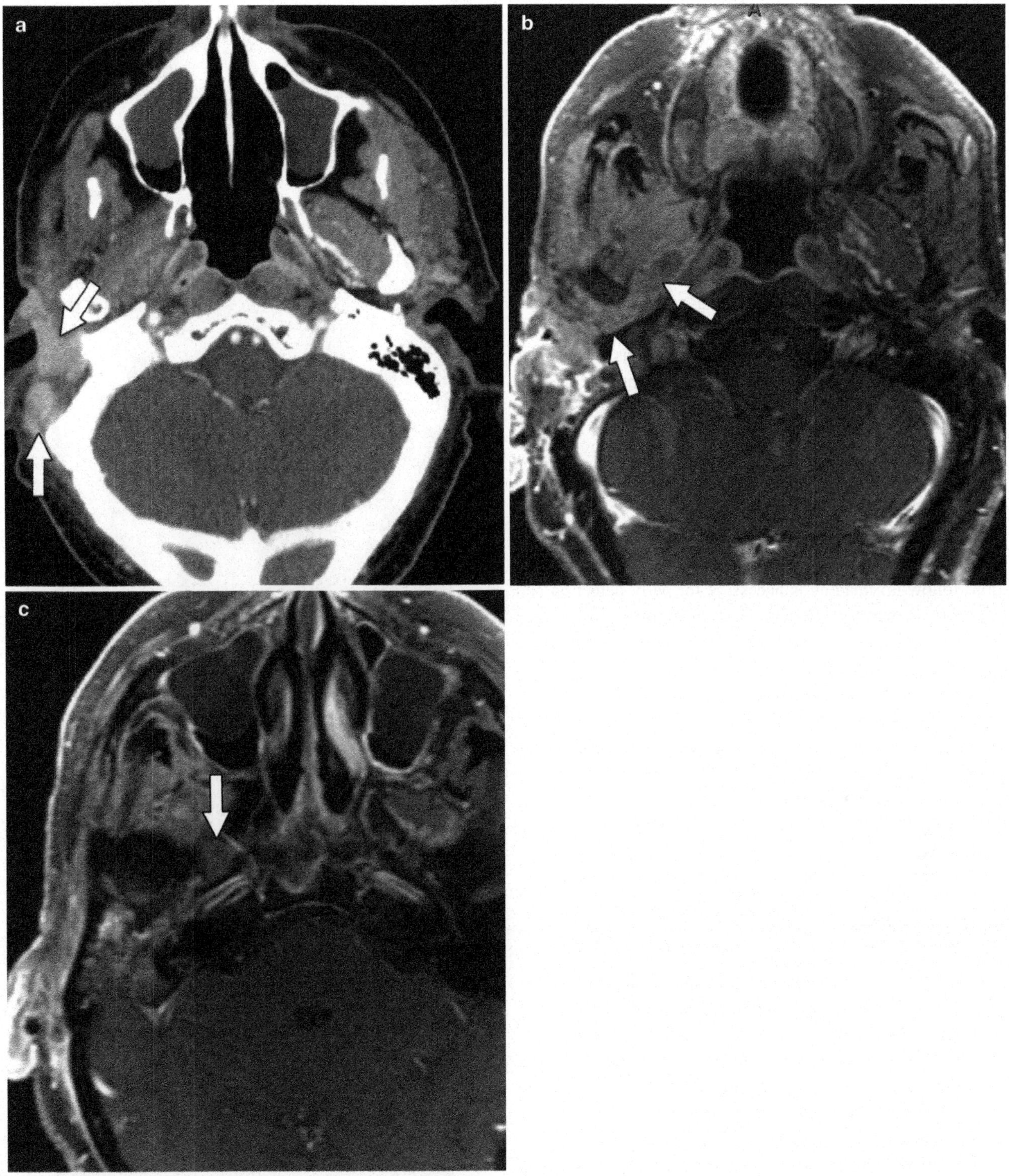

Fig. 3.12 A 65-year-old man with recurrent SCC following parotidectomy, lateral temporal bone resection (LTBR), and skin graft. (**a**) Axial CT with contrast, soft tissue window. Homogeneously enhancing recurrent tumor in the LTBR site and post-auricular region (arrows). (**b**) Axial T1-weighted MRI sequence with contrast, perineural spread along the auriculotemporal nerve in to the masticator space (arrows). (**c**) Axial T1-weighted MRI sequence with contrast. Further perineural spread through foramen ovale (arrow)

Imaging of Flap Reconstruction

For local regional control, aggressive tumors involving the temporal bone are often treated with lateral temporal bone resection (LTBR). LTBR involves the surgical removal of portions of the temporal bone and adjacent structures such as the parotid gland [47–49]. Reconstruction following LTBR may be performed with skin grafts and pedicled flaps. For extensive defects and cases where postoperative radiation is employed, free flaps are preferred [50]. On MRI, the muscular component of a myocutaneous flap has a striated appearance on T1-weighted pre-contrast sequences, may demonstrate some degree of enhancement [51, 52], and has hyperintensity that may decrease over time on T2-weighted sequences (Fig. 3.13) [51–54].

Recurrence After Flap Reconstruction

As tumor recurrence following LTBR and reconstruction can occur [55–57] and may not be evident on clinical examination, follow-up imaging is necessary for early detection and appropriate treatment. Early detection of tumor recurrence in patients who have undergone LTBR and reconstruction is often difficult owing to postoperative changes leading to loss of normal anatomic landmarks and to the bulkiness and heterogeneous appearance of the flaps that are needed for reconstruction. Following flap reconstruction, recurrent tumors may occur at the operative site (Fig. 3.12a) or remotely in the neck (Fig. 3.14). An enhancing mass at either site or loss of the normal muscular striations of the flap raises concern for tumor recurrence.

Radiation Effects

Following reconstructive surgery, radiation may be used as part of the treatment. Osteoradionecrosis of the bony structures in the radiation field is characterized by bone destruction that can be localized or extensive. Sequestrum within or surrounding necrotic bone and small collections of air within the bone or adjacent soft tissues may also be noted as are mastoid effusions (Fig. 3.15) [58, 59].

Radiation necrosis can also occur in the temporal lobes of the brain if included in the treatment field. The earliest sign of radiation necrosis is cerebral edema that may be extensive [60]. Enhancing lesions in the gray or white matter can also occur (Fig. 3.16) [60]. Disparity between the clinical and radiologic findings is highly suggestive of radiation necrosis [61]. When treated early with corticosteroids, patients can make a complete or near-complete recovery with only residual cerebral atrophy [60].

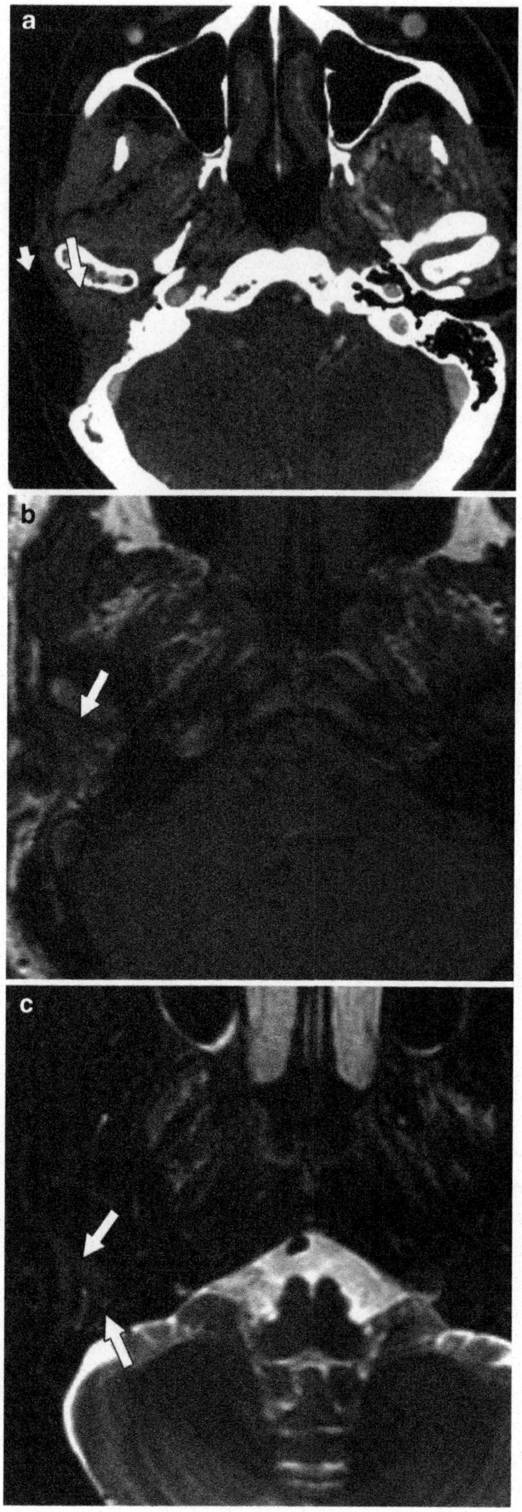

Fig. 3.13 A 73-year-old man with SCC of the right external auditory canal treated with lateral temporal bone resection and myocutaneous flap reconstruction (same patient as Fig. 3.3). (**a**) Axial CT with contrast, soft tissue window. The muscular (large arrow) and fat (small arrow) components of the flap. (**b**) Axial T1-weighted MRI sequence without contrast. Striated appearance of the muscular component of the flap (arrow). (**c**) Axial T2-weighted MRI sequence. Hyperintense appearance of the flap (arrows)

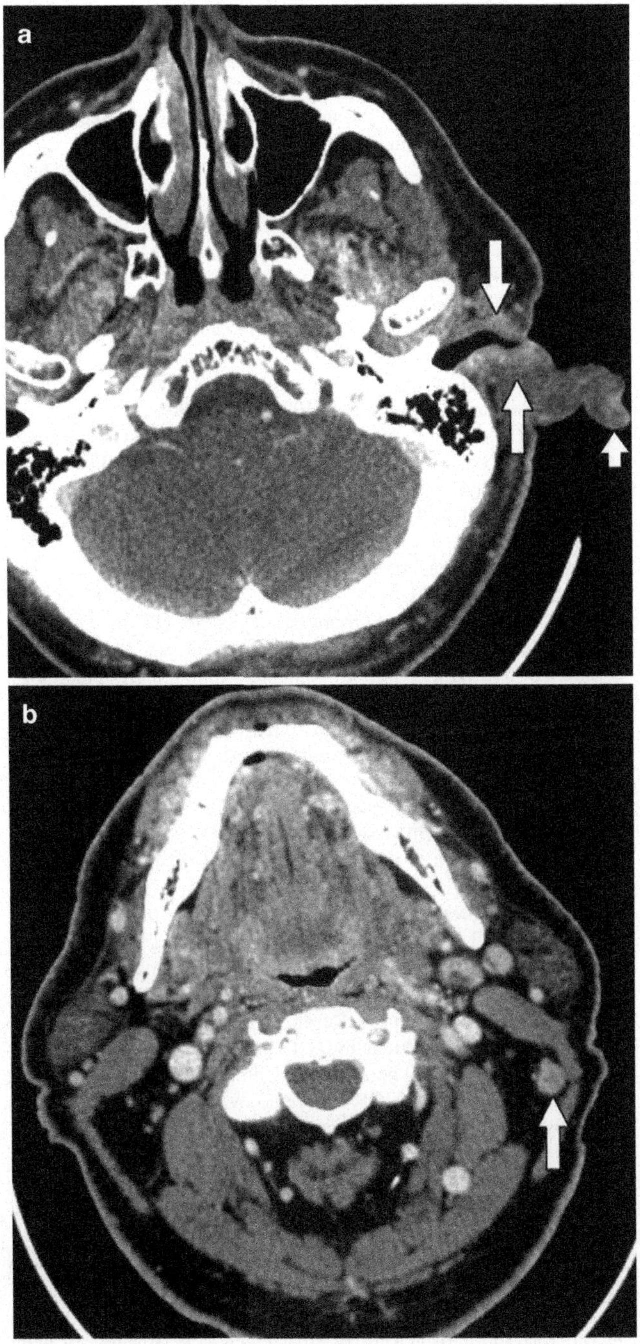

Fig. 3.14 A 67-year-old man with left helix and external auditory canal SCC. (**a**) Axial CT with contrast, soft tissue window. Tumor in the left helix (small arrow) and external auditory canal (large arrows). (**b**) Axial CT with contrast, soft tissue window. Metastatic left neck node after resection and flap reconstruction (arrow)

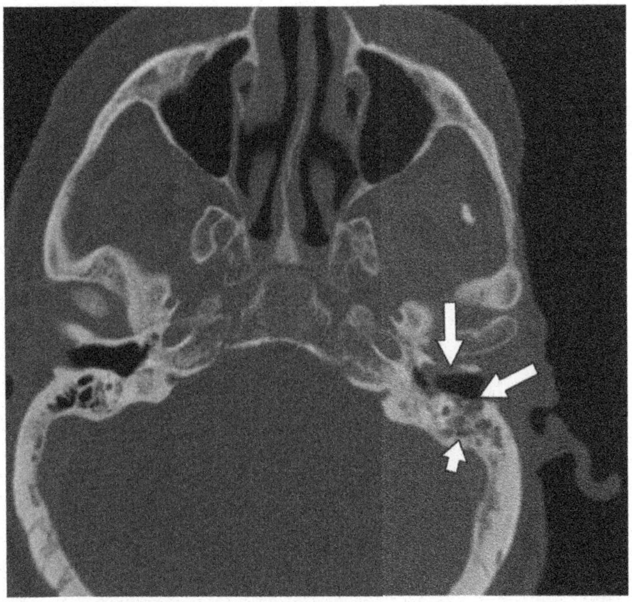

Fig. 3.15 Osteoradionecrosis. Axial CT with contrast, bone window. Destruction of the left anterior and posterior ear canal walls (large arrows) and a mastoid effusion (small arrow)

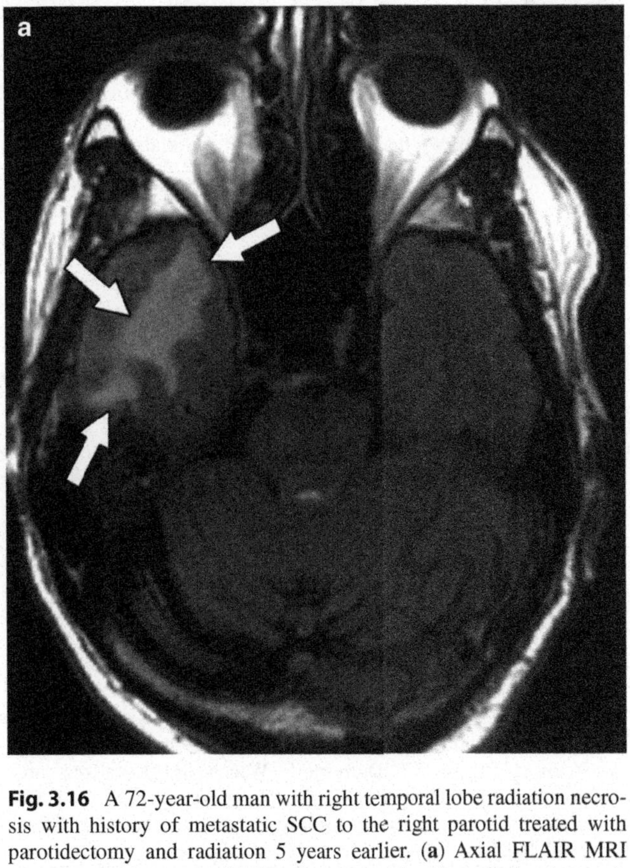

Fig. 3.16 A 72-year-old man with right temporal lobe radiation necrosis with history of metastatic SCC to the right parotid treated with parotidectomy and radiation 5 years earlier. (**a**) Axial FLAIR MRI sequence. Right temporal lobe edema related to the radiation (arrows). (**b**) Axial T1-weighted MRI sequence with contrast. Heterogeneously enhancing foci in the right temporal lobe (arrows)

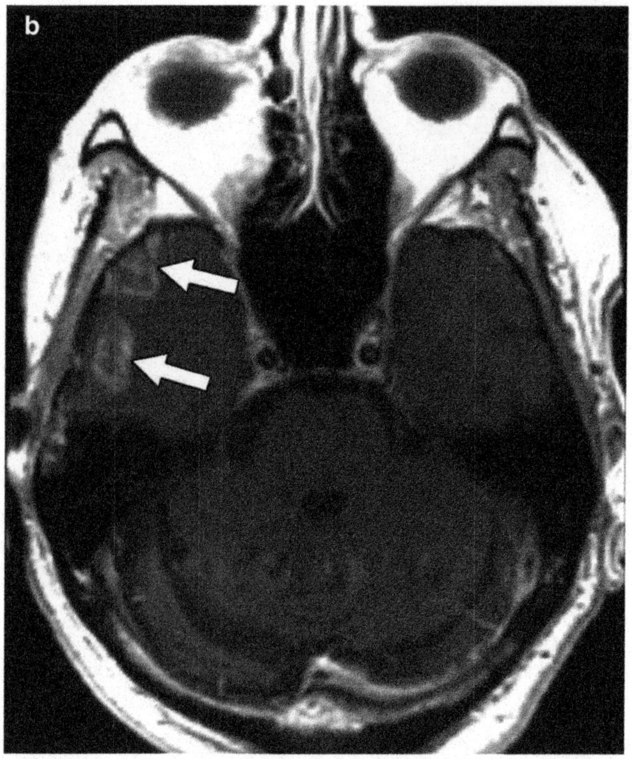

Fig. 3.16 (continued)

Acknowledgment We thank Bryan Tutt for editorial assistance with the chapter.

References

1. Lanka B, Turner M, Orton C, Carrington BM. Cross-sectional imaging in non-melanoma skin cancer of the head and neck. Clin Radiol. 2005;60:869–77.
2. Acartürk TO, Edington H. Nonmelanoma skin cancer. Clin Plast Surg. 2005;32:237–48.
3. Netscher DT, Leong M, Orengo I, Yang D, Berg C, Krishnan B. Cutaneous malignancies: melanoma and nonmelanoma types. Plast Reconstr Surg. 2011;127:37–56.
4. Brantsch KD, Meisner C, Schönfisch B, Trilling B, Wehner-Caroli J, Röcken M, et al. Analysis of risk factors determining prognosis of cutaneous squamous-cell carcinoma: a prospective study. Lancet Oncol. 2008;9:713–20.
5. Lee D, Nash M, Har-El G. Regional spread of auricular and periauricular cutaneous malignancies. Laryngoscope. 1996;106:998–1001.
6. Tavin E, Persky M. Metastatic cutaneous squamous cell carcinoma of the head and neck region. Laryngoscope. 1996;106:156–8.
7. Yoon M, Chougule P, Dufresne R, Wanebo HJ. Localized carcinoma of the external ear is an unrecognized aggressive disease with a high propensity for local regional recurrence. Am J Surg. 1992;164:574–7.
8. Thacker CA, Weiss GJ, Tibes R, Blaydorn L, Downhour M, White E. 18-FDG PET/CT assessment of basal cell carcinoma with vismodegib. Cancer Med. 2012;1:230–6.
9. Levell NJ, Igali L, Wright KA, Greenberg DC. Basal cell carcinoma epidemiology in the UK: the elephant in the room. Clin Exp Dermatol. 2013;38:367–9.
10. Williams LS, Mancuso AA, Mendenhall WM. Perineural spread of cutaneous squamous and basal cell carcinoma: CT and MR detection and its impact on patient management and prognosis. Int J Radiat Oncol Biol Phys. 2001;49:1061–9.
11. Breuninger H, Black B, Rassner G. Microstaging of squamous cell carcinomas. Am J Clin Pathol. 1990;94:624–7.
12. Arena S, Keen M. Carcinoma of the middle ear and temporal bone. Am J Otol. 1988;9:351–6.
13. Pensak ML, Gleich LL, Gluckman JK, Shumrick KA. Temporal bone carcinoma: contemporary perspectives in the skull base surgical era. Laryngoscope. 1996;106:1234–7.
14. Grandis JR, Hirsch B, Yu VL. Simultaneous presentation of malignant external otitis and temporal bone cancer. Arch Otolaryngol Head Neck Surg. 1993;119:687–9.
15. Al-Shihabi A. Carcinoma of temporal bone presenting as malignant otitis externa. J Laryngol Otol. 1992;106(10):908–10.
16. Moffat DA, Wagstaff SA, Hardy DG. The outcome of radical surgery and postoperative radiotherapy for squamous cell carcinoma of the temporal bone. Laryngoscope. 2005;115:341–7.
17. Wilson JS, Blake GB, Richardson AE, Westbury G. Malignant tumours of the ear and their treatment. II. Tumours of the external auditory meatus, middle ear cleft and temporal bone. Br J Plast Surg. 1974;27:77–91.
18. Bird CR, Hasso AN, Stewart CE, Hinshaw DB Jr, Thompson JR. Malignant primary neoplasms of the ear and temporal bone studied by high-resolution computed tomography. Radiology. 1983;149:171–4.
19. Leonetti JP, Smith PG, Kletzker GR, Izquierdo R. Invasion patterns of advanced temporal bone malignancies. Am J Otol. 1996;17:438–42.
20. Michaels L, Wells M. Squamous cell carcinoma of the middle ear. Clin Otolaryngol Allied Sci. 1980;5:235–48.
21. Conley J. Cancer of the middle ear. Ann Otol Rhinol Laryngol. 1965;74:555–72.
22. Goodwin WJ, Jesse RH. Malignant neoplasms of the external auditory canal and temporal bone. Arch Otolaryngol. 1980;106:675–9.
23. Malawer MM, Link MP, Donaldson SS. Sarcomas of bone. In: DeVita Jr VT, Hellman S, Rosenberg SA, editors. Cancer. 5th ed. Philadelphia, PA: Lipincott-Raven; 1997. p. 1789–852.
24. Nora FE, Unni KK, Pritchard DJ, Dahlin DC. Osteosarcoma of extragnathic craniofacial bones. Mayo Clin Proc. 1983;58:268–72.
25. Ogunlewe MO, Ajayi OF, Adeyemo WL, Ladeinde AL, James O. Osteogenic sarcoma of the jaw bones: a single institution experience over a 21-year period. Oral Surg Oral Med Oral Pathol Oral Radiol Endod. 2006;101:76–81.
26. Littrell LA, Wenger DE, Wold LE, Bertoni F, Unni KK, White LM, et al. Radiographic, CT, and MR imaging features of dedifferentiated chondrosarcomas: a retrospective review of 174 de novo cases. Radiographics. 2004;24:1397–409.
27. Murphey MD, Nomikos GC, Flemming DJ, Gannon FH, Temple HT, Kransdorf MJ. From the archives of AFIP. Imaging of giant cell tumor and giant cell reparative granuloma of bone: radiologic-pathologic correlation. Radiographics. 2001;21:1283–309.
28. Rock JP, Mahmood A, Cramer HB. Giant cell tumor of the skull base. Am J Otol. 1994;15:268–72.
29. Rhea JT, Weber AL. Giant-cell granuloma of the sinuses. Radiology. 1983;147:135–7.
30. Som PM, Lawson W, Cohen BA. Giant-cell lesions of the facial bones. Radiology. 1983;147:129–34.
31. Aralasmak A, Aygun N, Westra WH, Yousem DM. Giant cell reparative granuloma of the sphenoid bone. AJNR Am J Neuroradiol. 2006;27:1675–7.
32. Kashiwagi N, Dote K, Kawano K, Tomita Y, Murakami T, Nakanishi K, et al. MRI findings of mucoepidermoid carcinoma of the parotid gland: correlation with pathological features. Br J Radiol. 2012;85:709–13.

33. Christe A, Waldherr C, Hallett R, Zbaeren P, Thoeny H. MR imaging of parotid tumors: typical lesion characteristics in MR imaging improve discrimination between benign and malignant disease. AJNR Am J Neuroradiol. 2011;32:1202–7.
34. Curtin HD. CT of acoustic neuroma and other tumors of the ear. Radiol Clin N Am. 1984;22:77–105.
35. Schwartz RH, Movassaghi N, Marion ED. Rhabdomyosarcoma of the middle ear: a wolf in sheep's clothing. Pediatrics. 1980;65:1131–3.
36. Goepfert H, Cangir A, Lindberg R, Ayala A. Rhabdomyosarcoma of the temporal bone. Is surgical resection necessary? Arch Otolaryngol. 1979;105:310–3.
37. Sbeity S, Abella A, Arcand P, Quintal MC, Saliba I. Temporal bone rhabdomyosarcoma in children. Int J Pediatr Otorhinolaryngol. 2007;71:807–14.
38. Chevallier KM, Wiggins RH, Quinn NA, Gurgel RK. Differentiating pediatric rhabdomyosarcoma and langerhans cell histiocytosis of the temporal bone by imaging appearance. AJNR Am J Neuroradiol. 2016;37:1185–9.
39. Clayman GL, Lee JJ, Holsinger FC, Zhou X, Duvic M, El-Naggar AK, et al. Mortality risk from squamous cell skin cancer. J Clin Oncol. 2005;23:759–65.
40. Nijsten TE, Stern RS. Oral retinoid use reduces cutaneous squamous cell carcinoma risk in patients with psoriasis treated with psoralen-UVA: a nested cohort study. J Am Acad Dermatol. 2003;49:644–50.
41. Frierson HF Jr, Cooper PH. Prognostic factors in squamous cell carcinoma of the lower lip. Hum Pathol. 1986;17:346–54.
42. Garcia-Serra A, Hinerman RW, Mendenhall WM, Amdur RJ, Morris CG, Williams LS, et al. Carcinoma of the skin with perineural invasion. Head Neck. 2003;25:1027–33.
43. McCord MW, Mendenhall WM, Parsons JT, Flowers FP. Skin cancer of the head and neck with incidental microscopic perineural invasion. Int J Radiat Oncol Biol Phys. 1999;43:591–5.
44. Ginsberg LE. Imaging of perineural tumor spread in head and neck cancer. Semin Ultrasound CT MR. 1999;20:175–86.
45. Matzko J, Becker DG, Phillips CD. Obliteration of fat planes by perineural spread of squamous cell carcinoma along the inferior alveolar nerve. AJNR Am J Neuroradiol. 1994;15:1843–5.
46. Curtin HD. Detection of perineural spread: fat is a friend. AJNR Am J Neuroradiol. 1998;19:1385–6.
47. Essig GF, Kitipornchai L, Adams F, Zarate D, Gandhi M, Porceddu S, et al. Lateral temporal bone resection in advanced cutaneous squamous cell carcinoma: report of 35 patients. J Neurol Surg B Skull Base. 2013;74:54–9.
48. Medina JE, Park AO, Neely JG, Britton BH. Lateral temporal bone resections. Am J Surg. 1990;160:427–33.
49. Graham MD, Sataloff RT, Kemink JL, Wolf GT, McGillicuddy JE. Total en bloc resection of the temporal bone and carotid artery for malignant tumors of the ear and temporal bone. Laryngoscope. 1984;94:528–33.
50. Hanasono MM, Silva A, Skoracki RJ, Gidley PW, DeMonte F, Hanna EY, et al. Skull base reconstruction: an updated approach. Plast Reconstr Surg. 2011;128:675–86.
51. Chong J, Chan LL, Langstein HN, Ginsberg LE. MR imaging of the muscular component of myocutaneous flaps in the head and neck. AJNR Am J Neuroradiol. 2001;22:170–4.
52. Sedrak P, Lee PS, Guha-Thakurta N, Chang EI, Ginsberg LE, Esmaeli B, et al. MRI findings of myocutaneous and fasciocutaneous flaps used for reconstruction of orbital exenteration defects. Ophthal Plast Reconstr Surg. 2014;30:328–36.
53. Fox MG, Bancroft LW, Peterson JJ, Kransdorf MJ, Terkonda SP, O'Connor MI. MRI appearance of myocutaneous flaps commonly use in orthopedic reconstructive surgery. AJR Am J Roentgenol. 2006;187:800–6.
54. Naidich MJ, Weissman JL. Reconstructive myofascial skull-base flaps: normal appearance on CT and MR imaging studies. AJR Am J Roentgenol. 1996;167:611–4.
55. Morris LG, Mehra S, Shah JP, Bilsky MH, Selesnick SH, Kraus DH. Predictors of survival and recurrence after temporal bone resection for cancer. Head Neck. 2012;34(9):1231.
56. Dean NR, White HN, Carter DS, Desmond RA, Carroll WR, McGrew BM, et al. Outcomes following temporal bone resection. Laryngoscope. 2010;120:1516–22.
57. Mazonni A, Danesi G, Zanoletti E. Primary squamous cell carcinoma of the external auditory canal: surgical treatment and long-term outcomes. Acta Otorhinolaryngol Ital. 2014;34:129–37.
58. Huang XM, Zheng YQ, Zhang XM, Mai HQ, Zeng L, Liu X, et al. Diagnosis and management of skull base osteoradionecrosis after radiotherapy for nasopharyngeal carcinoma. Laryngoscope. 2006;116:1626–31.
59. Ahmed S, Gupta N, Hamilton JD, Garden AS, Gidley PW, Ginsberg LE. CT findings in temporal bone osteoradionecrosis. J Comput Assist Tomogr. 2014;38:662–6.
60. Chong VE, Fan YF. Radiation-induced temporal lobe necrosis. AJNR Am J Neuroradiol. 1997;18:784–5.
61. Glass JP, Hwang TL, Leavens ME, Libshitz HI. Cerebral radiation necrosis following treatment of extracranial malignancies. Cancer. 1984;54:1966–72.

Balloon Test Occlusion in Temporal Bone Tumors

4

Orlando M. Diaz, Brandon D. Liebelt,
and Robert A. Scranton

Abbreviations

ACA	anterior cerebral artery
BTO	balloon test occlusion
CBF	cerebral blood flow
EEG	electroencephalography
ICA	internal cerebral artery
LMA	leptomeningeal anastomoses
MCA	middle cerebral artery
PCA	posterior cerebral artery
PET	positron emission tomography
SPECT	single-photon emission computed tomography

Introduction

The surgical treatment of complex temporal bone tumors has a number of preoperative vascular considerations. Preoperative embolization may be considered for hypervascular tumors to reduce operative time and intraoperative blood loss. Some tumors may not have dedicated branches amenable to embolization, and carotid sacrifice may be considered. Tumors may also invade the carotid or be so adherent that gross total resection cannot be performed without carotid sacrifice or a carotid injury may be highly likely though not planned. To assist in the preoperative risk assessment and planning, advanced information regarding the patient's ability to tolerate sacrifice is desirable. Carotid artery ligation can result in significant neurological morbidity and mortality, as high as 41–54% and 32–60%, respectively, in one series [1]. If patients are unable to tolerate sacrifice, preoperative bypass may be considered. The ability to tolerate carotid ligation requires robust collateral circulation, usually through the circle of Willis. The gold standard test for evaluating the collateral circulation is the carotid balloon test occlusion (BTO) where flow through the ipsilateral internal carotid artery (ICA) is halted temporarily for assessment. Testing usually entails neurological examination combined with some other modality including advanced metabolic or blood flow imaging, angiography, Doppler ultrasonography, or electroencephalography (EEG). This chapter describes the relevant vascular anatomy, indications for BTO, endovascular technique, and how to evaluate the adequacy of the collateral circulation.

Intracranial Vascular Anatomy and Collateral Pathways

The circle of Willis comprises the normal pathway of blood flow through the internal carotid arteries and vertebral arteries to the brain and brainstem, ultimately being connected to one another by anterior communicating and posterior communicating arteries. While, in general, the major proximal vessels are common among most individuals, there is significant variability both in the caliber of proximal vessels as well as the exact distribution and branches of more distal vessels in the intracranial circulation. In addition to variability, an intact circle of Willis provides redundancy of blood flow in the event of a large vessel occlusion. However, internal carotid artery occlusion can result in unpredictable outcomes ranging from an asymptomatic patient to a large territorial infarct depending on the degree of collateral circulation [2].

The major avenues of collateral flow occur through the ophthalmic, anterior communicating, and posterior communicating arteries. However, a complete circle of Willis

O. M. Diaz, M.D. (✉) • R. A. Scranton, M.D.
Department of Radiology,
Houston Neurovascular Center, Houston, TX, USA
e-mail: ODiaz@hosutonmethodist.org;
rascranton@houstonmethodist.org

B. D. Liebelt, M.D.
Department of Neurosurgery,
Methodist Hospital, Houston, TX, USA
e-mail: dbliebelt@houstonmethodist.org

P. W. Gidley, F. DeMonte (eds.), *Temporal Bone Cancer*, https://doi.org/10.1007/978-3-319-74539-8_4

is present in only 21–52.3% of individuals, with variability between different races and geographic regions [3–5]. Intracranial vessels can be hypoplastic, duplicated, or atretic leading to an incomplete circle of Willis [4]. These alterations are likely genetically determined, occurring early in life, and predispose certain individuals to pathologic vascular processes [3, 4]. It is of the utmost importance to understand these common anatomic variations and to recognize them in patients who may undergo balloon test occlusion of the internal carotid artery, as certain anatomic scenarios may preclude the performance of balloon occlusion.

The most frequent anomaly present within the circle of Willis is a hypoplastic blood vessel, being reported to occur with a prevalence of 23–27% [5–7]. Hypoplasia most frequently occurs in one or both posterior communicating arteries, posterior cerebral arteries (PCA) (P1 segment), anterior communicating artery, and anterior cerebral arteries (ACA) (A1 segment) in descending order of prevalence [4]. The next most common anomaly is duplication or triplication of an artery. This is encountered most commonly in the anterior circulation with a duplicated or triplicated anterior communicating artery or a triplicated anterior cerebral artery. These anomalies have been reported in around 10.9–42% of the population [4, 8, 9]. Specifically, duplicated or triplicated anterior communicating arteries are more common than a triplicated anterior cerebral artery (median artery of Wilder) [4, 5, 8–12]. Congenital aberrations also occur in the posterior communicating artery region; a fetal origin of the posterior cerebral artery is present in 10–22% [3–5, 9]. In contrast, the posterior communicating artery can be absent in 3.8–6% of patients [5, 13].

In addition to normal variations in the circle of Willis, the ophthalmic artery and leptomeningeal collaterals also can provide supplemental flow in the event of a state of hypoperfusion [14]. Leptomeningeal collaterals, or leptomeningeal anastomoses (LMA), are pial arteries that serve as connecting branches between two different cortical areas [15]. These collaterals can be recruited in the setting of acute arterial insufficiency. LMAs can occur between distal cortical branches of the anterior cerebral artery (ACA) and middle cerebral artery (MCA), between MCA and posterior cerebral artery (PCA), and least commonly between the ACA and PCA. Dural pial collaterals from the extracranial carotid circulation can also form between the facial, maxillary, and middle meningeal artery to the ophthalmic artery as well as between the middle meningeal artery and the occipital artery (through the mastoid foramen or parietal foramen) [16].

The recruitment of these collateral pathways is influenced by the extent of the primary collateral circulation such as the caliber and flow in the anterior communicating and posterior communicating arteries. These primary collateral pathways serve as a source of direct, immediate flow to ischemic regions. Secondary collateral pathways may take time to fully develop under various pathologic processes [17]. The development of collaterals may be influenced in part by several factors, including stimulation by angiogenesis adjacent to ischemic regions [18] or secretion of angiogenic peptides within ischemic regions [19]. Various data from animal studies [20] as well as anecdotal experience demonstrate the temporal influence of chronic hypoperfusion and increased collateral development.

Carotid Balloon Test Occlusion: Indications

Endovascular carotid balloon test occlusion (BTO) is performed preoperatively in patients to provide a risk assessment prior to surgery or to aid in planning a tumor resection. The surgical strategy may necessitate carotid artery sacrifice in the case of hypervascular tumors with significant feeding vessels from the internal carotid artery that are not amenable to embolization. Alternatively, a highly malignant or aggressive tumor may encase the carotid to a significant degree that the vessel may need to be sacrificed to complete a safe or maximal resection. In these instances it is desirable to occlude the vessel prior to resection, avoiding excessive surgical blood loss.

Preoperative carotid BTO is also helpful in assessing a patient's potential for neurological injury if there were an inadvertent carotid injury during surgery. This would not be performed routinely given the risk inherent to the BTO procedure. However, in cases where the preoperative plan is carotid preservation but there is a high-risk for injury, it can provide the surgeon with more information to manage a potentially catastrophic situation. Some injuries may be repairable through direct means, patching, or grafting, possibly even through stenting. Unfortunately some form of anticoagulation, antiplatelet agent, or a combination of the two may be needed to prevent thrombus or embolic complications after repair. This is undesirable in a patient with a fresh surgical wound. If the surgeon knows that the patient can tolerate carotid occlusion in advance, the risk of anticoagulants and antiplatelet medications could be avoided. Alternatively the patient can be apprised of the risk before surgery if repair is needed.

Carotid Balloon Test Occlusion: Technique

The goal of carotid BTO is to determine if the patient has adequate collateral circulation to tolerate occlusion without neurological deficit [21]. To achieve this end, the patient's physiologic parameters during the test should be documented and attempts made to match what can reasonably be expected after occlusion. The patient's blood pressure while under general anesthesia is usually lower than their individual baseline, so matching this during carotid BTO with a relative hypotension may make the test more reliable [22–24]. A radial arterial line is placed for accurate blood pressure assessment throughout the procedure.

The endovascular technique for balloon test occlusion is best performed under local anesthetic beginning with sheath placement in both femoral arteries. Dual access is necessary to simultaneously occlude the ipsilateral carotid while injecting the contralateral internal carotid artery (ICA) and ipsilateral vertebral for evaluation of collateral flow through the anterior communicating and posterior communicating arteries, respectively. In patients with difficult vascular access where only one sheath can be placed, manual carotid compression can be used during the diagnostic portion as an alternative but is not optimal. Following sheath placement a complete diagnostic angiogram is performed including selective injections of the external carotid, internal carotid, and vertebral arteries bilaterally. Examination of the patient's MRI and angiogram will help decide the optimal location for balloon placement, but typically the balloon is inflated in the ipsilateral ICA just proximal to the ophthalmic segment. The goal is to inflate at the site of planned ligation distal to the tumor, but any unexpected collaterals that may be discovered during the diagnostic portion must be taken into consideration.

Once the diagnostic portion has been completed and the location for balloon placement has been selected, the patient is given 5000 units heparin. In our practice we prefer to use a double lumen nondetachable balloon (Scepter balloon, Microvention, California). Once inflated, contrast is injected proximal to the balloon to ensure adequate occlusion and stasis of the contrast; normal saline with heparin is then continuously flushed at a low rate via a pump proximal and distal to the balloon to prevent thrombus formation. The occlusion is timed and maintained over a period of 20 min unless the patient is unable to tolerate. The angiogram is then repeated in the ipsilateral common carotid, vertebral, and contralateral internal carotid arteries to assess for cross-filling and collateral circulation.

Evaluation of BTO

The adequacy of redundant cerebral circulation during balloon test occlusion can be performed in a number of ways including angiographic, single-photon emission computed tomography (SPECT), Doppler ultrasonography, electroencephalography (EEG), neurological exam, or a combination of any of the above. Our preferred method is a combination of angiographic interpretation, SPECT perfusion, and continuous neurological examination. There may be subtle defects seen on single-photon emission computed tomography (SPECT) scan or large drops detected by Doppler, but it is ultimately the clinical exam that matters most. In our opinion assessment other than through neurological exam becomes more valuable in patients that cannot tolerate a procedure under local anesthetic such as children, the cognitively impaired, or those requiring mechanical ventilation, often in patients being assessed following aneurysmal rupture rather than for tumors.

Angiographic evaluation includes assessing flow via the anterior communicating artery, posterior communicating artery, and rarely external carotid collaterals. The concept of synchronous venous filling refers to timing the delay in opacification of the cortical veins between the patent and occluded side following contrast bolus into the patent side [25–28]. Significant delays suggest inadequate blood flow through the collaterals. We consider a delay greater than 1 s to indicate failure [29] while some advocate delays up to 2 s to be safe [27]. A series by van Rooij et al. found a delay less than 0.5 s has a 98% positive predictive value for passing BTO without clinical symptoms or ischemic lesions on post-occlusion MRI [25]. The synchronous venous filling of less than 0.5 s delay was further evaluated in a small series using magnetic resonance arterial spin labeling to evaluate cerebral blood flow and found no significant difference between occluded and patent territories [26].

Cerebral blood flow (CBF) has also been evaluated using SPECT and positron emission tomography (PET), though the latter can be very expensive and cumbersome given the resources and protocols involved. PET scanning has the advantage of being able to measure CBF, oxygen extraction fraction, and the cerebral metabolic rate of oxygen consumption [30]. It is unclear whether this additional information from PET imaging has enough clinical impact to justify the difficulty and expense involved. SPECT scanning uses a gamma-ray-emitting tracer, usually ^{99m}Tc-hexamethylpropyleneamine (HMPAO) or dime ^{r99m}TC-ethylene cysteine dimer (ECD), which is injected into the patient [31–33]. Specific protocols vary but all are looking for perfusion defects. Typically the tracer is injected during the occlusion at the moment a patient shows symptomatic neurological deficit (while simultaneously deflating the balloon) or at the end of the occlusion period if no deficit occurs [33]. The patient is then taken to the head scanner within a couple of hours of receiving the tracer, and if no perfusion defect is seen, a baseline scan is not needed [34]. However, if a perfusion defect is seen or suspected, a baseline scan is performed to determine if it is a preexisting defect [35]. If the patient has a symptomatic neurologic deficit, baseline scanning is not necessary as the patient has already failed the test on clinical grounds.

Patients may also be evaluated with Doppler ultrasonography based on the decrease in flow velocity of the ipsilateral middle cerebral artery during occlusion when compared to prior to the procedure. This method is advantageous in patients who require general anesthesia during BTO, but the test requires good windows for Doppler evaluation and precise positioning of the probe without drifting for meaningful interpretation. Sorteberg et al. described using this method in retrospective series of 136 patients where patient-specific headsets were used to fix the probe position during recordings taken prior to BTO, during BTO lasting around 90 s, and after carotid ligation, if needed [36]. The authors reported that drops in ipsilateral MCA flow velocity during BTO to less than 55% of baseline correlated with infarction, whereas flow velocity 65% or greater was well tolerated. Flow velocities between these two values required careful interpretation of pulsatility [36]. The reported complication rate was comparable to standard diagnostic angiography, likely because of the brief occlusion period of 90 s. Doppler ultrasonography can also be valuable in guiding postoperative blood pressure management in patients requiring carotid ligation. This group of patients may be very sensitive to hypotension, and cerebral autoregulation may not function appropriately in the acute phase following ligation. Ipsilateral MCA flow velocities may be used to guide titration of blood pressure to maintain adequate perfusion [36–38]. Despite the information this method provides and the low complication rate, it is impossible to definitively compare with other methods. In our opinion, continuous neurological examination during prolonged occlusion with a hypotensive challenge remains more reliable than Doppler ultrasonography.

The person performing the procedure must examine the patient prior to BTO to have a clear understanding of the patient's neurological baseline. While the balloon is inflated the patient should be examined almost continuously. In the case of anterior circulation BTO, as is relevant to this chapter, the exam should focus on motor and speech functions [39]. The motor exam should take into account the development of a pronator drift as a subtle sign of impairment. If any deficit occurs, the balloon should be deflated immediately. During balloon occlusion trial, [<Dr. Diaz, is this acceptable?] the occlusion time extends for a minimum of 20 min. The neurological exam may be supplemented with any of the other techniques described above. Silent ischemia can produce subtle neurocognitive effects. Although the results of clinical examination are most important, CBF should be evaluated in some other manner to minimize the risk of missing silent ischemia that could not be detected during the test period.

Case Illustrations

Incomplete Circle of Willis

Ultimately balloon test occlusion is the assessment of the adequacy of all of the previously mentioned collateral pathways to compensate for primary occlusion of the internal carotid artery. The absence of adequate primary collateral pathways is one scenario that would preclude safe diagnostic testing. Figure 4.1a illustrates a case in which the right ICA fills both ACAs via the anterior communicating artery. A left ICA injection shows angiographic absence of the left A1 segment and a fetal origin of the posterior cerebral artery (Fig. 4.2b). In the setting of right ICA occlusion, compensatory flow through the contralateral anterior communicating artery would not occur due to the absent left A1. Further, left vertebral injection shows absence of the left P1 segment (Fig. 4.3). Occlusion of the left ICA would likely lead to a PCA stroke in this patient as they have a fetal origin of the PCA with no P1 segment. Additionally, left ICA occlusion would also lead to hypoperfusion in the left MCA territory due to left A1 absence. This case emphasizes the point of

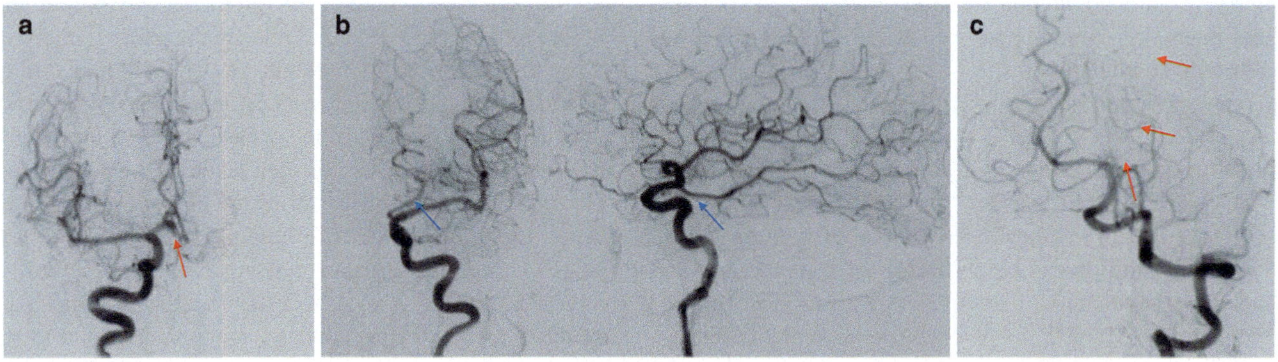

Fig. 4.1 (**a**) Illustrates a case in which the right ICA fills both ACAs via the anterior communicating artery (*arrow*). A left ICA injection shows angiographic absence of the left A1 segment (*red arrow*) and a fetal origin of the posterior cerebral artery (*blue arrow*) (**b**). In the setting of right ICA occlusion, compensatory flow through the contralateral anterior communicating artery would not occur due to the absent left A1. Further, left vertebral injection shows absence of the left P1 segment (*red arrows*) (**c**). Occlusion of the left ICA would likely lead to a PCA stroke in this patient as they have a fetal origin of the PCA with no P1 segment. Additionally, left ICA occlusion would also lead to hypoperfusion in the left MCA territory due to left A1 absence

performing and analyzing a routine cerebral angiogram in order to assess the safety of balloon occlusion testing as this patient would not be an ideal candidate.

Equivocal Testing

The following case depicts a situation with borderline results and poses a diagnostic dilemma regarding the safety in sacrificing the carotid artery. Pre-occlusion, the left ICA injection shows filling of the left MCA and ACA with a small but patent A1 segment (Fig. 4.2a). After the balloon is inflated, a right ICA injection reveals cross-filling through the anterior communicating artery to the left ACA and MCA (Fig. 4.2b). A right vertebral injection also shows some primary collateral flow through the posterior communicating artery to the MCA branches (Fig. 4.2c). The patient tolerated test occlusion for 30 min with no changes in neurologic exam or on continuous EEG. However, SPECT scan indicated a slightly reduced perfusion to the posterior left temporal lobe at the watershed region between the MCA and PCA (Fig. 4.2d). In cases where reduced perfusion is encountered on SPECT scan, it is important to look at the quantitation of brain perfusion ratio comparing relative blood flow between the two hemispheres. In this patient the ratio was 0.91; typically a ratio greater than 0.90 is predictive of a good clinical outcome with permanent occlusion.

Robust Primary Collaterals

One final case example will illustrate robust primary collaterals through the communicating arteries. This patient presented with tumor of the salivary gland encasing the left

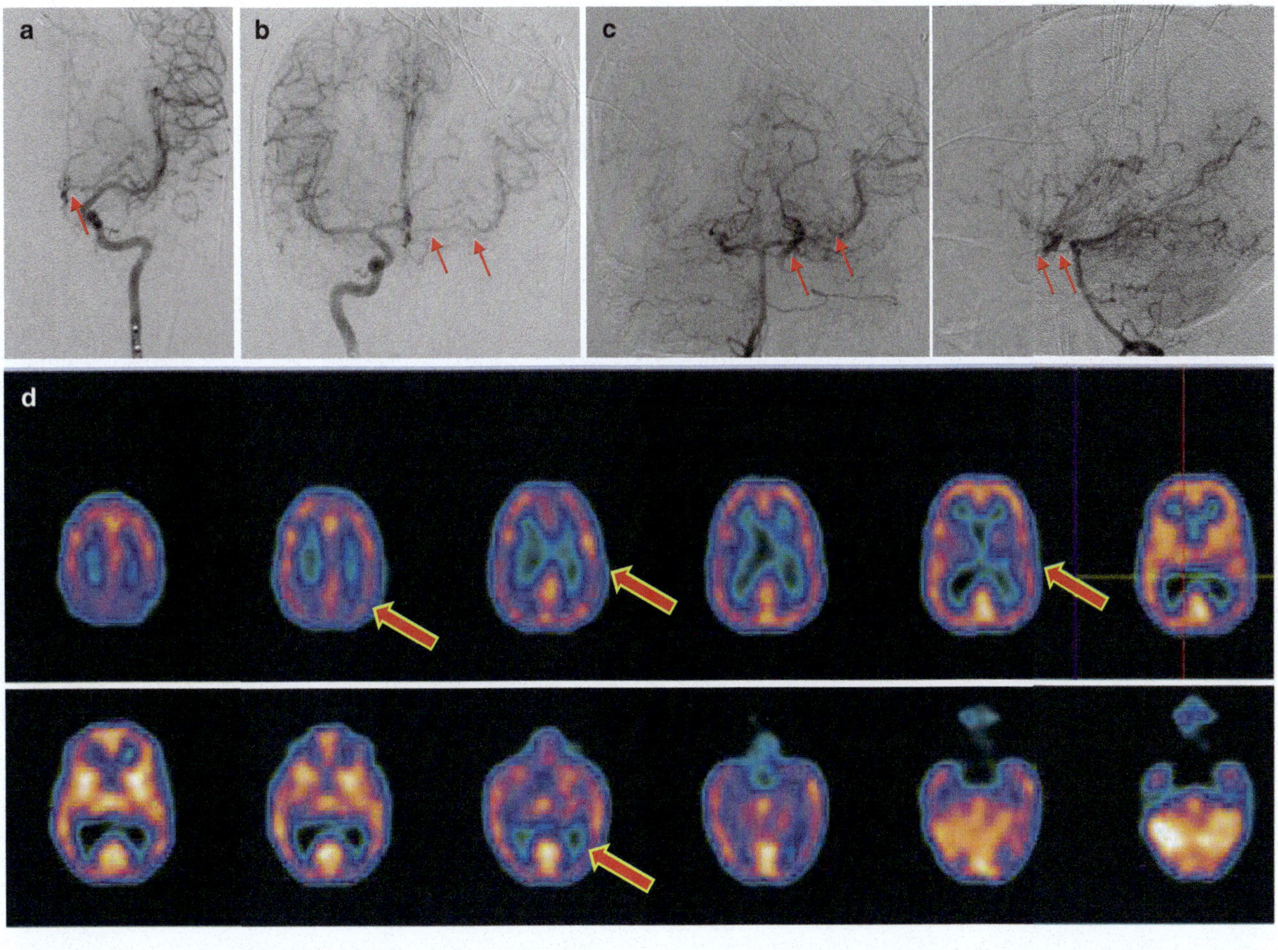

Fig. 4.2 The following case depicts a situation with borderline results and poses a diagnostic dilemma regarding the safety in sacrificing the carotid artery. Pre-occlusion, the left ICA injection shows filling of the left MCA and ACA with a small but patent A1 segment (*arrow*) (**a**). After the balloon is inflated, a right ICA injection reveals cross-filling through the anterior communicating artery to the left ACA and MCA (*arrows*) (**b**). A right vertebral injection also shows some primary collateral flow through the posterior communicating artery to the MCA branches (*arrows*) (**c**). The patient tolerated test occlusion for 30 min with no changes in neurologic exam or on continuous EEG. (**d**) SPECT scan indicated a slightly reduced perfusion to the posterior left temporal lobe at the watershed region between the *left* MCA and PCA (Fig. 4.2d). In this patient the ratio was 0.91; typically a ratio greater than 0.90 is predictive of a good clinical outcome with permanent occlusion

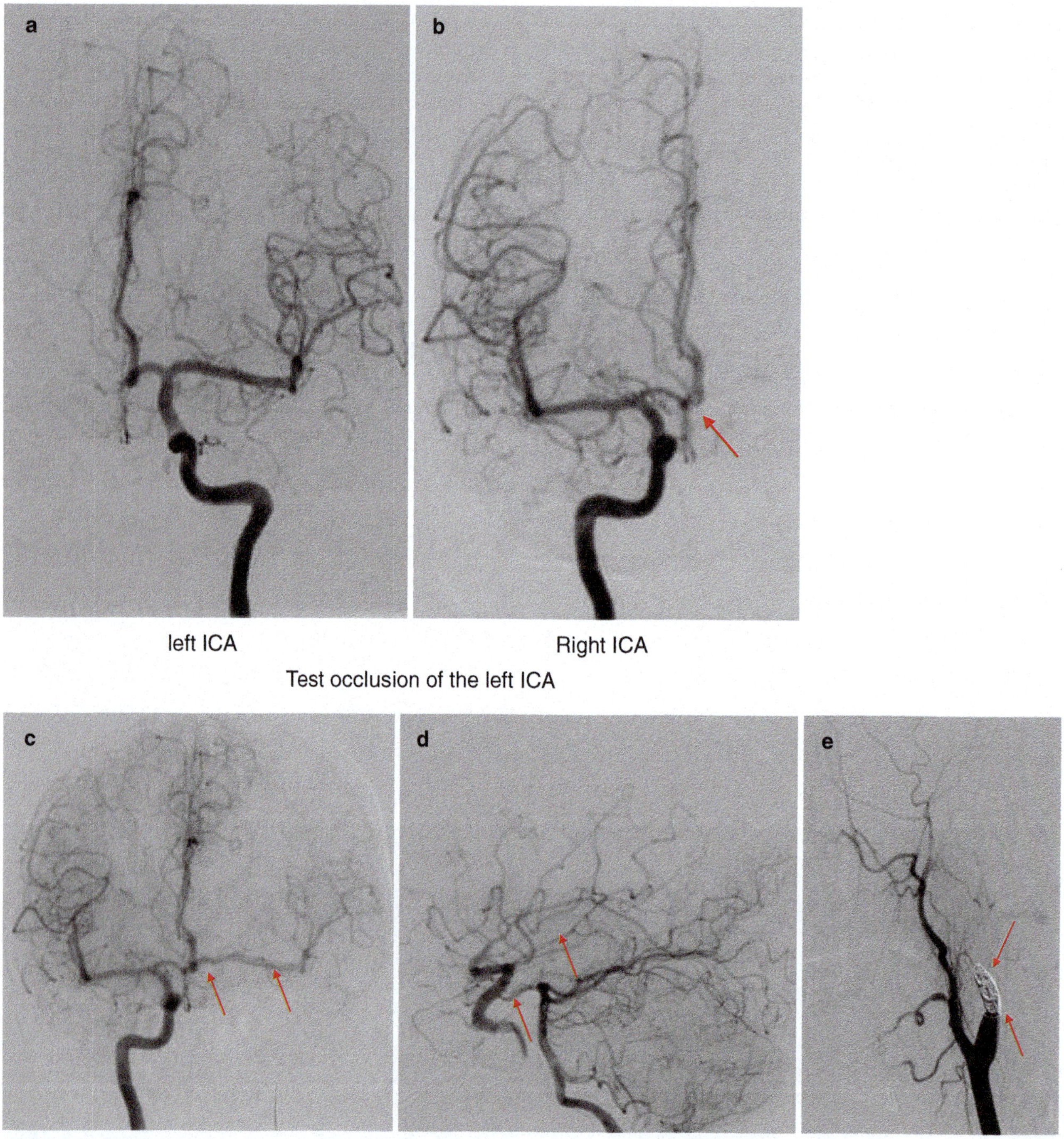

Fig. 4.3 Case illustrating robust primary collaterals through the communicating arteries. (**a**) Left carotid injection shows pre-occlusion filling status in the ICA distribution as well as cross-filling through the anterior communicating artery from right to left to fill distal left ACA branches (*arrow*) (**b**). During test occlusion, the right ICA injection is shown with robust cross-filling of not only the contralateral ACA but also the contralateral MCA (*arrows*) (**c**). Vertebral injection also shows good flow through the posterior communicating artery to fill branches of the MCA (*arrows*) (**d**). The patient tolerated 30 min of balloon occlusion without neurologic change in exam and underwent endovascular occlusion of the left cervical ICA during the same procedure (*arrows* showing coils) (**e**)

cervical segment of the internal carotid artery. Left carotid injection shows pre-occlusion filling status in the ICA distribution (Fig. 4.3a) as well as cross-filling through the anterior communicating artery from right to left to fill distal left ACA branches (Fig. 4.3b). During test occlusion, the right ICA injection is shown with robust cross-filling of not only the contralateral ACA but also the contralateral MCA (Fig. 4.3c). Vertebral injection also shows good flow through the posterior communicating artery to fill branches of the MCA. The patient tolerated 30 min of balloon occlusion without neurologic change in exam and underwent endovascular occlusion of the left cervical ICA during the same procedure (Fig. 4.3d).

References

1. Razack MS, Sako K. Carotid artery hemorrhage and ligation in head and neck cancer. J Surg Oncol. 1982;19(4):189–92.
2. Miralles M, Dolz JL, Cotillas J, Aldoma J, Santiso MA, Giménez A, et al. The role of the circle of willis in carotid occlusion: assessment with phase contrast MR angiography and transcranial duplex. Eur J Vasc Endovasc Surg. 1995;10(4):424–30.
3. Riggs HE, Rupp C. Variation in form of circle of Willis: the relation of the variations to collateral circulation: anatomic analysis. Arch Neurol. 1963;8:8–14.
4. Iqbal S. A comprehensive study of the anatomical variations of the circle of willis in adult human brains. J Clin Diagn Res. 2013;7(11):2423–7.
5. Alpers BJ, Berry RG, Paddison RM. Anatomical studies of the circle of Willis in normal brain. AMA Arch Neurol Psychiatry. 1959;81(4):409–18.
6. Kamath S. Observations on the length and diameter of vessels forming the circle of Willis. J Anat. 1981;133(Pt 3):419–23.
7. Fetterman GH, Moran TJ. Fetterman: Anomalies of the circle of Willis in relation… - Google Scholar: Arch Pathol; 1941.
8. Fawcett E, Blachford JV. The Circle of Willis: an Examination of 700 Specimens. J Anat Physiol. 1905;40(Pt 1):63.2.
9. Milenković Z, Vučetić R, Puzić M. Asymmetry and anomalies of the circle of willis in fetal brain. Microsurgical study and functional remarks. Surg Neurol. 1985;24(5):563–70.
10. Puchades Orts A, Nombela Gomez M, Ortuño Pacheco G. Variation in form of circle of willis: some anatomical and embryological considerations. Anat Rec. 1976;185(1):119–23.
11. Baptista AG. Studies on the arteries of the brain: II. The anterior cerebral artery: some anatomic features and their clinical implications. Neurology. 1963;13(10):825.
12. Perlmutter D, Rhoton AL Jr. Microsurgical anatomy of the anterior cerebral-anterior communicating-recurrent artery complex. J Neurosurg. 2009;45(3):259–72.
13. Ozaki T, Handa H, Tomimoto K, Hazama F. Anatomical variations of the arterial system of the base of the brain. Nihon geka hokan Archiv fur japanische Chirurgie. 1977;46(1):3–17.
14. McVerry F, Liebeskind DS, Muir KW. Systematic review of methods for assessing leptomeningeal collateral flow. Am J Neuroradiol. 2012;33(3):576–82.
15. Brozici M, van der Zwan A, Hillen B. Anatomy and functionality of leptomeningeal anastomoses. Stroke. 2003;34(11):2750–62.
16. Liebeskind DS. Collateral circulation. Stroke. 2003;34(9):2279–84.
17. Meyer JS, Denny-Brown D. The cerebral collateral circulation: 1. Factors influencing collateral blood flow. Neurology. 1957;7(7):447.
18. Wei L, Erinjeri JP, Rovainen CM, Woolsey TA. Collateral growth and angiogenesis around cortical stroke. Stroke. 2001;32(9):2179–84.
19. Manoonkitiwongsa PS, Jackson-Friedman C, McMillan PJ, Schultz RL, Lyden PD. Angiogenesis after stroke is correlated with increased numbers of macrophages: the clean-up hypothesis. J Cereb Blood Flow Metab. 2001;21(10):1223–31.
20. Coyle P, Heistad DD. Development of collaterals in the cerebral circulation. J Vasc Res. 1991;28:183–9.
21. Lesley WS, Rangaswamy R. Balloon test occlusion and endosurgical parent artery sacrifice for the evaluation and management of complex intracranial aneurysmal disease. J Neurointerv Surg. 2009;1(2):112–20.
22. Standard SC, Ahuja A, Guterman LR, Chavis TD, Gibbons KJ, Barth AP, et al. Balloon test occlusion of the internal carotid artery with hypotensive challenge. AJNR Am J Neuroradiol. 1995;16(7):1453–8.
23. Wong GK, Poon WS, Chun Ho Yu S. Balloon test occlusion with hypotensive challenge for main trunk occlusion of internal carotid artery aneurysms and pseudoaneurysms. Br J Neurosurg. 2010;24(6):648–52.
24. Dare AO, Gibbons KJ, Gillihan MD, Guterman LR, Loree TR, Hicks WL Jr. Hypotensive endovascular test occlusion of the carotid artery in head and neck cancer. Neurosurg Focus. 2003;14(3):e5.
25. van Rooij WJ, Sluzewski M, Slob MJ, Rinkel GJ. Predictive value of angiographic testing for tolerance to therapeutic occlusion of the carotid artery. AJNR Am J Neuroradiol. 2005;26(1):175–8.
26. Gevers S, Heijtel D, Ferns SP, van Ooij P, van Rooij WJ, van Osch MJ, et al. Cerebral perfusion long term after therapeutic occlusion of the internal carotid artery in patients who tolerated angiographic balloon test occlusion. AJNR Am J Neuroradiol. 2012;33(2):329–35.
27. Abud DG, Spelle L, Piotin M, Mounayer C, Vanzin JR, Moret J. Venous phase timing during balloon test occlusion as a criterion for permanent internal carotid artery sacrifice. Am J Neuroradiol. 2005;26(10):2602–9.
28. van Rooij WJ, Sluzewski M, Metz NH, Nijssen PC, Wijnalda D, Rinkel GJ, et al. Carotid balloon occlusion for large and giant aneurysms: evaluation of a new test occlusion protocol. Neurosurgery. 2000;47(1):116–21; discussion 22.
29. Sanna M, Piazza P, Ditrapani G, Agarwal M. Management of the internal carotid artery in tumors of the lateral skull base: preoperative permanent balloon occlusion without reconstruction. Otol Neurotol. 2004;25(6):998–1005.
30. Kawai N, Kawanishi M, Shindou A, Kudomi N, Yamamoto Y, Nishiyama Y, et al. Cerebral blood flow and metabolism measurement using positron emission tomography before and during internal carotid artery test occlusions: feasibility of rapid quantitative measurement of CBF and OEF/CMRO(2). Interv Neuroradiol. 2012;18(3):264–74.
31. Eckard DA, Purdy PD, Bonte FJ. Temporary balloon occlusion of the carotid artery combined with brain blood flow imaging as a test to predict tolerance prior to permanent carotid sacrifice. AJNR Am J Neuroradiol. 1992;13(6):1565–9.
32. Lorberboym M, Pandit N, Machac J, Holan V, Sacher M, Segal D, et al. Brain perfusion imaging during preoperative temporary balloon occlusion of the internal carotid artery. J Nucl Med. 1996;37(3):415–9.
33. Mathews D, Walker BS, Purdy PD, Batjer H, Allen BC, Eckard DA, et al. Brain blood flow SPECT in temporary balloon occlusion of carotid and intracerebral arteries. J Nucl Med. 1993;34(8):1239–43.
34. Monsein LH, Jeffery PJ, van Heerden BB, Szabo Z, Schwartz JR, Camargo EE, et al. Assessing adequacy of collateral circulation during balloon test occlusion of the internal carotid artery with 99mTc-HMPAO SPECT. AJNR Am J Neuroradiol. 1991;12(6):1045–51.
35. Peterman SB, Taylor A Jr, Hoffman JC Jr. Improved detection of cerebral hypoperfusion with internal carotid balloon test occlusion and 99mTc-HMPAO cerebral perfusion SPECT imaging. AJNR Am J Neuroradiol. 1991;12(6):1035–41.
36. Sorteberg A, Bakke SJ, Boysen M, Sorteberg W. Angiographic balloon test occlusion and therapeutic sacrifice of major arteries to the brain. Neurosurgery. 2008;63(4):651–60; dicussion 60–1.
37. Sorteberg A, Sorteberg W, Bakke SJ, Lindegaard KF, Boysen M, Nornes H. Cerebral haemodynamics in internal carotid artery trial occlusion. Acta Neurochir. 1997;139(11):1066–73.
38. Sorteberg W, Sorteberg A, Lindegaard KF, Boysen M, Nornes H. Transcranial Doppler ultrasonography-guided management of internal carotid artery closure. Neurosurgery. 1999;45(1):76–87; discussion 87–8.
39. Morris P. Practical neuroangiography. 3rd ed. Philadelphia, PA: Lippincott Williams & Wilkins; 2013. xiii, 511 p.

Pathology of Malignant Neoplasms of the Ear and Temporal Bone

5

Diana Bell

Introduction

The chapter is dedicated to cancers of the temporal bone; therefore, very common benign temporal bone tumors (e.g., paraganglioma, meningioma, schwannoma) will not be discussed.

Tumors of the ear can be divided into external auditory canal (EAC) and pinna tumors, middle ear tumors, and inner ear tumors. Tumors of the middle and inner ear are grouped together, as their sites of origin cannot always be determined.

Tumors of the EAC and Pinna

Basal Cell Carcinoma

Basal cell carcinoma (BCC) is a slow growing, locally infiltrative malignant neoplasm of the skin and subcutaneous adnexal tissue; BCC represents the most common cutaneous malignancy. More common in men than in women, BCC is commonly seen in the seventh decade of life. The sun-exposed areas are the most frequent sites of occurrence (e.g., pinna). BCCs of the external auditory canal although uncommon usually have extensive subcutaneous involvement, which clinically is not obvious. Initially, BCC appears as a raised papule or nodule with telangiectasia. With time, the central portion ulcerates and is surrounded by raised borders ("rodent ulcer") [1–6]. BCC may be inherited in nevoid BCC syndrome (autosomal dominant disorder caused by mutations in PTCH tumor suppressor gene on 9q22.3p31). The histology OF EAC BCC is similar to that of BCC occurring elsewhere in the body (Fig. 5.1a–c).

D. Bell, M.D.
Departments of Pathology and Head and Neck Surgery, The University of Texas M.D. Anderson Cancer Center, Houston, TX, USA
e-mail: diana.bell@mdanderson.org

Squamous Cell Carcinoma

Squamous cell carcinoma (SCC) of the EAC or pinna affects about 1 million people [7], usually between the ages of 55 and 65 years. In general, SCC has an overall predominance in women; however, pinna tumors tend to occur more frequently in men [8].

Actinic overexposure and frostbite are recognized etiologies for pinna tumors, whereas chronic inflammation and radiation are possible etiologic factors for EAC tumors [7, 9–11]. Papillomas in this region rarely transform into SCC [12].

On clinical examination, pinna tumors appear as excoriated or ulcerated masses. Usual symptoms at presentation are otitis externa, otitis media, pain, hearing changes, and cholesteatomas; nerve symptoms have later onset.

Macroscopically, EAC SCCs are warty, exophytic masses that occlude the EAC and invade the tympanic membrane. The histology of EAC SCC is similar to that of SCCs occurring elsewhere in the body, with spindle and acantholytic, but rarely verrucous variants (Fig. 5.2a, b); desmoplastic response and inflammation are frequently seen (Fig. 5.2c, d).

EAC SCC is aggressive. The disease frequently involves vital structures, often recurs locally, and can metastasize to the lymph nodes. Poor prognosis is linked to high clinical stage, tumor depth, and lymphovascular and perineural invasion [7, 9, 13–16].

Malignant Melanoma

Malignant melanoma, although relatively rare, is the third most common malignancy of the external ear, accounting for 7–16% of all head and neck melanoma [17]. Similar to the other actinically related neoplasms, there is a 2:1 male-to-female ratio with a mean age at diagnosis of 72 years [17]. Malignant melanoma can be pigmented, amelanotic, nodular, ulcerated. Histologically known as "the great mimicker," it may show a poorly differentiated epithelioid

P. W. Gidley, F. DeMonte (eds.), *Temporal Bone Cancer*, https://doi.org/10.1007/978-3-319-74539-8_5

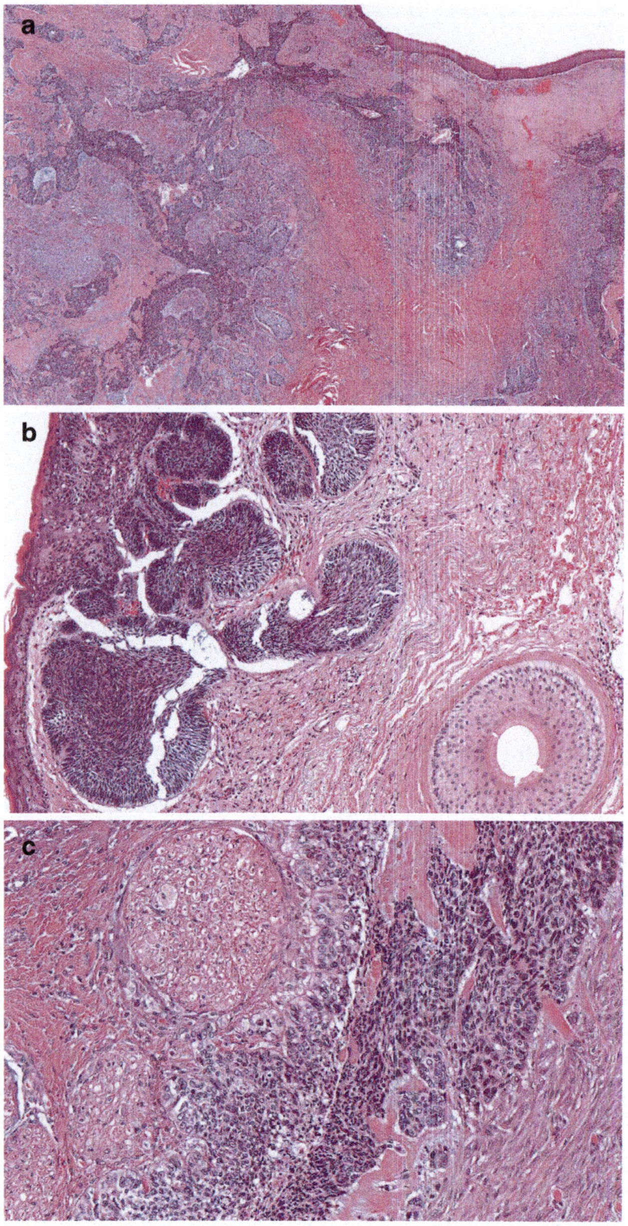

Fig. 5.1 Basal cell carcinoma (BCC). Hematoxylin and eosin stain, (**a**) low power (4×) with a deeply infiltrative growth pattern; high-power (10×) (**b**) conventional, nodular-type BCC with characteristic peripheral clefting and (**c**) BCC with perineural invasion

or sarcomatoid neoplasm, with immunoperoxidase studies paramount to the differential diagnosis (Fig. 5.3a–c). S-100, melanoma cocktail (HMB-45, tyrosinase A), MiTF5, and SOX10 are valuable and specific antibodies in the immunohistochemical work-up for melanoma. [Primary melanoma has to be distinguished from dermal and mucosal metastasis. Treatment varies according to anatomic location: melanoma of the pinna is amenable to wide local excision/amputation, while melanoma of the external ear canal may require extensive surgery including partial temporal bone resection. Similar to other cutaneous sites, the prognosis is linked to depth of invasion].

Atypical Fibroxanthoma

Atypical fibroxanthoma (AFX) is a pleomorphic, dermal mesenchymal tumor with predilection on actinic-damaged cutaneous sites of elderly individuals (75% of cases) or occasionally in younger patients (25% of cases). AFX is also known historically as low-grade malignant fibrous histiocytoma (MFH), pseudosarcoma of the skin, and pseudosarcomatous dermatofibroma. AFX presents as a solitary nodule often ulcerated, with possible bleeding, pruritus, or pain. Histology shows an unencapsulated spindle cell neoplasm centered in the dermis, with a spectrum of spindle shaped to pleomorphic cells with hyperchromatic nuclei and bizarre multinucleated cells (Fig. 5.4a, b). Foamy histiocytes, increased mitotic figures (including atypical mitoses), and a storiform pattern can be seen. The differential diagnosis includes spindle cell squamous carcinoma, melanoma spindled type, and leiomyosarcoma. Immunohistochemistry is helpful, with AFX reactivity for anti-CD68 and negative for carcinoma, melanoma, and muscle markers. Complete surgical excision is the treatment of choice, with excellent prognosis.

Ceruminous Gland Adenocarcinoma

Ceruminous gland adenocarcinomas, also known as ceruminal adenocarcinomas, cylindromas, and ceruminomas, are malignant neoplasms that arise from the apocrine ceruminous glands of the EAC. They are rare, accounting for <2.5% of EAC tumors [18–20]. Ceruminous gland adenocarcinomas can mimic adenoid cystic carcinomas, mucoepidermoid carcinomas, and adenocarcinomas not otherwise specified.

The tumors occur in the outer half of the EAC, which excludes the possibility of direct extension from the parotid [18–20], complemented by imaging studies. They occur in women and men at a ratio of 1.5:1. Patients tend to be middle-aged or older at presentation [18, 21–23] and typically present with a mass, hearing changes, drainage, pain, and neurologic deficits, such as facial nerve paralysis. Imaging studies are used to define tumor extent and exclude direct extension from the parotid or nasopharynx.

Grossly, the tumors have a polypoid appearance and are up to 3 cm in diameter. Histologically, these tumors are unencapsulated and invasive, infiltrating soft tissue and bone with various architectural patterns, such as solid, cystic, cribriform, glandular, and single-cell patterns; perineural invasion and comedonecrosis are appreciated (Fig. 5.5a). Hypercellularity, moderate to severe nuclear pleomorphism,

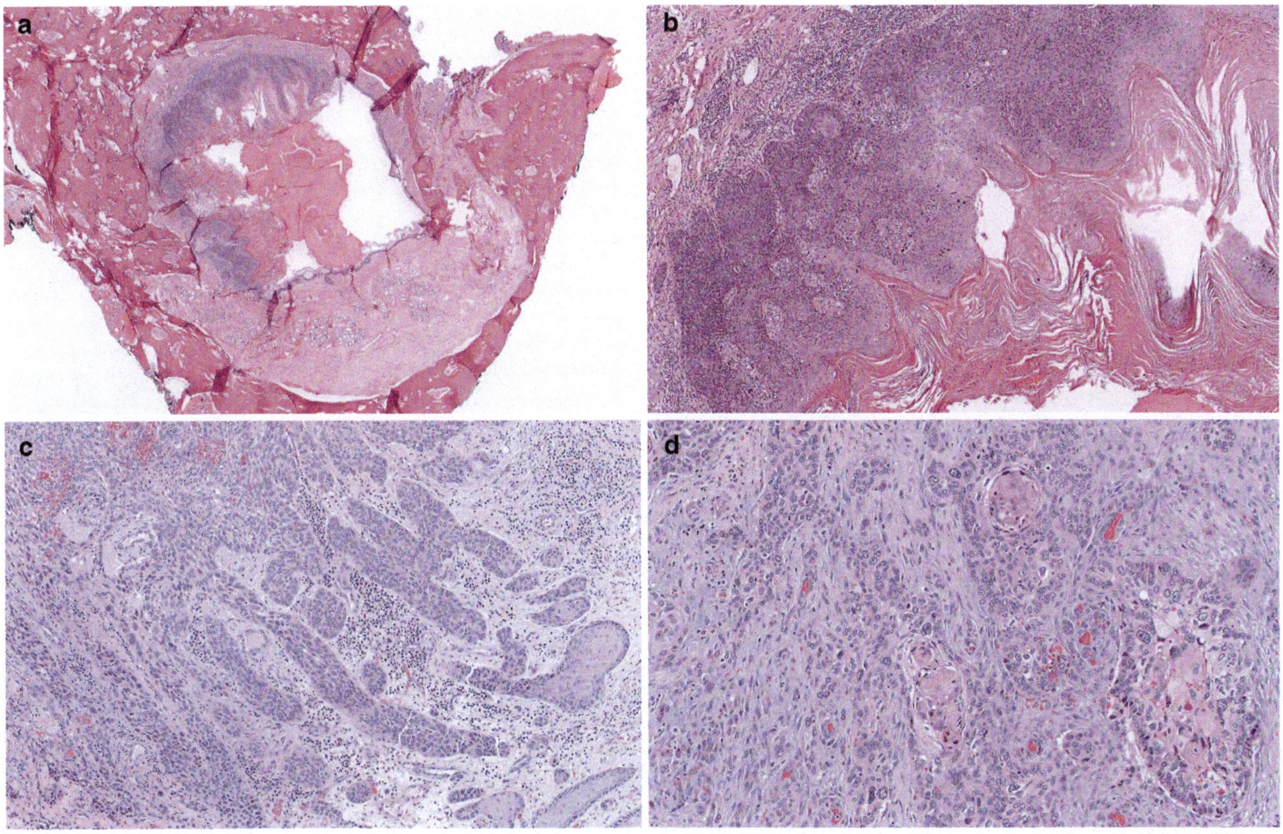

Fig. 5.2 Squamous cell carcinoma (SCC) of the ear canal. Hematoxylin and eosin stain, (**a**) low scanning power and (**b**) high power (10×) of verrucous-type carcinoma with abundant keratinization and bulbous and pushing rete pegs and (**c**) low magnification (4×) and (**d**) higher magnification (10×) of conventional-type SCC showing infiltrative cords and islands of keratinizing cells, in a background of desmoplasia and solar elastosis

and increased mitotic figures are present. Ceroid pigment is absent. Ceruminous adenocarcinomas are recognized by the eosinophilic character of their cells; apocrine-type secretions and a myoepithelial layer are less frequent in these tumors than in benign ceruminous adenomas (Fig. 5.5b). Ceruminous adenoid cystic carcinoma and ceruminous mucoepidermoid carcinoma are histologically identical to salivary gland carcinomas. Adenoid cystic carcinomas are widely infiltrative, with characteristic perineural spread (Fig. 5.6a–d). Immunohistochemistry highlights biphasic composition with CK7- and CD117-positive luminal cells and p63-, S100-, and CK14-positive abluminal cells [18, 24, 25]. Similar to salivary carcinomas, ceruminous adenoid cystic carcinomas bear the t(6;9) translocation with the MYB-NFIB fusion transcript [26, 27]. Mucoepidermoid carcinoma, myoepithelial carcinoma, and acinic cell carcinoma have been seen on rare occasions. It is very important to exclude direct invasion from a primary parotid gland and metastasis.

The prognosis is variable and depends on the extent of the disease. Recurrence, which is associated with positive surgical margins and high-grade histology, is common; patients with destruction of local vital structures or with distant metastases, which occur more commonly in the lungs than in the lymph nodes, have dismal outcomes [18–20, 28].

Rhabdomyosarcoma

Rhabdomyosarcoma (RMS) is the most common malignant tumor of the ear in children, accounting for 7% of ear tumors [21]. Common presentation is a mass in the auditory canal. Extensive bone destruction is present on imaging. RMS types are similar to those at other locations: botryoid/embryonal (frequent), alveolar, solid/pleomorphic, and spindled. On histology the malignant cells are small, dark, spindled in a loose myxoid background. Rhabdoid and striated cells can be seen occasionally and facilitate the diagnosis (Fig. 5.7a–d). The major differential diagnosis is with aural polyp (Fig. 5.7e). Immunophenotyping with lineage-specific markers (desmin, myogenin, MyoD1) is part of the work-up.

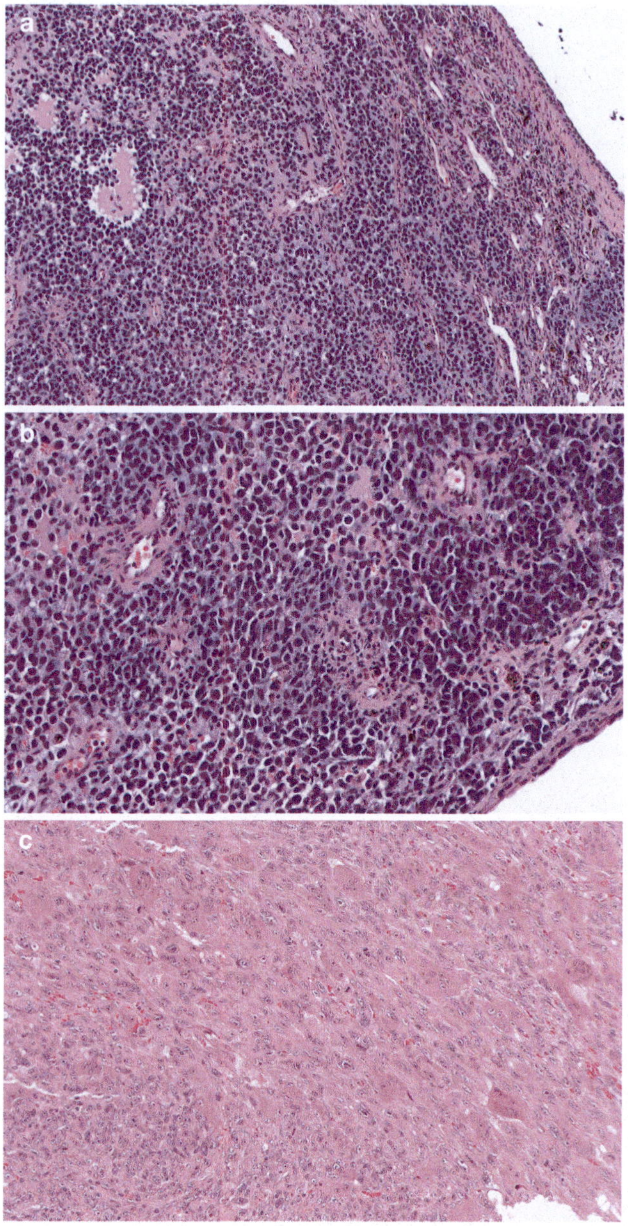

Fig. 5.3 Melanoma. Hematoxylin and eosin stain, (**a**) low (4×) and (**b**) high (10×) power—small round cell malignant morphology, with perivascular arrangement and prominent hyperchromatic, eccentric nuclei. The differential diagnosis is broad including the vast category of small round cell malignant tumors, with immunophenotyping being paramount in diagnosis. (**c**) Malignant melanoma with spindled/epithelioid morphology and associated multinucleated giant cells

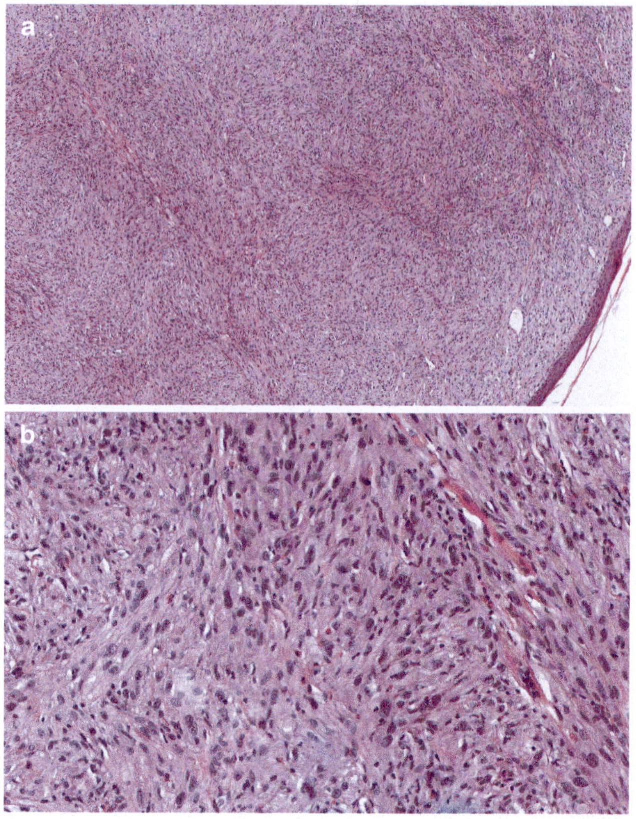

Fig. 5.4 Atypical fibroxanthoma (AFX). Histology shows an unencapsulated spindle cell neoplasm centered in the dermis (**a**), with a spectrum of spindle shaped to pleomorphic cells with hyperchromatic nuclei and bizarre multinucleated cells (**b**)

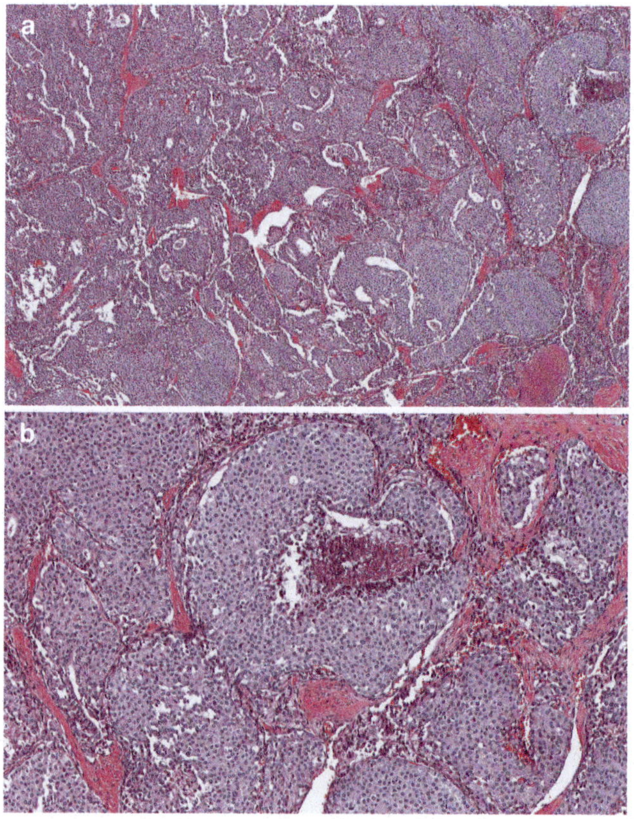

Fig. 5.5 Ceruminous gland adenocarcinoma. (**a**) Hematoxylin and eosin stain, low power (4×) morphologically; ceruminous adenocarcinomas are identical to the similar tumors arising in salivary glands, with variably irregular gland formation and significant infiltrative growth. (**b**) Hematoxylin and eosin stain, high-power (10×) cellular pleomorphism, prominent nucleoli, mitoses, and comedo-type necrosis are present in this high-grade adenocarcinoma

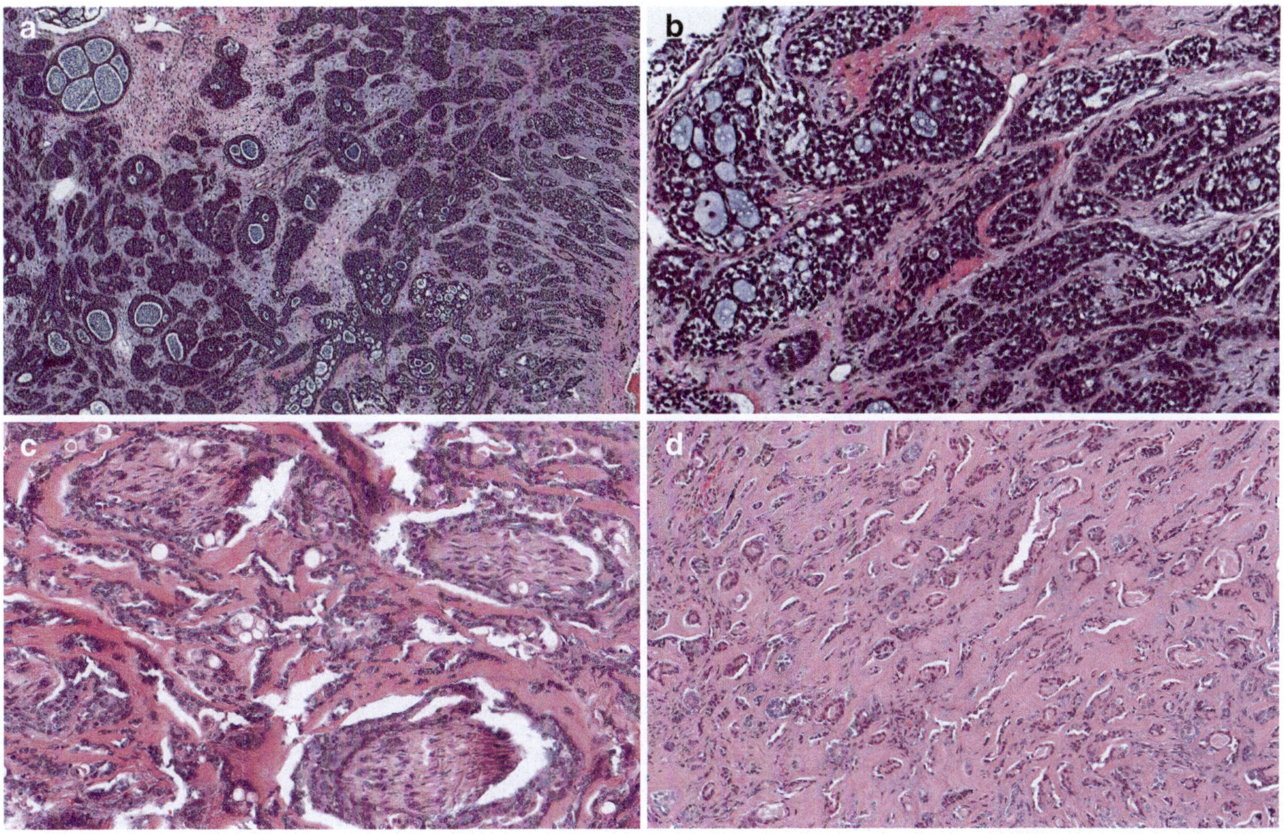

Fig. 5.6 Ceruminous adenoid cystic carcinoma (ACC). Hematoxylin and eosin. The morphology is similar to the tumors seen in major and minor salivary glands, with dual composition of epithelial and myoepithelial cells arranged in a cribriform and tubular patterns (**a**, **b**) and extensive perineural invasion (**c**). The sclerosing type ACC is rarely seen (**d**)

Tumors of the Middle and Inner Ear

Squamous Cell Carcinoma

SCC in the middle ear is rare. The mean age of patients with middle ear SCC at presentation is 60 years, and the disease has a predilection for men [29]. Chronic otitis may be a predisposing factor [30]. The tumors may originate in the middle ear or extend from SCC in the EAC. Direct spread into the inner ear, usually along cranial nerve VIII, is uncommon [31]. Prognosis is poor owing to advanced disease at presentation and delayed diagnosis. SCC of the external ear, ear canal, and middle ear is histologically identical.

Neuroendocrine adenomatoid tumor of the Middle Ear [32]

Neuroendocrine adenomatoid tumor of the middle ear is a neuroendocrine neoplasm that have been described by many names, including carcinoid tumors, middle ear adenomas, adenomatous tumors of the middle ear, adenocarcinoids, and amphicrine tumors.

These tumors are very rare, accounting for <2% of ear tumors. They have an equal gender distribution and typically occur in the fifth decade of life [33–36]. Symptoms at presentation include decreased hearing acuity, a feeling of fullness or pressure in the ear, and tinnitus. Otoscopy usually reveals an intact tympanic membrane and a brown reddish structure immediately beyond. The tumors occasionally extend into the EAC or mastoid bone. Histologically, they are unencapsulated, with variable cellularity and various architectural patterns [33, 34, 37]. The dominant glandular pattern consists of duct-like structures with "back-to-back" gland configuration; minor components include trabeculae, festooning, anastomosing cords, and solid sheets (Fig. 5.8a, b). The cytoplasm is eosinophilic, and the nuclei tend to be round to oval and plasmacytoid with minimal pleomorphism and salt-and-pepper chromatin distribution. Immunophenotypically, the tumors are positive for keratins and neuroendocrine markers, including chromogranin, synaptophysin, and neuron-specific enolase (Fig. 5.8c, d) [33, 34, 37]. The differential diagnosis

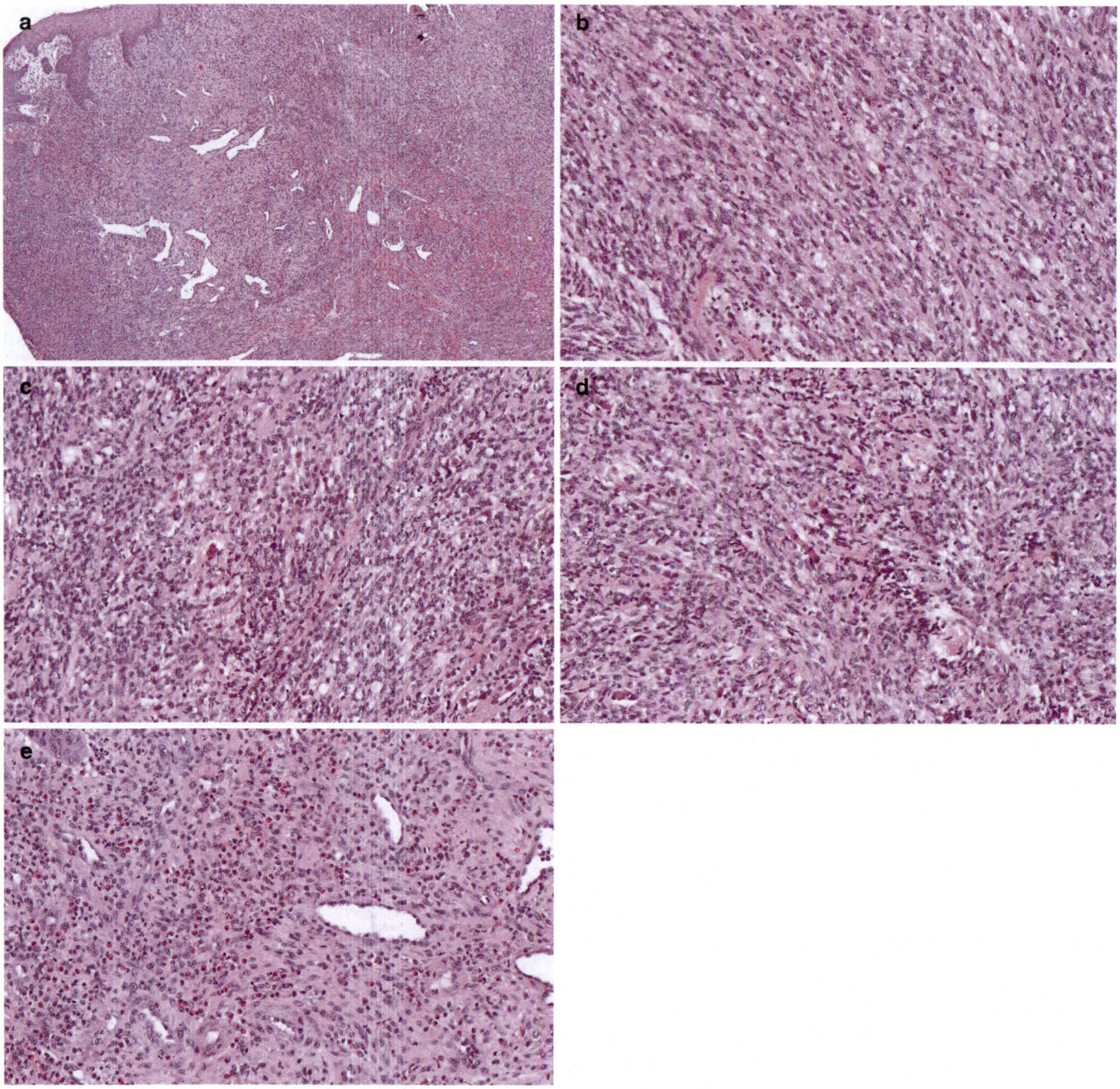

Fig. 5.7 Rhabdomyosarcoma (RMS). On histology the malignant cells are small, dark, spindled in a loose myxoid background (**a**, **b**). Rhabdoid and striated cells can be seen occasionally and facilitate the diagnosis (**c**, **d**). The major differential diagnosis is with aural polyp (**e**)

includes ceruminous adenoma, meningioma, paraganglioma, and metastatic adenocarcinoma [33, 35, 37].

The treatment of choice for middle ear adenocarcinomas with neuroendocrine features is complete surgical removal, including removal of the ossicles. Most adenocarcinomas with neuroendocrine features are excised in a piecemeal fashion (<1 cm) owing to the confined anatomic space [33, 34, 37]. About 15–20% of patients have recurrence [33, 36, 38]. Facial nerve paralysis may occur and is due to mass-related compression rather than invasion [33, 36, 38]. Unreported institutional experience (MD Anderson Cancer Center) indicates that the disease can metastasize to the lymph nodes and liver.

Aggressive Papillary Tumor (aka Endolymphatic SAC Tumor, Low-Grade Adenocarcinoma of Endolymphatic SAC Origin)

The endolymphatic sac tumor (ELST) is a rare lesion of the skull base for which an endolymphatic sac origin is supported by early manifestations of vestibular disease, radiographic evidence of a tumor in the posterior-medial petrous ridge, identification of an in situ tumor, and morphophenotypical similarities to normal endolymphatic sac epithelium. Historically, first series was described by Gaffey

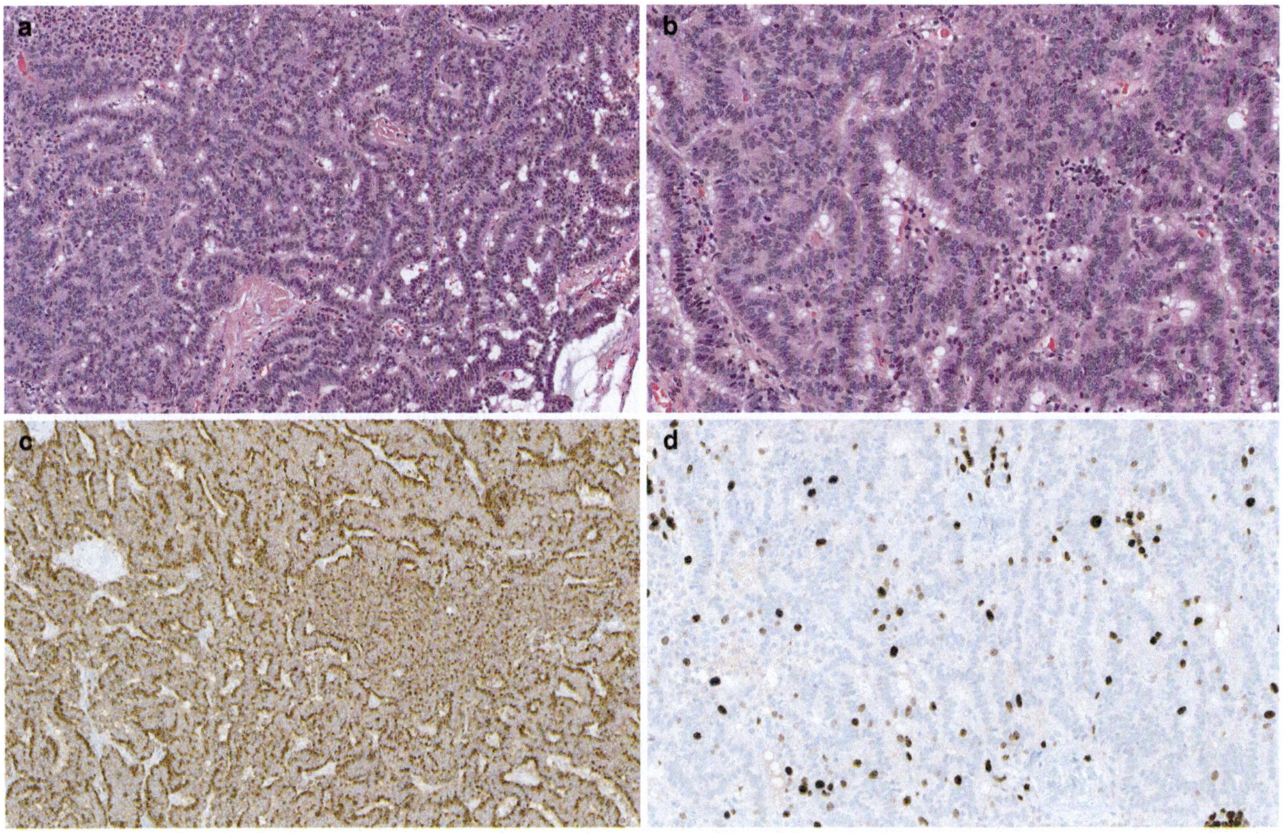

Fig. 5.8 Middle ear adenocarcinomas with neuroendocrine features. The histologic architectural patterns may be solid, glandular, or trabecular (**a**—hematoxylin and eosin stain, low power 4×); the tumor cells are uniform, with a moderate amount of acidophilic cytoplasm and nuclei with "salt-and-pepper" chromatin pattern (**b**—hematoxylin and eosin stain, high power 10×). Neuroendocrine markers are usually positive (**c**—immunoperoxidase study with anti-synaptophysin antibody, brown membranous reactivity pattern), and the proliferation rate is low to intermediate (**d**—immunoperoxidase study with anti-Ki-67 antibody, brown nuclear reactivity pattern)

et al. in 1988, reporting a series of ten cases of an aggressive papillary middle ear tumor (APMET) characterized by a locally aggressive papillary growth pattern, bone destruction, and frequent endolymphatic sac invasion, thus establishing an entity separate from middle ear adenoma [39]. A year later, Heffner reported 20 cases of an identical tumor and proposed an endolymphatic sac origin [40]. Prior to this, Hassard et al. had described intraoperatively a tumor adherent to the endolymphatic sac while performing decompression surgery for presumed Ménière's disease [41].

The endolymphatic sac is derived from neuroectoderm and is located subjacent to the posteromedial surface of the temporal bone. The distal part is ensheathed by two layers of dura mater, and the intermediate rugose part lies within the vestibular canal. It is from the latter part that ELST is suspected to originate [40, 42]. This anatomic location is important as it explains the propensity of the tumor to involve the petrous portion of the temporal bone as well as cerebellopontine angle (CPA) structures [43]. There are four potential vectors for tumor extension: posteromedially into the cerebellopontine angle, laterally toward the middle ear, superiorly toward the middle cranial fossa, and anteromedially along the petrous ridge to the cavernous and sphenoid sinuses [43]. Patients present with hearing loss, tinnitus, and vertigo; facial nerve paralysis occurs less commonly. Large tumors with growth along the posteromedial vector may cause symptoms secondary to cerebellopontine angle extension. An indolent clinical course and long-standing symptom history is typical. A diagnosis of ELST should prompt the clinician to consider the possibility of von Hippel-Lindau (VHL) disease, but this is not a prerequisite for diagnosis as these tumors also occur sporadically. Patients with VHL disease are more likely to have bilateral ELSTs. The histopathological appearance of ELST is that of a papillary, cystic, and glandular neoplasm. Interdigitating complex papillary processes are embedded in sheets of dense fibrous stroma. The papillary processes are lined with a single layer of low columnar-to-cuboidal epithelial cells, resembling those of the normal endolymphatic sac, middle ear, and mastoid sinuses (Fig. 5.9a–c). Nuclear pleomorphism and mitotic figures are inconspicuous. The histopathologic differential diagnosis includes metastatic carcinomas from the thyroid, lung, kidney and breast; paraganglioma; choroid plexus papilloma; meningioma; and middle ear adenoma. The precise location of the tumor as defined by preoperative imaging studies and intraoperative surgical observation, together with

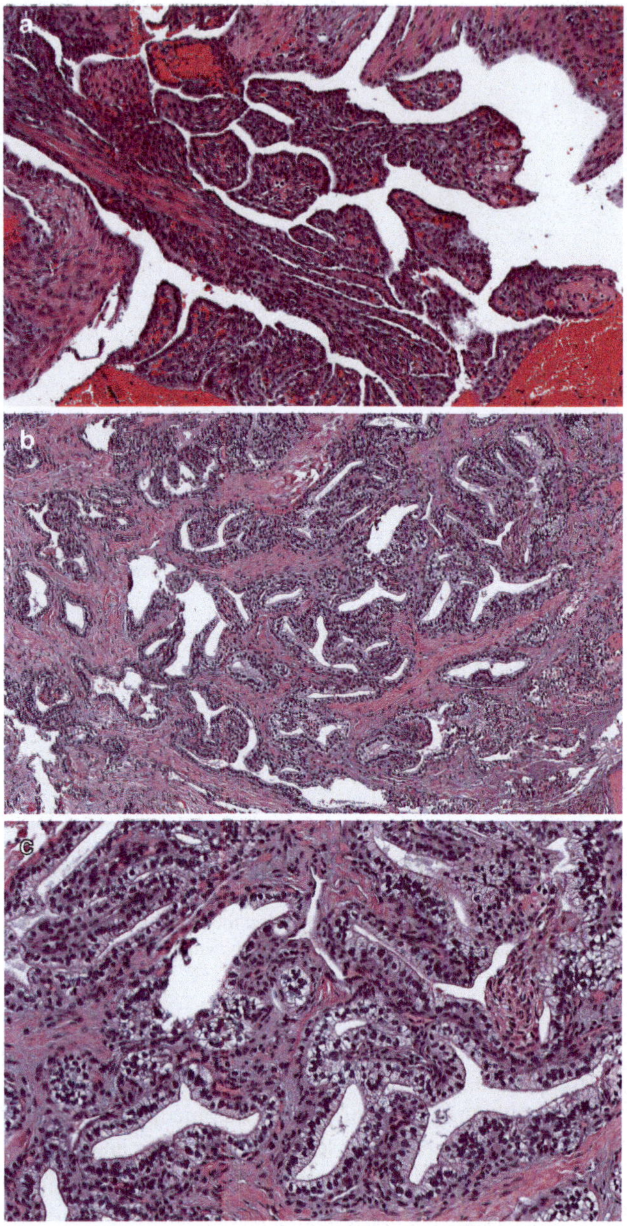

Fig. 5.9 Endolymphatic sac tumor (ELST). The histopathological appearance of ELST is that of a papillary, cystic, and glandular neoplasm. Interdigitating complex papillary processes are embedded in sheets of dense fibrous stroma (**a**, **b**—hematoxylin and eosin stain, low power 4×). The papillary processes are lined with a single layer of low columnar-to-cuboidal epithelial cells, resembling those of the normal endolymphatic sac, middle ear, and mastoid sinuses (**c**—hematoxylin and eosin stain, high power 10×)

the use of immunohistochemical markers (Table 5.1), helps to differentiate ELST from mimics [43]. Choroid plexus papillomas (CPPs) typically express transthyretin (prealbumin), which is not characteristic of the ELST immunophenotype. Of note, other differentiation markers, such as glial fibrillary acidic protein (GFAP) and synaptophysin (associated with central nervous system tumors), may also be expressed by ELSTs, in keeping with the embryonic origin of the endolymphatic sac from the neural crest. A history of VHL disease or other tumors associated with the VHL disease spectrum, or of bilateral ELST, facilitates correct diagnosis [39, 44]. Metastatic renal clear cell carcinoma can still be a diagnostic consideration since it occurs in patients with VHL disease, and both ELSTs and clear cell carcinomas of the kidney may occur in the same patient. The imaging hallmark of ELST is the presence of a retrolabyrinthine mass associated with osseous erosion. ELST presents a diagnostic challenge at all levels of presentation. Clinically, patients often initially receive a misdiagnosis of Méniére's disease. Metastases from ELST have rarely been reported in the literature [45, 46]. The following ELST grading system was proposed by Bambakidis et al. [47]: grade I lesions are confined to the temporal bone, middle ear, and external auditory meatus; grade II lesions have extension into the posterior fossa; grade III lesions involve the posterior and middle cranial fossae; and grade IV lesions (very rare, 2–4% ELSTs) extend to the clivus or sphenoid wing. Surgery is the treatment of choice for small ELST [38]. Remission may last for years, but local recurrence after surgery, likely secondary to incomplete resection, can occur. Radiotherapy has a 50% success rate with large or residual tumors.

A mouse model for ELST has been described recently [48]; the tumors also expressed mutant EGFR and downstream targets Akt, mTOR, and ERK1/2. The good response to EGFR inhibitors cetuximab and erlotinib suggests that EGFR inhibitors may be potential alternatives in the treatment of ELST [48].

Other Malignant Tumors of the Middle Ear and Temporal Bone

Osteosarcoma

Osteosarcomas of the skull (including temporal bone) are exceedingly rare (1% of all osteosarcomas) [49–51]. Paget disease of the bone, fibrous dysplasia, and postradiation therapy are the usual setting for osteosarcomas in this location. New osteoid matrix production (Fig. 5.10a) is mandatory for the diagnosis in all histological types of osteosarcoma: osteoblastic (Fig. 5.10b), chondroblastic, fibroblastic, telangiectatic, and small cell type. Osteosarcomas of the skull are aggressive, with lung and brain metastasis and with a dismal 5-year survival [52–54].

Chondrosarcoma

The region of the spheno-petrous synchondrosis is the most commonly reported site for chondrosarcoma of temporal bone [55]. Similar to other locations, chondrosarcomas are morphologically classified as conventional (most common) (Fig. 5.11a, b) [55], mesenchymal, clear cell, dedifferentiated. Grading according to a three-tier system (I, II, III

Table 5.1 Immunophenotype of middle ear and temporal bone glandular neoplasms

	Neuroendocrine (synapto/chromo/NSE)	Keratins	S100	Mucin	Prealbumin (transthyretin)	PSA	TTF-1 and thyroglobulin	Vimentin and RCC	GFAP
NAME	+	+	–	+	–	–	–	–	–
ELST	+/–	+	+/–	–	–	–	–	–	+
Choroid plexus papilloma	–	+	+	–	+	–	–	–	–
Metastatic thyroid carcinoma		+	–	–	–	–	+	–	–
Metastatic renal cell carcinoma		+	–	–	–	–	–	–	–
Metastatic prostate carcinoma		+	–	–	–	+	–	+	–

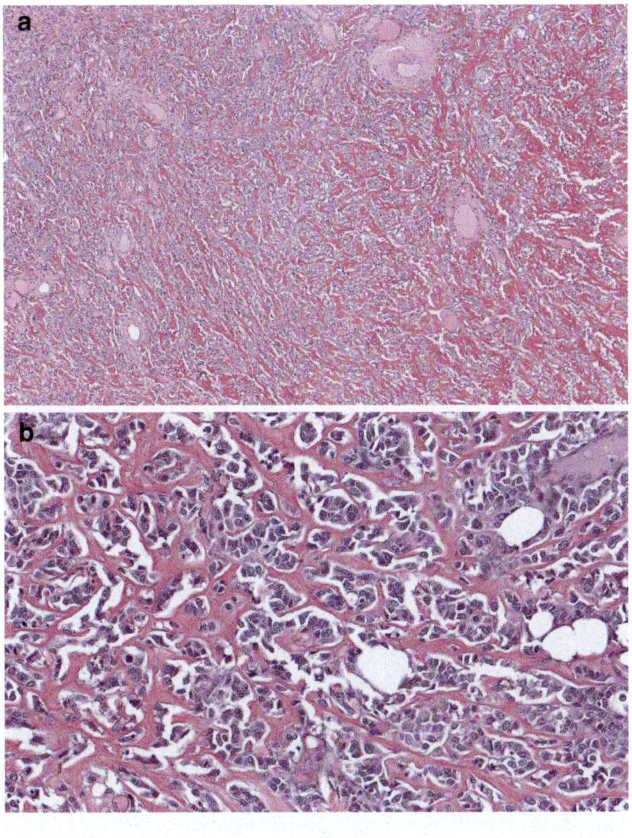

Fig. 5.10 Osteosarcoma. New osteoid matrix production (**a**) is mandatory for the diagnosis in all histological types of osteosarcoma. (**b**) Osteosarcoma, osteoblastic type

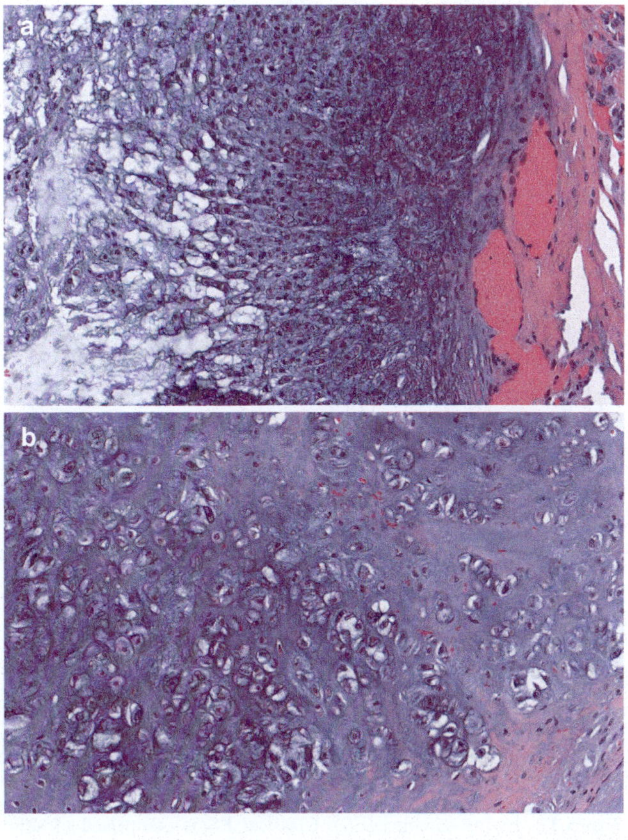

Fig. 5.11 Chondrosarcoma, conventional type (**a**) and low grade (**b**) showing disorganized chondrocytic architecture, increased cellularity and cellular pleomorphism, and scattered hyperchromatic nuclei

corresponding to well/moderately/poorly differentiated) is an important prognosticator. Surgery with radiotherapy is the treatment of choice.

Ewing Sarcoma

Ewing sarcoma (ES) is the second most common primary malignant bone tumor in children and adolescents, following osteosarcoma. The majority of ES arise in the bone and up to 30% in soft tissue [56]. Six cases have been reported in the literature, with a primary ES of the petrous temporal bone [57–59].

ES is a histologically diverse group of tumors with varying degrees of neural differentiation. Traditionally, ES is divided into three major histologic subtypes: classical ES, primitive neuroectodermal tumor (PNET), and atypical ES [56]. Classical ES is comprised of solid sheets or vague lobules of uniform small cells; majority of ES show classical morphology. Tumors with evidence of neural differentiation are classified as primitive neuroectodermal tumors (PNET); rosettes and neural differentiation highlighted on phenotyping are supporting the diagnosis. Atypical ES (large cell ES) category describes tumors that deviate from classical ES;

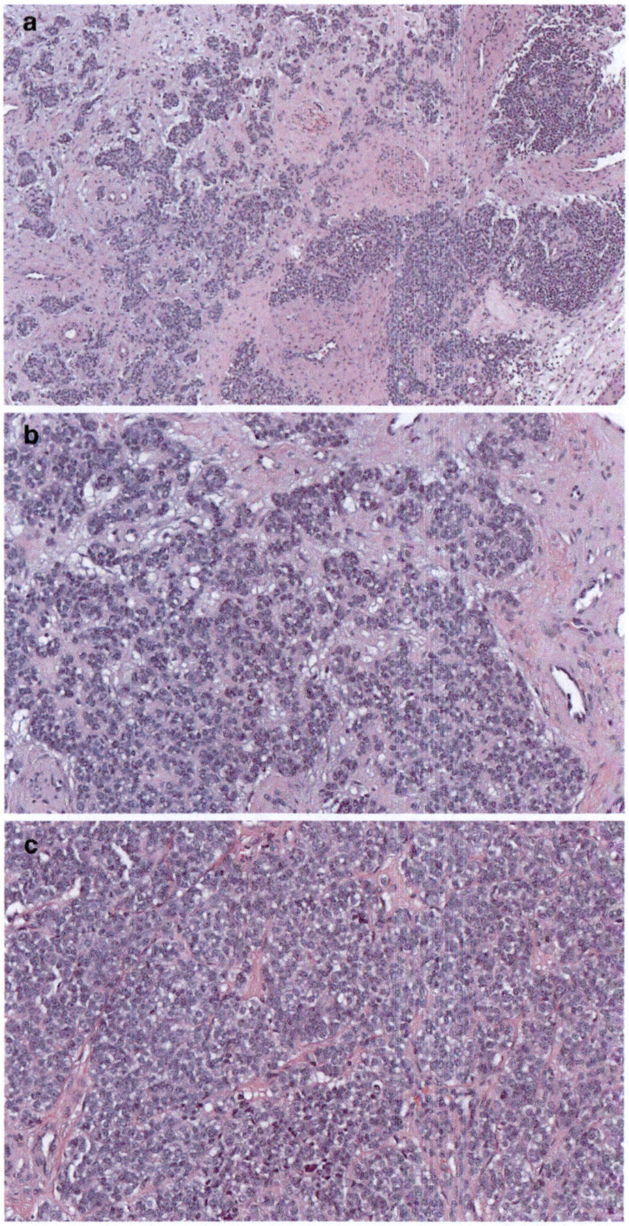

Fig. 5.12 Ewing sarcoma (ES). Classical ES is comprised of solid sheets or vague lobules of uniform small cells. Low (4×) (**a**) and high power (10×) (**b**, **c**)

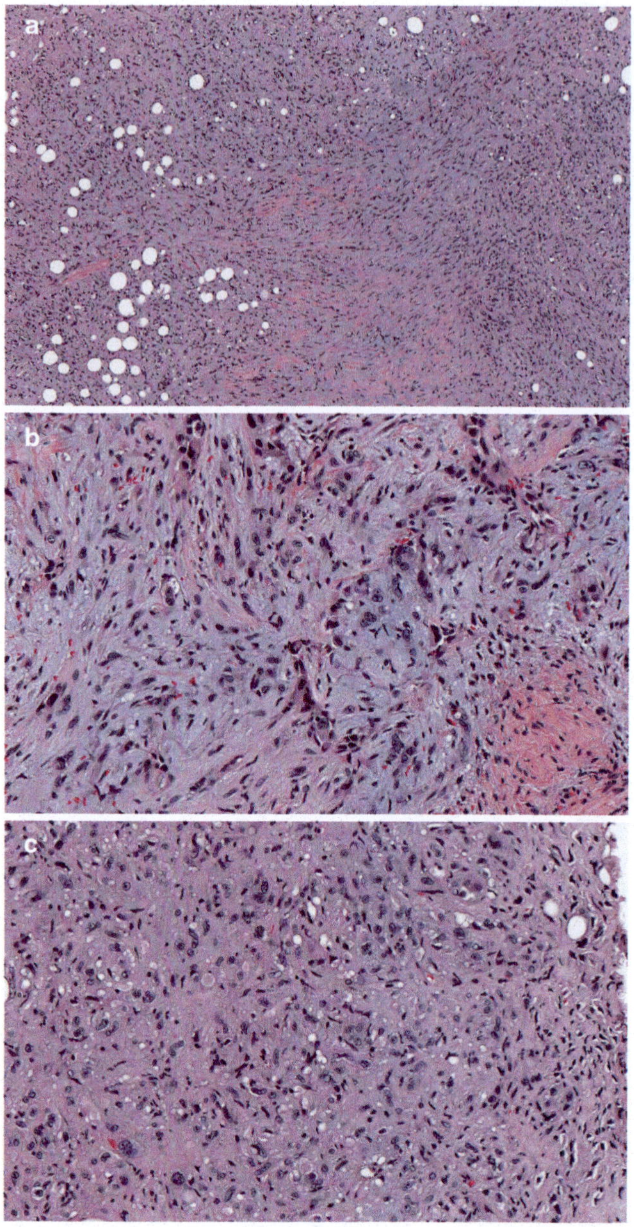

Fig. 5.13 Epithelioid hemangioendothelioma (EHE). Low-to-intermediate-grade mesenchymal neoplasm characterized by short cords and nests of epithelioid tumor cells with endothelial differentiation set in a myxohyaline matrix (**a**, **b**, **c**)

adamantinoma-like ES is a relatively newer described entity. ES is genetically defined by a balanced translocation that involves the *EWSR1* gene (locus22q12) and a member of the *ETS* family of transcription factors, most frequently *FLI1* or *ERG*. Eighty-five percent of ES harbor a t(11;22)(q24;q12) resulting in *EWSR1-FLI1* gene fusion [56]. [Diana, where do you want to place Fig. 5.12a–c?]

Hemangioendothelioma/Epithelioid Hemangioendothelioma

Epithelioid hemangioendothelioma (EHE) is a rare low-to-intermediate-grade mesenchymal neoplasm (Fig. 5.13a) characterized by short cords and nests of epithelioid tumor cells with endothelial differentiation set in a myxohyaline matrix (Fig. 5.13b, c) [60]. Primary sites include the skin, superficial and deep soft tissues, visceral organs, and bone [60]. Anecdotal cases of primary hemangioendothelioma of the temporal bone have been described [61–64]. Although the majority behave in an indolent fashion, there is about 20% risk of widespread metastasis and death from disease [60]. The diagnosis of EHE may be challenging particularly on limited biopsy, with several mimickers such as metastatic carcinoma and myoepithelial and chondroid neoplasms.

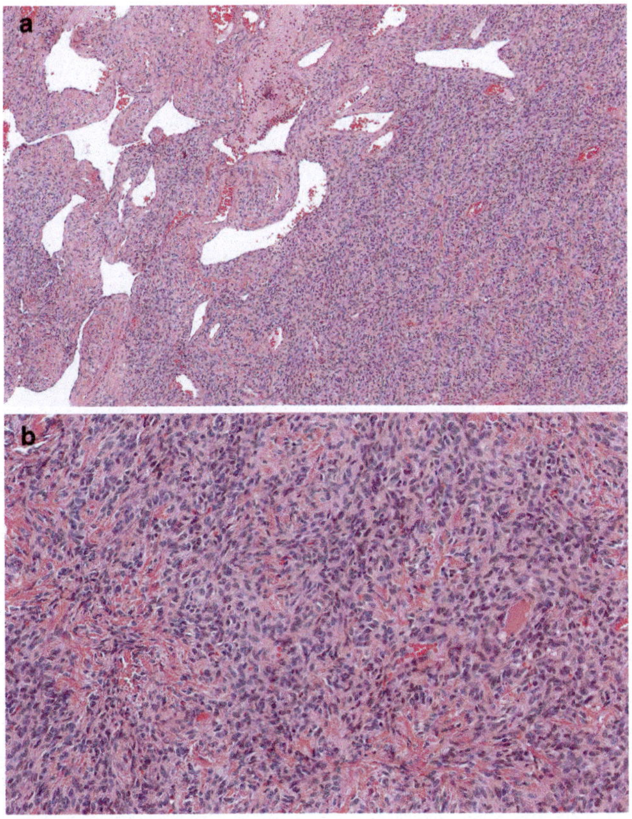

Fig. 5.14 Hemangiopericytoma/solitary fibrous tumor. The tumors are uniformly cellular with numerous thin branching vessels with gaping sinusoidal spaces (staghorn configuration) (**a**); hyalinization, myxoid changes, and fibrosis can be present (**b**)

EHE of the bone and extra-skeletal sites has a highly specific recurrent translocation, t(1;3)(p36.3;q23–25), resulting in a *WWTR1-CAMTA1* fusion transcript [60].

Hemangiopericytoma/Solitary Fibrous Tumor

Hemangiopericytoma (HPC) coined in 1924 by Stout and Murray was described as a distinctive soft tissue neoplasm, presumably of pericytic origin, exhibiting a characteristic "staghorn" branching vascular pattern [65]. Over the years, it became more obvious that this growth pattern is shared by several unrelated benign and malignant lesions and that HPC was better considered as a diagnosis of exclusion. Up to 15% of soft tissue neoplasms show HPC-like features, at least focally [65]. Solitary fibrous tumors (SFT) can be allocated to the group of HPC-like neoplasms [65]. Solitary fibrous tumor is considered by many to form a spectrum with hemangiopericytoma. Microscopically, the tumors are uniformly cellular with numerous thin branching vessels with gaping sinusoidal spaces (staghorn configuration) (Fig. 5.14a); hyalinization, myxoid changes, and fibrosis can be present (Fig. 5.14b). Molecular studies have discovered a NAB2-STAT6 fusion gene in up to 100% of HPC/SFT. Recent studies demonstrated that STAT6 immunohistochemistry is a reliable surrogate for the detection of the fusion gene. Nuclear STAT6 immunoreactivity is highly sensitive and specific marker of SFTs and can be helpful when diagnosis is inconclusive by conventional methods [66]. HPC/SFT has been reported to involve the temporal bone and temporal fossa [67–74].

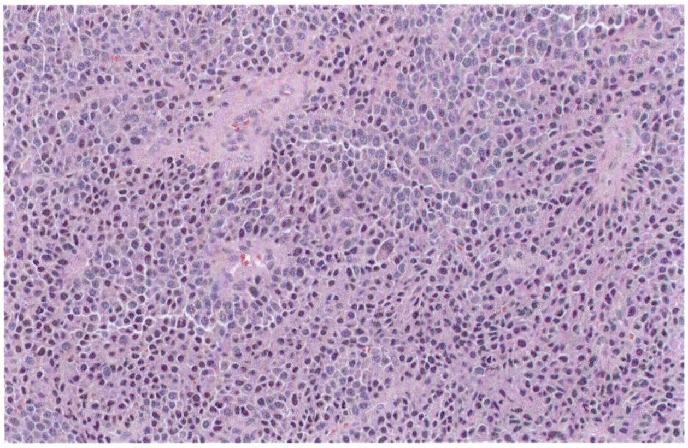

Fig. 5.15 Extramedullary plasmacytoma. Monotonous (clonal) proliferation of plasma cells with eccentric nuclei (hematoxylin and eosin)

Hematolymphoid Neoplasms

Non-Hodgkin and Hodgkin lymphomas, leukemias, and plasma cell dyscrasias (Fig. 5.15) can secondary involve the middle ear and temporal bone in the setting of primary disease elsewhere [55].

Metastatic Tumors to the Middle Ear and Temporal Bone (Secondary Tumors)

Metastasis to the middle ear and temporal bone may originate from virtually every site, most frequently of breast, head and neck, lungs, and prostate origin [75–78]. Beside hematogenous spread, direct extension from nearby primary tumors (squamous cell carcinoma) and leptomeningeal extension from intracranial tumors and meningeal carcinomatosis are other possible routes of middle ear/temporal bone involvement.

References

1. Farley RL, Manolidis S, Ratner D. Aggressive basal cell carcinoma with invasion of the parotid gland, facial nerve, and temporal bone. Dermatol Surg. 2006;32:307–15; discussion 15.
2. Goldman NC, Hardcastle B. Partial temporal bone resection for basal cell carcinoma of the external auditory canal with preservation of facial nerve and hearing. Laryngoscope. 1974;84:84–9.
3. Gussack GS, Schlitt M, Lushington A, Woods KE. Invasive basal cell carcinoma of the temporal bone. Ear Nose Throat J. 1989;68:605–6, 9–11.

4. Lasso JM, Garcia-Tutor E, Bazan A. Aggressive basal cell carcinoma of the temporal region in a patient with Gorlin-Goltz syndrome. Ann Plast Surg. 2000;44:429–34.
5. Nelson WR, Kell JF Jr, Kay S. Temporal bone resection and radical neck dissection for basal cell carcinoma with metastases. Surg Gynecol Obstet. 1962;115:585–92.
6. Parkin JL, Stevens MH. Basal cell carcinoma of the temporal bone. Otolaryngol Head Neck Surg. 1979;87:645–7.
7. Ouaz K, Robier A, Lescanne E, Bobillier C, Moriniere S, Bakhos D. Cancer of the external auditory canal. Eur Ann Otorhinolaryngol Head Neck Dis. 2013;130:175–82.
8. Johns ME, Headington JT. Squamous cell carcinoma of the external auditory canal. A clinicopathologic study of 20 cases. Arch Otolaryngol. 1974;100:45–9.
9. Fleiner F, Jumah M, Goktas O. Cancer of the external auditory canal-diagnostic and treatment. Ind J Otolaryngol Head Neck Surg. 2009;61(4):270.
10. Lo WC, Ting LL, Ko JY, Lou PJ, Yang TL, Chang YL, et al. Malignancies of the ear in irradiated patients of nasopharyngeal carcinoma. Laryngoscope. 2008;118:2151–5.
11. Shu MT, Lin HC, Lee JC, Chen BF. Radiation-induced squamous cell carcinoma of the external auditory canal. Otol Neurotol. 2011;32:e24–5.
12. Miah MS, Crawford M, White SJ, Hussain SS. Malignant transformation from benign papillomatosis of the external auditory canal. Otol Neurotol. 2012;33:643–7.
13. Clark RR, Soutar DS, Hunter KD. A retrospective analysis of histological prognostic factors for the development of lymph node metastases from auricular squamous cell carcinoma. Histopathology. 2010;57:138–46.
14. Mazzoni A, Danesi G, Zanoletti E. Primary squamous cell carcinoma of the external auditory canal: surgical treatment and long-term outcomes. Acta Otorhinolaryngol Ital. 2014;34:129–37.
15. Nyrop M, Grontved A. Cancer of the external auditory canal. Arch Otolaryngol Head Neck Surg. 2002;128(7):834.
16. Wermker K, Kluwig J, Schipmann S, Klein M, Schulze HJ, Hallermann C. Prediction score for lymph node metastasis from cutaneous squamous cell carcinoma of the external ear. Eur J Surg Oncol. 2015;41:128–35.
17. Bono A, Bartoli C, Maurichi A, Moglia D, Tragni G. Melanoma of the external ear. Tumori. 1997;83:814–7.
18. Crain N, Nelson BL, Barnes EL, Thompson LD. Ceruminous gland carcinomas: a clinicopathologic and immunophenotypic study of 17 cases. Head Neck Pathol. 2009;3:1–17.
19. Jan JC, Wang CP, Kwan PC, Wu SH, Shu HF. Ceruminous adenocarcinoma with extensive parotid, cervical, and distant metastases: case report and review of literature. Arch Otolaryngol Head Neck Surg. 2008;134(6):663.
20. Perzin KH, Gullane P, Conley J. Adenoid cystic carcinoma involving the external auditory canal. A clinicopathologic study of 16 cases. Cancer. 1982;50:2873–83.
21. Dehner LP, Chen KT. Primary tumors of the external and middle ear. Benign and malignant glandular neoplasms. Arch Otolaryngol. 1980;106:13–9.
22. Lynde CW, McLean DI, Wood WS. Tumors of ceruminous glands. J Am Acad Dermatol. 1984;11:841–7.
23. Michel RG, Woodard BH, Shelburne JD, Bossen EH. Ceruminous gland adenocarcinoma: a light and electron microscopic study. Cancer. 1978;41:545–53.
24. Ito K, Ito T, Tsukuda M, Kanisawa M. An immunohistochemical study of adenoid cystic carcinoma of the external auditory canal. Eur Arch Otorhinolaryngol. 1993;250:240–4.
25. Lott Limbach AA, Hoschar AP, Thompson LD, Stelow EB, Chute DJ. Middle ear adenomas stain for two cell populations and lack myoepithelial cell differentiation. Head Neck Pathol. 2012;6:345–53.
26. Persson M, Andren Y, Mark J, Horlings HM, Persson F, Stenman G. Recurrent fusion of MYB and NFIB transcription factor genes in carcinomas of the breast and head and neck. Proc Natl Acad Sci U S A. 2009;106:18740–4.
27. Persson M, Andren Y, Moskaluk CA, Frierson HF Jr, Cooke SL, Futreal PA, et al. Clinically significant copy number alterations and complex rearrangements of MYB and NFIB in head and neck adenoid cystic carcinoma. Genes Chromosomes Cancer. 2012;51:805–17.
28. Mansour P, George MK, Pahor AL. Ceruminous gland tumours: a reappraisal. J Laryngol Otol. 1992;106:727–32.
29. Gidley PW, Roberts DB, Sturgis EM. Squamous cell carcinoma of the temporal bone. Laryngoscope. 2010;120:1144–51.
30. Hu XD, Wu TT, Zhou SH. Squamous cell carcinoma of the middle ear: report of three cases. Int J Clin Exp Med. 2015;8:2979–84.
31. Michaels L, Wells M. Squamous cell carcinoma of the middle ear. Clin Otolaryngol Allied Sci. 1980;5:235–48.
32. Bell D, El-Naggar AK, Gidley PW. Middle ear adenomatous neuroendocrine tumor: a 25-year experience at MD Anderson Cancer Center. Virchow Arch. 2017. 471:667–72. PMID 28547535.
33. Torske KR, Thompson LD. Adenoma versus carcinoid tumor of the middle ear: a study of 48 cases and review of the literature. Mod Pathol. 2002;15:543–55.
34. Agaimy A, Lell M, Schaller T, Markl B, Hornung J. 'Neuroendocrine' middle ear adenomas: consistent expression of the transcription factor ISL1 further supports their neuroendocrine derivation. Histopathology. 2015;66:182–91.
35. Dogru S, Wilkinson EP, Robinson RA, Smith RJ. Middle ear adenoma with neuroendocrine differentiation (MEA-ND) in the pediatric population. Int J Pediatr Otorhinolaryngol. 2009;73:895–8.
36. Pelosi S, Koss S. Adenomatous tumors of the middle ear. Otolaryngol Clin N Am. 2015;48:305–15.
37. Saliba I, Evrard AS. Middle ear glandular neoplasms: adenoma, carcinoma or adenoma with neuroendocrine differentiation: a case series. Cases J. 2009;2:6508.
38. Duderstadt M, Forster C, Welkoborsky HJ, Ostertag H. Adenomatous tumors of the middle ear and temporal bone: clinical, morphological and tumor biological characteristics of challenging neoplastic lesions. Eur Arch Otorhinolaryngol. 2012;269:823–31.
39. Gaffey MJ, Mills SE, Fechner RE, Intemann SR, Wick MR. Aggressive papillary middle-ear tumor. A clinicopathologic entity distinct from middle-ear adenoma. Am J Surg Pathol. 1988;12:790–7.
40. Heffner DK. Low-grade adenocarcinoma of probable endolymphatic sac origin A clinicopathologic study of 20 cases. Cancer. 1989;64:2292–302.
41. Hassard AD, Boudreau SF, Cron CC. Adenoma of the endolymphatic sac. J Otolaryngol. 1984;13:213–6.
42. Stendel R, Suess O, Prosenc N, Funk T, Brock M. Neoplasm of endolymphatic sac origin: clinical, radiological and pathological features. Acta Neurochir. 1998;140:1083–7.
43. Bell D, Gidley P, Levine N, Fuller GN. Endolymphatic sac tumor (aggressive papillary tumor of middle ear and temporal bone): sine qua non radiology-pathology and the University of Texas MD Anderson Cancer Center experience. Ann Diagn Pathol. 2011;15:117–23.
44. Gaffey MJ, Mills SE, Boyd JC. Aggressive papillary tumor of middle ear/temporal bone and adnexal papillary cystadenoma. Manifestations of von Hippel-Lindau disease. Am J Surg Pathol. 1994;18:1254–60.
45. Bambakidis NC, Rodrigue T, Megerian CA, Ratcheson RA. Endolymphatic sac tumor metastatic to the spine. Case report. J Neurosurg Spine. 2005;3:68–70.
46. Tay KY, Yu E, Kassel E. Spinal metastasis from endolymphatic sac tumor. AJNR Am J Neuroradiol. 2007;28:613–4.

47. Bambakidis NC, Megerian CA, Ratcheson RA. Differential grading of endolymphatic sac tumor extension by virtue of von Hippel-Lindau disease status. Otol Neurotol. 2004;25:773–81.
48. Kawabata S, Hollander MC, Munasinghe JP, Brinster LR, Mercado-Matos JR, Li J, et al. Epidermal growth factor receptor as a novel molecular target for aggressive papillary tumors in the middle ear and temporal bone. Oncotarget. 2015;6:11357–68.
49. Iemoto Y, Ushigome S, Ikegami M, Koide K. Case report 648: parosteal osteosarcoma arising from the right temporal bone. Skelet Radiol. 1991;20:59–61.
50. Nora FE, Unni KK, Pritchard DJ, Dahlin DC. Osteosarcoma of extragnathic craniofacial bones. Mayo Clin Proc. 1983;58:268–72.
51. Sanal HT, Kilickesmez O, Can C. Radiology quiz case 2. Classic osteosarcoma of the temporal bone. Arch Otolaryngol Head Neck Surg. 2005;131:922, 6.
52. Huvos AG, Sundaresan N, Bretsky SS, Butler A. Osteogenic sarcoma of the skull. A clinicopathologic study of 19 patients. Cancer. 1985;56:1214–21.
53. Sundaresan N, Galicich JH, Rosen G, Huvos AG. Primary osteogenic sarcoma of the skull. Five-year disease-free survival following surgery and high dose methotrexate therapy. N Y State J Med. 1985;85:598–9.
54. Sundaresan N, Huvos AG, Rosen G, Galicich JH. Combined-modality treatment of osteogenic sarcoma of the skull. J Neurosurg. 1985;63:562–7.
55. Kakkar A, Nambirajan A, Suri V, Sarkar C, Kale SS, Singh M, et al. Primary bone tumors of the skull: spectrum of 125 cases, with review of literature. J Neurol Surg B Skull Base. 2016;77:319–25.
56. Choi EY, Gardner JM, Lucas DR, McHugh JB, Patel RM. Ewing sarcoma. Semin Diagn Pathol. 2014;31:39–47.
57. Carroll R, Miketic LM. Ewing sarcoma of the temporal bone: CT appearance. J Comput Assist Tomogr. 1987;11:362–3.
58. Pfeiffer J, Boedeker CC, Ridder GJ. Primary Ewing sarcoma of the petrous temporal bone: an exceptional cause of facial palsy and deafness in a nursling. Head Neck. 2006;28:955–9.
59. Souviron Encabo R, Arenas Britez O, Gil R, Perez-Luengo E, Scola Yurrita B. Primitive neuroectodermal tumor/extraosseus Ewing sarcoma of the temporal bone. Acta Otorrinolaringol Esp. 2005;56:38–40.
60. Hart JL, Edgar MA, Gardner JM. Vascular tumors of bone. Semin Diagn Pathol. 2014;31:30–8.
61. Chen F, Hu H, Li J, Yang W. A case of temporal bone epithelioid hemangioendothelioma. Zhonghua Er Bi Yan Hou Tou Jing Wai Ke Za Zhi. 2014;49:603–4.
62. Eliashar R, Saah D, Osin P, Sichel JY. Hemangioendothelioma of the temporal bone in a child. Int J Pediatr Otorhinolaryngol. 1997;40:67–71.
63. Goldstein WS, Bowen BC, Balkany T. Malignant hemangioendothelioma of the temporal bone masquerading as glomus tympanicum. Ann Otol Rhinol Laryngol. 1994;103:156–9.
64. Ibarra RA, Kesava P, Hallet KK, Bogaev C. Hemangioendothelioma of the temporal bone with radiologic findings resembling hemangioma. AJNR Am J Neuroradiol. 2001;22:755–8.
65. Gengler C, Guillou L. Solitary fibrous tumour and haemangiopericytoma: evolution of a concept. Histopathology. 2006;48:63–74.
66. Yoshida A, Tsuta K, Ohno M, Yoshida M, Narita Y, Kawai A, et al. STAT6 immunohistochemistry is helpful in the diagnosis of solitary fibrous tumors. Am J Surg Pathol. 2014;38:552–9.
67. Chin LS, Rabb CH, Hinton DR, Apuzzo ML. Hemangiopericytoma of the temporal bone presenting as a retroauricular mass. Neurosurgery. 1993;33:728–31; discussion 31–2.
68. Coca-Pelaz A, Llorente-Pendas JL, Vivanco-Allende B, Suarez-Nieto C. Solitary fibrous tumor of the petrous bone: a successful treatment option. Acta Otolaryngol. 2011;131:1349–52.
69. Colia V, Provenzano S, Hindi N, Casali PG, Stacchiotti S. Systemic therapy for selected skull base sarcomas: chondrosarcoma, chordoma, giant cell tumour and solitary fibrous tumour/hemangiopericytoma. Rep Pract Oncol Radiother. 2016;21:361–9.
70. Cross DL, Mixon C. Temporal bone hemangiopericytoma. Otolaryngol Head Neck Surg. 1996;114:631.
71. Heiser MA, Waldron JS, Tihan T, Parsa AT, Cheung SW. Temporal fossa hemangiopericytoma: a case series. Otol Neurotol. 2009;30:985–9.
72. Kamrava B, Mukherjee A, Weaver M, Roehm PC. Temporal malignant solitary fibrous tumor. Otol Neurotol. 2016;37:e185–6.
73. Magliulo G, Terranova G, Cordeschi S. Hemangiopericytoma and temporal bone. An Otorrinolaringol Iberoam. 1999;26:67–74.
74. Tewfik TL, Finlayson M, Attia EL. Hemangiopericytoma of the temporal bone. J Otolaryngol. 1981;10:72–7.
75. Grubbe Gregersen K, Hansen S. Metastasis to the temporal bone may cause acute peripheral vestibular syndrome and impaired hearing. Ugeskr Laeger. 2013;175:1576–7.
76. Jalava-Karvinen P, Kemppainen J, Saario R, Kotilainen P. Metastasis in the temporal bone mimicking temporal arteritis. J Clin Rheumatol. 2010;16:19–21.
77. Vize G. Laryngeal metastasis to the temporal bone causing facial paralysis. J Laryngol Otol. 1974;88:175–7.
78. Wu C, Kaga K, Ohira Y, Suzuki J. Histopathology of multiple temporal bone metastasis from pancreatic adenocarcinoma: a case showing bilateral hearing loss and Bechterew's phenomenon. Otolaryngol Head Neck Surg. 2000;122:613–5.

Auricular and Periauricular Skin Cancers

6

Blair Barton and Brian Moore

Introduction

Cutaneous malignancy is the most common cancer worldwide and has been estimated to account for approximately one million new cases each year in the United States alone [1]. Basal cell carcinoma (BCC) makes up the overwhelming majority of these cases, accounting for 80%. The remainder is made up by squamous cell carcinoma (SCC), melanoma, and Merkel cell carcinoma (MCC) [2]. Approximately 80–90% of these malignancies appear on sun-exposed areas of the head and neck [3, 4].

The National Comprehensive Cancer Network (NCCN) has published comprehensive guidelines recommending patients with advanced cutaneous tumors seek consultation from a multidisciplinary tumor board [5]. Historically, cutaneous tumors of the auricle were thought to have similar malignant potential as other subsites. However, SCC of the auricle has been shown to have a greater metastatic potential than other subsites, potentially related to its different histologic behavior with sun exposure compared to the rest of the body [6]. A study found the ratio of SCC to BCC on the head and neck to be 4:1; however, when isolated to the auricle, the ratio dropped to 1.3:1 [7]. A landmark study by Rowe et al. demonstrated that the metastatic rate of SCC of the auricle is much higher when compared to other subsites in the body and granted special surgical considerations, prompting an update to the American Joint Committee on Cancer (AJCC) staging for nonmelanoma skin cancer (NMSC) [8]. The converse has been shown in melanoma of the auricle. Though originally associated with a poorer prognosis, recent literature provides that survival outcomes of melanoma of the auricle are similar to those at other subsites of the body [9–12]. Due to its prominent location, the functionality and cosmetic appearance of the auricle require special attention to these unique anatomical features.

B. Barton, M.D. • B. Moore, M.D. (✉)
Department of Otorhinolaryngology — Head and Neck Surgery,
Ochsner Health System, New Orleans, LA, USA

Epidemiology

In 2006, an estimated 3.5 million people in the United States (US) were diagnosed with NMSC. Despite an increase in public awareness, this number is projected to increase by 50% by 2030 [13]. The true incidence of skin cancer is hard to estimate, as NMSC is significantly underreported to national cancer registries; however, it has been estimated at 850,000 cases per year, affecting approximately 3.4 million patients [4, 14].

To date, the Survival Epidemiology and End Results (SEER) has no published data on NMSC; rather, it publishes reports on cutaneous melanoma. Melanoma of the auricle is a rare cutaneous malignancy, accounting for up to 1–4% of all cutaneous melanoma, with the most common location being on the helix [9, 15]. The reported incidence of distant metastasis from cutaneous SCC has been quoted as less than 1%, whereas the metastatic rate from the external ear has been estimated to be 5–18% [6, 16]. The difference in these rates has been attributed to the proximity of the auricle to embryonic fusion plates and the skull base, thin overlying skin, close proximity to cartilage, lack of subcutaneous adipose tissue, and multiple lymph node drainage basins [6, 10, 15].

The estimated economic burden of skin cancer reportedly exceeds $29 billion dollars directly, with an additional $10 billion lost to productivity [17]. The SEER database reported over 76,000 new cases of cutaneous melanoma in 2016 in the United States, with melanoma deaths accounting for 70–75% of deaths from skin cancer and 1.7% of all cancer deaths [18]. Typically, skin cancers present in Caucasian men during their sixth to seventh decades of life [16]. Melanoma, like NMSC, is more common in Caucasian males and has a median age of 64 at diagnosis [19].

BCC is a malignant neoplasm of keratinocytes residing in the basal layer of the epidermis and is classically thought to be a locally aggressive form of skin cancer, with extremely low rates of metastasis estimated to be 0.0028–0.5% [20, 21]. SCC also derives its neoplastic processes from keratinocytes and has a higher chance for perineural invasion (PNI), with

P. W. Gidley, F. DeMonte (eds.), *Temporal Bone Cancer*, https://doi.org/10.1007/978-3-319-74539-8_6

greater potential for regional metastasis [22]. Merkel cell carcinoma is a neuroendocrine tumor of epithelial cells that form a complex with sensory neurons at the epidermal-dermal junction [23]. MCC, like other cutaneous malignancies, has shown increased incidence with UV exposure, immunosuppression, and increasing age. Recently, however, a Merkel cell polyomavirus has been detected, suggesting viruses may play a role in MCC propagation [24, 25].

Ultraviolet radiation (UVR) contributes overwhelmingly to both the formation of NMSC and melanoma, with the incidence increasing with age, history of blistering sunburns, and cumulative sun exposure [13, 26]. Despite increasing public awareness of sun exposure increasing the chance of cutaneous malignancy, evidence has shown that sun-seeking activities release behavior rewarding beta-endorphins and may be hardwired in our evolutionary pathway, possibly explaining these potentially dangerous habits [27].

Risk Factors and Pathogenesis

Ultraviolet Radiation (UVR)

Exposure to UV-A (320–400 nm) and UV-B (290–320 nm) is the single greatest risk factor for the development of NMSC [17, 22]. UVR has reportedly also played a causative role in the development of head and neck cutaneous melanoma [28]. Similarly, BCC has been linked to increased UV-B exposure. In BCC, UVR causes activation of the Hedgehog signaling pathway allowing for unregulated proliferation of epidermal basal cells [13]. The p53 tumor suppressor gene, which is estimated to be inactive in 90% of cSCC, is a key modulator in the induction of apoptosis after UVR damage. UV-B induces pyrimidine dimer formation that begins a cascade toward tumor formation [17]. The link between skin cancer and artificial UV-B exposure found in tanning beds was previously investigated and found to increase the risk for melanoma by 15%, squamous cell carcinoma by 125%, and basal cell carcinoma by 3%, when compared to those who did not use tanning beds [29].

Immunosuppression

In contrast to immune competent individuals, SCC is the most common skin cancer in transplant recipients, occurring 65–250 times more commonly than in the general population [30, 31]. BCC is still ten times more common in immunosuppressed patients—emphasizing the need to stay vigilant in screening for cancer in this unique patient population [30]. This unusual reversal of trends is believed to be due to the lack of major histocompatibility complex-I in BCC, allowing SCC to go unregulated [32]. A 2006 study published a 0% 2-year survival rate for SCC in immune-compromised patients, compared to an 87% 2-year survival rate in immune competent individuals [33]. Immunosuppressed patients due to transplants can be further stratified by solid-organ transplant type, with lung and heart transplant patients more likely to develop NMSC versus patients with kidney or liver transplants [34, 35]. A possible explanation for these differences is that lung and heart transplant patients require more immunosuppression than other solid-organ transplant subtypes [31, 36].

The human immunodeficiency virus (HIV) has been shown to increase the risk of both SCC and BCC in earlier studies [17, 30]. However, a recent study showed that a group of patients with HIV, unlike other immunocompromised groups, did not experience increased NMSC with extensive subclinical spread, possibly explaining the discrepancy in a previous study by Batra et al. [35, 37]. These findings do not question the validity of the association between HIV and NMSC but instead raise the possibility that treatment of NMSC in HIV positive individuals may not need to be as aggressive as other immunosuppressed individuals.

Both NMSC and melanoma are complex diseases influenced by both the external environment and multiple genetic factors. Familial cancer syndromes that predispose individuals to BCC include basal cell nevus syndrome (formally known as Gorlin syndrome) and Rombo syndrome, a rare genetic disorder that predisposes to the development of BCC around the age of 35. Basal cell nevus syndrome is an autosomal dominant disorder characterized by multiple BCC, rhabdomyosarcomas, meningiomas, plantar pits, falx cerebri calcifications, and coarse faces. Basal cell nevus syndrome has been linked to the loss of heterozygosity at chromosome 9q22 [38].

Xeroderma pigmentosum is another autosomal recessive disorder that causes a defect in DNA repair, allowing hypersensitivity to the DNA-damaging effects of UVR with patients developing NMSC or melanoma within the first decade of life [38]. Similarly, familial syndromes are also present for melanoma; familial melanoma/dysplastic nevus syndrome is a syndrome in which patients develop malignant melanoma much earlier than patients with sporadic melanoma [39]. Table 6.1 summarizes risk factors for developing skin cancer in the head and neck.

Anatomy

The ear can be divided into defined subunits: helix, antihelix, tragus, antitragus, lobule, concha bowl, and scapha. The conchal bowl is divided into the concha cavum and concha cymba. The scapha can similarly be further divided by the upper and lower crus of the antihelix to form the fossa triangularis [40] (Fig. 6.1).

Table 6.1 Risk factors for developing skin cancer of the head and neck

Melanoma and NMSC	Melanoma	NMSC
Childhood sun exposure	Family history of melanoma	Ionizing radiation
Intermittent sun exposure	Preexisting pigmented lesions	Genodermatoses
Severe sunburns	Large congenital nevi	Albinism
Fair complexion	Sporadic dysplastic nevi	Xeroderma pigmentosum
Blond or red hair	Lentigo maligna	Basal cell nevus syndrome
Blue or green eyes	–	Bazex syndrome
Fitzpatrick class 1–2	–	Actinic keratoses
–	–	Immunosuppression
–	–	Organ transplantation
–	–	Chronic lymphocytic leukemia
–	–	Lymphoma
–	–	Chemical exposures
–	–	Polycyclic hydrocarbons
–	–	Arsenic
–	–	Coal tar
–	–	Psoralens
–	–	Human papillomavirus infection
–	–	Chronic irritation
–	–	Burn scars
–	–	Prior skin cancer (including melanoma)
–	–	Bowen's disease
–	–	Bowenoid papulosis
–	–	Epidermodysplasia verruciformis

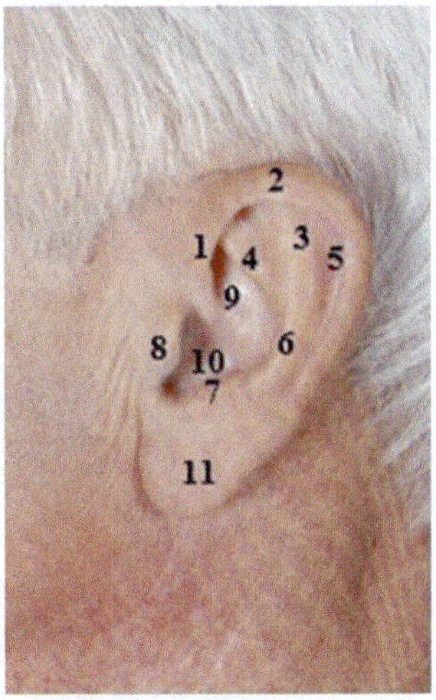

Fig. 6.1 Anatomic picture of the ear. 1. Helical crus. 2. Helix. 3. Superior crus of the antihelix. 4. Inferior Crus of the antihelix. 5. Scaphoid fossa. 6. Antihelix. 7. Antitragus. 8. Tragus. 9. Concha cymba. 10. Concha cavum. 11. Lobule

The embryological development of the ear delineates the natural pathways of spread; therefore, it is important to fully understand all anatomical relations. The ear is derived from six hillocks of His that undergo differentiation around the fourth week of gestational age. The overlying skin of the posterior (or medial) auricle is much more loosely attached to the underlying fibroelastic cartilage, which allows for easier contiguous spread [41]. Conversely, the anterior skin of the ear is more adherent to the perichondrium, which provides some resistance to direct spread [25]. While not directly thought of as part of the auricle, the external auditory canal (EAC) has two defects located on the anterior inferior canal wall, Santorini's fissures and the foramen of Huschke. These defects could potentially lead to direct invasion into the parotid parenchyma or deeper intracranially [41, 42].

Patient Evaluation

History and Physical Examination

A comprehensive history and physical examination is paramount in any initial patient evaluation. Risk factors for cutaneous malignancy of the auricle and periauricular region are summarized in Table 6.1. Pertinent questions about the lesion itself include preexisting lesions, rate of growth, change in characteristics, presence of formication (sense of insects crawling over skin), and decreased sensation in the surrounding skin.

Patients with a prior history of treated skin cancer may present up to several years later with either a neck or parotid mass. Due to the complex lymphatic drainage of the scalp, face, and auricle, both parotid and periauricular lymph nodes are common locations for metastatic lesions of both NMSC and melanoma [43]. Given these findings, it is imperative to inquire about prior treatment of ipsilateral cutaneous malignancies or any kind of skin lesion, in the head and neck, as patients may underestimate the magnitude of previous skin treatments.

Though a complete head and neck physical exam is routinely performed on all cancer patients, certain adjunctive measures are helpful in the clinical assessment of a periauricular lesion. Close examination of the lesion with detailed measurements and palpation of depth is critical for both NMSC lesions and melanoma, as NMSC greater than 2 cm diameter is at an increased risk for metastatic potential [8, 44]. Melanoma of the auricle can vary on physical exam from flat-pigmented lesions to exophytic lesions with bleeding and ulceration [9]. Mobility of the lesion over the underlying perichondrium or deeper layers provides a clinical suggestion of depth and aggressiveness. Dermoscopy has recently been found to make the diagnosis of melanoma 9–15 times more likely than clinical evaluation alone [45]. Otoscopy and binocular microscopy can elucidate involvement of the external auditory canal, tympanic membrane, or middle ear. Historically, because of its location in the H-zone, lesions of the auricle and periauricular region tend to have a higher recurrence rate and propensity for deeper invasion [46] (Fig. 6.2).

Cranial nerve examination can also lead to some key physical examination findings due to the close association of the fifth (trigeminal) and seventh (facial) cranial nerves with the cutaneous skin of the head and neck. Perineural invasion (PNI) is reported to be present in less than 5% of skin cancers, although often it is incidentally reported pathologically in a patient without any evidence of cranial neuropathy [47]. However, perineural spread (PNS) is a more symptomatic description of gross invasion of tumor into larger caliber nerves that either present radiologically or clinically with symptoms or signs of cranial nerve neuropathy [48]. Pain and numbness in one of the branches of the trigeminal nerve or paralysis in one or more branches of the facial nerve are classic signs of PNS that are associated with worse overall survival at 5 years, compared to patients without PNS [48].

The primary lymphatic drainage basins of the auricle and periauricular regions include the parotid gland and periparotid nodes along the external jugular vein, level II lymph nodes, and retroauricular and suboccipital lymph nodes [17]. Posterior scalp lesions are more likely to involve level V nodes, whereas anterior scalp lesions more commonly involve levels I–III, loosely adhering to a vertical line of demarcation through the external auditory meatus [49]. The auricle represents a watershed region, so both anterior and posterior metastases are possible. Therefore, focused examination of the parotid glands and the full cervical chain is critical in the physical examination of any patient presenting with a suspicious lesion on or around the ear.

Biopsy

Any lesion that is suspicious for malignancy should undergo biopsy for histopathologic diagnosis. Lesions that are suspicious for NMSC should undergo incisional or excisional biopsy that adequately assesses the full depth of the skin—this may be achieved with either a 2, 3, or 4 mm punch biopsy or even a shave technique. Care should be taken over the cartilage to preserve the perichondrium, as this site may be allowed to heal by secondary intention. Pathology templates are commonly used for melanoma, and there is increasing interest in such detailed templates in NMSC [50].

Pigmented lesions that are suspicious for melanoma should also be evaluated by a full-thickness biopsy. Excisional biopsy with 1–2 mm margins is the preferred method for histologic diagnosis, allowing for full evaluation of the lesion with preservation of the lymphatics should further management be needed, although this may not be possible on the auricle given the tight relationship between the skin and the cartilage—a smaller punch biopsy may be taken in such a cosmetically sensitive area. Shave biopsies play less of a role in the workup of pigmented lesions, as they rarely provide an adequate sample for full-thickness evaluation. Nevertheless, the widespread use of shave biopsy has been shown to minimally impact outcome, providing an accurate diagnosis in 97% of cases, and can be used to plan treatment without the need for rebiopsy [51]. Treatment recommendations based on a shave biopsy must consider the potential for

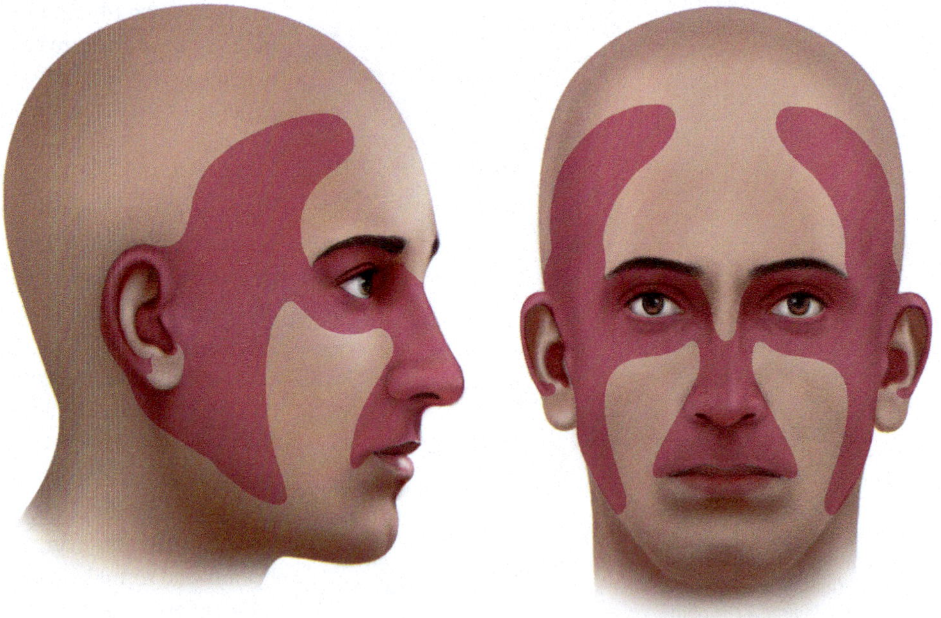

Fig. 6.2 The H-zone. Cutaneous cancers arising from this area are at a higher risk for local recurrence (reprinted with permission from Baker SR, Swanson NA, Grekin RC. An interdisciplinary approach to the management of basal cell carcinoma of the head and neck. J Dermatol Surg Oncol. 1987;12(10):1096)

an underestimation of lesion depth. In comparison to NMSC, melanoma has a structured report format of major histopathological prognostic factors—these are summarized in Table 6.2, along with ideal reported features for NMSC [52].

Imaging

Routine use of radiographic imaging in the workup of NMSC has limited indications. Physical exam findings that are concerning for a deep lesion with gross invasion of underlying structures may warrant a computed tomography (CT) with intravenous contrast for evaluation of cartilage invasion, external auditory canal extension, or temporal bone invasion. CT may assist with staging of aggressive lesions and facilitate preoperative planning. Specifically, lesions of the auricle and periauricular regions have the potential to invade the parotid gland either by lymphatic metastasis or by direct spread from the external auditory canal through the fissures of Santorini. CT scans are helpful in identifying potentially involved or suspicious lymph nodes in the parotid or cervical lymphatic basins [53] (Fig. 6.3).

Magnetic resonance imaging (MRI) with neurography protocol is typically used in patients with suspected PNS [48]. MRI and CT examinations provide complementary information, with CT better demonstrating temporal bone involvement or widening of neural foramina and MRI providing better information on PNS or intracranial invasion. The use of positron emission tomography (PET) has been well documented in the workup for mucosal SCC; however, its use in cutaneous malignancy remains controversial [54]. PET has shown use in the workup of metastatic and recurrent melanoma; however, its use for early-stage melanoma is limited [55]. The use of PET in the workup of Merkel cell carcinoma changed the management of 37% of MCC patients and altered the stage of 22%, with the authors advocating its routine use in MCC [56]. PET has also been shown to be beneficial in the post-therapy evaluation [57].

Table 6.2 Components of a thorough pathology report

NMSC	Melanoma
Histologic type	Histologic type
Differentiation	Depth of invasion
Depth of invasion	Clark level
Clark level	Breslow thickness (mm)
Breslow thickness (mm)	Patterns of growth
Perineural invasion	Vertical phase present/absent
Lymphovascular invasion	Radial phase present/absent
Inflammation	Ulceration
Margins	Perineural invasion
Lesion size	Regression
–	Margins
–	Satellitosis
–	**Special stains**
–	S-100
–	MARTI
–	HMB-45

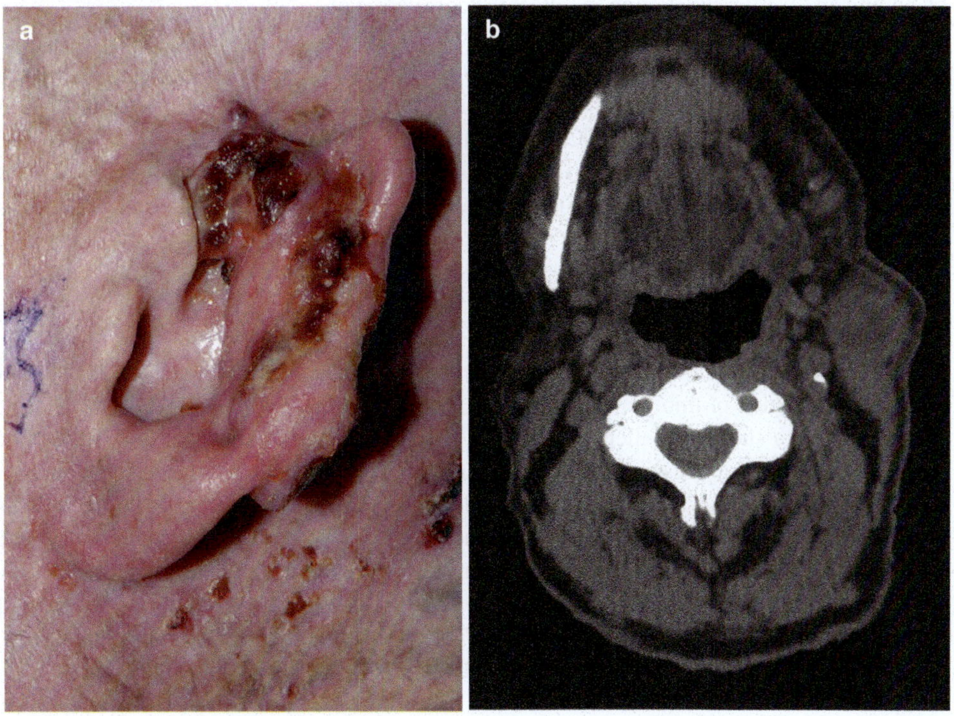

Fig. 6.3 (**a**) SSC of the left auricle. Loss of the upper helix and antihelix, with gross extension into the external auditory canal. (**b**) CT in axial plane at the level of the mandibular angle showing left auricular SCC with evidence of periauricular lymphadenopathy

Staging

The American Joint Committee on Cancer (AJCC) recently updated its tumor, node, metastases (TNM) staging system and introduced updates to both NMSC and malignant melanoma. This structural guide focuses on the greatest diameter of the primary lesion, its involvement of adjacent tissues, the status of regional lymph nodes, and the presence of distant metastases. The TNM system serves as a guide on which to base clinical decisions; however, it has its limitations and is an ever-evolving system, with a new eighth edition published in 2017.

cSSC

For the first time, the AJCC separated cSCC from NMSC, which reflects the specific natural history and stage-specific prognostic outcome of cSCC [58]. The updates also make the cSCC staging system similar to the TMN criteria used for staging other head and neck cancers, which allows for a more uniform language. All other NMSC (except MCC) will be staged according to the cSCC staging system. Table 6.3 demonstrates the current staging system for cSCC. The AJCC not only includes the tumor size correlating to T stage, but it also includes the T stage based on high-risk factors where T1 has less than two and T2 has two or more risk factors. Strong consideration was given to the inclusion of immunosuppression due to the strong correlation with the development of NMSC; however, the AJCC decided against this inclusion and recommended that centers collect this data by adding an "I" after the staging to reflect the correlation of immunosuppression with the development of NMSC [58]. The AJCC also updated the staging system by adding the auricle (and nonglabrous lip) as a high-risk subsite due to its increased metastatic potential. MCC was completely separated into its own staging system. Table 6.4 reflects these new updates with the new MCC staging system.

Table 6.3 Clinical TNM staging of nonmelanoma skin cancer adapted from the 2010 American Joint Committee on Cancer System

Primary tumor (T)	
Tx	Primary tumor cannot be assessed
T0	No evidence of primary tumor
Tis	Carcinoma in situ
T1	Tumor 2 cm or less in greatest dimension with fewer than two high-risk features[a]
T2	Tumor more than 2 cm in greatest dimension or tumor in any size with two or more high-risk features[a]
T3	Tumor with invasion of maxilla, mandible, orbit, or temporal bone
T4	Tumor with invasion of skeleton (axial or appendicular) or perineural invasion of skull base
Regional lymph nodes (N)	
Nx	Regional lymph nodes cannot be assessed
N0	No regional lymph node metastases
N1	Metastasis in single ipsilateral lymph node, less than or equal to 3 cm in greatest dimension
N2	Metastasis in single ipsilateral lymph node, greater than 3 cm but not greater than 6 cm in greatest dimension; in multiple ipsilateral lymph nodes, none greater than 6 cm in greatest dimension; or in bilateral or contralateral lymph nodes, none greater than 6 cm in greatest dimension
N2a	Metastasis in single ipsilateral lymph node, greater than 3 cm but no greater than 6 cm in greatest dimension
N2b	Metastasis in single ipsilateral lymph node, greater than 3 cm but no greater than 6 cm in greatest dimension
N2c	Metastasis in bilateral or contralateral lymph nodes, none greater than 6 cm in greatest dimension
N3	Metastasis in lymph node, greater than 6 cm in greatest dimension
Distant metastases (M)	
Mx	Distant metastases cannot be assessed
M0	No distant metastases
M1	Distant metastases

[a]High-risk features for the primary tumor (T) staging: depth/invasion, >2 mm thickness, Clark level ≥ IV or perineural invasion; anatomic location, primary site ear or primary site non-hair-bearing lip; differentiation, poorly differentiated or undifferentiated

Melanoma

Updates to the melanoma staging system include amendments to the staging of thin melanomas (<1 mm). The goal was to identify a subset of patients who are at an increased risk of developing aggressive clinical behavior. Mitotic rate has replaced Clark's level of invasion in defining pT1b melanoma, as it was found to be an independent adverse predictor of survival [59, 60]. Also included in the updates are recommendations to offer sentinel lymph node biopsy (SLNB) to patients with melanoma of stage pT1b [41, 61]. Table 6.5 is an updated AJCC seventh edition for staging of cutaneous melanoma. Due to an increase in public awareness, the majority of diagnosed melanomas are thin (<1 mm) and have a favorable survival outcome if managed early and appropriately [62].

Management of the Primary Lesion

A multitude of destructive and excisional modalities have been described for the treatment of both auricular and periauricular cutaneous malignancies. A variety of specialties (otolaryngologists, dermatologists, general surgeons, and plastic surgeons) have contributed to the treatment of cutaneous tumors located on the external ear, each having their own preference. Surgical specialists typically prefer excision, whereas dermatologists use both surgical

Table 6.4 Clinical TNM staging of Merkel cell carcinoma adapted from the 2010 American Joint Committee on Cancer System

Primary tumor (T)	
Tx	Primary tumor cannot be assessed
T0	No evidence of primary tumor
Tis	In situ primary tumor
T1	Less than or equal to 2 cm maximum tumor dimension
T2	Greater than 2 cm but not more than 5 cm maximum tumor dimension
T3	Over 5 cm maximum tumor dimension
T4	Primary tumor invades the bone, muscle, fascia, or cartilage
Regional lymph nodes (N)	
Nx	Regional lymph nodes cannot be assessed
N0	No regional lymph node metastases
cN0	Nodes negative by clinical exam[a]
pN0	Nodes negative by pathologic exam
N1	Metastasis in regional lymph node(s)
N1a	Micrometastasis[b]
N1b	Macrometastasis[c]
N2	In-transit metastasis[d]
Distant metastases (M)	
Mx	Distant metastases cannot be assessed
M0	No distant metastasis
M1	Metastasis beyond regional lymph nodes
M1a	Metastasis to the skin, subcutaneous tissues, or distant lymph nodes
M1b	Metastasis to the lung
M1c	Metastasis to all other visceral sites

[a]Clinical detection of nodal disease may be via inspection, palpation, and/or imaging
[b]Micrometastases are diagnosed after sentinel or elective lymphadenectomy
[c]Macrometastases are defined as clinically detectable nodal metastases confirmed by therapeutic lymphadenectomy or needle biopsy
[d]In-transit metastasis: a tumor distinct from the primary lesion and located either (1) between the primary lesion and the draining regional lymph nodes or (2) distal to the primary lesion

Table 6.5 Staging of cutaneous melanoma adapted from the 7th edition American Joint Committee on Cancer melanoma staging system

Primary tumor (T)	
Tx	Primary tumor cannot be assessed
T0	No evidence of primary tumor
Tis	Melanoma in situ
T1	Tumor ≤1.0 mm thick
T1a	Without ulceration and mitosis less than 1/mm^2
T1b	With ulceration or mitosis greater than or equal to 1/mm^2
T2	Tumor 1.01–2.0 mm thick
T2a	Without ulceration
T2b	With ulceration
T3	Tumor 2.01–4.0 mm thick
T3a	Without ulceration
T3b	With ulceration
T4	Tumor >4.0 mm thick
T4a	Without ulceration
T4b	With ulceration
Regional lymph nodes (N)	
Nx	Regional lymph nodes cannot be assessed
N0	No regional lymph node metastases
N1	One positive lymph node
N1a	Micrometastasis
N1b	Macrometastasis
N2	Two or three positive lymph nodes
N2a	Micrometastases
N2b	Macrometastases
N2c	In-transit metastases/satellites without metastatic nodes
N3	Four or more positive nodes, matted nodes, or in-transit/satellite nodes with metastatic node(s)
Distant metastases (M)	
Mx	Distant metastases cannot be assessed
M0	No distant metastases
M1	Distant metastases
M1a	Distant skin, subcutaneous, or lymph node metastasis
M1b	Lung metastasis
M1c	All other visceral metastases or any distant metastasis with an elevated serum LDH

LDH, lactate dehydrogenase

excision with Mohs micrographic technique and less invasive options such as electrodesiccation and topical therapy. Complete surgical resection with negative margins is associated with better outcomes and constitutes the mainstay in management [63, 64].

Topical Therapy

There are a variety of topical therapies for the treatment of NMSC. Imiquimod is an agonist for the toll-like receptors 7 and 8 present on neutrophils, macrophages, and dendritic cells that promote release of tumor necrosis factor-alpha [65]. The Food and Drug Administration (FDA) approved 5% imiquimod to treat non-facial biopsy-confirmed superficial BCC. Imiquimod's role in the treatment of SCC in situ lesions is limited; more often it is used in patients who are poor surgical candidates or wish to not undergo surgery [12].

Diclofenac is a topical nonsteroidal anti-inflammatory drug (NSAID) that has been FDA approved for the treatment of precancerous lesions known as actinic keratosis (AK). Its mechanism of action likely is related to the inhibition of cyclooxygenase-2 that has been found to be upregulated in NMSC lesions [12, 64]. Fluorouracil (5-FU) is an antineoplastic pyrimidine analogue that has been shown to be efficacious against AK and superficial BCC only [65]. Major limitations have been described with topical therapies, the most concerning being the inability to assess for complete tumor clearance with evaluation of margins. There are currently no US FDA-approved topical therapies for the treatment of melanoma; however, imiquimod has been shown to have some use in the treatment of melanoma in situ, particularly for patients unable or unwilling to undergo surgical resection [66].

Photodynamic Therapy (PDT)

PDT is a decades-old treatment that involves a two-part application of a photosensitizing drug, such as aminolevulinic acid or methyl-aminolevulinic acid and oxygen combined to produce an antitumor effect [65]. PDT has potential advantages over other topical therapies, such as improved patient compliance and the potential to reduce other signs of photodamage.

Cryotherapy and Electrodesiccation and Curettage (ED&C)

The application of liquid nitrogen to select premalignant and low-risk NMSC has shown clearance rates of 94–99%. Tumor cells are more sensitive to cryotherapy due to their high water content, higher metabolism, and microcirculation in comparison to non-dysplastic cells [67]. Cryotherapy causes rapid irreversible intracellular destruction and inflammation, and it is often performed in conjunction with other noninvasive methods. In ED&C, the bulk of the tumor is first removed by vigorous curettage followed by light electrodesiccation of the base of the lesion [67]. Indications for ED&C are smaller BCC (<2 cm in diameter), small SCC in situ, and well-differentiated SCC (<1 cm in diameter) [67]. Like treatment with topical therapies, PDT, cryotherapy, and ED&C does not allow histologic confirmation of tumor clearance and is to be avoided in invasive malignancy, except in rare situations.

Mohs Micrographic Surgery (MMS)

Due to the unique cosmetic aspects of the ear, complete surgical resection with minimal tissue loss is the ideal situation. The topography of the auricle can disorient and confuse assessment of tumor boundaries, potentially confounding complete margin assessment with the least amount of tissue loss [68]. MMS is the preferred modality for NMSC with biopsy-proven PNI, showing recurrent rates of approximately 3% in the auricular region versus almost 11% by standard excision [8, 69]. Although MMS has been described for melanoma in the literature, its role for excision of auricular melanoma exhibits an unacceptably high rate of recurrence of 30% when compared to other modalities [15].

Wide Local Excision (WLE)

MMS is not indicated for surgical resection in advanced, aggressive disease or for a tumor that invades deeper underlying structures, such as cartilage. With thin skin overlying cartilage, lesions on the lateral aspect of the ear often require resection of the skin and the underlying cartilage. The NCCN guidelines recommend taking 4–6 mm margins for low-risk SCC and over 10 mm for high-risk tumors [2, 5]. The use of comprehensive *en face* frozen sections for NMSC may deliver local control with recurrence rates comparable to MMS [70]. Table 6.6 shows the current margins proposed by the NCCN for management of cutaneous melanoma, NMSC, and MCC.

There are no specific guideline modifications for auricular NMSC or melanoma, and strict guideline adherence often results in a more radical resection, including total auriculectomy.

Due to the close proximity of the cartilage to the skin, there has been significant debate regarding the management of auricular lesions. As proposed by some authors, auricular cartilage can be preserved if there is no gross invasion of the cartilage [71]. Excision of the skin alone has comparable survival to more aggressive composite resections, without altering cosmesis and function of the auricle [10, 71–73].

When cartilage is grossly involved, one author advocates for resection of the grossly involved cartilage and preservation of either the anterior or posterior skin and reconstruction with a full-thickness skin graft. Using 1.5 cm margins and this technique, no local recurrences with acceptable cosmetic outcomes were achieved [74] (Fig. 6.4).

Simple wedge excision with primary closure may be pursued for smaller helical or antihelical lesions or if the cutaneous lesion violates both the anterior and posterior auricular skin. If the superior aspect of the helix and helical root can be safely preserved, patients may be able to support glasses with the remnant.

Due to prominence of the ear, consideration must be given to the cosmetic deformity after surgical management.

Table 6.6 Recommended surgical guidelines for cutaneous melanoma, BCC, SCC, and MCC, based on the National Comprehensive Cancer Network and adapted from Porceddu et al.

Cutaneous melanoma		
Tumor stage	Tumor thickness	Surgical margin
Tis	In situ	0.5–1.0 cm
T1	≤1.0 mm	1.0 cm
T2	1.01–2.0 mm	1.0–2.0 cm
T3	2.01–4.0 mm	2.0 cm
T4	>4.0 mm	2.0 cm
Cutaneous squamous cell carcinoma [2]		
Tumor type	Surgical margin	
Low risk	4–6 mm	
High risk	10 mm	
Cutaneous basal cell carcinoma [2]		
Tumor type	Surgical margin	
Low risk	2–4 mm	
High risk	4–10 mm	
Merkel cell carcinoma		
Tumor stage	Tumor thickness	Surgical margin
Tis	In situ	1.0 cm
T1	≤2 cm	1.0 cm
T2	>2 cm–<5 cm	2.0 cm
T3	>5 cm	2.0 cm

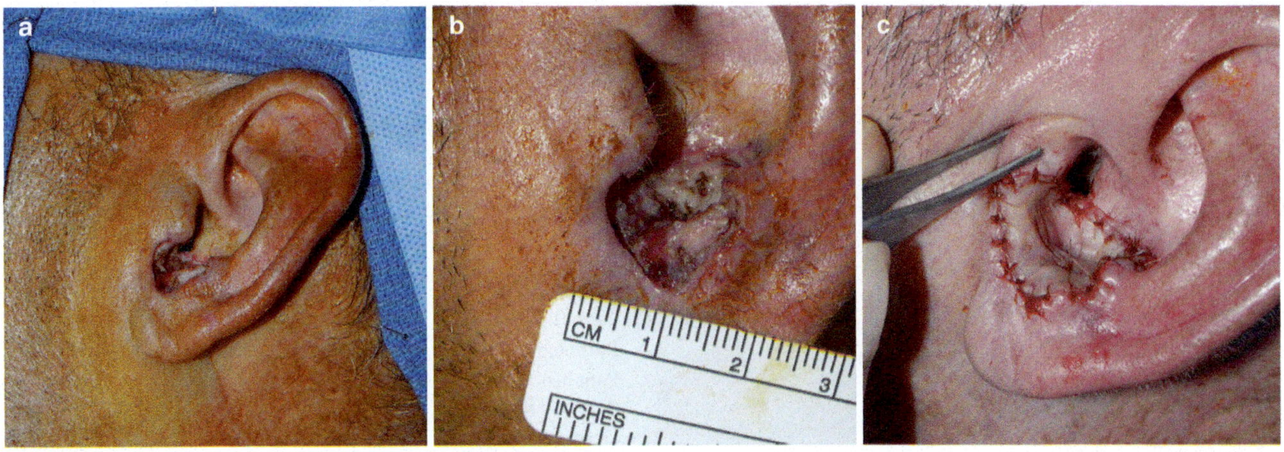

Fig. 6.4 (**a**) SCC of the left auricle, involving the tragus, the antitragus, and the conchal bowl. (**b**) Postexcision defect following negative margin surgery. (**c**) Reconstruction of the defect using a split-thickness skin graft after preservation of posterior skin

However, reconstructive concerns, even for complex or important areas, should not take precedence over oncologic considerations in periauricular malignancy. Although a wedge resection and repair is a modestly straightforward approach, other options for auricular reconstruction exist and are discussed elsewhere in this text. With that in mind, it is best to perform an oncologically sound resection with appropriate margins and then convert the defect to a wedge as appropriate—do not limit the reconstructive options by performing a wedge resection. Reconstruction of the auricle is a complex task and should be managed primarily by a reconstructive-trained surgeon.

Total Auriculectomy and Lateral Temporal Bone Resection (LTBR)

When tumors occupy the majority of the external ear or external ear canal (EAC), radical surgical resection via total auriculectomy with or without removal of portion of the temporal bone is considered the first choice for management. The *en bloc* LTBR includes removal of the cartilaginous and bony EAC, including the tympanic membrane, periauricular soft tissues, and parotid and neck lymph nodes [75]. The technique of lateral temporal bone resection will be described elsewhere in the text. Although the auricular superstructure can occasionally be saved in external auditory canal primaries, a total auriculectomy is often required in conjunction with lateral temporal bone resection for advanced auricular malignancy—this is typically performed in conjunction with a parotidectomy and posterolateral neck dissection.

Radiation Therapy

Radiation therapy remains an option for patients who are not able to tolerate surgery, if the ablative procedure will cause significant cosmetic defects, or for patients who refuse surgical intervention. There is currently no evidence to support radiation therapy for primary, curative treatment of malignant melanoma; however, it can remain an option for treatment of metastatic melanoma to the brain and melanoma in situ [66, 76].

For the management of NMSC, radiation therapy can be used for recurrent disease, perineural invasion, and positive margins. The NCCN supports radiation therapy as an option for primary monotherapy for patients older than 60 years for low-risk lesions in the H area and for high-risk lesions that are <1.5 cm and located in the H area or <2.0 cm and located in the M area (cheeks, forehead, neck, and scalp) with minimal cosmetic deformity [5, 77]. Patients who have inoperable, aggressive disease, generally accepted as intracranial extension beyond the geniculate or trigeminal ganglion, may be managed by palliative radiation therapy alone [69].

Management of Regional Metastases

Elective Parotidectomy

The role of an elective parotidectomy is controversial for auricular primaries with a clinically negative parotid and neck. The true incidence of parotid involvement in auricular cancers is unknown and hard to estimate as most studies include tumors of the EAC which skews the true rate of parotid involvement in isolated auricular malignancies [41]. The estimated rate of metastatic SCC of the auricle is 7.9–11%, higher than other areas, but still is below the 15–20% accepted risk to offer all patients treatment to their regional lymph node basins [6, 78] (Fig. 6.5) .

A recent study recommended elective superficial parotidectomy for SCC lesions greater than 2 cm, with vascular or perineural invasion located in the temporal region, as almost 25% of their patients had occult parotid disease [79].

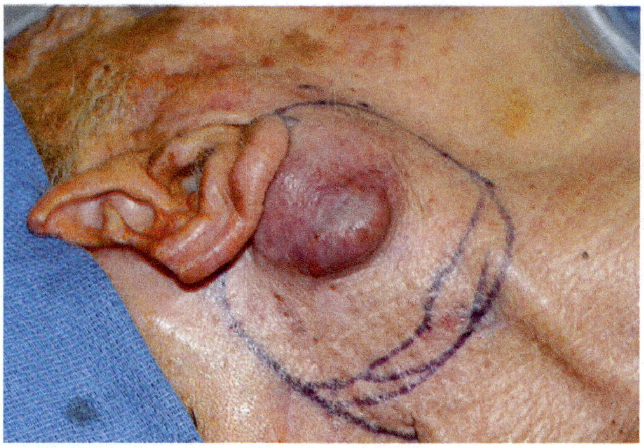

Fig. 6.5 Regional recurrence of a previously treated SCC of the right auricle

Table 6.7 Features of aggressive nonmelanoma and melanoma skin cancer

NMSC	Melanoma
Clinical features	Clinical features
Recurrent lesion size >2.0 cm	Ulceration of primary
Depth > 4.0 mm	Patient age <60 years
Invasion to subcutaneous tissues	–
Preexisting scar	–
Ear or lip location	–
Pathologic features	**Pathologic features**
Poor histologic differentiation	Vertical growth phase present
Desmoplastic SCC	Infiltrative tumor strands
Spindle cell SCC	Histologic type other than superficial spreading
Basosquamous carcinoma	Breslow thickness (continuous variable)
Infiltrative BCC	Clark level > III
Perineural invasion	Acantholysis
Lymphovascular invasion	Lymphovascular invasion
Inflammation	Single cell infiltration

Sentinel Lymph Node Biopsy (SLNB)

There are no current recommendations for the use of SLNB in the management of auricular or periauricular NMSC. Due to the low rate of metastasis of low-risk NMSC (well differentiated, less than 2 cm, slow growing), the use of SLNB remains under investigation, but the increased risk of regional metastases from auricular sites makes it a logical consideration. The highly aggressive subtypes of NMSC (Table 6.7) theoretically provide a potential application of SLNB in the staging of NMSC, potentially avoiding the morbidity associated with elective neck dissections (END) and parotidectomy [80]. A recent systematic review demonstrated 100% successful identification of the SLN, paralleling that of SLNB for cutaneous melanoma and another study showing the false omission rate of around 7% [81, 82].

SLNB does pose some unique difficulties in the head and neck. First, due to the close proximity of the lymph nodes in question to the injection site, lymphatic drainage may be difficult to visualize due to a "shine-through" effect [83]. Sentinel nodes may be located in sites that are not easily accessible or are located in more than one drainage basin [83]. Despite these challenges, sentinel lymph node biopsy plays an important role in the workup of intermediate-thickness melanoma and, increasingly, stage I and II MCC. The value of SLNB in melanoma and Merkel cell carcinoma has led some authors to extrapolate its application to cSCC as well [60, 80, 82–84].

Sentinel lymph node biopsy is an integral part of the workup of cutaneous melanoma in a clinically N0 neck. Due to the low rate of nodal metastasis in thin (<0.75 mm) melanomas, sentinel lymph node biopsy is not typically employed in thin melanomas [85]. However, SLNB for intermediate-size (1–4 mm) melanoma offers some benefit, as approximately 15% have histologically positive nodes in a clinically N0 neck [85]. Some recent studies looking at thin melanoma have identified a select subset of patients who may benefit from SLNB versus the traditional elective lymph node dissection [86]. Kesmodel et al. showed that patients with a melanoma tumor thickness >0.75 mm and mitotic rate >0 have a 12.3% rate of nodal disease, with others arguing that SLNB should be offered to all patients with tumor thickness >0.75 mm [87, 88] (Fig. 6.6).

The Multicenter Selective Lymphadenectomy Trial-I (MSLT-I) opened in January, 1994 and was designed to confirm the accuracy of nodal staging based on SNLB, proving that SNLB positivity correlated with disease-free survival and melanoma-specific survival [89–91]. The MSLT-I confirmed that after positive SLNB, patients should be treated with completion lymph node dissection (CLND) [89].

The MSLT-II was generated from the MSLT-I data that showed that after a SLNB that found a single positive node, 88% of patients would have no other positive nodes after CLND. The MSLT-II opened in 2005 and, at the time of writing this chapter, is currently still collecting data. Its objective is to look at melanoma-specific survival in patients who undergo SLNB and CLND versus SLNB with conservative management of lymph nodes with ultrasound evaluation [89].

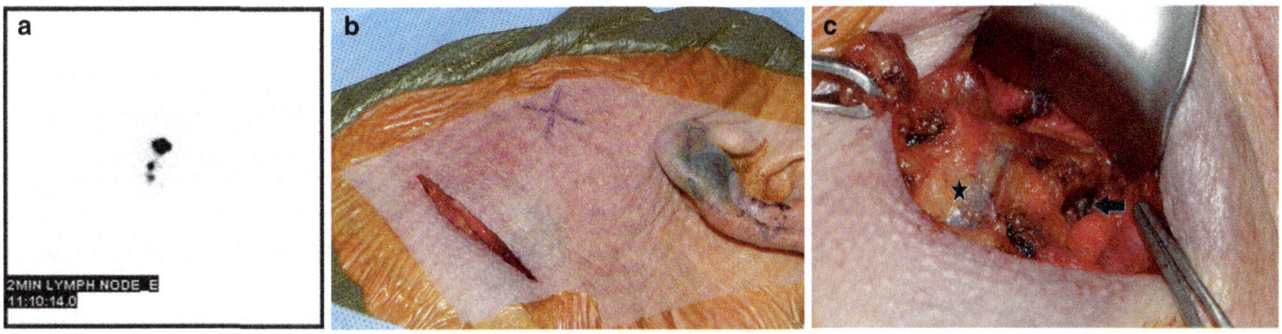

Fig. 6.6 Sentinel lymph node biopsy for auricular melanoma. (**a**) Preoperative lymphoscintigraphy revealing uptake at the primary site and in two adjacent lymph nodes, likely in the tail of parotid or external jugular group. (**b**) Intraoperative injection of methylene blue dye and radiolocalization of sentinel node (marked X). (**c**) Intraoperative identification of sentinel node. Black star marks the external jugular vein, and black arrow marks site of sentinel lymph node

Management of Clinically Positive Nodal Disease

The principles of managing regional metastases are similar for both melanoma and nonmelanoma skin cancer of the auricle and periauricular region. In the presence of a positive SLNB, clinical or radiographic neck nodes, or documented cervical node or parotid gland involvement, management of the primary lesion should also include a parotidectomy with neck dissection [16]. All attempts should be made to preserve a functioning facial nerve when a plane may be developed between the nerve and tumor, as this has not been shown to negatively impact prognosis. Direct or symptomatic invasion of the facial nerve necessitates facial nerve sacrifice, immediate nerve grafting, and possibly total parotidectomy [92]. Patients with advanced perineural invasion may originally be misdiagnosed with Bell's palsy or even tic douloureux [93].

While most surgeons perform a superficial parotidectomy with facial nerve preservation for metastatic SCC to the parotid followed by postoperative radiation therapy, some authors suggest a more aggressive total parotidectomy (Fig. 6.7) [43]. Approximately 25% of the lymph nodes are contained within the deep lobe of the parotid - leaving these nodes in place potentially has the risk of leaving occult metastatic disease within the parotid [43]. The study by Thom et al. found positive lymph deep lobe nodes in 26% of their population with SCC, approaching the frequency of cervical metastasis and supporting total parotidectomy in the setting of clinical extension or metastases [43].

In managing a clinically negative neck with parotid involvement, selective neck dissection of levels II and III is sufficient for anterior scalp and auricular primaries and levels II to V for posterior scalp and neck primaries. Studies have found 35–50% rate of subclinical metastases in nodes after pathological evaluation [21, 94, 95]. Tumors that are anterior to the EAC require removal of levels II to IV, while tumors posterior to the EAC require removal of levels II to V, including the suboccipital and retroauricular lymph nodes, also known as a posterolateral neck dissection [17, 96]. Oftentimes, the watershed location of the auricle may mandate both a parotidectomy and a posterolateral neck dissection, particularly in the postradiation salvage setting.

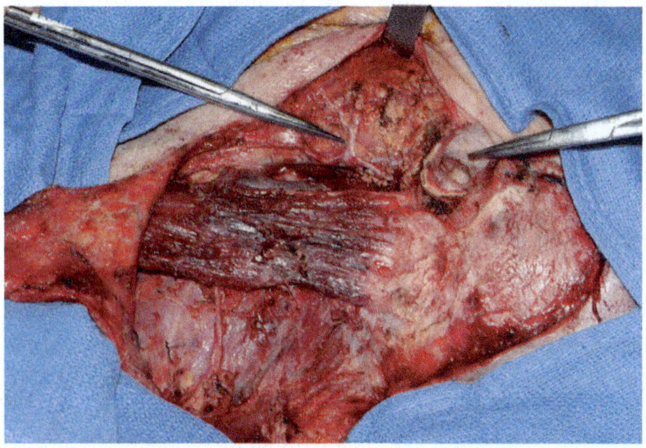

Fig. 6.7 Intraoperative periauricular lymph node dissection and preservation of the facial nerve

Adjuvant Therapy

Postoperative Radiation Therapy (PORT)

Both early-stage NMSC and melanoma (stages I and II) can be managed with WLE, provided negative margins; and PORT may not be required. In close or positive margins that are not favorable for re-excision, PORT may be implemented [17]. Other pathological factors that should be treated with PORT are multiple positive lymph nodes, extracapsular spread, PNI, lymphovascular invasion, and involvement of a named nerve.

The use of PORT after therapeutic lymphadenectomy for patients with melanoma at high risk of further lymph node field and distant recurrence is controversial. PORT has been shown to improve disease control in patients at high risk of lymph node field relapse after therapeutic lymphadenectomy for metastatic melanoma; however, regional failure is a harbinger of distant disease, and these patients are prone to distant failure [97, 98].

Adjuvant Chemotherapy

High-dose interferon α-2b (IFNa-2b) is the only adjuvant treatment approved by the FDA to minimize the chance of recurrence and metastasis in stage IIB to III melanoma. Unfortunately, the high-dose regimen is associated with significant toxicities including constitutional symptoms, fatigue, headache, nausea, weight loss, depression, hepatic injury, and myelosuppression, but, with dose modification, most patients are able to complete the proscribed course.

Systemic Therapy for Metastatic Disease

Systemic chemotherapy has limited use in the management of NMSC: 5-FU, cisplatin, vincristine, bleomycin, and methotrexate have all been described in the treatment of SCC and BCC [91, 99]. However, with the emergence of targeted molecular therapy, there seems to be more encouraging evidence to support its use over classical chemotherapeutic agents. The epidermal growth factor receptor (EGFR) inhibitor, cetuximab, has been shown to improve locoregional control and overall survival when added to radiotherapy versus radiotherapy alone [12, 99]. Cetuximab acts by blocking the extracellular domain of the EGFR that has been found to be overexpressed in SCC, as well as other malignancies. The oral tyrosine kinase inhibitors such as erlotinib and gefitinib, which also target EGFR, have early supporting data and are currently undergoing large multicenter trials [100].

Vismodegib, a Hedgehog signaling pathway inhibitor, was FDA approved for the treatment of locally advanced and metastatic BCC based on a phase II clinical trial (ERIVANCE) [2, 30, 101]. Cetuximab has also been shown to be effective in small case reports for the treatment of BCC where platinum-based chemotherapy previously failed, and studies have shown that the EGFR is present in 30–38% of BCC [102].

The use of systemic therapy for the treatment of MCC remains unclear, with MCC being thought of as a radiosensitive tumor. Chemotherapy has been reserved for advanced disease or palliative therapy, choosing drugs based on similar neuroendocrine tumors, like small cell carcinoma of the lung [23]. Evidence suggests that MCC may initially be chemosensitive with some studies showing partial response to platinum-based therapy. However, despite these encouraging findings, recurrence develops soon after initiation of chemotherapy and has been found to have no improvement in overall survival [103]. Despite these findings, research into targeted molecular therapies for MCC may prove to be beneficial in the future.

Historically, chemotherapy has had little success in cutaneous melanoma. Patients with stage IIB, IIC, and III melanoma are at high risk of systemic metastases and subsequent death [104]. Dacarbazine was approved by the FDA in the 1970s as first-line treatment for metastatic melanoma. This alkylating agent was shown to produce a partial response in approximately 25% of patients and a complete response in 5% with metastatic melanoma [104].

High-dose IFNa-2b was the only adjuvant treatment approved by the US Food and Drug Administration (FDA) to minimize the chance of recurrence and metastasis in stage IIB to III melanoma. Targeted immunotherapy has been shown to be more useful in the treatment of cutaneous melanoma. With 50% of all metastatic melanomas carrying the BRAF V600E kinase mutation, causing activation of the mitogen-activated protein kinase (MAPK), targeted immunotherapy seemed an ideal therapy [20]. Vemurafenib, an inhibitor of the BRAF V600E, was shown to be superior in treatment of primary untreated metastatic melanoma versus dacarbazine alone, showing the overall response rate to be 53% [20, 105]. Ipilimumab, an IgG monoclonal antibody against the T-CTLA-4 receptor, present on activated T-cells, allows for increased T-cell survivability and activity against melanoma tumor cells [104].

In general, patients with stage IV disease have a poor prognosis, with 5–20% 5-year survival. Treatment for stage IV melanoma is limited; however, a prospective clinical trial investigating the safety and efficacy of combining local RT with systemic ipilimumab immunotherapy in patients with metastatic melanoma shows encouraging results [106].

There are a multitude of other targeted molecular therapies that have shown great promise in the treatment of melanoma, including NRAS inhibitors, Rac1 inhibition, MEK inhibitors, and KIT inhibitors. An exhaustive list of targeted therapies is beyond the scope of this chapter.

Conclusions

Although the majority of NMSC and melanoma can be treated successfully if identified early, both auricular and periauricular skin cancers present many unique clinical and pathological characteristics. Due to the complex anatomy of the ear and prominent aesthetic location, there are practical considerations in managing local disease, but the oncologic outcome should not be sacrificed for cosmetic concerns. The ear and periauricular region constitute a high-risk subsite for regional metastases, and careful consideration should be given to elective parotidectomy in advanced cases or sentinel lymph node biopsy in high-risk situations. The potential for regional and distant metastases demands a multidisciplinary approach to cutaneous lesions of the ear and periauricular region.

Bibliography

1. American Cancer Society. 2010, cited 2016 June. Available from http://cancer.org.
2. Porceddu SV, Veness MJ, Guminski A. Nonmelanoma cutaneous head and neck cancer and merkel cell carcinoma: current concepts, advances, and controversies. J Clin Oncol. 2015;33(29):3338–45.
3. Rogers HW, Weinstock MA, Harris AR, et al. Incidence estimate of nonmelanoma skin cancer in the United States, 2006. Arch Dermatol. 2010;146:283–7.
4. Alam M, Ratner D. Cutaneous squamous-cell carcinoma. N Engl J Med. 2001;344(3):975–83.
5. National Comprehensive Cancer Network. NCCN clinical practice guidelines in oncology: Basal cell and squamous cell skin cancers.
6. Clark RR, Soutar DS. Lymph node metastases from auricular squamous cell carcinoma. A systematic review and meta-analysis. J Plast Reconstr Aesthet Surg. 2008;61(10):1140–7.
7. Ahmad I, Das Gupta AR. Epidemiology of basal cell carcinoma and squamous cell carcinoma of the pinna. J Laryngol Otol. 2001; 115(2):85–6.
8. Rowe DE, Carroll RJ, Day CL Jr. Prognostic factors for local recurrence, metastasis, and survival rates in squamous-cell carcinoma of the skin, ear, and lip. J Am Acad Dermatol. 1992;26(6):976–90.
9. Mondin V, Rinaldo A, Shaha AR, et al. Malignant melanoma of the auricle. Acta Otolaryngol. 2005;125(11):1140–4.
10. Toia F, Garbo G, Tripoli M, et al. A systematic review on external ear melanoma. J Plast Reconstr Aesthet Surg. 2015;68(7):883–94.
11. Lachiewicz AM, Berwick M, Wiggins CL, et al. Survival differences between patients with scalp or neck melanoma and those with melanoma of other sites in the Surveillance, Epidemiology, and End Results (SEER) program. Arch Dermatol. 2008;144(4):515–21.
12. Ravin AG, Pickett N, Johnson JL, et al. Melanoma of the ear: treatment and survival probabilities based on 199 patients. Ann Plast Surg. 2006;57(1):70–6.
13. Dubas LE, Ingraffea A. Nonmelanoma skin cancer. Facial Plast Surg Clin North Am. 2013;21(1):43–53.
14. Rodgers HW, Weinstock MA, Feldman SR, et al. Incidence estimate of nonmelanoma skin cancer (keratinocyte carcinomas) in the U.S. population, 2012. JAMA Dermatol. 2015;151(10):1081–8.
15. Jones TS, Jones EL, Gao D, et al. Management of external ear melanoma: the same of something different? Am J Surg. 2013; 206(3):307–13.
16. Lee D, Nash M, Har-El G. Regional spread of auricular and periauricular cutaneous malignancies. Laryngoscope. 1996;106(8):998–1001.
17. Gurudutt VV, Genden EM. Cutaneous squamous cell carcinoma of the head and neck. J Skin Cancer. 2011;2011:502723.
18. National Cancer Institute. SEER Stat Fact Sheets: Melanoma of the Skin. Cited 2016 June. Available from http://seer.cancer.gov/statfacts/html/melan.html.
19. Golger A, Young DS, Ghazarian D, et al. Epidemiological features and prognostic factors of cutaneous head and neck melanoma. Arch Otolaryngol Head Neck Surg. 2007;133(5):442–7.
20. Kolk A, Wolff KD, Kesting M, et al. Melanotic and non-melanotic malignancies of the face and external ear – a review of current treatment concepts and future options. Cancer Treat Rev. 2014;40(7):819–37.
21. Danial C, Lingala B, Balise R, et al. Markedly improved overall survival in 10 consecutive patients with metastatic basal cell carcinoma. Br J Dermatol. 2013;169(3):255–61.
22. Mydlardz WK, Weber RS, Kupferman ME. Cutaneous malignancy of the head and neck. Surg Oncol Clin N Am. 2015;24(3): 593–613.
23. Saini AT, Miles BA. Merkel cell carcinoma of the head and neck: pathogenesis, current and emerging treatment options. Onco Targets Ther. 2015;8:2157–67.
24. Chen MM, Roman SA, Sosa JA, et al. The role of adjuvant therapy in the management of head and neck merkel cell carcinoma. JAMA Otolaryngol Head Neck Surg 2015;141(2):137–41.
25. Feng H, Shuda M, Chang Y, et al. Clonal integration of a polyomavirus in human Merkel cell carcinoma. Science. 2008;319(5866): 1096–100.
26. Gandhi SA, Kampp J. Skin cancer epidemiology, detection, and management. Med Clin N Am. 2015;99(6):1323–35.
27. Merlino G, Herlyn M, Fisher DE, et al. The state of melanoma: challenges and opportunities. Pigment Cell Melanoma Res. 2016;29(4):404–16.
28. Shain AH, Bastian BC. From melanocytes to melanomas. Nat Rev Cancer. 2016;16(6):345–58.
29. IARC. Exposure to Artificial UV Radiation and Skin Cancer. Lyon, France:IARC Working Group on Risk of Skin Cancer and Exposure to Artificial Ultraviolet Light, International Agency for Research on Cancer, World Health Organization; 2005. [Online]. Available from http://www.iarc.fr/en/publications/pdfs-online/wrk/wrk1/ArtificialUVRad&SkinCancer.pdf.
30. Marzuka AG, Book SE. Basal cell carcinoma: pathogenesis, epidemiology, clinical features, diagnosis, histopathology, and management. Yale J Biol Med. 2015;88(2):167–79.
31. Chockalingam R, Downing C, Tyring SK. Cutaneous squamous cell carcinomas in organ transplant recipients. J Clin Med. 2015;4(6):1229–39.
32. Walter A, Barysch MJ, Behnke S. Cancer-testis antigens and immunosurveillance in human cutaneous squamous cell and basal cell carcinomas. Clin Cancer Res. 2010;16(14):3562–70.
33. Southwell KE, Chaplin JM, Eisenberg RL, et al. Effect of immunocompromise on metastatic cutaneous squamous cell carcinoma in the parotid and neck. Head Neck. 2006;28(3):244–8.
34. Zwald FO, Brown M. Skin cancer in solid organ transplant recipients: advances in therapy and management. Part I: Epidemiology of skin cancer in solid organ transplant recipients. J Am Acad Dermatol. 2011;65(2):253–61.
35. Song SS, Goldenberg A, Ortiz A, et al. Nonmelanoma skin cancer with aggressive subclinical extension in immunosuppressed patients. JAMA Dermatol. 2016;152(6):683–90.
36. Ducroux E, Boillot O, Ocampo MA, et al. Skin cancers after liver transplantation: retrospective single-center study on 371 recipients. Transplantation. 2014;98(3):335–40.
37. Batra RS, Kelley LC. Predictors of extensive subclinical spread in nonmelanoma skin cancer treated with Mohs micrographic surgery. Arch Dermatol. 2002;138(8):1043–51.
38. Jaju PD, Batra RS, Kelley LC. Familial skin cancer syndromes: increased risk of nonmelanotic skin cancers and extracutaneous tumors. J Am Acad Dermatol. 2016;74(3):437–51.
39. Ransohoff KJ, Jaju PD, Tang JY, et al. Familial skin cancer syndromes: increased melanoma risk. J Am Acad Dermatol. 2016;74(3):423–34.
40. Sajic D, Archibald J, Murray C. Surface anatomy of the ear. J Cutan Med Surg. 2014;18(2):137–40.
41. Osborne RF, Shaw T, Zandifar H, et al. Elective parotidectomy in the management of advanced auricular malignancies. Laryngoscope. 2008;118(12):2139–45.
42. Sand M, Sand D, Brors D, et al. Cutaneous lesions of the external ear. Head Face Med. 2008;4:2.

43. Thom JJ, Moore EJ, Price DL, et al. The role of total parotidectomy for metastatic cutaneous squamous cell carcinoma and malignant melanoma. JAMA Otolaryngol Head Neck Surg. 2014;140(6):548–54.
44. Brantsh KD, Meisner C, Schonfish B, et al. Analysis of risk factors determining prognosis of cutaneous squamous-cell carcinoma: a prospective study. Lancet Oncol. 2008;9(8):713–20.
45. Butler TD, Matin RN, Affleck AG, et al. Trends in dermoscopy use in the UK: results from surveys in 2003 and 2012. Dermatol Pract Concept. 2015;5(2):29–38.
46. Netterville JL, Sinard RJ, Bryant GL, et al. Delayed regional metastasis from midfacial squamous carcinomas. Head Neck. 1998;20(4):328–33.
47. Mendenhall WM, Amdur RJ, Williams LS, et al. Carcinoma of the skin of the head and neck with perineural invasion. Head Neck. 2002;24(1):78–83.
48. Warren TA, Nagle CM, Bowman J, et al. The natural history and treatment outcomes of perineural spread of malignancy within the head and neck. J Neurol Surg B Skull Base. 2016;77(2):107–12.
49. Pan WR, le Roux CM, Levy SM, et al. Lymphatic drainage of the external ear. Head Neck. 2011;33(1):60–4.
50. Stratigos A, Garbe C, Lebbe C, et al. Diagnosis and treatment of invasive squamous cell carcinoma of the skin: European consensus-based interdisciplinary guideline. Eur J Cancer. 2015;51(14):1989–2007.
51. Zager JS, Hochwald SN, Marzban SS, et al. Shave biopsy is a safe and accurate method for the initial evaluation of melanoma. J Am Coll Surg. 2011;212(4):454–60.
52. Scolyer RA, Judge MJ, Evans A, et al. Data set for pathology reporting of cutaneous invasive melanoma: recommendations from the international collaboration on cancer reporting (ICCR). Am J Surg Pathol. 2013;37(12):1797–814.
53. Eisenmenger LB, Wiggins RH. Imaging of head and neck lymph nodes. Radiol Clin N Am. 2015;53(1):115–32.
54. Duncan JR, Carr D, Kaffenberger BH. The utility of positron emission tomography with and without computed tomography in patients with nonmelanoma skin cancer. J Am Acad Dermatol. 2016;75(1):186–96.
55. Kumar R, Alavi A. Clinical applications of fluorodeoxyglucose – positron emission tomography in the management of malignant melanoma. Curr Opin Oncol. 2005;17(2):154–9.
56. Siva S, Byrne K, Seel M, et al. 18F-FDG PET provides high-impact and powerful prognostic stratification in the staging of Merkel cell carcinoma: a 15-year institutional experience. J Nucl Med. 2013;54(8):1223–9.
57. Byrne K, Siva S, Chait L, et al. 15-year experience of 18F-FDG PET imaging in response assessment and restaging after definitive treatment of Merkel cell carcinoma. J Nucl Med. 2015;56(9):1328–33.
58. Farasat S, Yu SS, Neel VA, et al. A new American Joint Committee on Cancer staging system for cutaneous squamous cell carcinoma: creation and rationale for inclusion of tumor (T) characteristics. J Am Acad Dermatol. 2011;64(6):1051–9.
59. Chu VH, Tetzladd MT, Torres-Cabala CA, et al. Impact of the 2009 (7th edition) AJCC melanoma staging system in the classification of thin cutaneous melanomas. Biomed Res Int. 2013;2013:898719.
60. Alex JC. The application of sentinel node radiolocalization to solid tumors of the head and neck: a 10-year experience. Laryngoscope. 2004;114(1):2–19.
61. Caldarella A, Fancelli L, Manneschi G, et al. How staging of thin melanoma is changes after introduction of TMN 7th edition: a population-based analysis. J Cancer Res Clin Oncol. 2016;142(1):73–6.
62. Smithers BM, Hughes MC, Beesley VL, et al. Prospective study of patterns of surgical management in adults with primary cutaneous melanoma at high risk spread, in Queensland, Australia. J Surg Oncol. 2015;112(4):359–65.
63. Lansbury L, Bath-Hextall F, Perkins W, et al. Interventions for non-metastatic squamous cell carcinoma of the skin: systematic review and pooled analysis of observational studies. BMJ. 2013;347:f6153.
64. Chren MM, Linos E, Torres JS, et al. Tumor recurrence 5 years after treatment of cutaneous basal cell carcinoma and squamous cell carcinoma. J Invest Dermatol. 2013;133(5):1188–96.
65. McGillis ST, Fein H. Topical treatment strategies for non-melanoma skin cancer and precursor lesions. Semin Cutan Med Surg. 2004;23(3):174–83.
66. Erickson C, Miller SJ. Treatment options in melanoma in situ: topical and radiation therapy, excision, and Mohs surgery. Int J Dermatol. 2010;49(5):482–91.
67. Ermertcan AT, Hellings PW, Cingi X. Nonmelanoma skin cancer of the head and neck, nonsurgical treatment. Facial Plast Surg Clin North Am. 2012;20(4):445–54.
68. Niparko JK, Swanson NA, Baker SR, et al. Local control of auricular, periauricular and external canal cutaneous malignancies with Mohs surgery. Laryngoscope. 1990;100(10 Pt 1):1047–51.
69. Gupta A, Veness M, De'Ambrosis B, et al. Management of squamous cell and basal cell carcinomas of the head and neck with perineural invasion. Australas J Dermatol. 2016;57(1):3–13.
70. Baddour HM, Magliocca KR, Chen AY. The importance of margins in head and neck cancer. J Surg Oncol. 2016;113(3):248–55.
71. Craig ES, Nagarajan P, Lee ES, et al. The perichondrium in auricular melanomas: implications for surgical management. Otolaryngol Head Neck Surg. 2013;148(3):431–5.
72. McCarty MA, Lentsch EJ, Cerrati EW, et al. Melanoma of the ear: results of a cartilage-sparing approach to resection. Eur Arch Otorhinolaryngol. 2013;270(11):2963–7.
73. Jahn V, Breuninger H, Garbe C, et al. Melanoma of the ear: prognostic factors and surgical strategies. Br J Dermatol. 2006;154(2):310–8.
74. Yenidunya MO. Surgical treatment of auricular malignancies when the anterior or posterior skin is intact. J Craniofac Surg. 2013;24(2):350–3.
75. Mazzoni A, Zanoletti E, Marioni G, et al. En bloc temporal bone resections in squamous cell carcinoma of the ear. Technique, principles, and limits. Acta Otolaryngol. 2016;135(6):425–32.
76. Kahn MK, Kahn N, Almasan A, et al. Future of radiation therapy for malignant melanoma an era of newer, more effective biological agents. Onco Tragets Ther. 2011;4:137–48.
77. Mendenhall WM, Amdur RJ, Hinerman RW, et al. Radiotherapy for cutaneous squamous and basal cell carcinomas of the head and neck. Laryngoscope. 2009;119(10):1994–9.
78. Clark RR, Soutar DS, Hunter KD. A retrospective analysis of histological prognostic factors for the development of lymph node metastases from auricular squamous cell carcinoma. Histopathology. 2010;57(1):138–46.
79. Kadakia S, Ducic Y, Marra D, et al. The role of elective superficial parotidectomy in the treatment of temporal region squamous cell carcinoma. Oral Maxillofac Surg. 2016;20(2):143–7.
80. Michl C, Starz H, Bachter D, et al. Sentinel lymphonodectomy in nonmelanoma skin malignancies. Br J Dermatol. 2003;149(4):763–9.
81. Ahmed MM, Moore BA, Schmalbach CE. Utility of head and neck cutaneous squamous cell carcinoma sentinel node biopsy: a systematic review. Otolaryngol Head Neck Surg. 2014;150(2):180–7.
82. Durham AB, Lowe L, Malloy KM, et al. Sentinel lymph node biopsy for cutaneous squamous cell carcinoma on the head and neck. JAMA Otolaryngol Head Neck Surg. 2016;142:1171–6. https://doi.org/10.1001/jamaoto.2016.1927.
83. Shpitzer T, Gutman H, Barnea Y, et al. Sentinel node-guided evaluation of drainage patterns for melanoma of the helix of the ear. Melanoma Res. 2007;17(6):365–9.

84. Valsecchi ME, Silbermins D, de Rosa N, et al. Lymphatic mapping and sentinel lymph node biopsy in patients with melanoma: a meta-analysis. J Clin Oncol. 2011;29(11):1479–87.
85. Patel SG, Coit DC, Shaha AR, et al. Sentinel lymph nose biopsy for cutaneous head and neck melanomas. Arch Otolaryngol Head Neck Surg. 2002;128(3):285–91.
86. Balch CM, Soong SJ, Bartolucci AA, et al. Efficacy of an elective regional lymph node dissection of 1 to 4 mm thick melanomas for patients 60 years of age and younger. Ann Surg. 1996;224(3):255–63.
87. Kesmodel SB, Karakousis GC. Botbyl, et al. Mitotic rate as a predictor of sentinel lymph node biopsy in thin melanomas. Ann Surg Oncol. 2005;12(6):449–58.
88. Phan GQ, Messina JL, Sondak VK, et al. Sentinel Lymph node biopsy for melanoma: indications and rationale. Cancer Control. 2009;16(3):234–9.
89. Morton DL. Overview and update of the phase III multicenter selective lymphadenectomy trials (MSLT-I and MSLT-II) in melanoma. Clin Exp Metastasis. 2012;29(7):699–706.
90. Morton DL, Thompson JF, Cochran AJ, et al. Final trial report of sentinel-node biopsy versus nodal observation in melanoma. N Engl J Med. 2014;370(7):599–609.
91. Main BG, Coyle MJ, Godden A, et al. The metastatic potential of head and neck cutaneous malignant melanoma: is sentinel node biopsy useful? Br J Oral Maxillofac Surg. 2014;52(4):340–3.
92. Khurana VG, Mentis DH, O'Brien CJ, et al. Parotid and neck metastases from cutaneous squamous cell carcinoma of the head and neck. Am J Surg. 1995;170(5):446–50.
93. Turner SJ, Morgan GJ, Palme CE, et al. Metastatic cutaneous squamous cell carcinoma of the external ear: a high-risk cutaneous subsite. J Laryngol Otol. 2010;124(1):26–31.
94. Veness MJ, Morgan GJ, Palme CE, et al. Surgery and adjuvant radiotherapy in patients with cutaneous head and neck squamous cell carcinoma metastatic to lymph nodes: combined treatment should be considered best practice. Laryngoscope. 2005;155(5):870–5.
95. O'Hara J, Ferlito A, Takes RP. Cutaneous squamous cell carcinoma of the head and neck metastasizing to the parotid gland – a review of current recommendations. Head Neck. 2011;33(12):1789–95.
96. Medina JE. Posterolateral neck dissection. Oper Tech Otolaryngol. 2004;15:176–9.
97. Burmeister BH, Henderson MA, Ainslie J, et al. Adjuvant radiotherapy versus observation alone for patients at risk of lymph-node field relapse after therapeutic lymphadenectomy for melanoma: a randomised trial. Lancet Oncol. 2012;13(6):589–97.
98. Mathen P, Debenham BJ, Voroney JP, et al. Clinical outcomes in stage III cutaneous melanoma treated with adjuvant radiation therapy. Int J Radiat Biol Phys. 2016;96(2S):E714.
99. Soura E, Chasapi V, Strarigos AJ. Pharmacologic treatment options for advanced epithelial skin cancer. Expert Opin Pharmacother. 2015;16(10):1479–93.
100. Rudnick EW, Thareja S, Cherpelis B. Oral therapy for nonmelanoma skin cancer in patients with advanced disease and large tumor burden: a review of the literature with focus on a new generation of targeted therapies. Int J Dermatol. 2016;55(3):249–58.
101. Sekulic A, Migden MR, Lewis K, et al. Pivotal ERIVANCE basal cell carcinoma (BCC) study: 12-month update of efficacy and safety of vismodegib in advanced BCC. J Am Acad Dermatol. 2015;72(6):1021–6.
102. Bonner JA, Harari PM, Giralt J, et al. Radiotherapy plus cetuximab for squamous-cell carcinoma of the head and neck. N Engl J Med. 2006;354(6):567–78.
103. Pectasides D, Pectasides M, Psyrri A, et al. Cisplatin-based chemotherapy for Merkel cell carcinoma of the skin. Cancer Investig. 2006;24(8):780–5.
104. Davey RJ, van der Westhuizen A, Bowden NA. Metastatic melanoma treatment: combining old and new therapies. Crit Rev Oncol Hematol. 2016;98:242–53.
105. Sharma A, Shah SR, Illum H, et al. Vemurafenib: targeted inhibition of mutated BRAF for treatment of advanced melanoma and its potential in other malignancies. Drugs. 2012;72(17):2207–22.
106. Hiniker SM, Reddy SA, Maecker HT, et al. A prospective clinical trial combining radiation therapy with systemic immunotherapy in metastatic melanoma. Int J Radiat Oncol Biol Phys. 2016;96(3):578–88.

Squamous Cell Carcinoma and Basal Cell Carcinoma of the Ear Canal and Temporal Bone

7

Paul W. Gidley

Introduction

The most common primary tumor of the ear canal and temporal bone is squamous cell carcinoma. It accounts for approximately 60–70% of all tumors affecting the temporal bone. Basal cell carcinoma of the ear canal is in a distant second place compared to squamous cell carcinoma.

Primary temporal bone carcinoma is very rare, and it accounts for only 0.2% of tumors in the head and neck [1, 2]. A myriad of tumor types affects the temporal bone [3]. The literature on temporal bone cancer is difficult to interpret since many papers combine multiple tumor types or multiple primary sites (ear canal, auricular, periauricular, or parotid) in order to demonstrate a substantial clinical volume [4–14]. Different tumor histologies have very different natural histories and survival outcomes. Squamous cell carcinoma (SCC), for example, has a much worse prognosis than either adenocarcinoma or basal cell carcinoma [8]. Additionally, most papers contain small numbers of patients, which prohibit drawing impactful conclusions, or survey long-time periods, over which diagnostic imaging and surgical techniques vary [15]. Some papers combine cases with different staging systems, e.g., the Pittsburgh staging system and the AJCC system for cutaneous or parotid malignancies [4, 16]. While these published reports do contain important observations, conclusions drawn must be tempered by remembering that these are tumors with widely varying natural histories, and these staging systems have widely varying criteria (e.g., a T2 parotid tumor is not equal to a T2 non-melanoma cutaneous malignancy nor is it equal to a T2 temporal bone tumor). As far as possible, this chapter will attempt to tease out the important clinical facts regarding squamous cell carcinoma and basal cell carcinoma in the ear canal and temporal bone.

P. W. Gidley, M.D., F.A.C.S.
Department of Head and Neck Surgery, The University of Texas M.D. Anderson Cancer Center, Houston, TX, USA
e-mail: pwgidley@mdanderson.org

Incidence

In general, the cancer incidence rate is the number of new cancers at a specific site occurring in a specified population during a year. Exact numbers for the incidence of middle ear and temporal bone cancer have been elusive. From the University of Michigan at Ann Arbor, Furstenberg in 1924 made an extensive literature search and gathered 75 cases; he estimated the incidence of temporal bone cancer to be 1 case in 20,000 cases of aural conditions [17]. Tabb et al. reported 9 patients with cancer of the ear canal among 8500 consecutive otologic patients admitted to Charity Hospital in New Orleans over a 15-year period [18].

Lodge et al. estimated an incidence of 6/1,000,000 in 1955 [19]. This number was based on their experience with six cases over a 3-year period of time in Halifax, England, two men and four women, with ages ranging from 36 to 65 years. Despite these figures being over 60 years old, they are repeated frequently throughout the literature and often with incorrect citation.

In 1984, Morton et al. calculated the incidence of middle ear and mastoid cancers in the UK at around 1/1,000,000 persons per year [20]. The incidence of middle ear cancer is estimated at 1 case per 8,000–10,000 patients hospitalized with otologic disease [21, 22]. The incidence of aural cancer in otologic practice has been reported to be 1 in 20,000 patients [19]. These older series include many different tumor types, including paraganglioma. Although these papers are frequently cited, their results must be viewed with caution by contemporary readers.

Arena and Keen (1988) reported that the estimated incidence of temporal bone and middle ear cancer in the US is 0.08 cases/100,000 US standard population [23]. Their incidence is based on SEER data. Their paper makes note of a decline in the number of temporal bone resections performed: 3.8/year in the 1960s and 1970s and 1.2/year in the 1980s. They offered several possible explanations for the decline: decreased incidence of chronic suppurative otitis media, decreased use of head and neck radiation for benign

P. W. Gidley, F. DeMonte (eds.), *Temporal Bone Cancer*, https://doi.org/10.1007/978-3-319-74539-8_7

disease, and an increase in fellowship-trained head and neck surgeons, leading to a dilution of cases.

In 1998, Mandolis et al. reported an updated report on the SEER database, revealing that there are roughly 200 new cases of temporal bone cancer per year in the US [14]. Manolidis et al. reported the incidence of temporal bone malignancy to be 1 in every 432 new patients seen by a mature skull base group and that tumors of epithelial origin were 1 in every 1167 new cases seen by the group [14]. Their series contained patients with many different tumor histologies and many different primary locations.

Contemporary twenty-first century data place the incidence of temporal bone cancer between 1 and 2 cases/1,000,000 persons/year. Chee et al. reported that the incidence is slightly higher at 2.1 cases/million population/year in Singapore [24]. A nationwide, retrospective study from Denmark of primary external ear canal and middle ear cancers published in 2008 revealed an incidence of 1.3 cases per million people per year [8]. While it is a small country (population 5.3 million at the time of publication), this represents the most accurate and up-to-date incidence in the literature.

The incidence of temporal bone cancer increases in patients who have received head and neck radiation. Lo et al. found an incidence of 0.15% (11 patients) of external auditory canal cancer in a cohort of nasopharyngeal cancer patients ($N = 7442$) who had received radiotherapy as part of treatment for nasopharyngeal tumor [25]. This rate is 1000 times higher than in the general population.

Squamous cell cancer of the middle ear is exceedingly rare. In a large, single institution review, Gidley et al. found only 3 cases of middle ear SCC out of 71 cases of SCC of the ear canal and temporal bone [5]. Using the Surveillance, Epidemiology, and End Results (SEER) database, Gurgel et al. reported on 135 patients with middle ear SCC over a 32-year span (or roughly 4 cases/year) [26].

Etiology

The exact etiology of cancers in the ear canal and temporal bone remains elusive. Unlike traditional head and neck cancer, smoking and alcohol use are not strong etiologic factors for development of ear canal and temporal bone cancer [27]. While both squamous cell and basal cell carcinomas are known to be caused by sun exposure, this cause surely could not account for cancers within the canal or middle ear.

Chronic otitis externa and malignant otitis externa have been linked to the development of SCC [28, 29]. Nyrop et al. reported that 30% of their patients had a prior history of chronic otitis externa [12]. Yin et al. reported that 12.6% of their patients had recurrent or long-term otitis externa and otitis media [30].

SCC developing in mastoid cavities has been documented in a few case series [31–33]. Monem et al. reported a case of SCC developing in a mastoid cavity of a person who used a chlorinated disinfectant (Eusol—Edinburgh Solution of Lime) to irrigate his mastoid cavity and theorized that this chemical compound might be a carcinogenic etiologic agent [34]. Meiteles and Conley described a case of SCC arising in a fenestration cavity [35].

Long-standing otorrhea (averaging 20 years or more in duration) is reported frequently in association with SCC and has been implicated as a potential cause of middle ear and temporal bone cancer [19, 21, 36–41]. Bradley and Maxwell (1954) found 35 cases of carcinoma in 7287 cases of chronic otitis media, i.e., 1 in 208 cases [42]. Chronic otitis media and externa have been reported in 7–61% of patients with SCC of the ear canal, middle ear or mastoid (Fig. 7.1) [2, 39, 43–48].

Cholesteatoma has been associated with squamous cell carcinoma of the middle ear and mastoid in a few case reports and small case series [31, 49, 50]. Intermittent chronic drainage of long-standing duration was common in these patients. Many patients did not seek additional treatment until facial paralysis prompted consultation with an otologist [31, 41]. Vikram et al. studied 3 cases of middle ear SCC out of 225 cases of chronic suppurative otitis media (CSOM) in India, and they found cholesteatoma associated with 2 of these cases and another presenting with aural polyp. Their report highlights the fact that cancer should be suspected when CSOM is suddenly associated with new symptoms such as severe earache, bleeding, or facial palsy [51]. A case of squamous cell carcinoma arising from external auditory canal cholesteatoma has been reported in the Japanese literature [52].

More recently, there has been research into the presence of human papillomavirus (HPV) in middle ear and temporal bone cancers [53, 54]. Jin et al. first reported the presence of HPV-16 in 11 of 14 patients with middle ear squamous cell carcinoma [55]. A history of long-term (more than 20 years) chronic otitis media with otorrhea was present in 13 of these patients. It should be noted that HPV DNA has been found in 36% of middle ear cholesteatomas [56]. Masterson et al. identified high-risk human papillomavirus (HPV16, 18, 31, and 45) in 3 of 14 patients with squamous cell carcinoma of the temporal bone [57]. The presence of HPV was not shown to produce a difference in disease-specific survival when compared to other temporal bone cancer patients without HPV.

Radiation is a known cause of malignancy. Exposure to radium in watch dial painters has been described in two case reports [58, 59]. Therapeutic radiation to the head and neck can produce secondary temporal bone malignancies [60]. Both squamous cell carcinoma and sarcomas are described as occurring in the temporal bone following radiation [25, 39, 60–64]. Goh et al. reported on seven patients who had nasopharyngeal cancers treated with radiotherapy who later developed a temporal bone cancer (five SCC, one osteogenic sarcoma, and one chondrosarcoma) [63]. Lo et al. reported that 0.19% of their nearly 8000 patients with nasopharyngeal cancer developed a temporal bone malignancy [25]. This indicates a relative incidence of 15 cases/10,000 patients,

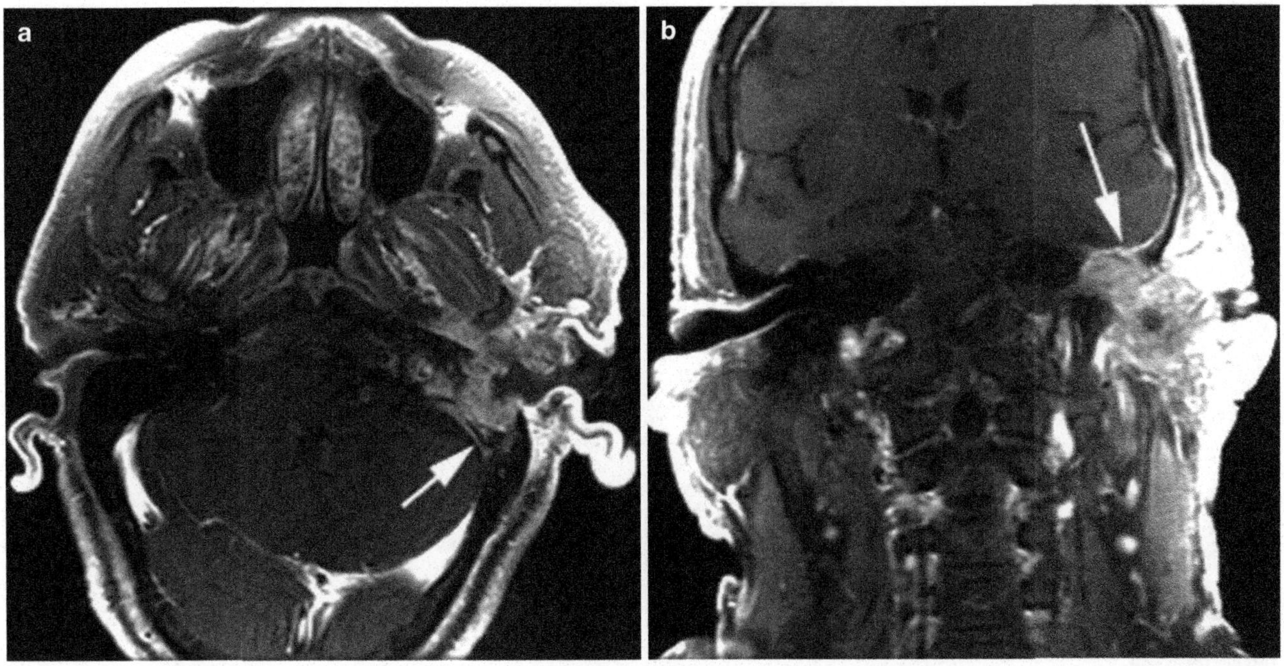

Fig. 7.1 Squamous cell carcinoma arising in a mastoid cavity. This 59-year-old man suffered from lifelong chronic otorrhea. Contrast-enhanced axial T1 MRI clearly showing dural enhancement (arrow) marking advanced-stage disease. (**a**) Axial. (**b**) Coronal

which is considerably higher (1500×) than the background incidence. Lambert et al. reported 13 cases of radiation-associated malignancy (RAM) involving the ear canal and temporal bone; 10 patients had SCC, while 3 had sarcoma [60]. Several reports include patients with a distant, prior history of radiotherapy [24, 47, 65].

Epidemiology

Squamous cell carcinoma of the ear canal, middle ear, and temporal bone typically occurs in older patients. Most large number studies have a mean age in the seventh decade of life. Depending on the study, the age can range from 21 to 92 years [5, 66]. Men are typically more commonly affected than women, but this finding does vary among recent studies. Higgins and Moody looked at 21 studies covering 348 patients, and they found an average age of 61.9 years [67]. In their study, the percentages of men to women were 60–40%, respectively [67].

Clinical Presentation

Cancers of the ear canal and temporal bone present with common symptoms such as otorrhea (24–100%), otalgia (19–81%), and hearing loss (2–75%) [5, 8, 15, 39, 46, 68–70]. The classic triad of otorrhea, otalgia, and hearing loss is found in only 10% of patients with cancer of the temporal bone. Other symptoms, such as trismus, facial weakness, dysphagia, and hoarseness, are seen much less commonly and are usually associated with advanced-stage disease.

Given that these symptoms are commonplace and usually caused by infection, many patients demonstrate symptoms for many months prior to diagnosis [5, 71]. Madsen et al. reported symptom duration was on average present for 13 months (range 1–74 months, median 6 months) [8]. Gidley et al. reported symptoms were present for 1–120 months prior to presentation, with ear pain having a shorter time to presentation (mean 5 months) than facial paralysis (mean 6 months), otorrhea (mean 9 months) or hearing loss (mean 37 months) [5]. Chang et al. reported symptom duration median of 12 months, with a range of 2–60 months [6]. Only four (out of 12) of their patients had a history of chronic otitis media [6].

Squamous cell carcinoma involving the ear canal will have an exophytic or ulcerated appearance (Fig. 7.2a) and can be mistaken for erythematous skin and granulation tissue. Basal cell carcinoma typically has an ulcerated appearance with rolled edges (Fig. 7.2b). Adenoid cystic carcinoma in its early stage is often subcutaneous and easily missed on a cursory ear examination (Fig. 7.2c). Melanoma in the ear canal is usually amelanotic (Fig. 7.2d).

These signs and symptoms can be confused with benign disease, such as otitis externa, otitis media, or cholesteatoma [72]. The differential diagnosis for disease in the ear canal should include osteomyelitis of the skull base (also called malignant otitis externa), pseudoepitheliomatous hyperplasia, and carcinoma [73, 74]. The differential diagnosis of a mass lesion in the ear canal includes benign lesions, such as adenoma or papilloma, and malignant lesions, such as squamous cell carcinoma, basal cell carcinoma, adenoid cystic carcinoma, mucoepidermoid carcinoma, adenocarcinoma,

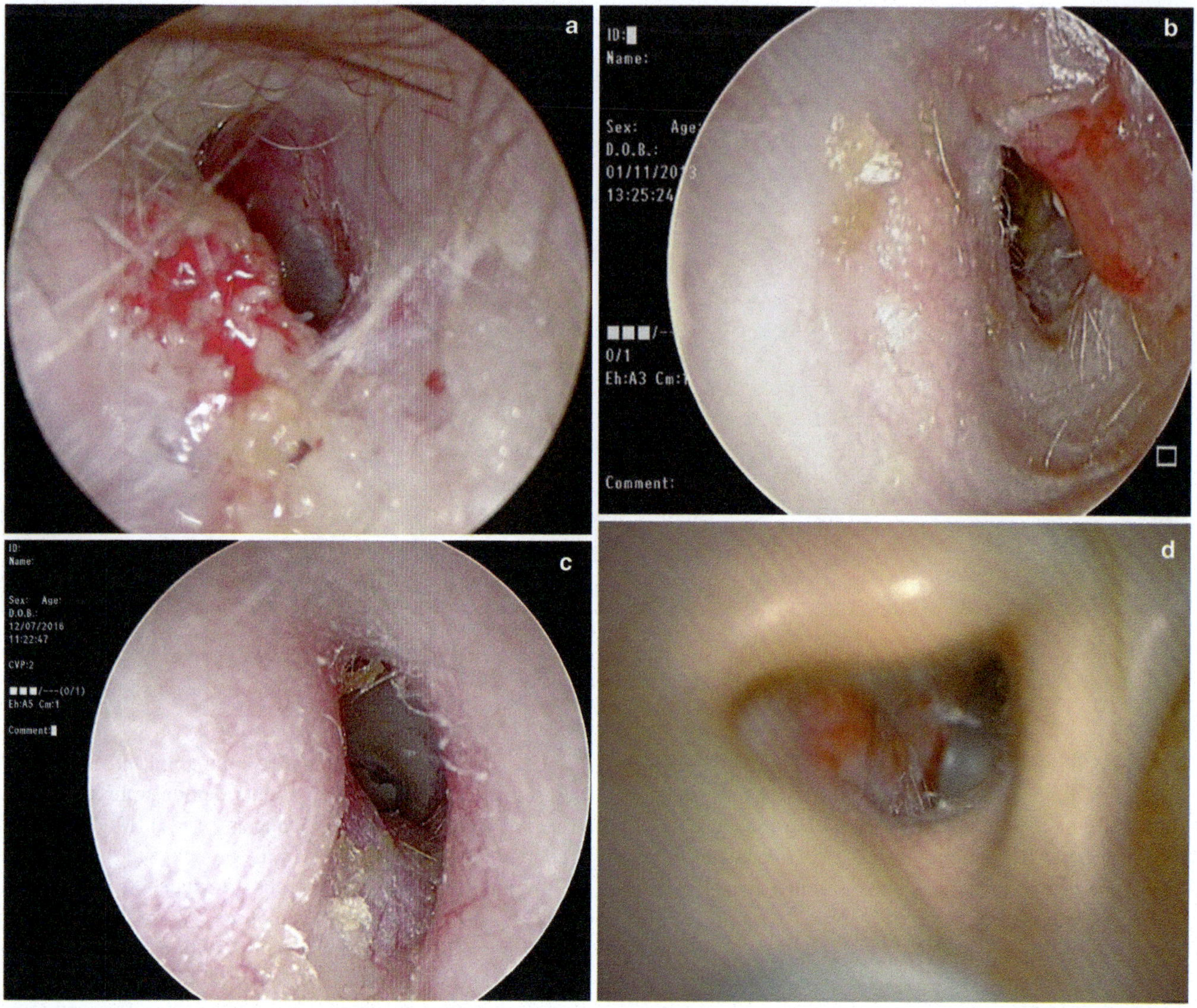

Fig. 7.2 Various cancers of the external auditory canal. (**a**) Squamous cell carcinoma of the left ear canal. (**b**) Basal cell carcinoma of the left ear canal. (**c**) Adenoid cystic carcinoma of the left ear canal. (**d**) Melanoma of the left ear canal

and melanoma. The malignant transformation of a benign papilloma to a squamous cell carcinoma in the ear canal has been described [75]. The temporal bone and ear canal are rare locations for metastatic cancers, usually from sites such as the breast, lung, prostate, or kidney [76–79].

The majority of patients with otitis externa or otitis media will respond to aural cleaning and eardrops or systemic antibiotics. Suspicion should arise when patients with these symptoms do not respond to standard therapy [72]. If patients with these symptoms do not respond to standard therapy, then any suspicious tissue should be sampled and sent for pathologic evaluation.

Only three cases of SCC isolated to the tympanic membrane have been reported in the English literature [80–82]. The classic clinical presentation is chronic drainage in an ear with granulation tissue on the tympanic membrane. Biopsy is essential but might only reveal dysplasia. In all three cases, definitive diagnosis was not established until surgical resection was performed.

Facial paralysis, when it occurs, is a very ominous sign and is linked with a poor prognosis [16, 46, 67]. The facial nerve generally becomes involved in one of the three ways: (1) extensive disease into the parotid to involve the nerve at the stylomastoid foramen, (2) erosion through the posterior canal wall into the mastoid or vertical segment of the nerve, and (3) erosion through the middle ear and along the middle fossa to involve the tympanic segment of the facial nerve [68]. All three modes indicate a large and aggressive tumor.

The incidence of facial nerve involvement ranges from 4% to 64% [5, 27, 45, 46, 69]. Gidley et al. reported a 15.5% incidence of facial nerve dysfunction at presentation in patients with SCC of the temporal bone which was present for an average of 6 months prior to presentation [5]. The incidence of facial paralysis is particularly high in patients with middle ear squamous cell carcinoma. Jia et al. found that patients with middle ear squamous cell carcinoma had a 55% incidence of facial paralysis [2].

Generally, right and left sides are equally affected. Gaudet et al. in a small study of only ten patients found that seven had left-sided tumors [83]. Gidley et al. in a study of 71 SCC of the temporal bone tumors found that 55% were on the left side and 45% on the right side [5]. In a study of 45 cases of SCC of the temporal bone, Bacciu identified a slight right-sided predominance, 57.8% right side versus 42.2% left side [46].

Thankfully, most cases of ear canal or middle ear SCC are unilateral. The earliest report of bilateral middle ear carcinoma was by Juby in 1957 [84]. Since then, there have been at least 23 case reports in the world literature of bilateral SCC of the ear canal and temporal bone [65, 85–105]. Most of these cases occur in patients with a prior history of chronic otitis media, and the tumors usually appear in a sequential and not simultaneous fashion.

Cervical Lymph Nodes

Cervical lymphadenopathy is a particularly poor prognostic sign associated with worse survival. The lymphatic drainage from the outer ear and ear canal is anteriorly to the parotid lymph nodes, posteriorly to mastoid lymph nodes, and inferiorly to levels II and III [108–112]. First echelon of nodes is the parotid gland and intraparotid lymph nodes [39, 113, 114]. Lymphatic drainage from the middle ear is poor [41] and runs to the mastoid and deep cervical nodes [82].

Level II is the most commonly involved neck nodes [5, 115]. Level III is a secondary drainage basin and usually does not become involved until level II has already been affected. Levels I, IV, and V are typically not involved from ear canal or temporal bone primaries [5, 114]. Level V nodes may become involved when tumors involve the postauricular skin. Submental lymph nodes are not involved.

Incidence of cervical lymph node metastasis has been reported to range between 10% and 23% [30, 45, 47, 113, 116–118]. In a large literature review, Rinaldo et al. reviewed 18 papers covering 491 patients and found an overall lymph node metastasis rate of 17.7% [114]. This finding refutes the claim that this tumor seldom metastasizes. Mazzoni et al. reported pathologically positive nodes 9 of 33 patients who underwent neck dissection. Their report highlights the fact that 5/29 clinically N0 necks had occult nodal metastasis [33].

Cervical nodal disease is an indicator of the aggressive nature of these tumors. Arriaga et al. reported 7/39 patients with positive lymph nodes [119]. In their series, patients with positive lymph nodes had only a 29% 2-year survival rate. In several series, patients with lymph node metastasis at presentation died of disease, usually within 24 months of diagnosis [39, 45, 120, 121]. Therefore, the presence of lymph node metastasis increases the staging so that T1-T3N1 is considered stage IV disease on the Pittsburgh staging system.

While death from temporal bone cancer is usually from local recurrence, cervical nodal disease is an important prognostic indicator of advanced and aggressive disease [114, 116]. Moffat et al. reported on a series of 39 patients with SCC of the temporal bone; 9 patients (23%) presented with lymph node metastasis, and all died within 27 months (mean 12.7 months). Of the remainder, 50% were alive and free of disease at a mean follow-up of 87 months [39]. It is important to note that patients with cervical nodal disease died of local recurrence and not regional or distant disease in their series.

Gillespie et al. reported that CT scan was typically adequate to detect nodal metastases; however, occult disease within the parotid gland was harder to detect [70, 122]. Choi et al. examined the rates of parotid and cervical lymph node metastasis and parotid invasion [123]. They studied 11 SCC and 10 adenoid cystic carcinomas of the external ear canal. They found that only two SCC (stages III and IV) involved parotid lymph nodes, and adenoid cystic carcinoma did not. SCC of the ear canal caused direct parotid invasion only in advanced-stage disease (stages III and IV), whereas 60% of patients with adenoid cystic carcinoma had direct parotid invasion, and it occurred with early-stage disease (stages I–IV) [123]. In their study, MRI missed direct parotid extension through the cartilaginous canal that was found on histologic study.

Diagnostic Imaging

Clinical examination is often limited by tumor filling the ear canal and obscuring the view of the tympanic membrane. Accurate imaging is necessary for staging and treatment planning. Computerized tomography (CT) and magnetic resonance imaging (MRI) each provides important information on tumor extent. Assessing tumor extent is essential since the main prognostic factor in temporal bone cancer is local extension [119]. Cross-sectional imaging (CT and MRI) are required for the staging of temporal bone cancers (Fig. 7.3). MRI and CT are often used in a complementary fashion [47, 69, 116, 124].

CT imaging has been correlated with pathologic findings in order to gauge the accuracy of the imaging. Arriaga et al. described that CT was accurate in 94 out of 96 comparisons [119]. They described one false negative, in which the CT did not diagnose soft tissue extension without bony erosion through the anterior canal wall, and one false positive, in which the CT predicted otic capsule involvement but mucosal biopsy was negative for tumor [119].

There are limitations of CT. CT cannot differentiate fluid and inflamed mucosa from tumor in the middle ear and mastoid [24, 68, 69]. Additionally, CT cannot distinguish inflammation from tumor when there is no adjacent bony erosion [68]. Anterior canal erosions less than 2 mm might be missed on CT [24, 125, 126]. However, bony canal defects greater than 2 mm are usually associated with tumor invasion through the bone and into anterior soft tissues [125]. CT scan

can miss microscopic extension of tumor from the anterior ear canal to the parotid gland [127]. When CT alone is used, radiographic underestimation and overestimation of disease has been reported. Leonetti et al. concluded that radiographic imaging underestimated disease in the middle ear and mastoid mucosa, tegmen tympani, middle fossa dura, and carotid canal [128]. Gillespie et al. found that CT underestimated disease anteriorly and felt that CT findings correlated best with advanced disease (T3 or T4) than with early-stage disease (T1 or T2) [70].

MRI has improved soft tissue detail and is essential for tumors that are producing nerve weakness or that invade the dura [70, 115, 124]. It has better resolution of disease affecting the parotid, temporomandibular joint, and petrous apex [70, 129].

PET/CT is important for patients with high-stage tumors (T3 or T4), since these patients are at higher risk of distant

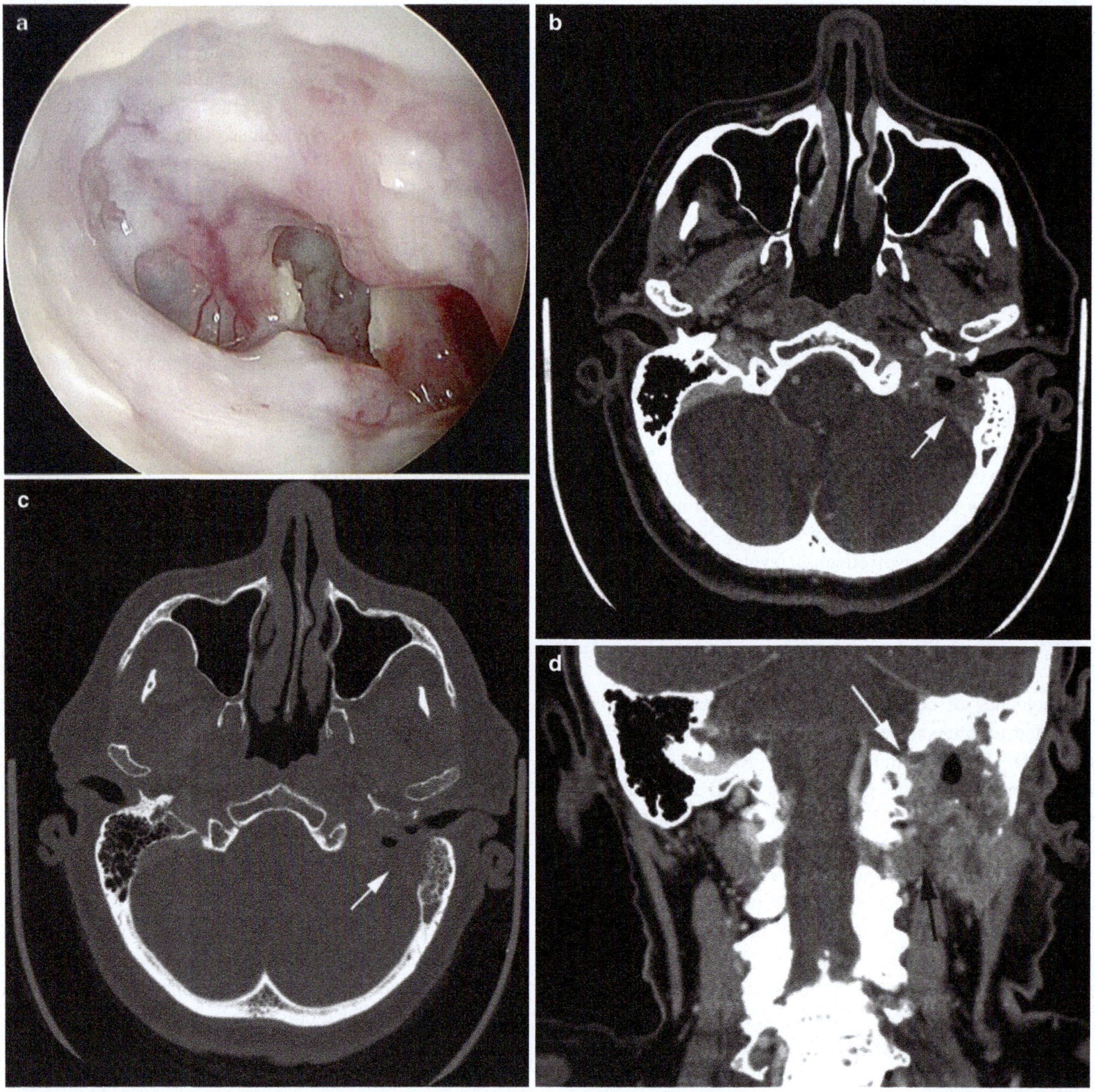

Fig. 7.3. Squamous cell carcinoma of the middle ear and temporal bone (stage IV) in an 82-year-old man. (**a**) Oto-endoscopic view. (**b**) Axial CT showing the mass filling the mastoid and middle ear. Note destruction of the posterior petrous bone (arrow). (**c**) Bone window CT showing the bony destruction from this tumor. (**d**) Coronal CT showing extension into the neck. White arrow marks hypoglossal canal. Black arrow marks disease at paraspinous muscles. (**e**) Contrast-enhanced axial T1 MRI at the same level as image (**b**). (**f**) Contrast-enhanced coronal T1 MRI showing no enhancement along the middle fossa dura at the same level as (**c**)

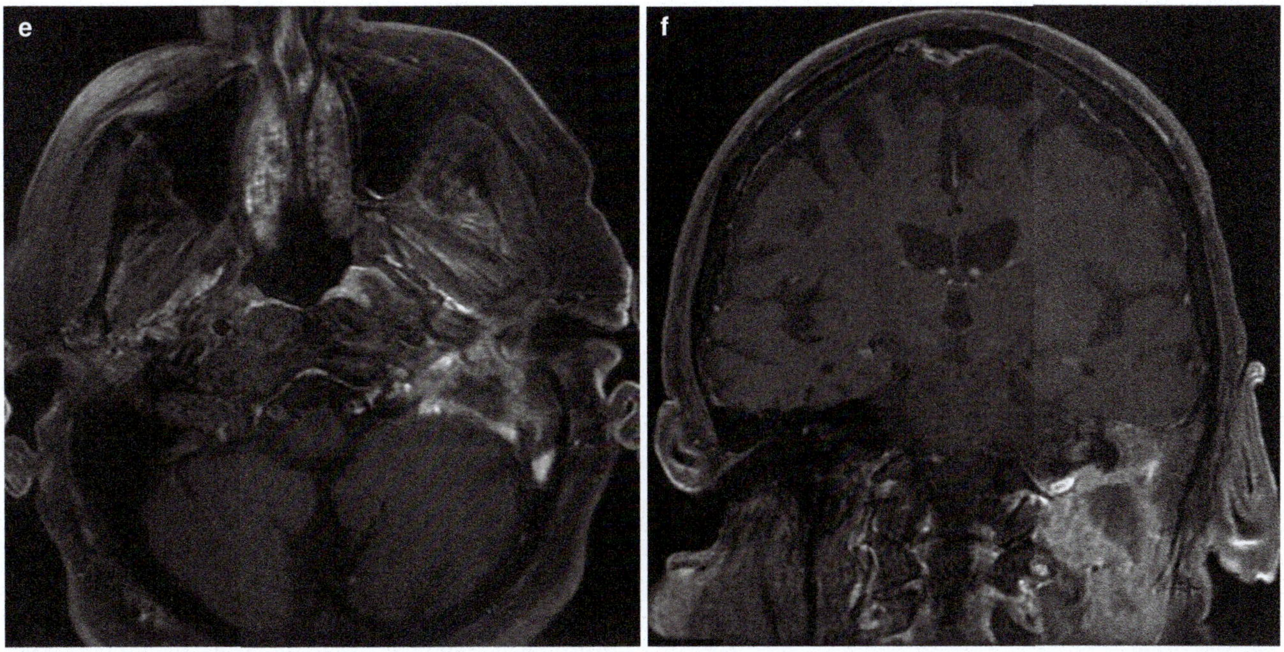

Fig. 7.3 (continued)

metastasis [69]. If distant disease was discovered on PET/CT, then primary surgery would not be offered. Instead, these patients are treated with neoadjuvant chemotherapy followed by concurrent chemoradiation therapy to the primary site.

Natural History and Directions of Spread

The bone of the ear canal and the eardrum is an early defense against the spread of SCC arising in the canal or outer ear. Once the ear canal and eardrum are penetrated, the tumor is able to spread anteriorly into the TMJ; inferiorly along the jugular vein, carotid artery, and lower cranial nerves; medially into the middle ear and mastoid; superiorly into the middle fossa and temporal lobe; and posteriorly into the sigmoid sinus and cerebellum. The numerous nerve and vascular foramina of the temporal bone allow spread of disease [33]. While the bone of the ear canal is relatively thick, the bone of the mastoid and tegmen is relatively thin or occasionally dehiscent, offering little resistance to invasion. The bone plates over many structures like the jugular bulb, carotid, tegmen, fallopian canal, and the labyrinth are thin and are vulnerable to tumor erosion [126].

The ear canal has preformed pathways like the cartilaginous fissures of Santorini, the petrosquamous suture line, and the bony foramen of Huschke that can facilitate spread of tumor anteriorly (Fig. 7.4) [126]. Embryologically, the ossification centers of the ear canal fuse to complete the tympanic ring. By age 5 years, the bone of the ear canal is usually completely fused. This foramen of Huschke is a sign of

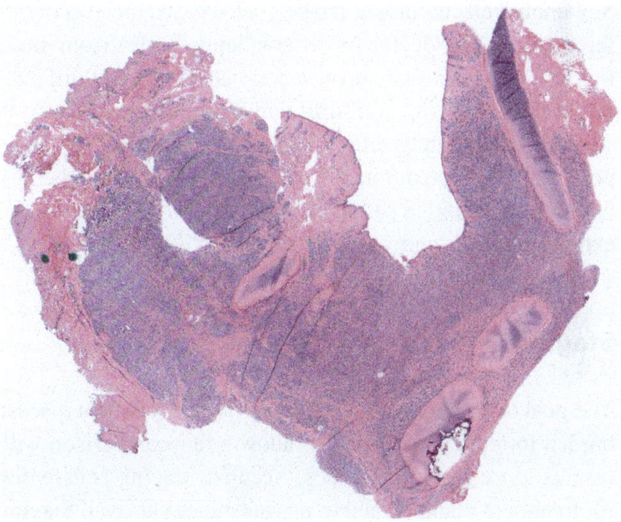

Fig. 7.4. Low-power photomicrograph of cancer spreading through the fissures of Santorini

incomplete fusion of the ossification centers in the developing tympanic bone. The foramen of Huschke is a pathway from the anterior ear canal at the level of the tympanic membrane to the soft tissues anterior to the ear canal [125]. Additionally, Haversian canals and angiolymphatic pathways are additional pathways for the spread of cancer [113].

The creation of canal wall down mastoidectomy cavities for cholesteatoma produces pathways for the spread of cancer. In the latter case, the fenestration procedure opens up the normally resistant inner ear and makes it more vulnerable to tumor invasion [35].

Leonetti et al. described the patterns of temporal bone invasions as (a) superiorly through the tegmen tympani into the middle cranial fossa, (b) anteriorly into the glenoid and infratemporal fossa, (c) inferiorly into the jugular foramen, (d) posteriorly into the mastoid air cells, and (e) medially into the middle ear, inner ear, and carotid canal [128]. In their study, CT and MRI underestimated disease in the mastoid mucosa, tegmen tympani, middle fossa dura, middle ear mucosa, and along the carotid canal. Underestimating disease preoperatively might lead to planning inadequate surgery. As a consequence, patients who later developed recurrence had radiographic underestimations in one or more of these locations.

Gidley et al. reported that extension anterior to the ear canal was present in 63% of patients [5]. They reported that tumor extended to involve the jugular foramen in 23%, the carotid artery in 11%, the infratemporal fossa in 11%, and the temporomandibular joint in 4% [5].

Histopathology

Squamous cell carcinoma can be graded based on level of differentiation. The degree of differentiation varies from study to study, and some authors have correlated degree of differentiation with survival. Well-differentiated tumors are found in 11–53%, moderately differentiated from 36% to 79%, and poorly differentiated from 4% to 36% [5, 39, 46, 48, 64, 129]. Gidley et al. reported perineural invasion in 7%, extracapsular extension in 2%, and vascular invasion in 4% [5].

Staging

The goal of staging is to sort patients with equivalent disease burden into the same group to allow a fair comparison with respect to treatment outcomes. Accurate staging is essential for treatment planning and to prognosticate survival. Staging is also necessary to counsel patients regarding treatment options and expected outcomes.

Accurate staging improves external validity and allows for analysis of the effects of specific disease characteristics, comorbidities, and treatment [67]. Staging must account for local disease extension, since this is the main determinant of survival [119]. Care must be exercised to avoid underestimating disease [70, 122]. Regional and distant disease must also be included. Given the complex anatomy of the temporal bone, clinical features alone are insufficient for accurate staging. Radiographic imaging and final pathologic findings are often necessary to complete staging [68, 130].

Several staging systems have been proposed over the years. Many of these early systems have just three stages, and they typically relied on physical examination findings. Prior to the development and refinement of cross-sectional, computerized imaging, surgeons relied on physical examination, plain film, and polytomography findings to assess extent of disease [131–135]. Goodwin and Jesse [88], Stell and McCormick [136], Pensak et al. [137], and Mandolis et al. [14] have all proposed different staging systems. These staging systems are reviewed in Chap. 2.

In 1990, Arriaga et al. published a landmark study in which CT radiographic findings were correlated with pathologic findings for squamous cell carcinoma of the external auditory meatus [119]. The authors excluded from consideration patients that had the ear canal involved secondarily from the external ear or parotid. They identified 12 anatomic areas to be assessed: external osseous meatus erosion anteriorly, posteriorly, inferiorly, and superiorly; infratemporal extension; middle ear involvement; otic capsule erosion; mastoid involvement; jugular fossa erosion; carotid canal erosion; tegmen erosion with middle fossa involvement; and posterior fossa involvement [119]. They reported a 98% concurrence between CT and pathologic extent of disease. This study highlights the fact that a careful and systematic review of CT scans is required for accurate prediction of disease extent. Their staging system ranks tumors by extent of local destruction (e.g., canal wall or soft tissue extension) and by involvement of medial structures (e.g., ear canal, middle ear/mastoid, inner ear involvement) and uses a TNM format for squamous cell carcinoma of the external auditory meatus. In their schema, any lymph node involvement was automatically considered a sign of advanced-stage disease; thus, Tl-3N+ and any T4 are considered stage IV [119]. This system has become known as the Pittsburgh staging system (PSS) and has undergone several amendments (Table 7.1).

Moody et al. modified the original PSS to move facial paresis or paralysis to T4, since a tumor that is affecting the facial nerve is either in the middle ear and eroding the medial wall (tympanic portion of the nerve), or has invaded the full thickness of the ear canal, or by involving tissue at the stylomastoid foramen (by definition >0.5 cm of soft tissue involvement) [68]. Facial nerve involvement, or its correlate facial paralysis, has been cited as an important prognostic feature in several papers [15, 113]; however, other papers have found that facial nerve involvement was not a significant factor [9, 116].

Higgins and Moody-Antonio performed a systematic review of the literature regarding outcomes for patients with or without facial paralysis in the setting of SCC of the ear canal and temporal bone [67]. Their study encompassed 21 studies covering 348 patients. They demonstrated that patient with facial paralysis had a significantly worse disease-specific survival and overall survival when compared to patients without facial paralysis. Furthermore, they showed that overall survival was worse for patients with facial

Table 7.1 Pittsburgh staging system, originally proposed by Arriaga et al. [119] with modification from Moody et al. [68]

T classification	
T1	Tumor limited to the EAC without bony erosion or evidence of soft tissue involvement
T2	Tumor limited to the EAC with bone erosion (not full thickness) or limited soft tissue involvement (<0.5 cm)
T3	Tumor eroding through the osseous EAC (full thickness) with limited soft tissue involvement (<0.5 cm) or tumor involvement in the middle ear and/or mastoid
T4	Tumor eroding the cochlea, petrous apex, medial wall of the middle ear, carotid canal, jugular foramen, or dura or with extensive soft tissue involvement (>0.5 cm), such as involvement of the TMJ or styloid process, or evidence of facial paresis
N classification	
N0	No regional nodes involved
N1	Single metastatic regional node <3 cm in size
N2a	Single ipsilateral metastatic node 3–6 cm in size
N2b	Multiple ipsilateral metastatic lymph nodes
N2c	Contralateral metastatic lymph node
N3	Metastatic lymph node >6 cm in size
Overall stage	
I	T1N0
II	T2N0
III	T3N0
IV	T4N0 and any T N+

Table 7.2 Proposed modification to the Pittsburgh staging system [33]

T classification	
T1	Tumor in the skin without bone involvement
T2	Tumor in the skin with bone/cartilage involvement, but not full thickness
T3a	Tumor extending <5 mm from cartilage to periauricular soft tissues or tumor strictly limited to the anterior bone wall and growing <5 mm into the parotid space
T3b	Same as for T3a, but extending >5 mm
T4a	Tumor growing into mastoid, without seventh paresis
T4b	Tumor growing into mastoid with facial paresis, or infratemporal space, or medial wall of tympanum, labyrinth, petrous bone (jugular foramen, internal carotid canal, petrous apex)

paralysis than those staged as Pittsburgh 2000 T3. There was no significant difference in overall survival between patients staged as Pittsburgh 2000 T4 and those with facial paralysis. From this analysis, they concluded that facial paralysis rightfully should be staged as T4 [67]. They also showed that the Pittsburgh 2000 staging was superior to the 1990 version and the Stell staging system by being able to discriminate overall survival in Stell T2 versus T3 disease and Pittsburgh T3 versus T4 disease.

Several studies have confirmed the correlation between Pittsburgh T stage and prognosis for squamous cell carcinoma [5, 8, 15, 39, 46, 113, 126, 130, 138], and this system has become the most frequently used for reporting results in contemporary literature [15]. A meta-analysis of the literature on squamous cell carcinoma of the temporal bone has shown that T classification is an independent factor for poor survival by Cox proportional hazard model (hazard ratio (HR) = 2.53, $p = 0.002$) [139]. Their multivariate analysis did not find that lymph node metastasis was a risk factor for survival (HR = 0.93, $p = 0.939$).

The Pittsburgh staging system has been applied to tumor histologies other than squamous cell carcinoma. Testa et al. applied the Pittsburgh staging system to describe 79 cancers of the external auditory canal, including SCC, basal cell carcinoma (BCC), and adenocarcinoma [118].

Gaudet et al. [83] used the Pittsburgh staging system for ten periauricular skin cancers. Their paper highlights the fact that large periauricular skin cancers might be staged as T4 by the prevailing AJCC system, but simultaneously, these tumors would be judged as T1 by the Pittsburgh staging system. Similarly, Essig and colleagues used the Pittsburgh staging system for large periauricular cancers that required lateral temporal bone resection [130].

Despite its popularity, problems with the Pittsburgh staging system have been identified, and changes have been suggested. Ito et al. state that extensive bone involvement correlates with prognosis, yet they do not define "extensive soft tissue involvement" [15]. Mazzoni et al. list four problems: "(1) The skin of the auditory canal. (2) Skin and bone and/or cartilage involvement, but not full thickness (the term 'full thickness' is appropriate for the anterior bone wall, while it needs to be defined for the other bone walls). (3) Anterior extension from anterior wall to parotid space, or from cartilage canal to periauricular soft tissues. (4) Extension from canal to mastoid and other sites of the temporal bone" [33]. They propose modifications to the PSS (Table 7.2).

Breau et al. proposed a modification to the Pittsburgh system for early-stage lesions based on the site of disease in the canal and less emphasis on the size of the primary tumor or degree of bony invasion [13].

Treatment Planning

Squamous cell carcinoma of the ear canal can require surgery, radiotherapy, and possibly chemotherapy. The complexity of treatment options emphasizes the role of the multidisciplinary team. Unfortunately, randomized trials do not exist to help guide treatment decisions. These patients should be seen by a number of consultants to arrive at the proper treatment. Consultations are typically sought from neurotology, head and neck surgery, radiation oncology, and medical oncology. Based on surgical requirements, consultations might be required from neurosurgery, oculoplastics, and plastic reconstructive surgery.

The Role of Surgery

Surgery has become a mainstay of treatment for cancers of the ear canal and temporal bone [46]. The extent of surgery has been a subject of debate and controversy. In a landmark study, Prasad and Janecka performed an early meta-analysis of 26 publications on temporal bone cancer covering 144 patients [140]. Their conclusion about surgical approach for temporal bone cancer was that patients who had tumors confined to the ear canal had similar survival rates whether they had mastoidectomy, lateral temporal bone resection, or subtotal temporal bone resection. This paper highlighted many of the deficiencies in the literature regarding temporal bone cancer and the surgical approaches to it. While some of its conclusions are no longer true, this paper launched better research and more rigorous outcome measures for this dreaded illness.

Up until the 1950s, radical mastoidectomy followed by radiotherapy was considered the treatment of choice for ear canal cancers. This approach is associated with high degree of recurrence and the potential for chronic drainage and osteoradionecrosis [141, 142]; however, Zhang et al. still promote this approach for SCC of the temporal bone [45]. Their philosophy is predicated on the belief that mastoidectomy causes less morbidity and mortality than temporal bone resection.

The goal of surgery is complete resection of the tumor with negative margins. Margin status is a clear prognostic indicator, and surgery must be conceived and designed in order to achieve a negative margin. Tumors that cannot be resected with negative margins are considered unresectable. Morris et al. reported close or positive margins in 38% of SCC ear canal. This number rose to 47% with T4 tumors [4]. Zhang et al. identified positive margins in 54% of early-stage (T1 and T2) tumors, and this finding prompted them to change from sleeve resection to lateral temporal bone resection for these early-stage tumors [127]. Rates of positive margins are quoted from 18% to 64% [5, 27, 30, 47, 68, 113, 130]. Clearly, achieving a negative margin is difficult in temporal bone cancer surgery.

Nomenclature of Surgical Procedures

The nomenclature surrounding surgical procedures has been confusing. Previous authors have named procedures such as wide local excision, sleeve resection, en bloc EAC resection, local canal resection, partial temporal bone resection, radical resection of the EAC, modified lateral temporal bone resection, and lateral temporal bone resection for procedures that excise lesions of the external auditory canal [6, 12, 70, 122, 138]. Medina et al. describe four types of lateral temporal bone resection [143].

Some authors have described "sleeve resection" where the skin of the ear canal and TM are removed and replaced with skin grafts [6]. The bone of the ear canal is left intact. The attractiveness of this approach is preservation of hearing and a lesser risk of neural or vascular injury.

The problems with this approach are a high rate of positive margins and a high recurrence rate. Goodwin and Jesse reported that sleeve resection for cancer of the external auditory meatus had a 41% recurrence rate [88]. Austin et al. reported that nine patients with T1 disease treated with local canal resection had a 5-year survival of 66%, and all failures were due to local recurrences [138]. Kunst et al. used local canal resection for T1 tumors, with a 25% recurrence rate [122]. Zhang et al. reported a recurrence rate of 46% and a positive margin rate of 54% with local canal resection [127].

A more recent study compared the results of local canal resection to lateral temporal bone resection for T1 and T2 temporal bone malignancies. This study showed a clear survival advantage and higher cure rate for patients who underwent LTBR with superficial parotidectomy over local canal resection [127].

Wide Local Excision

A clear distinction needs to be made about tumors located at the external auditory meatus versus tumors in the bony canal. Tumors that occupy the cartilaginous portions of the ear canal can be safely excised with surrounding soft tissues if the tumor does not extend medial to the bone-cartilage junction (Fig. 7.5). This procedure is more adequately termed "wide local excision" and is similar to other skin cancer excisions on the face and neck. Removing the underlying cartilage helps to ensure complete resection and to lower recurrence rate.

Tumors that extend medially into the canal past the bone-cartilage junction require lateral temporal bone resection for excision. The skin of the bony canal is quite thin, and an adequate margin of healthy skin is not present. Examining the ear with oto-endoscopes, in addition to the otomicroscope, is very helpful in making this determination.

Temporal Bone Resection

Lateral temporal bone resection is the workhorse of oncologic surgery for the temporal bone [4]. Lateral temporal bone resection (LTBR) is the en bloc removal of the ear canal, lateral to the facial nerve and stapes (Chap. 17). The procedure removes the bony ear canal, tympanic membrane, malleus, and incus. The stapes and inner ear are preserved. The facial nerve is generally preserved. LTBR can be combined with auriculectomy, parotidectomy, mandibulectomy, and neck dissection depending on the extent of disease.

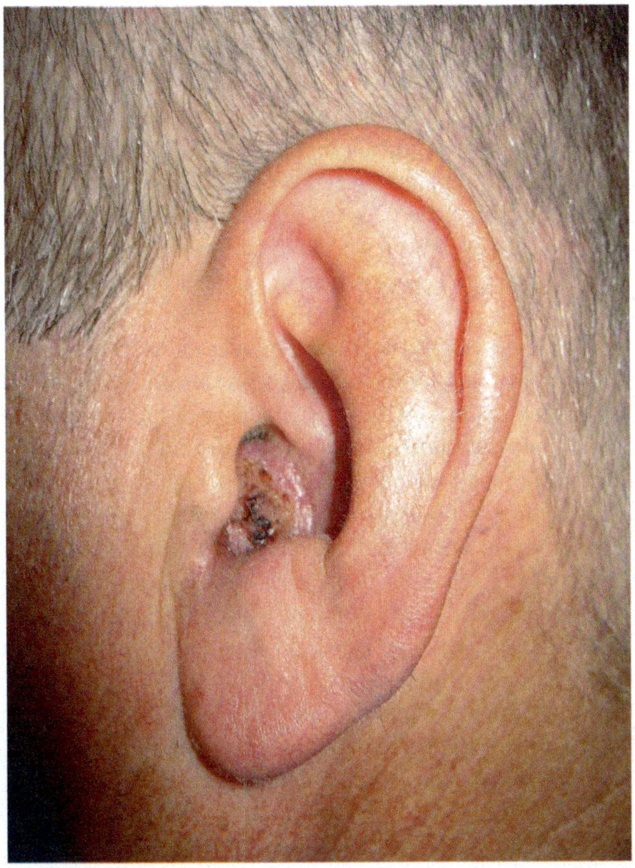

Fig. 7.5 Squamous cell carcinoma at the external auditory meatus, which was widely excised and reconstructed with a split thickness skin graft. The tumor did not extend into the bony ear canal and LTBR was not required

Limited dural resections can also be performed. Lateral temporal bone resection for Pittsburgh T1 is curative in 100% of patients [68].

Surgeons have devised procedures to remove the ear canal lateral to the tympanic membrane in an attempt to preserve hearing. Medina et al. first described this as "type I lateral temporal bone resection" [143]. Moody et al. describe this same procedure as "modified LTBR" [68].

On the other end of the spectrum, Moffat et al. recommend LTBR, total auriculectomy, mandibular condylectomy with superficial parotidectomy as a necessity for stage T1 and T2 tumors [39]. They justify this approach by citing the inability of radiographic studies to diagnose extent of disease into the TMJ and infratemporal fossa [39].

A subtotal temporal bone resection (STBR) is performed when disease extends past the tympanic membrane into the middle ear (Chap. 18). In this case, the labyrinth and cochlea are removed with a drill, and the disease is removed piecemeal. LTBR is usually a necessary first step to remove disease in the ear canal and to gain enough exposure for the middle ear, Eustachian tube, cochlea, and carotid artery. The margins of resection are the middle fossa dura superiorly, the carotid artery anteriorly, the jugular bulb inferiorly, and the sigmoid sinus and posterior fossa dura posteriorly. The internal auditory canal and anterior petrous apex are not removed. Dura is resected as dictated by frozen section and repaired with a dural graft. Microvascular free flap reconstruction is used for the majority of cases, since the surgical defect is too large for a temporalis flap. For tumors of the middle ear, Jia et al. showed that subtotal temporal bone resection had a higher survival rate than lateral temporal bone resection [2].

Total temporal bone resection (TTBR) expands the limits of the subtotal temporal bone resection to include the petrous apex and internal auditory canal. Again, dura resection is dictated by extent of disease as seen on frozen section pathology, and the dura is repaired with a dural graft. Microvascular free flap reconstruction is performed.

Both subtotal and total en bloc temporal bone resections have been described. Subtotal resection with piecemeal removal of disease beyond the limits of the subtotal temporal bone resection and postoperative radiotherapy is a reasonable option to total en bloc temporal bone resection [70]. Total en bloc temporal bone resection is fraught with increased morbidity and has not been shown to improve overall survival. In this setting of advanced disease, usually with carotid artery involvement, preoperative chemotherapy is emerging as likely the most efficacious approach. The interested reader is referred to Okada et al. for a description of subtotal and total en bloc temporal bone resection [144]. However, the introduction of chemotherapy for these large (T3 and T4) tumors has offered patients new hope without having to undergo such surgery.

Parotidectomy, Neck Dissection, Condylectomy, and Carotid Resection

The role of elective parotidectomy and neck dissection continues to be a source of controversy in the literature. Conley and Schuller in 1976 stated that the proclivity of ear canal cancers to metastasize to the parotid and cervical lymph nodes necessitates their inclusion in the treatment plan [43]. In 1977, Gacek and Goodman recommended that superficial parotidectomy be performed for all cases of en bloc temporal bone resection because of the proximity of the lymph nodes and to provide a more adequate margin of tissue anterior to the ear canal [145]. Parotidectomy is required where there is evidence of direct extension. Elective parotidectomy is recommended for accurate staging since many patients will have positive nodal metastases within the parotid. Chee et al. found direct extension to the parotid gland in only 1 of 14 cases of squamous cell carcinoma of the ear canal [24]. Morris et al. identified direct parotid invasion in 25% and parotid nodal metastasis in 43% of patients with SCC of the ear canal [4]. Parotid gland involvement has been noted as high as 62% of patients with stage IV disease [107]. Moffat et al. considered parotidectomy as a routine part of treatment for squamous cell carcinoma of the temporal bone [39].

Performing parotidectomy for ear canal cancer is not universal. Madsen et al. reported on a series of 68 ear canal cancers, and parotidectomy and mandibular condylectomy were not performed in any of their patients [8]. In their series, primary neck dissections were performed in only two patients.

Neck dissection for the N+ neck is essential when surgical treatment is being planned. Elective neck dissection continues to be a controversial subject. The incidence of positive lymph nodes varies between 10% and 20%. Selective neck dissection to include levels II and III is performed for adequate staging and to select appropriate patients for adjuvant therapy [5]. The morbidity of adding selective neck dissection is minimal in this setting. Regional lymph node recurrences have been reported in SCC of the temporal bone [5].

Resection of the mandibular condyle is also controversial. Moffat et al. consider mandibular condylectomy with LTBR, auriculectomy, and superficial parotidectomy as a necessity for stage T1 and T2 tumors [39]. Hosokawa et al. recommend condylectomy and removal of the soft tissues anterior to the ear canal in cases where preoperative CT scan shows an anterior bony canal wall erosion of 2 mm or greater [125]. Their study of 15 patients with ear canal carcinoma of differing histologies found tumor in the anterior soft tissues in every case where the anterior canal wall had more than 2 mm of erosion. Clearly, extent of resection for the mandible is guided by preoperative imaging and intraoperative findings, as determined by frozen section pathology.

Carotid involvement is a particularly poor survival indicator. Masterson et al. showed that all patients who underwent surgical resection and who had carotid involvement died before 2 years [47]. Moffat et al. reported that 8 out of 39 patients had carotid involvement from SCCa; only one was alive at the time of the manuscript, and that patient was only 9 months from surgery [39]. Since carotid resection carries with it such a poor outcome and the potential for significant morbidity (i.e., stroke), carotid sacrifice is not performed [116]. Therefore, carotid invasion is considered a sign of unresectability [64].

Absolute contraindications to surgery include cavernous sinus involvement, massive intracranial involvement, unresectable neck disease, distant metastasis, and poor general health [115]. Relative contraindications to surgery include carotid artery involvement and lower cranial nerve involvement [146].

Reconstruction

In the days where radical mastoidectomy was the norm for resection of squamous cell carcinoma, split thickness skin grafts were used. Split thickness skin grafts have been used to re-epithelialize the cavity resulting from LTBR with successful grafting in 83% of non-irradiated patients [147].

In the setting of postoperative radiotherapy, patients with such open cavities have a high risk of developing chronic otorrhea and osteoradionecrosis [142]. Reconstruction and obliteration are used to avoid an open cavity, as in a canal wall down mastoidectomy. Obliteration of the cavity using either a temporalis muscle flap or microvascular free flap is advisable.

The temporalis muscle flap provides an excellent reconstructive option when the surgical defect results from removal of the ear canal only. Larger defects, especially those that involve auriculectomy, mandibulectomy, dural resection, or exposure of the great vessels of the neck require microvascular free flap reconstruction [148, 149]. Some authors have used pedicled pectoralis flaps and scalp rotational flaps in addition to temporalis flaps [66], but the disadvantage of these flaps is the length of the pedicle to reach the temporal bone. Pedicled regional flaps, such as trapezius or pectoralis major, are avoided since the temporal bone is at the very limit of the arc of rotation [149].

Microvascular free flaps are also favored in patients that have previously been treated with radiotherapy. The anterolateral thigh (ALT) flap is the most frequent donor site, although many different donor sites are available depending on the size of the defect and donor site anatomy. The ALT flap has several advantages including low donor site morbidity, permitting a two-team operation, and the ability to harvest fascia lata grafts, nerve grafts, and even vein grafts from the same donor site incision and earlier mobilization [149].

In patients with normal preoperative facial function, immediate reconstruction with nerve grafting is recommended. Facial nerve recovery is not affected by age of patient or preoperative facial function or the use of postoperative radiotherapy [149, 150]. Facial nerve grafts can also be placed and result in return of function even if the proximal nerve margin is positive [151]. Additionally, placement of gold weight and fascial slings are helpful at protecting the eye and reestablishing some facial symmetry.

Preoperative consultation with an anaplastologist is important for patients who will require auriculectomy. Auricular prosthesis can be attached with either adhesives or osseointegrated implants.

A maximum conductive hearing loss is an expected outcome of LTBR. Only a few papers have reported hearing results following LTBR. Cristalli et al. included hearing results on their report of 17 patients with SCC of the ear canal. Their graph indicates on average a 20 dB change at 3 kHz and 30 dB change at 4 kHz in the five patients that did not receive radiotherapy. Hearing at 6 kHz was significantly worse for the patients that received postoperative radiotherapy [66].

Hearing rehabilitation is an integral part of the surgical planning for patients who have temporal bone surgery. Placement of an osseointegrated implant for cochlear stimulation is a reasonable option. A transcutaneous abutment is not placed with the first surgery to avoid complications with anticipated postoperative radiotherapy. Since radiotherapy has an effect on osseointegration, placement of the transcutaneous abutment is delayed. Planned second stage for placement of the abutment takes place 3 months later if no radiotherapy is given and 6 months later if radiotherapy is required [152]. This secondary procedure is usually scheduled along with free flap revision, if needed.

Surgical Complications

Surgical complications include facial paralysis, wound complications, cerebrospinal fluid leak, meningitis, lower cranial nerve deficits, stroke from carotid sacrifice, postoperative hemorrhage, pulmonary embolus, or microvascular free flap failure [47, 149]. Perioperative mortality rate in surgical series has been quoted from 0% to 6% [14, 68, 107, 109, 119, 130, 149].

The Role of Radiotherapy

Radiotherapy has been used as definitive or adjunctive therapy for SCC of the temporal bone. The outcomes for primary radiotherapy have been reported in only a few papers.

Birzgalis et al. (1992) reported the results of primary radiotherapy on 60 patients with tumors involving the middle ear and temporal bone [153]. Treatment dosages ranged from 45 to 55 Gy. None of the patients in their series had radical resection of the primary tumor. They staged patients into two broad categories: early and late, where late indicated bony erosion, facial paralysis, multiple cranial nerve deficits, or nodal metastasis (Stell T2 and T3). They reported an overall 5-year survival of 32%.

Hashi et al. (2000) suggested that radiotherapy alone is sufficient for T1 tumors [154]. They treated five patients with Stell T1 tumors, and none of these patients experienced disease recurrence. Treatment doses were 65 Gy, and there were no long-term complications of radiotherapy. They also treated two Stell T2 tumors with radiotherapy alone (65 Gy and 75 Gy), and both patients developed disease recurrence and survived only 6 months [154].

Pemberton et al. (2006) reviewed the historic record of definitive radiotherapy for primary ear canal and middle ear squamous cell carcinoma in 123 patients performed at Christie Hospital, Manchester, UK. Twenty patients had radical mastoidectomy, but none had a radical resection of disease. Their paper used the Stell staging system. The clinical response to radiotherapy was complete resolution in 50%, partial resolution in 27%, and no response in 20% [117]. Recurrence was local in 18%, nodal in 15%, and distant in 5% [117]. DFS was 45% at 5 years; the mean time to recurrence was 1.6 years [117].

Generally, while a few papers have shown that definitive radiotherapy is adequate treatment for T1 tumors, most reports have indicated that radiotherapy is inadequate as primary therapy for SCC of the temporal bone [23, 138, 155]. The use of external beam radiotherapy as a postoperative adjunct to surgery was first put forth by Lederman and reinforced by Conley and Schuller [43, 86]. Most papers report using postoperative radiotherapy as part of multidisciplinary care. Surgery plus postoperative radiotherapy offers better survival than either one alone [30, 48, 138].

Indications for postoperative radiotherapy include positive margins, recurrent cancer, perineural invasion, bone invasion, lymph node metastasis, and advanced-stage disease [27, 68, 70, 116]. Doses between 60 and 66 Gy are typical for patients with negative margins. Dose is increased to between 68 and 72 Gy for patients with close or positive margins [156]. Recurrence in cervical lymph nodes has been reported in patients who did not receive postoperative radiotherapy [5].

Radiotherapy with doses around 60 Gy does show a survival benefit for tumors T2 tumors and higher [5, 16, 30, 68, 122, 157]. T1 tumors did not benefit in a statistically significant way with combined therapy [5]. In a meta-analysis, Moody et al. found that radiotherapy helped improve survival in patients with T3 and T4 tumors [68].

Postoperative radiotherapy can improve local control in patients with negative margins; however, Goodwin and Jesse found that radiotherapy was of no benefit when the tumor could not be completely excised [88]. Other authors have also commented that radiotherapy is not a substitute for achieving negative margins [119, 158].

Zhang et al. reported in 1999 their results for 33 patients with SCC of the temporal bone [45]. Eleven (11) patients with stage III and IV disease were treated with radiotherapy alone with a 5-year survival of 28.7%, but 20 patients with stage III and IV disease treated with combined surgery and radiotherapy at a 5-year survival of 59.6% [45].

Kitani et al. reported a 5-year survival rate of 51% using definitive radiotherapy with or without chemotherapy [159].

Ogawa et al. reviewed their experience treating 87 patients with radiotherapy and surgery and concluded that radiotherapy alone is reasonable for Stell stage T1 tumors, whereas combined surgery and radiotherapy was indicated for T2 and T3 tumors [155]. They found that patients with Stell T3 disease did significantly better with surgery and radiotherapy rather than radiotherapy alone [155]. Furthermore, they found that the timing of radiotherapy (preoperative, postoperative, or combined pre- and postoperative) when combined with surgery did not influence disease-free survival [155].

There is very little information on the results of brachytherapy for temporal bone cancer. In the 1930s and 1940s, Figi and Hempstead treated patients with radical mastoidectomy, electrodessication, and implantation of radium; their survival rate was around 32% [160]. Using a more modern approach, Mayer et al. used either low-dose-rate (LDR) or high-dose-rate (HDR) brachytherapy to treat seven patients postoperatively [161]. Four of these seven (57%) patients remained disease free 10 years after treatment [161].

Cristalli et al. employed intraoperative radiotherapy (IORT) in eight patients with SCC of the ear canal [66]. They delivered 12 Gy as the first dose of planned postoperative radiotherapy once frozen section margins were determined to be tumor free. They advocated its use on the basis of direct visualization of the tumor bed to minimize the risk of geographic miss.

Complications of radiotherapy include dermatitis, xerostomia, hearing loss, vestibular weakness, brain necrosis, and osteoradionecrosis [117, 156]. The mean time to bone or soft tissue necrosis is 4.6 years (range 0.8–13.7 s); the average dose was either 52.2 or 55 Gy [117].

Postoperative radiotherapy offers survival benefits to patients with T2 and higher-staged disease. Postoperative radiotherapy is indicated for patients with bone invasion, perineural spread, cervical lymphadenopathy, or recurrent disease. Definitive radiotherapy is an option for patients with limited, early-stage disease who either refuse surgery or are otherwise not candidates for surgery.

The Role of Chemotherapy

Chemotherapy has an increasingly important role in the management of ear canal and temporal bone cancer. While it is often reserved for large tumors (T3 and T4), the results of chemotherapy, with or without surgery and radiotherapy, have shown promise. Chemotherapy, as a systemic treatment, might also have implications for the rare patient with bilateral SCCa of the ear canal and temporal bone so that bilateral conductive hearing loss might be avoided.

In 2006, Nakagawa et al. published a retrospective review of 25 patients with primary SCCa of the external ear canal and middle ear. This early study of chemotherapy, combined with radiotherapy and surgery, used TS-1 (tegafur, gimeracil, and oteracil) and 5-FU or cisplatin (70 mg/m^2) and 5-FU (700 mg/m^2). Surgery (either LTBR or STBR) was performed on selected patients. T1 and T2 tumors were treated primarily with surgery, and these patients had 100% estimated 3-year survival. T3 and T4 patients were treated with surgery, radiotherapy, and chemotherapy. Several T4 patients were treated with chemoradiotherapy (CRT) alone. The 5-year estimated survival for T3 and T4 patients was 80% and 35%, respectively. They showed some effectiveness of concurrent CRT as stand-alone treatment for temporal bone SCCa; however, survival for T4 tumors was better with preoperative CRT and surgery than with CRT alone. They conjectured that preoperative CRT contributed to a higher rate of tumor-free margins in patients undergoing surgery for T4 tumors [129].

Shiga et al. reported the results of concurrent chemotherapy and radiotherapy in a group of 15 patients with SCC of the ear canal and temporal bone; 9 patients had stage IV disease [162]. Their protocol consisted of 5-FU continuous infusion 500–600 mg/M^2 on days 1–5, with docetaxel 50 mg/M^2 and cisplatin 60 mg/M^2 on day 2, and radiotherapy to total dose of 70 Gy. There were significant toxicities related to this therapy including grade 3 and 4 hematopoietic adverse events. Complete remission was achieved in eight of nine stage IV patients. They calculated a 67% 5-year disease-specific survival for patients with T4 disease.

In 2015, Shinomiya reported the results of CCRT in a group of ten patients treated with TPF protocol. Their 5-year overall survival rate was 60%. Even for T4 or unresectable tumors, the overall 5-year survival rate was 56% [163].

In 2015, Kitani et al. reported the results of combined chemotherapy and radiotherapy in a group of 13 patients with squamous cell carcinoma of the temporal bone [159]. Patients were staged according to the Pittsburgh system; tumors were stages II–IV. All patients were treated with definitive radiotherapy (2 Gy fractions to total dose of 70 Gy). Concurrent chemoradiotherapy (CRT) was given to patients under 75 years old and consisted of two cycles of 5-FU (1000 mg/M^2) and cisplatin (60 mg/M^2). Patients with renal disease received docetaxel (15 mg/M^2/week). Patients with unresectable disease received induction chemotherapy consisting of docetaxel 60 mg/m^2 on day 1, cisplatin 70 mg/m^2 on day 4, and 5-FU 1000 mg/m^2 on days 1–5 followed by concurrent chemoradiotherapy. Of note, three of five patients with stage II disease died of disease due to locoregional failure; two of these three patients received radiotherapy only. Using this protocol, patients with stage III disease fared much better with four out of five patients demonstrating long-term survival. None of the stage IV patients survived past 14 months, and all developed local recurrences. While the authors cite surgery as producing unfavorable quality of life due to facial paralysis and hearing loss, they do not report their patients' quality of life, hearing status, or facial nerve function following this combined chemoradiotherapy.

Takenaka et al. performed a meta-analysis of stage III and IV squamous cell carcinoma of the temporal bone and found that the 5-year overall survival rate between CRT and standard treatment (surgery with or without radiotherapy) equivalent (43.6% vs 53.3%, respectively, $p = 0.210$) [139]. Caution is required in interpreting these data since the CRT group contained patients that were surgically unresectable, and thus, these patients naturally had worse disease and prognosis.

When CRT and surgery were combined, the outcomes depended on the setting. Preoperative CRT patients (87.5%

5-year survival) had a slightly better outcome than patients who received CRT postoperatively (0% 5-year survival), but this difference was not statistically significant [139]. In a multivariate analysis using the Cox proportional hazard model, preoperative CRT was significantly associated with an improved overall survival (Hazard Radio (HR) 0.18, $p = 0.030$), while postoperative CRT did not affect survival (HR = 1.30, $p = 0.617$) [139]. They conclude that (1) preoperative CRT may improve survival in advanced external auditory canal SCC; (2) definitive CRT may be an effective alternative for surgical treatment; and (3) postoperative CRT may not be effective enough to salvage patients with worse prognoses [139].

In summary, chemotherapy has a role for advanced-stage disease (Pittsburgh III and IV) and surgically unresectable disease. Preoperative, multidrug protocols and radiotherapy seem to offer advanced-staged patients a better overall survival than conventional surgery and radiotherapy.

Intra-Arterial Chemotherapy

Theoretically, intra-arterial therapy has the advantage of delivering high-dose chemotherapy to the target tumor while avoiding systemic toxicity. In 1965, Tucker reported the original use of intra-arterial chemotherapy for six cases of ear canal and temporal bone cancer [21]. The role of super-selective intra-arterial chemotherapy was first introduced for head and neck cancer by Robbins et al. [164]. A protocol for temporal bone SCC was piloted by Ueda et al. [165]. In their protocol, patients were given one dose of IV cisplatin (100 mg/patient) with sodium thiosulfate 1 week prior to radiotherapy. Two or three intra-arterial doses of cisplatin were given during radiotherapy (60 Gy at 2 Gy/day fractions). In this preliminary report of four patients, all patients developed complete remission of disease with mean follow-up of 30 months [165]. They reported only one patient with significant sensorineural hearing loss during the study period, and no patients had any thromboembolic complication from angiography [165].

More recently, Sugimoto et al. [166, 167] reported results in 12 patients. In their protocol, patients received conventional once daily external beam radiation (60–70 Gy) in 2 Gy doses, followed by intra-arterial cisplatin (200–600 mg in 2–6 portions). Surgical salvage was performed in patients with persistent disease. For the 12 patients (6 patients T3 and 6 patients T4) treated by this protocol, mean survival was 41.4 months in 9 patients. Two died of local recurrence and one died of distant disease. The application of this treatment requires skilled neurovascular interventionalist who can administer superselective chemotherapy, and this requirement limits the overall usage of this protocol.

Clinical Follow-Up

There are no current clinical guidelines dictating the frequency or extent of follow-up evaluations. Clinical evaluation of patients following temporal bone resection is limited given the fact that most patients with ear canal or temporal bone cancer will have a flap covering the operative site. The physical examination of these patients is limited to general factors such as weight, overall health, cranial nerve, and neck examination. For these reasons, cross-sectional imaging is indispensable and medically necessary for managing these patients.

Masterson et al. clinically evaluated patients every 2 months for the first 2 years and then every 6 months until 5 years following surgery [47]. Imaging is reserved for patients that have clinical signs of recurrence.

Moffat et al. describe seeing patients every 2 months for the first year, every 3 months for the second year, and then to every 4 months until 5 years after treatment [39]. Routine imaging was not performed unless clinically indicated. They reasoned that microscopic disease recurrence is difficult to discern from posttreatment changes on diagnostic imaging.

Mazzoni et al. describe seeing patients every 3 months for the year, every 6 months for 4 years, and then annually. Their imaging schedule includes CT and MRI every 6 months for the first year and then annually until 10 years [33].

Zanoletti et al. use clinical examination and contrast-enhanced head and neck MRI every 2 months in the first year, every 4 months in the second year, and every 6 months in the third to fifth years [1].

In our center, patients are seen every 3 months for the first 2 years following completion of treatment. Clinical follow-up is spaced to every 6 months for years 2–5. Contrast-enhanced cross-sectional imaging (either CT or MRI) of the head and neck is performed at each visit. An annual chest X-ray is performed for patients with early-stage disease. Patients with higher stage disease have an annual PET/CT performed. This schedule is similar to that described by Leong et al. [107].

Following the fifth year of follow-up, patients are transitioned into our Survivorship Clinic, where they are seen annually; and the focus of the visit moves from the primary tumor management to management of treatment complications and surveillance of second primary tumors (e.g., prostate, colon, or breast).

Recurrence and Survival

Recurrence is an ominous sign in this patient population, and recurrence is the major cause of death for temporal bone cancer. The pattern for recurrence is often the return of local disease [8, 33, 140, 165]. Local recurrence is especially common when surgical excision is incomplete, and a positive tissue margin is present [12, 122, 168].

Recurrence rates vary from 11% to 53% overall, and the recurrence rate can be as high as 72% in T3 and T4 tumors [4, 27, 45, 46, 69, 113]. For this reason, achieving local control is of paramount importance. Obtaining a negative margin is so important that even if surgery is extensive (i.e., total temporal bone resection) and a positive margin remains, the 2-year survival can be 0% [119].

Recurrence typically occurs within the first year of completing therapy [1, 5, 27, 46, 68, 113, 169], although there are instances of recurrences up to 3 years following treatment [5, 33, 68, 109]. Bacciu et al. described a series of 45 patients with SCC of the temporal bone; 13 patients (29%) developed recurrence within 1–30 months (mean 8.3 months) [46]. Once disease recurs, the average interval from local recurrence to death can be as short as 3.6 months [119]. Bacciu et al. reported a mean survival time after recurrence was 4.2 months (range 1–21 months) [46]. The median survival for patients with recurrence is approximately 16 months [1].

In a large, retrospective review of definitive radiotherapy for SCCa of the ear canal and temporal bone, Pemberton et al. reported local recurrence in 18%, nodal recurrence in 15%, and distant metastasis in 5% [117]. DFS was 45% at 5 years; the mean time to recurrence was 1.6 years [117]. Gidley et al. reported that 52.2% recurrences were local, 13.5% were to regional lymph nodes, 8.7% were both local recurrences and lymph node involvement, and only 4.3% patients had a solitary distant metastasis [5]. Lobo et al. reported local recurrences in 37% and distant metastasis in 16% [64]. Ogawa et al. reported recurrence in 38 out of 87 patients, 34 patients with local recurrence, 3 patients with regional lymph node recurrence, and 1 patient with distant metastasis (lung) [155].

Zanoletti et al. describe a series of 41 patients with SCCa of the ear canal or temporal bone, and they excluded any periauricular cancers [113]. All patients had negative surgical margins. Radiotherapy was administered to 23 patients. Eighteen patients (41%) developed recurrence within the study follow-up period. Their findings highlight several points: (1) the difficulty in assessing margins in temporal bone cancer, (2) the indications for adjuvant radiotherapy for SCCa in the temporal bone, and (3) the limitations of surgery in controlling disease in the temporal bone.

Factors associated with recurrence are positive margins [30, 68, 69], anterior canal involvement [13], dural involvement [33, 68, 113], facial nerve sacrifice [113], direction of spread in T4 tumors (anterior vs all other directions) [113], lymph node involvement [33], and pathologic tumor grade [113]. Factors not associated with recurrence include parotidectomy, neck dissection, and postoperative radiotherapy [113]. Zanoletti et al. in a review of 47 patients, including patients who presented with positive neck node, did not recur within the neck but instead recurred locally [170].

Surgical salvage for patients with local recurrence has a poor outcome, and these patients might be better served with palliative chemotherapy [1].

Survival

Overall survival for temporal bone squamous cell carcinoma has improved tremendously since Conley and Novack published their large series in 1960 [171]. They calculated an 18% 5-year survival rate. Fifteen years later, Lewis published his personal series of 100 cases of cancers of the ear and reported a 25% 5-year survival rate [172].

Overall Survival

Overall survival (OS) is defined as the time from a patient's first appointment until the last date of contact or death. Authors report various ranges for overall survival such as 2-year [6, 173], 3-year [129, 138], and 5-year [64]. Survival statistics are hard to compare since many studies have small numbers of patients or contain multiple histologic types or use various time intervals (2-year, 3-year, or 5-year) of survival.

Moody et al. report survival on a series of 32 patients with SCCa of the external auditory canal. They quote 2-year survival for stages T1 to T4 as 100%, 80%, 50%, and 7%, respectively [68].

More recent papers have seen increased survival in temporal bone cancer and used the standard 5-year survival statistic. Yin et al. reported an overall 5-year survival of 66.8% for their cohort of 95 patients. Stage I and II tumors had 100% 5-year survival, stage III tumors had 67.2%, and stage IV tumors had 29.5% 5-year survival [30].

Survival heavily depends on extent of disease. Gidley et al. found that overall survival was primarily affected by staging: Pittsburgh T stage (early T1 and T2 versus T3 and T4) [5]. Early-stage tumors (Pittsburgh stages 1 and 2) tend to have excellent 5-year survival. Late-stage tumors have much worse prognosis, but this has improved over time. The reported 5-year overall survival rate has risen from 57.5% to 72.5% for T3 cases and from 22.9% to 35.8% for T4 patients [174].

Prasad et al., in a literature review, found overall 5-year survival ranges from 80% to 100% for T1 tumors, 46–100% for T2 tumors, 17–100% for T3 tumors, and 14–54% for T4 tumors [126].

Takenaka et al. performed a meta-analysis of temporal bone squamous cell carcinoma [139]. Their study included 28 papers covering 752 cases. Their review showed an overall 5-year survival rate of 20–90% [139]. The weighted estimate of 5-year survival using a random effect model was 57% (95% confidence interval, 50–63%).

Their analysis showed that Pittsburgh T classification is an independent factor for poor survival by Cox proportional hazard model (hazard ratio (HR) = 2.53, $p = 0.002$) [139]. Their multivariate analysis did not find that lymph node metastasis was a risk factor for survival (HR = 0.93, $p = 0.939$) [139]. They report that patients with lymph node metastasis had worse survival compared to N0 patients (37.1 vs 47.8), but this was not statistically significant ($p = 0.372$) [139].

For patients with T3 or T4 disease, the overall 5-year survival was 72.5% and 35.8%, respectively, based on a subset analysis of 174 cases [139]. Their meta-analysis of these patients with T3 and T4 SCC of the EAC found that preoperative chemoradiation therapy followed by surgery improved overall 5-year survival rate to 85.7%, compared with surgery with or without radiation (53.5%), definitive CRT (43.6%), and postoperative CRT (0%) [139].

The survival rate for patients with positive margins is poor despite postoperative radiotherapy [68]. Takenaka et al. conjecture that these patients might fare better with preoperative CRT since postoperative treatment does not appear to improve overall survival [139].

Several studies have tried to tease out factors associated with overall survival. Masterson et al. in their multivariate analysis found that positive lymph nodes, poorly differentiated histology, and carotid involvement were indicators of poor prognosis [47]. Chi et al. found that survival was worse with poorly differentiated pathology [48]. Leong et al. found that patients with poorly differentiated tumors had significantly worse overall survival than patients with either well- or moderately differentiated tumors [107]. Others have not found histologic differentiation to affect overall survival.

For middle ear SCC, Gurgel et al. examined the SEER database and calculated a 23.9% 5-year observed survival rate for 135 reported cases [26]. For patients with localized middle ear disease, 5-year survival was slightly better for patients treated with surgery alone than with radiotherapy alone. For patients with regional disease, 5-year survival was better with surgery alone than with radiotherapy alone or combined surgery and radiotherapy [26].

Disease-Free Survival

Disease-free survival (DFS) measures the time from end of treatment until a locoregional recurrence is identified. In a large retrospective review of SCC of the temporal bone, Gidley et al. found that DFS was 60% [5]. Mazzoni et al. report an overall DFS of 49%. When divided into early- and late-stage tumors, they report a DFS for T1 and T2 tumors of 67%, and for T3 and T4 tumors the DFS is 41% [33].

Several factors have been found to affect DFS: positive margins [46], dura mater involvement [113], facial nerve sacrifice [16, 113], direction of spread in T4 tumors (anterior vs all other directions) [113], pathologic tumor grade [39, 113], Pittsburgh staging [5, 106, 130], and positive lymph nodes [64]. In a multivariate analysis, only dura mater involvement and nodal status were found to be independent factors affecting DFS [113].

Factors not associated with DFS include parotidectomy, neck dissection, and postoperative radiotherapy [113]. Essig et al. found that preoperative facial nerve palsy was not significantly correlated with disease-free survival [130]. Lobo et al. found that tumor histology did not make a significant difference in disease-free survival, but their study had only 19 patients [64].

Disease-Specific Survival

Disease-specific survival (DSS) is measured from the date of diagnosis until the last follow-up. The reported 5-year DSS for SCC of the temporal bone is 19–68% [5, 7, 8, 33, 46, 67, 175]. Mazzoni et al. further divided survival data based on early- and late-stage tumors. They found a DSS for T1 and T2 tumors of 92%, and for T3 and T4 tumors, the DSS is 48% [33]. Large tumors (Pittsburgh stage 3 and 4) have disease-specific survival ranging from 18% to 65% [69].

Several factors have been found to affect DSS: positive margins [46, 130], dura mater involvement [46, 113], facial nerve involvement or nerve sacrifice [46, 67, 113], direction of spread in T4 tumors (anterior vs all other directions) [113], pathologic tumor grade [113], Pittsburgh T stage [46, 67, 130], erosion of the medial wall of the middle ear [46], jugular bulb invasion [46], and TMJ invasion [46].

Higgins and Moody-Antonio performed a systemic review assessing 348 patients with temporal bone squamous cell carcinoma and found that DSS and overall survival were much worse for patients presenting with facial palsy compared to patients without facial weakness [67].

Factors not associated with DSS include parotidectomy, neck dissection, and postoperative radiotherapy [113]. Masterson et al. found that salvage surgery and brain involvement were not significant factors for disease-specific survival [47]. Essig et al. found that preoperative facial nerve palsy was not a significant correlation to disease-specific survival [130].

Bacciu et al. in a multivariate analysis found that only dural involvement was an independent predictor of DSS [46].

Zanoletti et al. found a significant difference in disease-free survival (DFS) based on the clinical and pathologic PSS by T stage, by lymph node involvement, and pathologic tumor grade [113].

Future Directions

Biomarkers

The family of signal transducers and activators of transcription (STAT) convey signals from extracellular stimuli and are important in inflammation, cell survival, differentiation, and proliferation. STAT3 has an important role in cancer development as an oncogene. STAT3 has been reported in head and neck cancers; however, STAT3 showed no significant correlation with survival in patients with temporal bone SCC [176].

Marioni et al. explored the expression of maspin in 29 archived squamous cell carcinomas of the temporal bone to determine patterns of recurrence and survival rates [106]. Cytoplasmic maspin (mammary serine protease inhibitor) is a tumor-suppressor protein. Their research found higher levels of maspin in patients who did not have a recurrence of SCCa of the temporal bone cancer. Additionally, they found that nuclear localization of maspin was also associated with significantly longer DFS [106].

Since bone invasion is an important prognostic factor for SCC of the temporal bone, Sugimoto et al. explored the factors that are responsible for epithelial-mesenchymal transition (EMT) [177]. EMT is determined based on histopathology. Their research showed an increase in vimentin expression in areas of bone invasion. They opined that increased EMT expression on biopsy might be a biomarker of propensity for bony invasion and thus a sign of poor prognosis.

Verrucous Carcinoma

Verrucous carcinoma is a variant of squamous cell carcinoma that is frequently seen in the oral cavity and larynx and only rarely has it been reported in the ear canal and temporal bone. To date, there have been only 18 cases reported in the English literature (Fig. 7.6) [178–182].

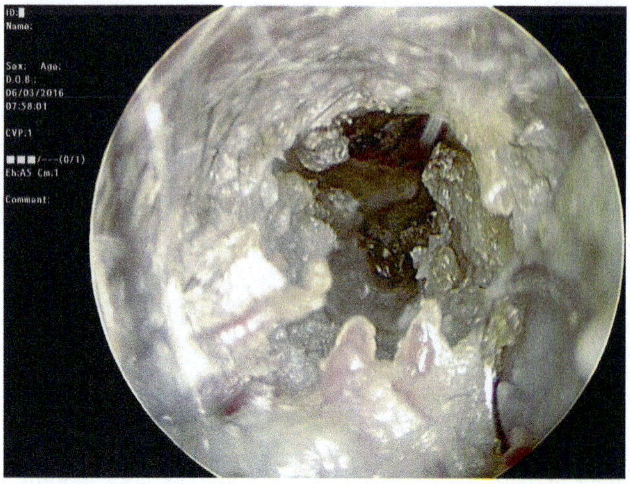

Fig. 7.6 Verrucous carcinoma of the ear canal. This tumor was staged as T1 and excised with lateral temporal bone resection. Postoperative radiotherapy was not indicated

Unlike SCC, chronic irritation and smoking seem to be causally linked to the development of verrucous carcinoma [180]. Long-term, chronic (more than 60 years in one case [181]) otorrhea has been reported in a majority of cases.

Diagnosis can be delayed due to the benign appearance of biopsy material [180]. A superficial biopsy might only show a well-differentiated, extensively keratinizing squamous epithelium with blunt pushing margins and without cytological atypias microscopically [182]. Macroscopically, these tumors are superficially growing and fungating, papillomatous masses with well-demarcated borders. Multiple biopsies paired with clinically invasive behavior help to formulate the diagnosis [180, 182].

This tumor can be widely invasive throughout the temporal bone, including the petrous apex; however, the bony labyrinth, the facial canal, and the internal auditory canal can be spared from destruction [181]. This tumor type does not metastasize either to regional lymph nodes or distantly.

Surgical excision is the primary treatment modality. The goal of achieving negative margins is emphasized for this tumor type, since adjuvant therapy has not improved outcomes.

The role of radiotherapy is controversial. Earlier reports indicated a potential dedifferentiation of tumor with radiation; however, more recent reports do not support this claim [182]. Radiotherapy was not helpful in preventing recurrences in patients with late-stage disease [178].

Radiation and chemotherapy have been linked with poorer prognosis, but this might be due to disease presenting at a later stage. For an inoperable tumor, chemotherapy consisting of vinblastine (2 mg/12 h IV, day 1), methotrexate (50 mg/8 h IV, day 2), and bleomycin (15 mg/6 h IV, days 2 and 3) as induction followed by three cycles with radiation (64 Gy in 2 Gy daily fractions) produced long-term survivor in one case [182].

Fully one-third of patients die within a year of diagnosis [180]. A few patients are reported to have long-term survival (4–10 years) [178]. These patients had complete resection of the tumor with negative margins and were treated with surgery alone. With such few cases reported, survival data is largely lacking.

Basal Cell Cancer

BCC of the ear canal and temporal bone is much rarer than SCC, but it represents the second most common tumor of the ear canal [8, 10, 12, 13, 118, 135, 137, 183, 184].

BCC also tends to have a better overall survival and prognosis than SCC [83, 88]. While the Pittsburgh staging system was devised for squamous cell carcinoma of the temporal bone, it has been applied to other tumor histologies that affect this site [118]. Beyond stage 1 and 2, Testa et al. demonstrate that SCC has a significantly worse prognosis than similar staged BCC.

BCC has a propensity for recurrence, even with negative margins. Vandeweyer et al. reported results of six patients with BCCa of the external canal. Their patients presented with local recurrences even after radical surgery with negative margins; therefore, they considered BCCa an aggressive tumor with a poor prognosis [185].

Gaudet reports three patients with extensive periauricular BCCa [83]. Their study indicated that BCCa could be managed with surgery alone, but none of their patients had high-risk pathologic features.

In the MD Anderson series of temporal bone cancers, 42 patients had BCC involving the ear canal. The mean age was 67 years, and 83% were men. The most common presenting symptoms were hearing loss (36%) and otorrhea (26%). Recurrent lesions accounted for 60% of this patient population [186]. The tumor was confined to the cartilaginous canal in 52%. The bony ear canal was involved in 29%. Two patients (5%) had disease in the middle ear. Disease extended into the parenchyma of the parotid gland in 38%. Two patients developed regional nodal disease. Ten patients were able to be managed with wide local excision of the external auditory meatus and were reconstructed with a split thickness skin graft (Fig. 7.7). The remainder required lateral temporal bone resection, usually with total auriculectomy for advanced disease.

Parotidectomy was performed in 26 patients, and 62% of these patients had either direct tumor extension or metastatic disease within the gland (Fig. 7.8). Metastatic disease was only found in intraparotid and level II lymph nodes.

Fifty-five percent (55%) of patients received postoperative radiotherapy as indicated by recurrent tumor, perineural invasion, metastatic disease, or bony invasion.

The 5-year disease-specific survival was 100% with an overall survival of 84% and a 5-year disease-free survival of 77%.

Vismodegib, a hedgehog pathway inhibitor, can be used for locally advanced and metastatic basal cell carcinoma. This drug is especially useful for patients with basal cell nevus syndrome. This drug, however, does not produce durable disease remission. Surgical resection and radiotherapy are usually required for definitive treatment.

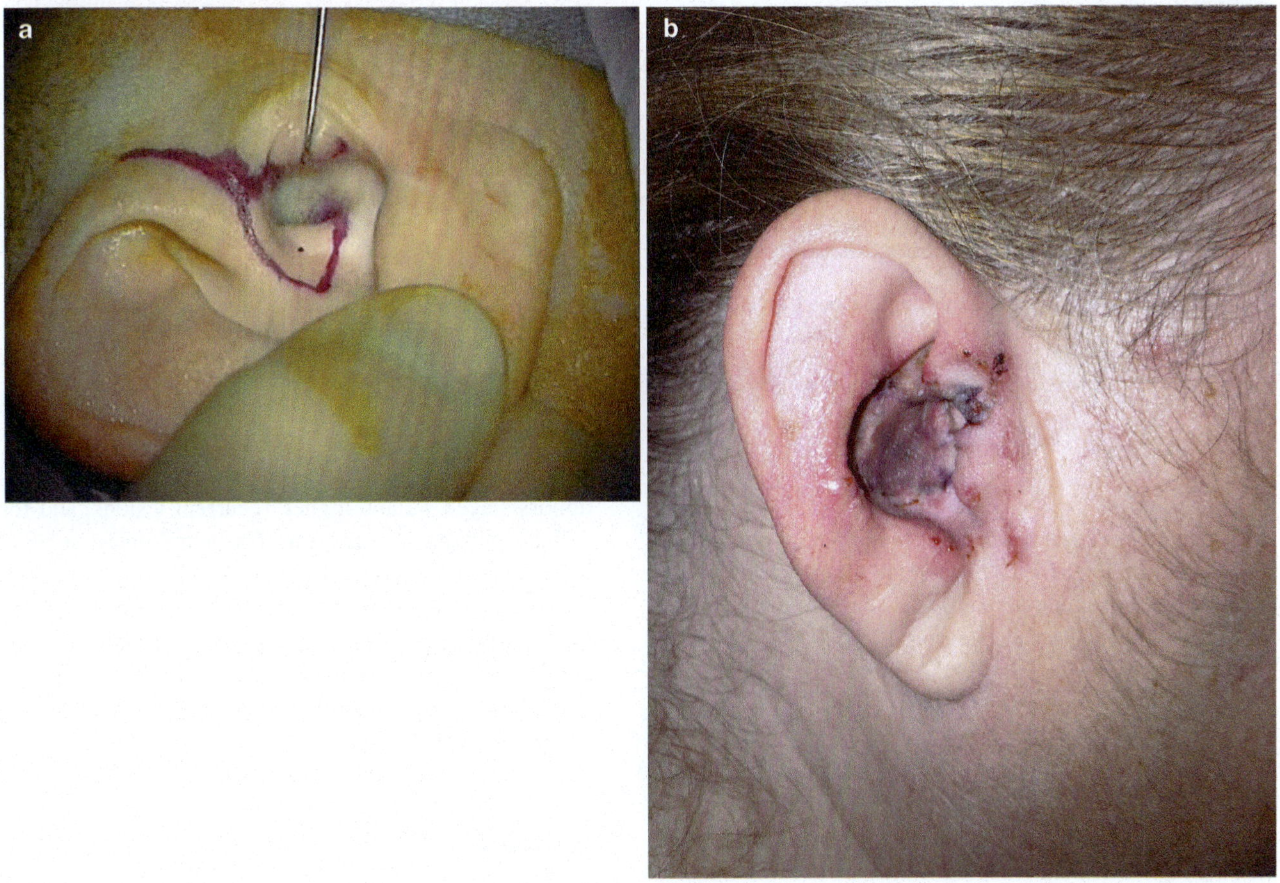

Fig. 7.7 Recurrent BCC of the right ear canal. (**a**) Endaural incision is performed to help with visualizing the ear canal portion. Additional tissues laterally and inferiorly were taken to achieve a final negative margin. (**b**) Nine days postoperative view of split thickness skin graft

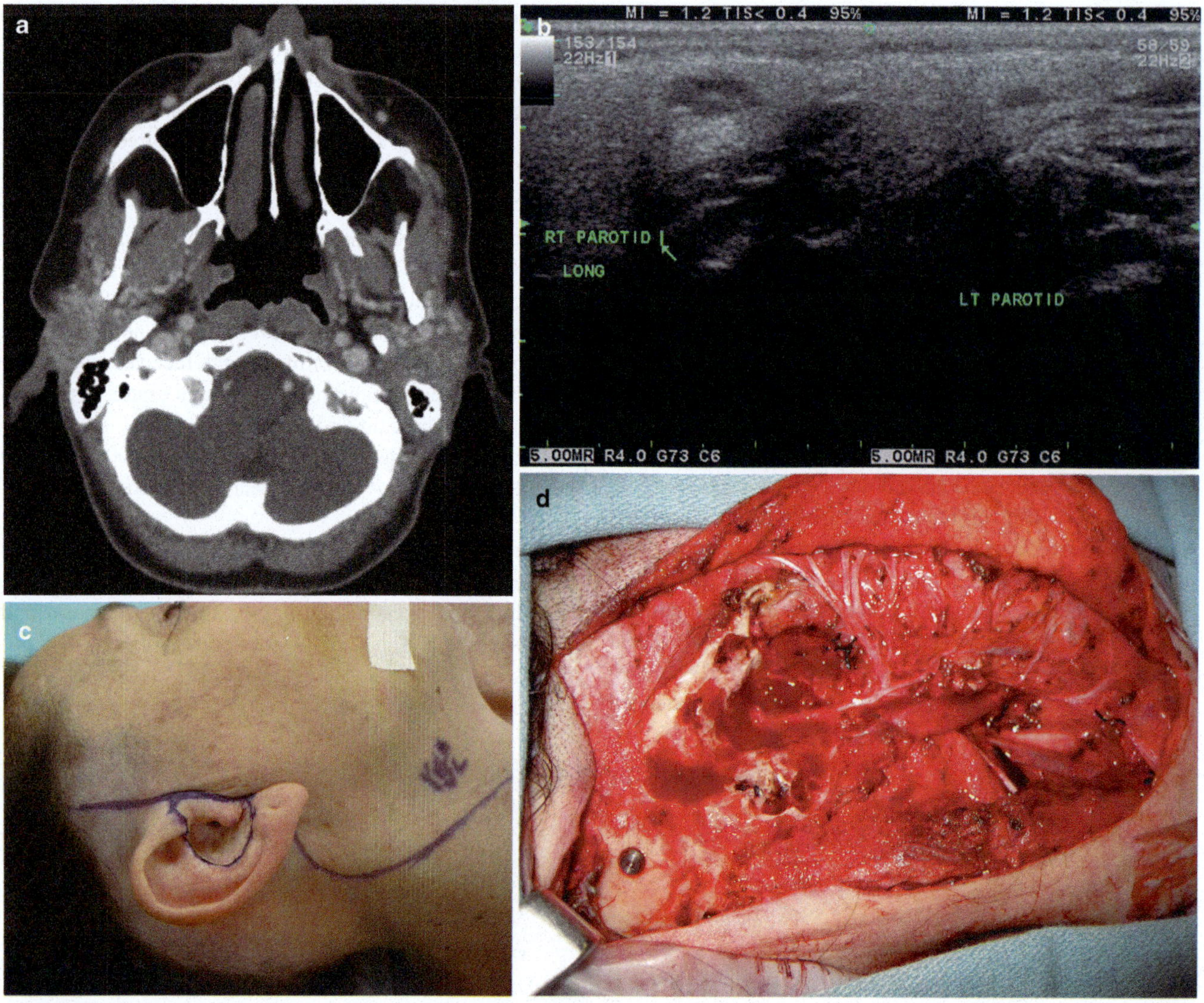

Fig. 7.8 Multiply recurrent BCC of the right ear. Lateral temporal bone resection was required. Final pathology revealed extensive perineural disease and metastatic lymph nodes in the parotid gland. (**a**) Preoperative CT showing disease within the right parotid gland. (**b**) Ultrasound-guided FNA confirmed BCC in the parotid. (**c**) Incisions marked. (**d**) Surgical defect following for lateral temporal bone resection, parotidectomy, and neck dissection. Osseointegrated implant is placed. Reconstruction performed with microvascular free flap

Conclusion

Squamous cell carcinoma is the most common malignant tumor of the ear canal, middle ear, and temporal bone. Basal cell carcinoma is the second most common tumor of the ear canal. Hearing loss, otalgia, and otorrhea are the classic triad of symptoms; however, this combination is seen in only 10% of cases. Squamous cell carcinoma of the ear canal is often mistaken for otitis externa or media until biopsy is performed, confirming the diagnosis. Cross-sectional imaging, either CT, MRI, or both, is required to evaluate the extent of disease. The Pittsburgh staging system is used, and it is a reliable predictor of survival. Surgery is the primary treatment for these tumors, especially for early-stage disease. Postoperative radiotherapy is indicated for tumors staged T2 and higher, recurrent lesions, and for patients with positive margins, perineural invasion, bone invasion, and lymph node metastasis. Preoperative chemotherapy and radiotherapy (CRT) has an emerging role for late-stage (T3 and T4) disease. The survival for temporal bone cancer has improved over the last 50 years, but overall survival still remains relatively low for advanced-stage disease.

References

1. Zanoletti E, Marioni G, Franchella S, Lovato A, Giacomelli L, Martini A, et al. Recurrent squamous cell carcinoma of the temporal bone: critical analysis of cases with a poor prognosis. Am J Otolaryngol. 2015;36(3):352–5.

2. Jia X, Liang Q, Chi F. Treatment and outcome of middle ear cancer. Eur Arch Otorhinolaryngol. 2014;271(10):2675–80.
3. Gidley PW, Thompson CR, Roberts DB, DeMonte F, Hanna EY. The oncology of otology. Laryngoscope. 2012;122(2):393–400.
4. Morris LG, Mehra S, Shah JP, Bilsky MH, Selesnick SH, Kraus DH. Predictors of survival and recurrence after temporal bone resection for cancer. Head Neck. 2012;34(9):1231–9.
5. Gidley PW, Roberts DB, Sturgis EM. Squamous cell carcinoma of the temporal bone. Laryngoscope. 2010;120(6):1144–51.
6. Chang CH, Shu MT, Lee JC, Leu YS, Chen YC, Lee KS. Treatments and outcomes of malignant tumors of external auditory canal. Am J Otolaryngol. 2009;30(1):44–8.
7. Martinez-Devesa P, Barnes ML, Milford CA. Malignant tumors of the ear and temporal bone: a study of 27 patients and review of their management. Skull Base. 2008;18(1):1–8.
8. Madsen AR, Gundgaard MG, Hoff CM, Maare C, Holmboe P, Knap M, et al. Cancer of the external auditory canal and middle ear in Denmark from 1992 to 2001. Head Neck. 2008;30(10):1332–8.
9. Moore MG, Deschler DG, McKenna MJ, Varvares MA, Lin DT. Management outcomes following lateral temporal bone resection for ear and temporal bone malignancies. Otolaryngol Head Neck Surg. 2007;137(6):893–8.
10. Schmerber S, Righini C, Soriano E, Delalande C, Dumas G, Reyt E, et al. The outcome of treatments for carcinoma of the external auditory canal. Rev Laryngol Otol Rhinol (Bord). 2005;126(3):165–70.
11. Kollert M, Draf W, Minovi A, Hofmann E, Bockmuhl U. Carcinoma of the external auditory canal and middle ear: therapeutic strategy and follow up. Laryngorhinootologie. 2004;83(12):818–23.
12. Nyrop M, Grontved A. Cancer of the external auditory canal. Arch Otolaryngol Head Neck Surg. 2002;128(7):834–7.
13. Breau RL, Gardner EK, Dornhoffer JL. Cancer of the external auditory canal and temporal bone. Curr Oncol Rep. 2002;4(1):76–80.
14. Manolidis S, Pappas D Jr, Von Doersten P, Jackson CG, Glasscock ME 3rd. Temporal bone and lateral skull base malignancy: experience and results with 81 patients. Am J Otol. 1998;19(6 Suppl):S1–15.
15. Ito M, Hatano M, Yoshizaki T. Prognostic factors for squamous cell carcinoma of the temporal bone: extensive bone involvement or extensive soft tissue involvement? Acta Otolaryngol. 2009;129(11):1313–9.
16. Lassig AA, Spector ME, Soliman S, El-Kashlan HK. Squamous cell carcinoma involving the temporal bone: lateral temporal bone resection as primary intervention. Otol Neurotol. 2013;34(1):141–50.
17. Furstenberg AC. XLII. Primary adenocarcinoma of the middle ear and mastoid. Ann Otol Rhinol Laryngol. 1924;33(3):677–89.
18. Tabb HG, Komet H, McLaurin JW. Cancer of the external auditory canal: treatment with radical mastoidectomy and irradiation. Laryngoscope. 1964;74:634–43.
19. Lodge WO, Jones HM, Smith ME. Malignant tumors of the temporal bone. AMA Arch Otolaryngol. 1955;61(5):535–41.
20. Morton RP, Stell PM, Derrick PP. Epidemiology of cancer of the middle ear cleft. Cancer. 1984;53(7):1612–7.
21. Tucker WN. Cancer of the middle ear; a review of 89 cases. Cancer. 1965;18:642–50.
22. Kenyon GS, Marks PV, Scholtz CL, Dhillon R. Squamous cell carcinoma of the middle ear. A 25-year retrospective study. Ann Otol Rhinol Laryngol. 1985;94(3):273–7.
23. Arena S, Keen M. Carcinoma of the middle ear and temporal bone. Am J Otol. 1988;9(5):351–6.
24. Chee G, Mok P, Sim R. Squamous cell carcinoma of the temporal bone: diagnosis, treatment and prognosis. Singap Med J. 2000;41(9):441–6. 51
25. Lo WC, Ting LL, Ko JY, Lou PJ, Yang TL, Chang YL, et al. Malignancies of the ear in irradiated patients of nasopharyngeal carcinoma. Laryngoscope. 2008;118(12):2151–5.
26. Gurgel RK, Karnell LH, Hansen MR. Middle ear cancer: a population-based study. Laryngoscope. 2009;119(10):1913–7.
27. McRackan TR, Fang TY, Pelosi S, Rivas A, Dietrich MS, Wanna GB, et al. Factors associated with recurrence of squamous cell carcinoma involving the temporal bone. Ann Otol Rhinol Laryngol. 2014;123(4):235–9.
28. al-Shihabi BA. Carcinoma of temporal bone presenting as malignant otitis externa. J Laryngol Otol. 1992;106(10):908–10.
29. Grandis JR, Hirsch BE, Yu VL. Simultaneous presentation of malignant external otitis and temporal bone cancer. Arch Otolaryngol Head Neck Surg. 1993;119(6):687–9.
30. Yin M, Ishikawa K, Honda K, Arakawa T, Harabuchi Y, Nagabashi T, et al. Analysis of 95 cases of squamous cell carcinoma of the external and middle ear. Auris Nasus Larynx. 2006;33(3):251–7.
31. Coachman EH. Squamous cell carcinoma secondary to cholesteatoma. AMA Arch Otolaryngol. 1951;54(2):187.
32. Issing PR, Kempf HG, Schonermark M, Lenarz T. Carcinoma of the temporal bone – current diagnostic and therapeutic aspects. Laryngorhinootologie. 1995;74(11):666–72.
33. Mazzoni A, Danesi G, Zanoletti E. Primary squamous cell carcinoma of the external auditory canal: surgical treatment and long-term outcomes. Acta Otorhinolaryngol Ital. 2014;34(2):129–37.
34. Monem SA, Moffat DA, Frampton MC. Carcinoma of the ear: a case report of a possible association with chlorinated disinfectants. J Laryngol Otol. 1999;113(11):1004–7.
35. Meiteles LZ, Conley JJ. Squamous cell carcinoma of the temporal bone arising 43 years after fenestration procedure. Am J Otol. 1993;14(5):512–4.
36. Adams WS, Morrison R. On primary carcinoma of the middle ear and mastoid; its incidence, etiological factors and clinical course, with the results of treatment by surgery and radiotherapy. J Laryngol Otol. 1955;69(2):115–31.
37. Conley J. Cancer of the middle ear. Ann Otol Rhinol Laryngol. 1965;74:555–72.
38. Savic DL, Djeric DR. Malignant tumours of the middle ear. Clin Otolaryngol Allied Sci. 1991;16(1):87–9.
39. Moffat DA, Wagstaff SA, Hardy DG. The outcome of radical surgery and postoperative radiotherapy for squamous carcinoma of the temporal bone. Laryngoscope. 2005;115(2):341–7.
40. Atallah I, Karkas A, Righini CA, Lantuejoul S, Schmerber S. Rare case study of a primary carcinoma of the petrous bone and a brief literature review. Head Neck. 2015;37(4):E45–8.
41. Michaels L, Wells M. Squamous cell carcinoma of the middle ear. Clin Otolaryngol Allied Sci. 1980;5(4):235–48.
42. Bradley WH, Maxwell JH. Neoplasms of the middle ear and mastoid. Report of fifty-four cases. Laryngoscope. 1954;64(7):533-56.
43. Conley J, Schuller DE. Malignancies of the ear. Laryngoscope. 1976;86(8):1147–63.
44. Waldemar E, Sorensen T, Bretlau P, Hansen HS. Cancer in the middle ear and the auditory canal. Ugeskr Laeger. 1995;157(15):2139–42.
45. Zhang B, Tu G, Xu G, Tang P, Hu Y. Squamous cell carcinoma of temporal bone: reported on 33 patients. Head Neck. 1999;21(5):461–6.
46. Bacciu A, Clemente IA, Piccirillo E, Ferrari S, Sanna M. Guidelines for treating temporal bone carcinoma based on long-term outcomes. Otol Neurotol. 2013;34(5):898–907.
47. Masterson L, Rouhani M, Donnelly NP, Tysome JR, Patel P, Jefferies SJ, et al. Squamous cell carcinoma of the temporal bone: clinical outcomes from radical surgery and postoperative radiotherapy. Otol Neurotol. 2014;35(3):501–8.
48. Chi FL, Gu FM, Dai CF, Chen B, Li HW. Survival outcomes in surgical treatment of 72 cases of squamous cell carcinoma of the temporal bone. Otol Neurotol. 2011;32(4):665–9.
49. Lewis JS. Squamous carcinoma of the ear. Arch Otolaryngol. 1973;97(1):41–2.
50. Hu XD, Wu TT, Zhou SH. Squamous cell carcinoma of the middle ear: report of three cases. Int J Clin Exp Med. 2015;8(2):2979–84.

51. Vikram B, Saimanohar S, Narayanaswamy G. Is squamous cell carcinoma of middle ear a complication of chronic suppurative otitis media. Internet J Otolaryngol. 2007;6:10.
52. Aoki H, Matsumoto K. A case of squamous-cell carcinoma originating in external auditory canal cholesteatoma. J Nippon Med Sch. 2003;70(4):363–6.
53. Tsai ST, Li C, Jin YT, Chao WY, Su IJ. High prevalence of human papillomavirus types 16 and 18 in middle-ear carcinomas. Int J Cancer. 1997;71(2):208–12.
54. Marioni G, Altavilla G, Busatto G, Blandamura S, De Filippis C, Staffieri A. Detection of human papillomavirus in temporal bone inverted papilloma by polymerase chain reaction. Acta Otolaryngol. 2003;123(3):367–71.
55. Jin Y, Tsai S, Li C, Chang K, Yan J, Chao W, et al. Prevalence of human papillomavirus in middle ear carcinoma associated with chronic otitis media. Am J Pathol. 1997;150(4):1327–33.
56. Bergmann K, Hoppe F, He Y, Helms J, Muller-Hermelink HK, Stremlau A, et al. Human-papillomavirus DNA in cholesteatomas. Int J Cancer. 1994;59(4):463–6.
57. Masterson L, Winder D, Marker A, Sterling JC, Sudhoff H, Moffat D, et al. Investigating the role of human papillomavirus in squamous cell carcinoma of the temporal bone. Head Neck Oncol. 2013;5(2):22–9.
58. Aub JC, Evans RD, Hempelmann LH, Martland HS. The late effects of internally-deposited radioactive materials in man. Medicine. 1952;31(3):221–329.
59. Beal DD, Lindsay JR, Ward PH. Radiation-induced carcinoma of the mastoid. Arch Otolaryngol. 1965;81:9–16.
60. Lambert EM, Garden AS, DeMonte F, Roberts DB, Gidley PW. Radiation-associated malignancies of the ear canal and temporal bone. Laryngoscope. 2015;125(5):1198–204.
61. Ruben RJ, Thaler SU, Holzer N. Radiation induced carcinoma of the temporal bone. Laryngoscope. 1977;87(10 Pt 1):1613–21.
62. Lustig LR, Jackler RK, Lanser MJ. Radiation-induced tumors of the temporal bone. Am J Otol. 1997;18(2):230–5.
63. Goh YH, Chong VF, Low WK. Temporal bone tumours in patients irradiated for nasopharyngeal neoplasm. J Laryngol Otol. 1999;113(3):222–8.
64. Lobo D, Llorente JL, Suarez C. Squamous cell carcinoma of the external auditory canal. Skull Base. 2008;18(3):167–72.
65. Elsurer C, Senkal HA, Zayyan E, Yilmaz T, Kaya S. Bilateral external auditory canal squamous cell carcinoma: a case report. Eur Arch Otorhinolaryngol. 2007;264(8):941–5.
66. Cristalli G, Manciocco V, Pichi B, Marucci L, Arcangeli G, Telera S, et al. Treatment and outcome of advanced external auditory canal and middle ear squamous cell carcinoma. J Craniofac Surg. 2009;20(3):816–21.
67. Higgins TS, Antonio SA. The role of facial palsy in staging squamous cell carcinoma of the temporal bone and external auditory canal: a comparative survival analysis. Otol Neurotol. 2010;31(9):1473–9.
68. Moody SA, Hirsch BE, Myers EN. Squamous cell carcinoma of the external auditory canal: an evaluation of a staging system. Am J Otol. 2000;21(4):582–8.
69. Lionello M, Stritoni P, Facciolo MC, Staffieri A, Martini A, Mazzoni A, et al. Temporal bone carcinoma. Current diagnostic, therapeutic, and prognostic concepts. J Surg Oncol. 2014;110(4):383–92.
70. Gillespie MB, Francis HW, Chee N, Eisele DW. Squamous cell carcinoma of the temporal bone: a radiographic-pathologic correlation. Arch Otolaryngol Head Neck Surg. 2001;127(7):803–7.
71. Dong F, Gidley PW, Ho T, Luna MA, Ginsberg LE, Sturgis EM. Adenoid cystic carcinoma of the external auditory canal. Laryngoscope. 2008;118(9):1591–6.
72. Zhang T, Dai C, Wang Z. The misdiagnosis of external auditory canal carcinoma. Eur Arch Otorhinolaryngol. 2013;270(5):1607–13.
73. Gacek MR, Gacek RR, Gantz B, McKenna M, Goodman M. Pseudoepitheliomatous hyperplasia versus squamous cell carcinoma of the external auditory canal. Laryngoscope. 1998;108(4 Pt 1):620–3.
74. Lim LH, Goh YH, Chan YM, Chong VF, Low WK. Malignancy of the temporal bone and external auditory canal. Otolaryngol Head Neck Surg. 2000;122(6):882–6.
75. Miah MS, Crawford M, White SJ, Hussain SS. Malignant transformation from benign papillomatosis of the external auditory canal. Otol Neurotol. 2012;33(4):643–7.
76. Nelson EG, Hinojosa R. Histopathology of metastatic temporal bone tumors. Arch Otolaryngol Head Neck Surg. 1991;117(2):189–93.
77. Sahin AA, Ro JY, Ordonez NG, Luna MA, Weber RS, Ayala AG. Temporal bone involvement by prostatic adenocarcinoma: report of two cases and review of the literature. Head Neck. 1991;13(4):349–54.
78. Cureoglu S, Tulunay O, Ferlito A, Schachern PA, Paparella MM, Rinaldo A. Otologic manifestations of metastatic tumors to the temporal bone. Acta Otolaryngol. 2004;124(10):1117–23.
79. Bakhos D, Chenebaux M, Lescanne E, Lauvin MA, Cormier B, Robier A. Two cases of temporal bone metastases as presenting sign of lung cancer. Eur Ann Otorhinolaryngol Head Neck Dis. 2012;129(1):54–7.
80. Gisselsson L. Squamous cell carcinoma of the tympanic membrane. Laryngoscope. 1952;62(7):736-40.
81. Somers T, Vercruysse JP, Goovaerts G, Govaerts P, Offeciers E. Isolated squamous cell carcinoma of the tympanic membrane. Otol Neurotol. 2002;23(5):808.
82. de Zoysa N, Stephens J, Mochloulis GM, Kothari PB. Persistent otorrhoea with an abnormal tympanic membrane secondary to squamous cell carcinoma of the tympanic membrane. J Laryngol Otol. 2011;125(3):318–20.
83. Gaudet JE, Walvekar RR, Arriaga MA, Dileo MD, Nuss DW, Pou AM, et al. Applicability of the Pittsburgh staging system for advanced cutaneous malignancy of the temporal bone. Skull Base. 2010;20(6):409–14.
84. Juby H. Bilateral malignant disease of the middle ear. J Laryngol Otol. 1957;71(10):700–2.
85. Hakata H, Ohashi T, Suzuki T. Bilateral carcinoma of the ears. Report of a case. Arch Otolaryngol. 1976;102(2):112–4.
86. Lederman J. Malignant tumors of the ear. J Laryngol Otol. 1965;79:85–119.
87. Schmidt PH, Verdonk GJ. Bilateral carcinoma of the ear. J Laryngol Otol. 1967;81(5):567–9.
88. Goodwin WJ, Jesse RH. Malignant neoplasms of the external auditory canal and temporal bone. Arch Otolaryngol. 1980;106(11):675–9.
89. Brookes GB. Bilateral middle ear carcinomas associated with Waldenström's Macroglobulinemia. Ann Otol Rhinol Laryngol. 1982;91(3):299–303.
90. Milford C, Violaris N. Bilateral carcinoma of the middle ear. J Laryngol Otol. 1987;101(07):711–3.
91. Fontanel J, Klossek J, Chauveau J, Daban A, de Larrard J, Babin P. Epidermoid carcinoma of the external auditory canal. Rev Laryngol Otol Rhinol. 1988;110(1):13–5.
92. Snyman J, Claasen A. Bilateral middle-ear squamous cell carcinoma. S Afr Med J. 1988;74(1):31–2.
93. Carlsoo B, Franzen L, Henriksson R, Lofroth PO, Schmidt SH. Bilateral squamous cell carcinoma of the middle ear. Int J Radiat Oncol Biol Phys. 1990;19(2):506–7.
94. Munk-Nielsen L, Hansen HS. Bilateral carcinoma of the external auditory meatus. J Laryngol Otol. 1991;105(2):112–4.
95. Murray E, Wiltshire C. Synchronous bilateral middle ear carcinoma. Clin Oncol. 1994;6(1):57.
96. Kuhel WI, Hume CR, Selesnick SH. Cancer of the external auditory canal and temporal bone. Otolaryngol Clin N Am. 1996;29(5):827–52.

97. Suzuki K, Takahashi M, Ito Y, Tsuge I, Motai H, Takeichi Y, et al. Bilateral middle ear squamous cell carcinoma and clinical review of an additional 5 cases of middle ear carcinomas. Auris Nasus Larynx. 1999;26(1):33–8.
98. Ohsako H, Haruta A, Tsuboi Y, Matsuura K, Komune S. Bilateral primary carcinoma of the external auditory meatus. Nippon Jibiinkoka Gakkai Kaiho. 2001;104(5):514–7.
99. Takano A, Takasaki K, Kumagami H, Higami Y, Kobayashi T. A case of bilateral middle-ear squamous cell carcinoma. J Laryngol Otol. 2001;115(10):815–8.
100. Knegt PP, Ah-See KW, Meeuwis CA, van der Velden LA, Kerrebijn JD, De Boer MF. Squamous carcinoma of the external auditory canal: a different approach. Clin Otolaryngol Allied Sci. 2002;27(3):183–7.
101. Wolfe SG, Lai SY, Bigelow DC. Bilateral squamous cell carcinoma of the external auditory canals. Laryngoscope. 2002;112(6):1003–5.
102. Thevarajah S, Carew J, Selesnick SH. Bilateral squamous cell carcinoma of the external auditory canal. Otolaryngol Head Neck Surg. 2005;132(6):960–2.
103. Shagdarsuren S, Schwaab M, Kissler M, Lautermann J, Sudhoff H. Bilateral auditory canal squamous cell carcinoma. HNO. 2006;54(1):41–5.
104. Bibas AG, Gleeson MJ. Bilateral squamous cell carcinoma of the temporal bones. Skull Base. 2006;16(4):213–8.
105. Vamvakidis T, Sengas J, Xenellis J. Bilateral carcinoma of the temporal bone: case report and literature review. J Craniomaxillofac Surg. 2010;38(6):473–6.
106. Marioni G, Zanoletti E, Stritoni P, Lionello M, Giacomelli L, Gianatti A, et al. Expression of the tumour-suppressor maspin in temporal bone carcinoma. Histopathology. 2013;63(2):242–9.
107. Leong SC, Youssef A, Lesser TH. Squamous cell carcinoma of the temporal bone: outcomes of radical surgery and postoperative radiotherapy. Laryngoscope. 2013;123(10):2442–8.
108. Stell P. Epithelial tumours of the external auditory meatus and middle ear. In: Booth J, editor. Otology Scott-Brown's otolaryngology, vol. 3. Oxford: Butterworth-Heinemann; 1987. p. 534–45.
109. Moffat DA, Grey P, Ballagh RH, Hardy DG. Extended temporal bone resection for squamous cell carcinoma. Otolaryngol Head Neck Surg. 1997;116(6 Pt 1):617–23.
110. Veness MJ, Palme CE, Smith M, Cakir B, Morgan GJ, Kalnins I. Cutaneous head and neck squamous cell carcinoma metastatic to cervical lymph nodes (nonparotid): a better outcome with surgery and adjuvant radiotherapy. Laryngoscope. 2003;113(10):1827–33.
111. Audet N, Palme CE, Gullane PJ, Gilbert RW, Brown DH, Irish J, et al. Cutaneous metastatic squamous cell carcinoma to the parotid gland: analysis and outcome. Head Neck. 2004;26(8):727–32.
112. Barzilai G, Greenberg E, Cohen-Kerem R, Doweck I. Pattern of regional metastases from cutaneous squamous cell carcinoma of the head and neck. Otolaryngol Head Neck Surg. 2005;132(6):852–6.
113. Zanoletti E, Marioni G, Stritoni P, Lionello M, Giacomelli L, Martini A, et al. Temporal bone squamous cell carcinoma: analyzing prognosis with univariate and multivariate models. Laryngoscope. 2014;124(5):1192–8.
114. Rinaldo A, Ferlito A, Suarez C, Kowalski LP. Nodal disease in temporal bone squamous carcinoma. Acta Otolaryngol. 2005;125(1):5–8.
115. Gidley PW, DeMonte F. Temporal bone malignancies. Neurosurg Clin N Am. 2013;24(1):97–110.
116. Moffat DA, Wagstaff SA. Squamous cell carcinoma of the temporal bone. Curr Opin Otolaryngol Head Neck Surg. 2003;11(2):107–11.
117. Pemberton LS, Swindell R, Sykes AJ. Primary radical radiotherapy for squamous cell carcinoma of the middle ear and external auditory cana – an historical series. Clin Oncol (R Coll Radiol). 2006;18(5):390–4.
118. Testa JR, Fukuda Y, Kowalski LP. Prognostic factors in carcinoma of the external auditory canal. Arch Otolaryngol Head Neck Surg. 1997;123(7):720–4.
119. Arriaga M, Curtin H, Takahashi H, Hirsch BE, Kamerer DB. Staging proposal for external auditory meatus carcinoma based on preoperative clinical examination and computed tomography findings. Ann Otol Rhinol Laryngol. 1990;99(9 Pt 1):714–21.
120. Wang CC. Radiation therapy in the management of carcinoma of the external auditory canal, middle ear, or mastoid. Radiology. 1975;116(3):713–5.
121. Chen KT, Dehner LP. Primary tumors of the external and middle ear. I. Introduction and clinicopathologic study of squamous cell carcinoma. Arch Otolaryngol. 1978;104(5):247–52.
122. Kunst H, Lavieille JP, Marres H. Squamous cell carcinoma of the temporal bone: results and management. Otol Neurotol. 2008;29(4):549–52.
123. Choi JY, Choi EC, Lee HK, Yoo JB, Kim SG, Lee WS. Mode of parotid involvement in external auditory canal carcinoma. J Laryngol Otol. 2003;117(12):951–4.
124. Imhof H, Henk CB, Dirisamer A, Czerny C, Gstottner W. CT and MRI characteristics of tumours of the temporal bone and the cerebello-pontine angle. Radiologe. 2003;43(3):219–26.
125. Hosokawa S, Mizuta K, Takahashi G, Okamura J, Takizawa Y, Hosokawa K, et al. Surgical approach for treatment of carcinoma of the anterior wall of the external auditory canal. Otol Neurotol. 2012;33(3):450–4.
126. Prasad SC, D'Orazio F, Medina M, Bacciu A, Sanna M. State of the art in temporal bone malignancies. Curr Opin Otolaryngol Head Neck Surg. 2014;22(2):154–65.
127. Zhang T, Li W, Dai C, Chi F, Wang S, Wang Z. Evidence-based surgical management of T1 or T2 temporal bone malignancies. Laryngoscope. 2013;123(1):244–8.
128. Leonetti JP, Smith PG, Kletzker GR, Izquierdo R. Invasion patterns of advanced temporal bone malignancies. Am J Otol. 1996;17(3):438–42.
129. Nakagawa T, Kumamoto Y, Natori Y, Shiratsuchi H, Toh S, Kakazu Y, et al. Squamous cell carcinoma of the external auditory canal and middle ear: an operation combined with preoperative chemoradiotherapy and a free surgical margin. Otol Neurotol. 2006;27(2):242–8; discussion 9.
130. Essig GF, Kitipornchai L, Adams F, Zarate D, Gandhi M, Porceddu S, et al. Lateral temporal bone resection in advanced cutaneous squamous cell carcinoma: report of 35 patients. Journal of neurological surgery Part B. Skull base. 2013;74(1):54–9.
131. Clark LJ, Narula AA, Morgan DA, Bradley PJ. Squamous carcinoma of the temporal bone: a revised staging. J Laryngol Otol. 1991;105(5):346–8.
132. Crabtree JA, Britton BH, Pierce MK. Carcinoma of the external auditory canal. Laryngoscope. 1976;86(3):405–15.
133. Kinney SE. Squamous cell carcinoma of the external auditory canal. Am J Otol. 1989;10(2):111–6.
134. Spector JG. Management of temporal bone carcinomas: a therapeutic analysis of two groups of patients and long-term followup. Otolaryngol Head Neck Surg. 1991;104(1):58–66.
135. Shih L, Crabtree JA. Carcinoma of the external auditory canal: an update. Laryngoscope. 1990;100(11):1215–8.
136. Stell PM, McCormick MS. Carcinoma of the external auditory meatus and middle ear. Prognostic factors and a suggested staging system. J Laryngol Otol. 1985;99(9):847–50.
137. Pensak ML, Gleich LL, Gluckman JL, Shumrick KA. Temporal bone carcinoma: contemporary perspectives in the skull base surgical era. Laryngoscope. 1996;106(10):1234–7.
138. Austin JR, Stewart KL, Fawzi N. Squamous cell carcinoma of the external auditory canal. Therapeutic prognosis based on a

proposed staging system. Arch Otolaryngol Head Neck Surg. 1994;120(11):1228–32.
139. Takenaka Y, Cho H, Nakahara S, Yamamoto Y, Yasui T, Inohara H. Chemoradiation therapy for squamous cell carcinoma of the external auditory canal: a meta-analysis. Head Neck. 2015;37(7):1073–80.
140. Prasad S, Janecka IP. Efficacy of surgical treatments for squamous cell carcinoma of the temporal bone: a literature review. Otolaryngol Head Neck Surg. 1994;110(3):270–80.
141. Isipradit P, Wadwongtham W, Aeumjaturapat S, Aramwatanapong P. Carcinoma of the external auditory canal. J Med Assoc Thail. 2005;88(1):114–7.
142. Nadol JB Jr, Schuknecht HF. Obliteration of the mastoid in the treatment of tumors of the temporal bone. Ann Otol Rhinol Laryngol. 1984;93(1 Pt 1):6–12.
143. Medina JE, Park AO, Neely JG, Britton BH. Lateral temporal bone resections. Am J Surg. 1990;160(4):427–33.
144. Okada T, Saito K, Takahashi M, Hasegawa Y, Fujimoto Y, Terada A, et al. En bloc petrosectomy for malignant tumors involving the external auditory canal and middle ear: surgical methods and long-term outcome. J Neurosurg. 2008;108(1):97–104.
145. Gacek RR, Goodman M. Management of malignancy of the temporal bone. Laryngoscope. 1977;87(10 Pt 1):1622–34.
146. Li W, Zhang T, Dai C. Temporal bone malignancies involving the jugular foramen: diagnosis and management. ORL J Otorhinolaryngol Relat Spec. 2014;76(4):227–35.
147. Renton JP, Wetmore SJ. Split-thickness skin grafting in postmastoidectomy revision and in lateral temporal bone resection. Otolaryngol Head Neck Surg. 2006;135(3):387–91.
148. Hanasono MM, Silva A, Skoracki RJ, Gidley PW, DeMonte F, Hanna EY, et al. Skull base reconstruction: an updated approach. Plast Reconstr Surg. 2011;128(3):675–86.
149. Hanasono MM, Silva AK, Yu P, Skoracki RJ, Sturgis EM, Gidley PW. Comprehensive management of temporal bone defects after oncologic resection. Laryngoscope. 2012;122(12):2663–9.
150. Gidley PW, Herrera SJ, Hanasono MM, Yu P, Skoracki R, Roberts DB, et al. The impact of radiotherapy on facial nerve repair. Laryngoscope. 2010;120(10):1985–9.
151. Wax MK, Kaylie DM. Does a positive neural margin affect outcome in facial nerve grafting? Head Neck. 2007;29(6):546–9.
152. Nader ME, Beadle BM, Roberts DB, Gidley PW. Outcomes and complications of osseointegrated hearing aids in irradiated temporal bones. Laryngoscope. 2015;126:1187–92.
153. Birzgalis AR, Keith AO, Farrington WT. Radiotherapy in the treatment of middle ear and mastoid carcinoma. Clin Otolaryngol Allied Sci. 1992;17(2):113–6.
154. Hashi N, Shirato H, Omatsu T, Kagei K, Nishioka T, Hashimoto S, et al. The role of radiotherapy in treating squamous cell carcinoma of the external auditory canal, especially in early stages of disease. Radiother Oncol. 2000;56(2):221–5.
155. Ogawa K, Nakamura K, Hatano K, Uno T, Fuwa N, Itami J, et al. Treatment and prognosis of squamous cell carcinoma of the external auditory canal and middle ear: a multi-institutional retrospective review of 87 patients. Int J Radiat Oncol Biol Phys. 2007;68(5):1326–34.
156. Prabhu R, Hinerman RW, Indelicato DJ, Morris CG, Werning JW, Vaysberg M, et al. Squamous cell carcinoma of the external auditory canal: long-term clinical outcomes using surgery and external-beam radiotherapy. Am J Clin Oncol. 2009;32(4):401–4.
157. Bibas AG, Ward V, Gleeson MJ. Squamous cell carcinoma of the temporal bone. J Laryngol Otol. 2008;122(11):1156–61.
158. Zieske LA, Johnson JT, Myers EN, Thearle PB. Squamous cell carcinoma with positive margins. Surgery and postoperative irradiation. Arch Otolaryngol Head Neck Surg. 1986;112(8):863–6.
159. Kitani Y, Kubota A, Furukawa M, Sato K, Nakayama Y, Nonaka T, et al. Primary definitive radiotherapy with or without chemotherapy for squamous cell carcinoma of the temporal bone. Eur Arch Otorhinolaryngol. 2016;273:1293–8.
160. Figi FA, Hempstead BE. Malignant tumors of the middle ear and the mastoid process. Arch Otolaryngol. 1943;37(2):149–68.
161. Mayer A, Polgar I, Poller I, Thalacker U. The brachytherapy of carcinoma of the external auditory canal. Strahlenther Onkol. 1992;168(3):162–4.
162. Shiga K, Ogawa T, Maki A, Amano M, Kobayashi T. Concomitant chemoradiotherapy as a standard treatment for squamous cell carcinoma of the temporal bone. Skull Base. 2011;21(3):153–8.
163. Shinomiya H, Hasegawa S, Yamashita D, Ejima Y, Kenji Y, Otsuki N, et al. Concomitant chemoradiotherapy for advanced squamous cell carcinoma of the temporal bone. Head Neck. 2016;38:E949–53.
164. Robbins KT, Storniolo A, Kerber C, Seagren S, Berson A, Howell SB. Rapid superselective high-dose cisplatin infusion for advanced head and neck malignancies. Head Neck. 1992;14(5):364–71.
165. Ueda Y, Kurita T, Matsuda Y, Ito S, Nakashima T. Superselective, intra-arterial, rapid infusion chemotherapy for external auditory canal carcinoma. J Laryngol Otol Suppl. 2009;31:75–80.
166. Sugimoto H, Hatano M, Yoshida S, Sakumoto M, Kato H, Ito M, et al. Efficacy of concurrent superselective intra-arterial chemotherapy and radiotherapy for late-stage squamous cell carcinoma of the temporal bone. Clin Otolaryngol. 2015;40(5):500–4.
167. Sugimoto H, Ito M, Yoshida S, Hatano M, Yoshizaki T. Concurrent superselective intra-arterial chemotherapy and radiotherapy for late-stage squamous cell carcinoma of the temporal bone. Ann Otol Rhinol Laryngol. 2011;120(6):372–6.
168. Pfreundner L, Schwager K, Willner J, Baier K, Bratengeier K, Brunner FX, et al. Carcinoma of the external auditory canal and middle ear. Int J Radiat Oncol Biol Phys. 1999;44(4):777–88.
169. Bai Y, Yin J, Zhang L. Adenoid cystic carcinoma of external auditory canal: a report of 7 cases. Lin Chuang Er Bi Yan Hou Ke Za Zhi. 2004;18(4):202–3.
170. Zanoletti E, Danesi G. The problem of nodal disease in squamous cell carcinoma of the temporal bone. Acta Otolaryngol. 2010;130(8):913–6.
171. Conley JJ, Novack AJ. Surgical treatment of cancer of the ear and temporal bone. Trans Am Acad Ophthalmol Otolaryngol. 1960;64:83–92.
172. Lewis JS. Temporal bone resection. Review of 100 cases. Arch Otolaryngol. 1975;101(1):23–5.
173. Xie B, Zhang T, Dai C. Survival outcomes of patients with temporal bone squamous cell carcinoma with different invasion patterns. Head Neck. 2015;37(2):188–96.
174. Zanoletti E, Lovato A, Stritoni P, Martini A, Mazzoni A, Marioni G. A critical look at persistent problems in the diagnosis, staging and treatment of temporal bone carcinoma. Cancer Treat Rev. 2015;41(10):821–6.
175. Barrs DM. Temporal bone carcinoma. Otolaryngol Clin N Am. 2001;34(6):1197–218, x.
176. Marioni G, Nucci R, Marino F, Cappellesso R, Pillon M, Zanoletti E, et al. Evaluation of the prognostic role of pSTAT3 expression in temporal bone squamous cell carcinoma. Otol Neurotol. 2013;34(8):1476–82.
177. Sugimoto H, Ito M, Hatano M, Kondo S, Suzuki S, Yoshizaki T. Roles of epithelial-mesenchymal transition in squamous cell carcinoma of the temporal bone. Otol Neurotol. 2011;32(3):483–7.
178. Miller ME, Martin N, Juillard GF, Bhuta S, Ishiyama A. Temporal bone verrucous carcinoma: outcomes and treatment controversy. Eur Arch Otorhinolaryngol. 2010;267(12):1927–31.
179. Edelstein DR, Smouha E, Sacks SH, Biller HF, Kaneko M, Parisier SC. Verrucous carcinoma of the temporal bone. Ann Otol Rhinol Laryngol. 1986;95(5 Pt 1):447–53.
180. Farrell ML, Dowe AC. Verrucous carcinoma of the temporal bone. Aust N Z J Surg. 1995;65(3):214–6.

181. Hagiwara H, Kanazawa T, Ishikawa K, Fujii T, Kitamura K, Noguchi Y, et al. Invasive verrucous carcinoma: a temporal bone histopathology report. Auris Nasus Larynx. 2000;27(2):179–83.
182. Strojan P, Soba E, Gale N, Auersperg M. Verrucous carcinoma of the temporal bone and maxillary antrum: two unusual presentations of a rare tumor. Onkologie. 2006;29(10):463–8.
183. Gabriele P, Magnano M, Albera R, Canale G, Redda MG, Krengli M, et al. Carcinoma of the external auditory meatus and middle ear. Results of the treatment of 28 cases. Tumori. 1994;80(1):40–3.
184. Dornhoffer JL, Gardner W, Breau RL. Malignancy of the temporal bone: a review of 32 cases at the University of Arkansas for medical sciences. Skull Base. 2001;11(Suppl 2):54–5.
185. Vandeweyer E, Thill MP, Deraemaecker R. Basal cell carcinoma of the external auditory canal. Acta Chir Belg. 2002;102(2):137–40.
186. Breen JT, Roberts DB, Gidley PW. Basal cell carcinoma of the temporal bone and external auditory canal. The Laryngoscope. 2017. doi:10.1002/lary.26785.

Melanoma of the Ear Canal and Temporal Bone

8

Paul W. Gidley

Introduction

Melanoma is a malignant tumor of melanocytes. Melanocytes are derived from neural crest cells and produce the pigment melanin. Melanoma affects the temporal bone both as a primary tumor and as a metastatic tumor. Skin cancer is the most common malignancy in the USA, and it affects nearly two million people annually. Melanoma accounts for just 5% of skin cancers, but it is associated with the highest rate of death. While elderly men are at highest risk, melanoma in the most common cancer in young adults aged 25–29 years [1].

This chapter is dedicated to primary and metastatic melanoma of the ear canal and temporal bone. There is very little literature on primary melanoma of the ear canal. Some papers include melanoma in a series of temporal bone cancer, and one cannot tease out the pertinent facts for melanoma alone [2–4].

Epidemiology

Globally, the incidence of melanoma has increased over the last 50 years [5, 6]. The incidence of melanoma has increased tenfold over this time period. It is estimated by the American Cancer Society that 75,000 persons will be diagnosed with a melanoma in 2016; and roughly 10,000 persons will die from melanoma (www.cancer.org). The estimated lifetime risk of developing melanoma is 1 in 62 [7].

Within the head and neck, the incidence of external ear melanoma has shown the greatest rise. Overall, 14.5% of melanomas occur in the head and neck, and the external ear accounts for 1% of all melanoma cases [7]. The external ear and ear canal account for 7–17% of melanomas in the head and neck [8, 9]. Independent predictors of survival for melanoma include tumor thickness, ulceration, vascular invasion, location, and nodal metastasis; and among locations, the external ear is known for having a particularly poor prognosis [10, 11].

Thankfully, melanoma of the ear canal and middle ear is very infrequent, but the disease has a dire prognosis.

Risk Factors

Sun exposure is the major cause of melanoma, especially in Caucasians [6]. Intermittent, rather than chronic or continuous, sun exposure is most strongly associated with melanoma risk [12]. The physical prominence of the external ear might account for the relative high incidence at that anatomic location, but sun exposure certainly would not explain the occurrence of melanoma within the ear canal or middle ear or Eustachian tube.

Approximately 5–10% of melanoma cases are familial; however, an identifiable germ-line mutation has eluded detection [12]. Skin pigmentation and iris color are both risk factors linked to melanoma. Several genes have been associated with melanoma, including CDKN2A/p16, ARF/p14, CDK4, and CDK6.

Other risk factors for melanoma development include multiple nevi and immunosuppression.

Primary Tumor Location

Primary melanoma can involve the external ear canal, middle ear, inner ear, or cerebellopontine angle [13–15]. External ear melanoma is relatively common compared to the rarity of melanoma in the external ear canal [3, 16]. Conley and Schuller reported melanoma accounted for 43.9% of 187 (82 patients) auricular tumors, 4.9% of 61 (3 patients) ear canal tumors, and 20% of 25 (5 patients) middle ear tumors [3]. They identified two cases of middle ear melanoma where the tumor involved both the middle ear and the "cushion of the

P. W. Gidley, M.D., F.A.C.S.
Department of Head and Neck Surgery, The University of Texas M.D. Anderson Cancer Center, Houston, TX, USA
e-mail: pwgidley@mdanderson.org

P. W. Gidley, F. DeMonte (eds.), *Temporal Bone Cancer*, https://doi.org/10.1007/978-3-319-74539-8_8

Eustachian tube." They remark that this clinical behavior was different from that of SCC of the middle ear and nasopharyngeal carcinoma, which tend to invade the skull base and cause cranial nerve deficits.

Langman et al. reported one case and performed a literature review identifying seven previous cases of external canal melanoma [17], but their report did not include the cases reported by Conley and Schuller. There have been less than a dozen case reports of ear canal melanoma [15, 16, 18–23].

Clinical Presentation

Melanoma of the ear canal is often confused clinically with squamous cell carcinoma, given that SCC is so much more common than melanoma [16]. Symptoms of melanoma of the middle ear include otalgia, otorrhea, aural fullness, and hearing loss [13, 24]. However, these tumors can be relatively symptom-free until they reach late stage [16].

Clinically, melanoma of the ear canal can present as an "inflammatory polyp" or polypoid mass [25–27] or with persistent otorrhea [19, 20]. Additionally patients with melanoma of the ear canal can present with facial palsy or abducens nerve palsy from petrous apex extension [25, 27].

Melanoma of the ear canal can present as a smooth, black mass blocking the ear canal [15, 28]. This mass can be quite friable and bleed easily when touched [19]. These tumors can also be amelanotic (Fig. 8.1). Initially pathology can be misleading and mistaken as inflammatory [20]. The case presented by Hannan et al. presented with cervical node involvement [28].

Benign intradermal nevus arising in the ear canal has been described as a large violaceous, dome-shaped, papillomatous lesion that can block the external canal and underlines the need to biopsy any pigmented lesion within the canal [29].

Less than a dozen cases of middle ear and mastoid melanoma, including a case of amelanotic melanoma, have been described [3, 24, 30–37]. Conley and Schuller appear to be the first to describe malignant melanoma of the middle ear and Eustachian tube [3]. Clinically melanoma of the middle ear presents as serous otitis media; and as the tumor grows, it pushes through the TM and can produce deep pain with otorrhea [35]. In the case of melanoma contained within the middle ear, patients are usually treated with repeated myringotomies and tubes until the tumor grows large enough to be seen or until bleeding occurs from the tumor [30]. Patients can present with involved cervical lymph nodes and disseminated disease, which raises the question of site of origin [35]. Full body evaluation and imaging, nowadays with PET/CT, is necessary to eliminate any other site of origin or involvement. Middle ear exploration shows a darkly pigmented lesion, and biopsy confirms the diagnosis [30, 37]. Despite surgery, radiotherapy, and chemotherapy, patients usually die within 6–12 months of diagnosis [24, 30].

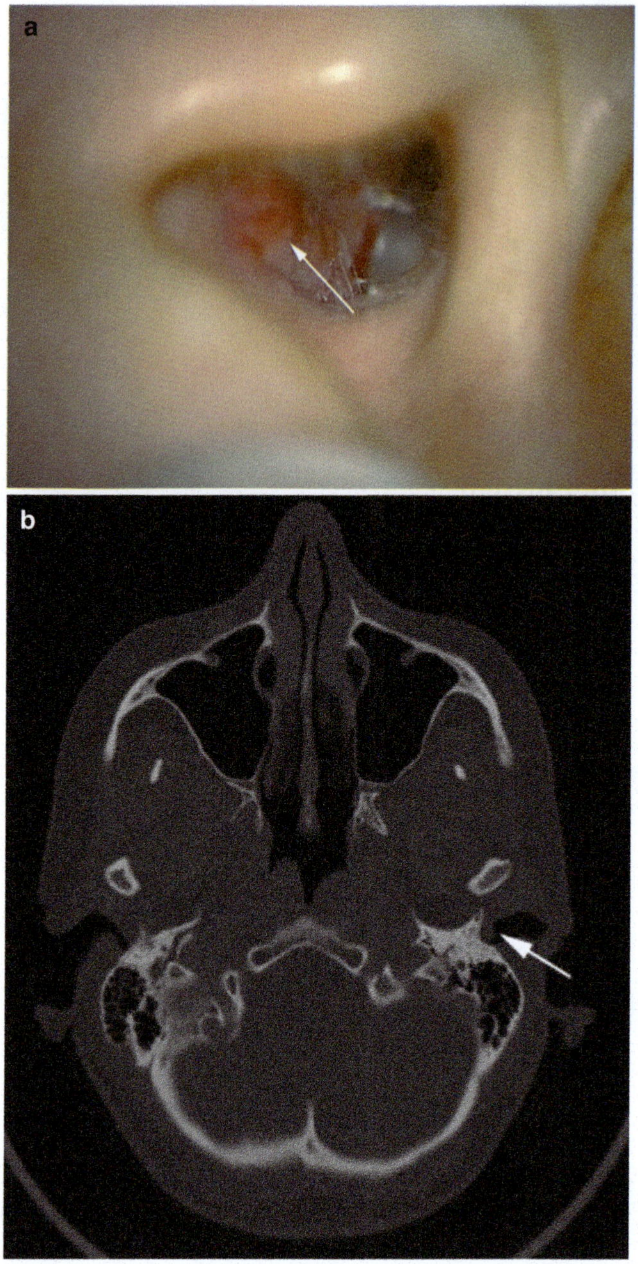

Fig. 8.1 Melanoma of the left ear canal. This 57-year-old woman presented with a 2-month history of itching and drainage from her left ear (**a**, white arrow). Punch biopsy revealed a 3.25 mm thick amelanotic melanoma. CT scan did not show bone erosion or cervical lymphadenopathy (**b**, white arrow points to lesion). She was treated with lateral temporal bone resection and temporalis muscle flap, followed by postoperative radiotherapy (30 Gy in 5 fractions). Pathologic staging pT4bcN0. She did well until 4.5 years later when she developed a left axillary lymph node metastasis. She is currently on pembrolizumab

Only a few cases of melanoma of the Eustachian tube have been reported [3, 38–41]; melanoma of the Eustachian tube needs to be differentiated from melanotic oncocytic metaplasia [42]. Melanoma of the Eustachian tube can present with cervical metastases [39]. Melanoma of the Eustachian tube is usually treated with radiotherapy, which seems to achieve local control. A single case of melanoma of the Eustachian tube has been treated with endoscopic surgery and postoperative radiotherapy [41]. Chemotherapy is used for patients with disseminated disease. Patients usually die of disseminated disease in less than 2 years.

Primary malignant melanoma of the CPA is exceedingly rare, with only a few case reports identified in the literature [14, 43, 44]. However, unilateral CPA metastasis has been described as the presenting sign of malignant melanoma [45].

Desmoplastic neurotropic melanoma (DNM) is an uncommon variant of melanoma that demonstrates properties of Schwann cells and extensive perineural invasion [46, 47]. DNM are often difficult to diagnose since they are often amelanotic. This variant shows an infiltrative growth pattern leading to aggressive local disease and frequent recurrences. Conversely, this variant has a lower rate of regional and distant metastasis and a better overall survival than conventional melanoma. A case of DNM involving the temporal bone as perineural spread has been described [46].

Lymph Node Metastasis

About 15–20% of head and neck patients will develop lymph node metastasis. The lymphatic drainage for melanoma of the external ear is well documented and is predicted to go to the parotid gland and to levels 1–5 [48, 49]. When the parotid gland is involved, the rate of pathologically positive nodes approaches 40% in the clinically negative neck [49]. Occasionally patients will have metastasis to postauricular nodes [48]. In the MD Anderson series, three patients were treated with ear canal melanoma. Only one of these patients presented with involved cervical lymph nodes, and these nodes were in level II (vide infra). However, data on the rate of positive lymph nodes for melanoma of the ear canal or middle ear is lacking in the literature.

Diagnostic Imaging

CT scan is useful to document the extent of disease and bone erosion. CT can underestimate the extent of disease from middle ear melanoma [30, 35]. Melanomas have been invasive of bone where this was not observed on CT imaging [30, 39]. Melanomas on MRI have hyperintense single of T1 and hypointense signal on T2.

Pathology

Melanomas are well known as histological pretenders, especially the amelanotic variants, and they are included in the differential diagnosis of many cutaneous lesions [50]. Several different types of melanoma have been described: superficial spreading, lentiginous, nodular, desmoplastic, and nevoid. The pathologic description of each of these types is beyond the scope of this chapter.

Immunohistochemistry has become critical in the evaluation of melanoma. These tumors are positive for S100, HMB-45, neuron-specific enolase, and vimentin. Amelanotic melanoma can be recognized by their labeling with several determinants, including S100, MART-1, PNL2, and MITF.

Genetic analysis of melanoma is recognized as an important part of pathologic analysis, since new drugs can target particular mutations. BRAF V600 has emerged as a genetic mutation that is an important target for chemotherapy. BRAF mutation has been identified in about 45% of patients with metastatic melanoma [51]. RAS gene mutations have been identified in about 30% of metastatic melanoma. RAS activates the MPK pathway and other pathways. The third most common genetic mutation is the NF1 tumor suppressor gene, which regulates RAS, and is present in about 14% of metastatic melanomas [52].

Sentinel Lymph Node Biopsy

Since its introduction in the early 1990s, sentinel lymph node biopsy (SLNB) has emerged as a reliable and safe procedure to identify nodal disease for cutaneous melanoma of the head and neck [17, 53–55]. The presence or absence of nodal disease, even in the form of micrometastases, has been found to be the most important prognostic factor in early-stage melanoma patients (AJCC stage I–II) [56]. The risk of nodal metastasis increases with tumor thickness; and most patients with thin or intermediate thickness tumors will not harbor nodal metastasis [57]. SLNB is the accepted method for staging patients with clinically node-negative cutaneous melanoma [58]. The false negative rate of 15% must be borne in mind and prompts efforts at improving tracers and intraoperative devices.

Sentinel lymph node biopsy can be performed for melanoma of the ear canal, and it provides useful information regarding lymph node metastasis (Fig. 8.2).

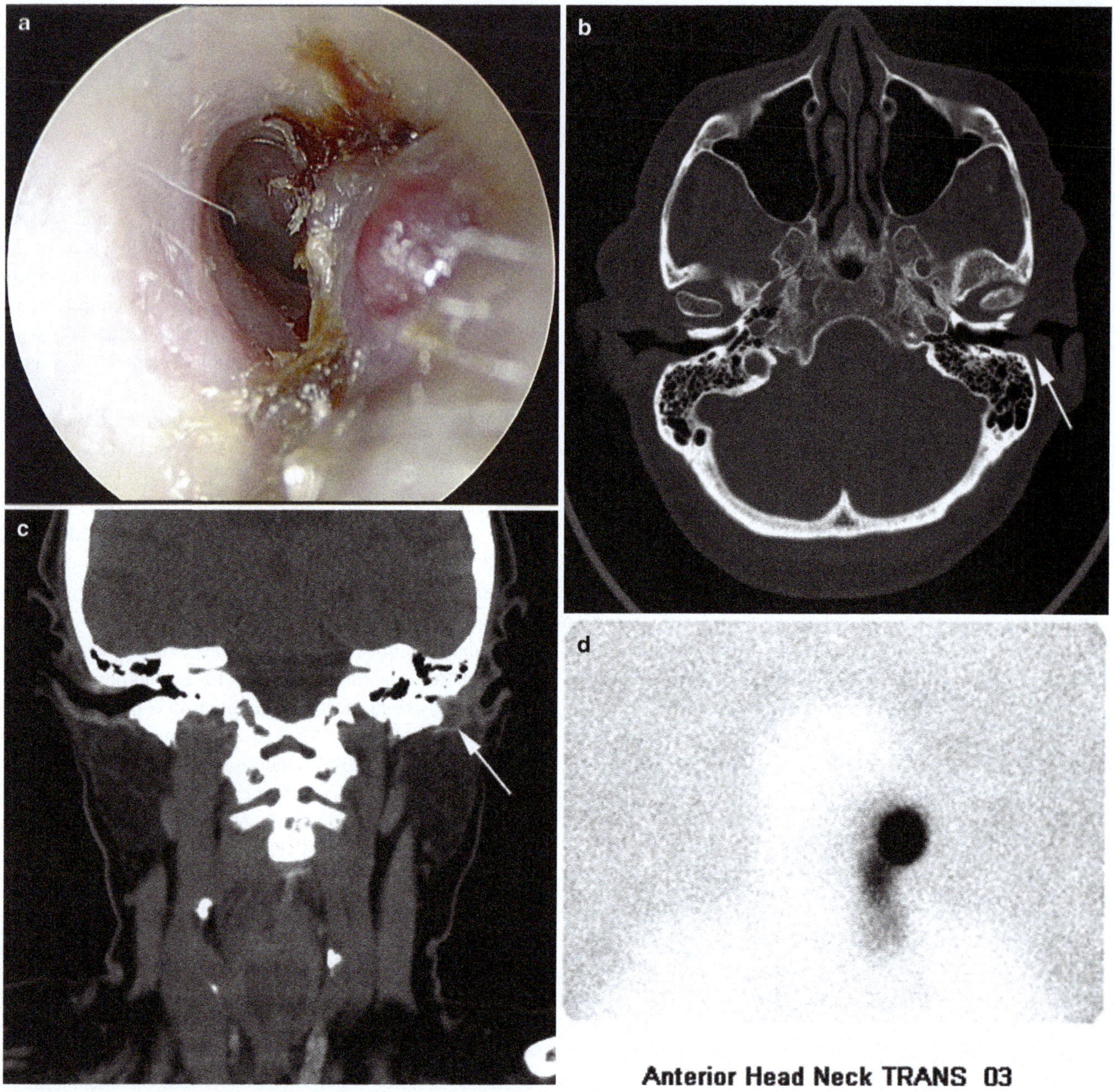

Fig. 8.2 This 75-year-old woman with left ear canal amelanotic melanoma. (**a**) Oto-endoscopic photograph of melanoma of the ear canal and axial (**b**) and coronal (**c**) CT scan with contrast showing soft tissue thickening in the left ear canal (arrows). There were no positive lymph nodes on CT or PET/CT. (**d**) Lymphoscintigraphy showing activity in the left neck. Sentinel lymph node biopsy was positive. She was treated with lateral temporal bone resection, parotidectomy, and neck dissection. Final pathology showed Breslow depth of 5.1 mm, microsatellitosis, 1 positive intraparotid lymph node and 2 positive level 2b lymph nodes, and bony invasion from this tumor (stage pT4b pN3 – pIIIc)

Staging

The staging for melanoma has undergone change over the last few years. A specific melanoma staging for ear canal or temporal bone tumors does not exist. The TNM staging by the American Joint Committee for Cancer (AJCC) is complex (Tables 8.1 and 8.2). This staging is largely based on tumor thickness, but mitotic rate and ulceration are denoted as "a" if they are lacking and "b" if they are present.

Metastatic Melanoma in the Ear Canal, Inner Ear, and Cerebellopontine Angle

Malignant melanoma has been rising in incidence for the last several decades. Melanoma is well known to produce distant metastasis. Metastatic melanoma involvement of the temporal bone may actually be quite common in patients who have widely disseminated disease (see references in Yang and Linthicum [59]).

Table 8.1 Cutaneous melanoma staging

Primary tumor (T)*	
TX	Primary tumor cannot be assessed
T0	No evidence of primary tumor
Tis	Melanoma in situ
T1	Melanomas 1.0 mm or less in thickness
T2	Melanomas 1.01–2.0 mm
T3	Melanomas 2.01–4.00 mm
T4	Melanomas more than 4.0 mm
Regional lymph nodes (N)**	
Nx	Patients in whom the regional nodes cannot be assessed
N0	No regional metastases detected
N1	1 node
N2	2–3 nodes
N3	4 or more metastatic nodes, or matted nodes, or in-transit metastases, satellites with metastatic nodes
Distant metastasis (M)	
M0	No detectable evidence of distant metastasis
M1a	Metastases to skin, subcutaneous, or distant lymph nodes
M1b	Metastases to lung
M1c	Metastases to all other visceral sites or distant metastases to any site combined with an elevated serum LDH

*a and b subcategories of T are assigned based on ulceration and number of mitoses per mm^2, as shown below

**a–c subcategories of N are assigned based on the presence of micrometastases (a), macrometastases (b), or in-transit metastases (c)

Table 8.2 Anatomic stage/prognostic groups

Clinical staging				Pathologic staging			
Stage 0	Tis	N0	M0	0	Tis	N0	M0
Stage IA	T1a	N0	M0	IA	T1a	N0	M0
Stage IB	T1b	N0	M0	IB	T1b	N0	M0
	T2a	N0	M0		T2a	N0	M0
Stage IIA	T2b	N0	M0	IIA	T2b	N0	M0
	T3a	N0	M0		T3a	N0	M0
Stage IIB	T3b	N0	M0	IIB	T3b	N0	M0
	T4a	N0	M0		T4a	N0	M0
Stage IIC	T4b	N0	M0	IIC	T4b	N0	M0
Stage III	Any T	≥N1	M0	IIIA	T1–4a	N1b	M0
					T1–4a	N2a	M0
				IIIB	T1–4b	N1a	M0
					T1–4b	N2a	M0
					T1–4a	N1b	M0
					T1–4	N2b	M0
					T1–4a	N2c	M0
				IIIC	T1–4b	N1b	M0
					T1–4b	N2b	M0
					T1–4b	N2c	M0
					Any T	N3	M0
Stage IV	Any T	Any N	M1	IV	Any T	Any N	M1

Melanoma can metastasize as satellite or in-transit metastases, as lymph node metastases, or as distant metastases. Satellite metastases occur when a metastatic nodule occurs within 2 cm of the primary tumor. In-transit metastasis occurs in the dermal and subdermal lymphatics before reaching the first regional lymph nodes. Satellite, in-transit, and lymph node metastases are considered locoregional metastases. Distant metastases occur beyond the regional lymph nodes and can involve the viscera, bone, or brain. Roughly two-thirds of metastases are locoregional and one-third are distant. The median time to development of these metastases is different: lymph node metastasis is 16 months, satellite or in-transit metastasis is 17 months, and distant metastasis is 25 months.

Three mechanisms have been described to explain the patterns of melanoma metastasis: the stepwise spread model, the simultaneous spread model, and the model of differential spread [60]. The stepwise model emphasizes that melanoma spreads initially via the lymphatic system to regional lymph nodes and then to systemic sites. This model is the basis for SLNB. This model does not explain the occurrence of hematogenous spread to distant sites without lymph node involvement. The simultaneous spread model states that both lymphatic and hematogenous spread occur at the same time. This model does not explain the fact that 30% of patients who undergo regional lymph node dissection do not develop distant disease. The model of differential spread proposes that melanoma cells have different aptitudes to spread either to only lymph nodes, only distantly, or to both sites.

At present, the most important factor to influence the different metastatic pathway is the anatomic location of the primary tumor. More than 30% of head and neck patients will develop satellite or in-transit metastasis; in contrast more than 30% of trunk or upper extremity will develop direct metastases. Gender and tumor thickness are also factors but with smaller influence.

The effect of genetic mutation on metastatic pathway is still poorly understood. BRAF-mutant tumors, and not NRAS-mutant tumors, are associated with a greater risk of nodal metastasis at diagnosis [60]. Further BRAF-mutant tumors have a higher incidence of brain metastasis than wild-type tumors.

Metastatic melanoma can affect the ear canal, inner ear, and cerebellopontine angle. The ear canal can be involved from either hematogenous metastasis or from tumor extension from nearby lymph nodes or the parotid gland. Hematogenous spread of melanoma to the ear canal has been reported as a polypoid mass [26, 27]. This author has seen one patient with metastatic melanoma in the ear canal, and this tumor was quite friable (Fig. 8.3).

The ear canal can also be involved secondarily from massive metastatic disease. Presumably due to metastatic lymph node involvement, rapidly growing melanoma tumors present as a large, painful tumor that can easily bleed (Figs. 8.4 and 8.5). The decision for surgery in this circumstance is predicated on locoregional control, decreased tumor burden, and symptom relief.

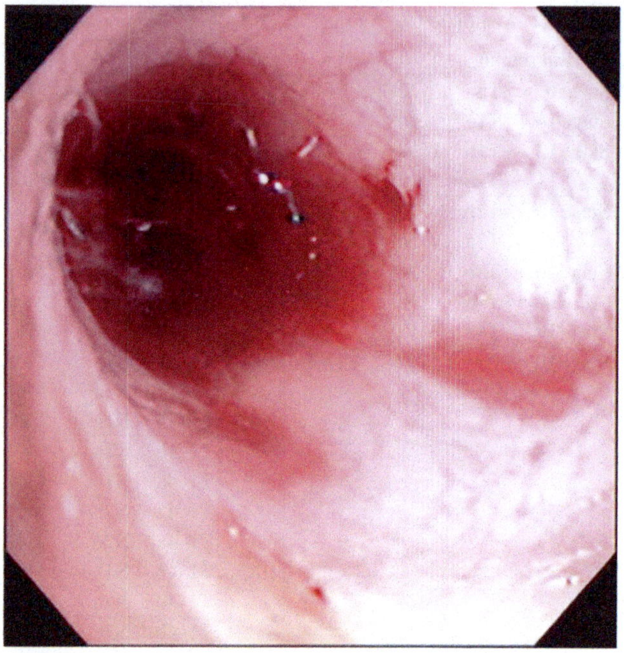

Fig. 8.3 Metastatic melanoma in the ear canal. This patient had a history of a right ear canal melanoma that was treated with a lateral temporal bone resection. He later developed melanoma in the left ear canal (pictured) along with distant disease

The inner ear can be involved with metastatic melanoma. Patients with extensive melanoma involvement of the inner ear can be asymptomatic [59, 61, 62]. Tumor can extend into the IAC and involve the modiolus and stria vascularis and Scarpa's ganglion [59, 61]. Involvement of the stria vascularis can be a striking characteristic of this tumor [63]. In the cochlea, inner and outer hair cell degeneration has been reported [63]. The middle ear mucosa, tensor tympani canal, bone marrow, and blood vessels of the temporal bone have also been described as involved with metastatic melanoma [59]. Melanoma can involve the facial, vestibular, or cochlear nerve [59, 61]. Conley et al. reported a single case of melanoma metastatic to the facial nerve extratemporally [64].

Melanoma has the highest risk of spread to the CNS of all common cancer types, even though in absolute numbers lung and breast cancer are much more prevalent [65]. Clinically, 40–60% of melanoma patients develop CNS metastasis, and autopsy studies reveal that CNS metastases occur in nearly 80% of patients with metastatic disease.

Suspicion of metastatic melanoma should be aroused when patients with a past history of melanoma present with rapid changes in cranial nerve function [66]. Individual case reports have mentioned tinnitus, vertigo, sensorineural hearing loss, facial weakness, and cerebellar signs in association with isolated metastatic melanoma to the CPA [45, 66]. Most patients present with symptoms that point to leptomeningeal disease (LMD) such as headache, visual disturbance, hearing loss, or lower cranial nerve deficit.

Metastatic malignant tumors account for only 0.2% of cerebellopontine angle tumors [14]. Malignant melanoma in the cerebellopontine angle mimics vestibular schwannoma [67]. Arriaga et al. present a case where the CPA tumor was the only focus of metastatic disease, and the patient lived for 5 years after resection, ultimately dying of widespread CNS disease [66].

A hallmark of metastatic melanoma is bilateral IAC metastases [63, 66, 68–72]. These metastases have been reported as late as 13 years following resection of the original primary tumor [68]. Kojima et al. described the findings of five temporal bones from three patients who had widely disseminated disease; two patients had bilateral internal auditory canal metastases [63].

MRI may not differentiate melanoma from schwannoma in the CPA. Radiographically, melanoma is hyperintense or hypointense on non-contrast T1 and hypointense on T2 imaging [14, 45]. These tumors enhance with gadolinium and thus mimic schwannoma [14, 45]. T2 imaging might show cerebellar edema in the case of metastatic melanoma, and this might be useful to differentiate it from schwannoma.

Median survival of metastatic melanoma to the CNS is 2–3 months. Several studies have examined the benefit of radiotherapy with a BRAF inhibitor for CNS metastasis [73]. Surgery improves survival. LMD has a median survival time of 3.6 months [14].

Treatment

Surgery

The treatment for primary cutaneous melanoma is surgery. Primary tumors need to be resected with wide margins. The definition of wide margin has varied over the years. For non-head and neck locations, 2 cm margins are considered reasonable for patients with melanomas thicker than 2 mm [74]. This recommendation may not apply for the head and neck where anatomic and functional structures like the nose, eye, or ear might preclude such a wide margin. In the head and neck margins, 2 cm or less are acceptable depending on the location of the tumor [75]. Unfortunately, due to the nature of melanoma, frozen section cannot be relied on for margin control.

Canal skin excision or "sleeve resection" is associated with local recurrence, since an adequate margin of tissue cannot be excised [19]. For malignant melanoma of the ear canal, lateral temporal bone resection, superficial parotidectomy, and selective neck dissection have been recommended and associated with long-term tumor control [15–17, 20]. In spite of best efforts, local, regional, and distant metastasis can occur within 8 months of such therapy [15].

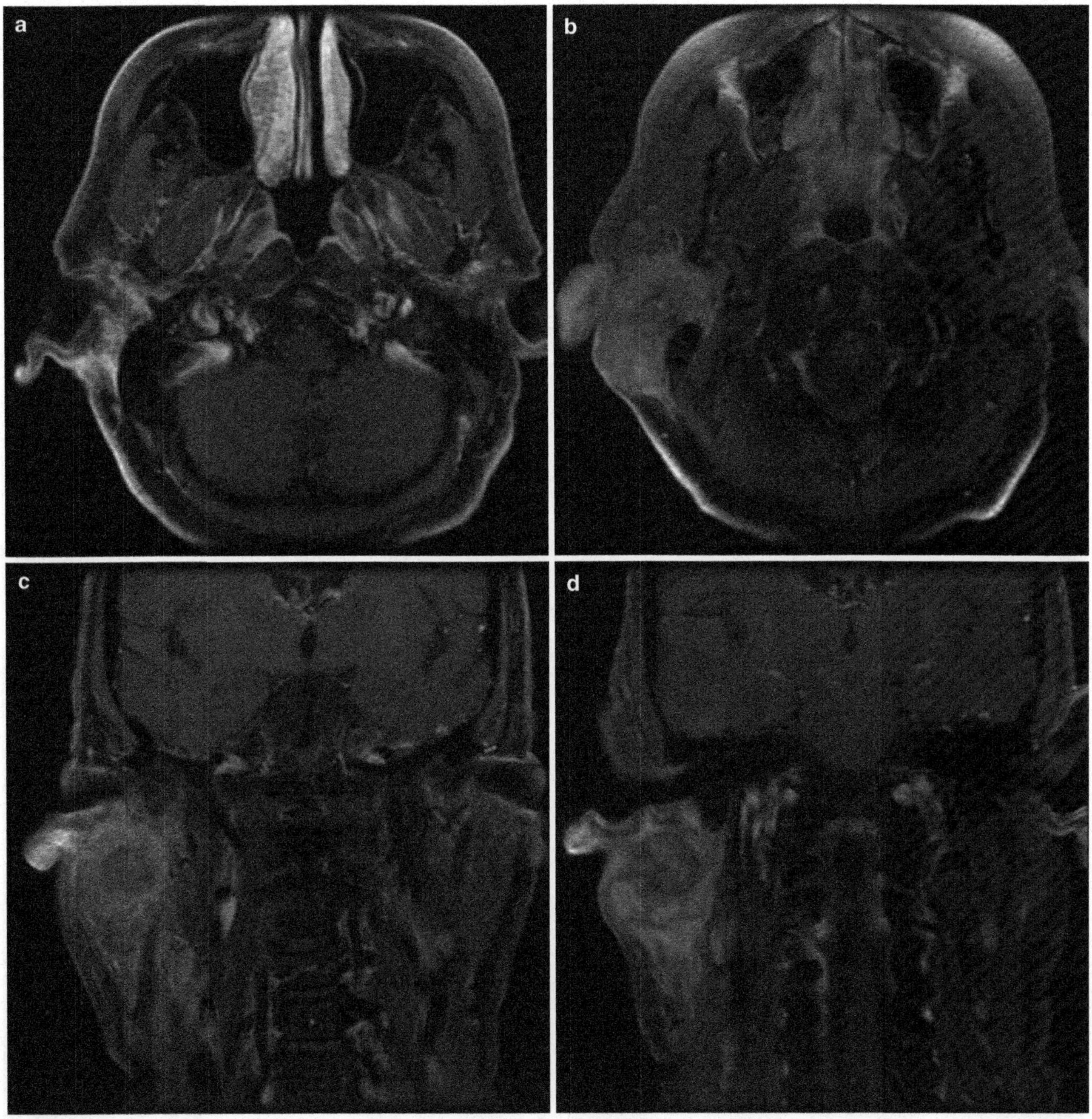

Fig. 8.4 Metastatic melanoma to right preauricular lymph node. This 52-year-old man presented with a large right preauricular neck mass that involved his ear canal. He had history of a pigmented lesion on his forehead 10 years prior. He underwent lateral temporal bone resection, parotidectomy, neck dissection, and free flap reconstruction. His pathology report showed metastatic melanoma in the soft tissues and 2/41 positive lymph nodes. He received postoperative radiotherapy of 30 Gy in 5 fractions. He remained cancer-free until his death 8.5 years later. Postcontrast (**a**, **b**) axial and (**c**, **d**) coronal MRI

Radiotherapy

Melanoma is generally considered to be radioresistant. Adjuvant radiotherapy to the primary site is controversial since only local control is improved and not overall survival. At MD Anderson, for patients with head and neck melanoma and N0 neck, a postoperative dose of 30 Gy is given in five fractions over 2.5 weeks [76]. Since 15–20% of patients will develop cervical nodal metastasis and since the regional recurrence rate after neck dissection is roughly 30–50%, radiotherapy can offer a positive impact on locoregional control [73].

Using this fraction scheme, a large retrospective study from MD Anderson examined the outcome of surgery alone versus surgery with postoperative radiotherapy of 615 patients [77]. Regional recurrence was 40.6% after surgery

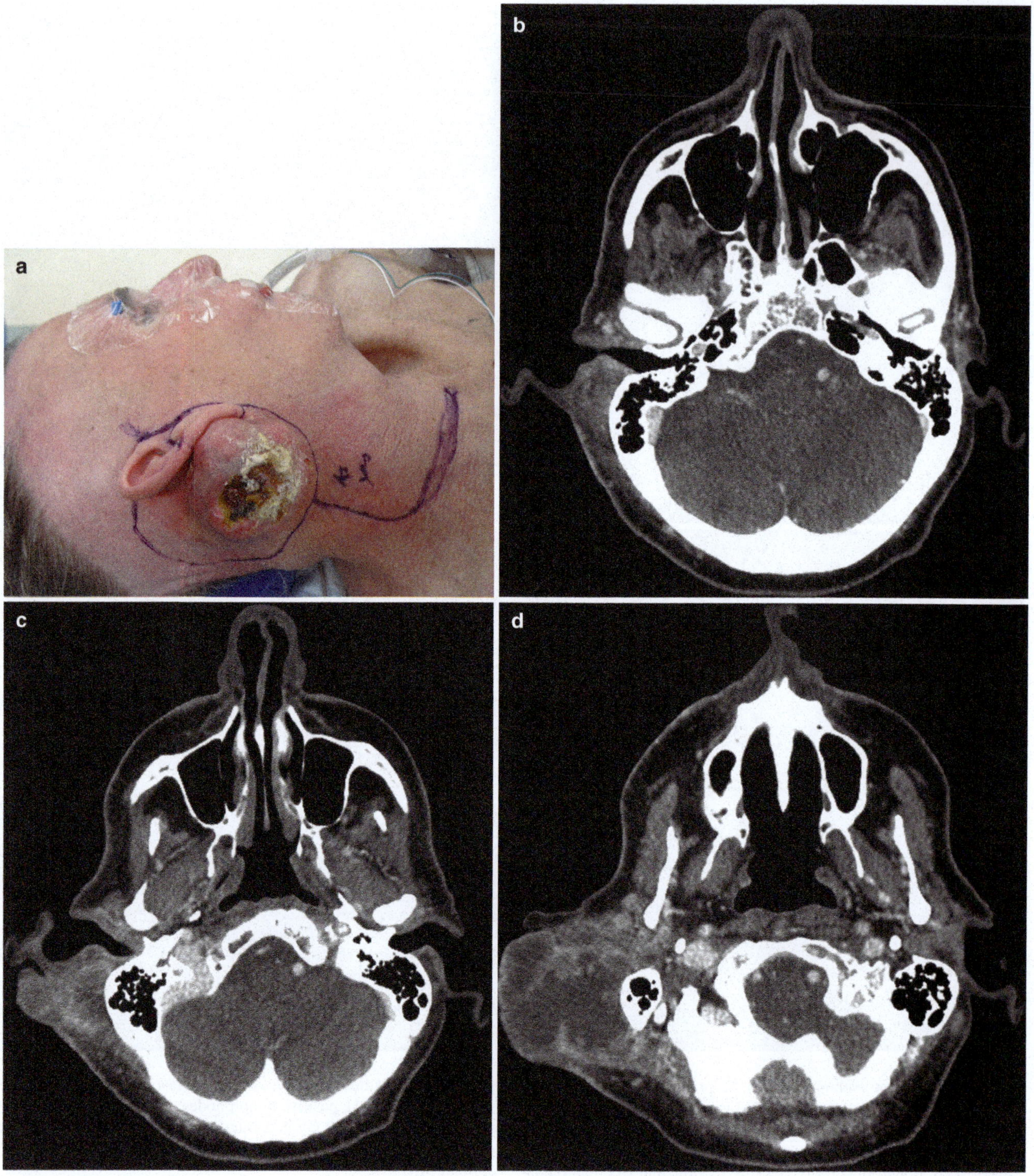

Fig. 8.5 Metastatic melanoma involving left ear canal. This 58-year-old man had a large right postauricular mass which increased in size while on a chemotherapy protocol of cisplatin, vinblastin, and dacarbazine. A primary tumor was never found. The decision for surgery was made for palliation and local tumor control. He underwent lateral temporal bone resection, parotidectomy, neck dissection, and free flap reconstruction. He then received postoperative radiotherapy 30 Gy in 5 fractions of 600 cGy. Three months later he developed lung and liver metastases, and he died 15 months after his surgery. (**a**) Intraoperative photo showing planned incisions to include total auriculectomy. (**b-d**) Postcontrast axial images

alone versus 10.2% after combined therapy. Local control rate was 90% in the combined therapy group versus 59.4% in the surgery only group. Smaller, prospective studies from Australia [78], MD Anderson [79], and University of Florida [80] have also reported positive effects from postoperative radiotherapy for local control.

Evidence is emerging that the combination of radiotherapy and immune checkpoint inhibitors is synergistic [81]. Radiotherapy might potentiate the antitumor effects of immune checkpoint inhibitors in both target and nontarget lesions.

Palliative radiotherapy to the temporal bone (40 Gy) has shown improvement in cranial nerve deficits, but distant disease usually develops [27].

Chemotherapy

Traditional therapies for metastatic melanoma have been based on dacarbazine or alpha interferon. Dacarbazine (DTIC) was the first drug approved for the treatment of metastatic melanoma and is still a standard to which modern treatment is compared. Interferons (IFN) are a class of glycoproteins that have antiproliferative and immune-modulatory effect causing tumor cells to be more susceptible to the immune system. However, analysis of randomized control trials did not demonstrate a benefit from alpha interferon in melanoma patients [82]. Previously at MD Anderson, a protocol consisting of DTIC, cisplatin, vinblastine, interferon, and interleukin-2 has been used for metastatic melanoma, and 21% of patients achieved a complete remission with a median survival time of 6 months [83]. This regimen, however, was accompanied by significant constitutional, hemodynamic, and myelosuppressive side effects. Analysis of eight randomized control trials comparing DTIC alone versus DTIC with IFN showed moderate improvement in the complete response rate but with increased adverse effect, and this combination had no significant effect on 1- and 3-year survival [84].

A chemotherapy protocol consisting of dacarbazine (110 mg/day × 5 days), intra-arterial cisplatin (20 mg/day × 3 days), and oral tamoxifen citrate (20 mg/day) has been tried for middle ear melanoma [35].

The management of melanoma has changed considerably since the introduction of immune checkpoint inhibitors (ICI) and targeted therapy. ICI are monoclonal antibodies that block co-inhibitory molecules. Examples of co-inhibitory molecules are cytotoxic T-lymphocyte-associated antigen-4 (CTL-4), programmed death-1 (PD1), and its ligand PDL1. CTL-4 is expressed on activated CD4+ and CD8+ effector T cells and regulatory T cells. PD1 is expressed on dendritic cells, activated T cells, and tumor cells. Ipilimumab (Yervoy), nivolumab (Opdivo), and pembrolizumab (Keytruda) are examples of ICI. Ipilimumab is an anti-CTL4 monoclonal antibody. Nivolumab and pembrolizumab target PD1 and have shown greater efficacy than ipilimumab [85].

Targeted therapy for melanoma has been aimed at the mitogen-activated protein kinase (MAPK) pathway. In normal cells, activation of MAPK pathway leads to cell growth and differentiation. In cells with the BRAF V600 mutation, the normal negative feedback inhibition does not exist leading to permanent MAPK pathway activation and uncontrolled cellular proliferation [86]. Vemurafenib (Zelboraf) and dabrafenib (Tafinlar) are specific for the BRAF V600 mutation and are effective for melanoma. One of the most severe adverse effects of these medications is secondary skin cancer. While these drugs are initially effective, tumors develop resistance in 6–7 months. Other medications, such as trametinib (Mekinist) and cobimetinib (Cotellic), block the downstream signaling molecule MEK, which inactivates the MAPK pathway. MEK inhibitors improve the effectiveness of BRAF inhibitors and reduce the incidence of secondary skin cancers [85].

The simultaneous inhibition of BRAF and MEK appears to have a longer progression-free survival (PFS) than anti-CTL4 or anti-PD1 antibodies alone and to be the most effective treatment for melanomas that harbor BRAF V600 mutation, while anti-PD1 antibodies is less toxic [85]. Therefore, the combination of a BRAF inhibitor and MEK inhibitor is considered current standard of care for inoperable stage IIIC/IV BRAF-mutated melanoma [52].

Conclusion

Malignant melanoma makes up only 5% of cutaneous malignancy, but it accounts for significant proportion of skin cancer mortality. Melanoma can affect any part of the ear canal and temporal bone, including the internal auditory canal and cerebellopontine angle. The evaluation and management of these tumors is described. Surgery is the main treatment for primary cutaneous melanomas. Adjuvant radiotherapy has a role in improving local control of disease. Targeted agents and immune checkpoint inhibitors are emerging as successful treatments for systemic disease.

References

1. Board PDQATE. Melanoma treatment (PDQ(R)): Health professional version. PDQ cancer information summaries. National Cancer Institute: Bethesda; 2017.
2. Schmerber S, Righini C, Soriano E, et al. [The outcome of treatments for carcinoma of the external auditory canal]. Rev Laryngol Otol Rhinol (Bord). 2005;126(3):165–70.
3. Conley J, Schuller DE. Malignancies of the ear. Laryngoscope. 1976;86(8):1147–63.
4. Altuna Mariezkurrena X, Henriquez Alarcon M, Vea Orte JC, Algaba Guimera J. [Malignant tumors of external ear. Review of cases in 1991-2001]. An Otorrinolaringol Ibero Am. 2003;30(1):83–94.
5. Stang A, Pukkala E, Sankila R, Soderman B, Hakulinen T. Time trend analysis of the skin melanoma incidence of Finland from 1953 through 2003 including 16,414 cases. Int J Cancer. 2006;119(2):380–4.
6. Green AC, Kimlin M, Siskind V, Whiteman DC. Hypothesis: hair cover can protect against invasive melanoma on the head and neck (Australia). Cancer Causes Control. 2006;17(10):1263–6.

7. Ravin AG, Pickett N, Johnson JL, Fisher SR, Levin LS, Seigler HF. Melanoma of the ear: treatment and survival probabilities based on 199 patients. Ann Plast Surg. 2006;57(1):70–6.
8. Ringborg U, Afzelius LE, Lagerlof B, et al. Cutaneous malignant melanoma of the head and neck. Analysis of treatment results and prognostic factors in 581 patients: a report from the Swedish Melanoma Study Group. Cancer. 1993;71(3):751–8.
9. Fisher SR. Cutaneous malignant melanoma of the head and neck. Laryngoscope. 1989;99(8 Pt 1):822–36.
10. Thorn M, Ponten F, Bergstrom R, Sparen P, Adami HO. Clinical and histopathologic predictors of survival in patients with malignant melanoma: a population-based study in Sweden. J Natl Cancer Inst. 1994;86(10):761–9.
11. Byers RM, Smith JL, Russell N, Rosenberg V. Malignant melanoma of the external ear. Review of 102 cases. Am J Surg. 1980;140(4):518–21.
12. Hawkes JE, Truong A, Meyer LJ. Genetic predisposition to melanoma. Semin Oncol. 2016;43(5):591–7.
13. Ozturk O, Baglam T, Uneri C, Kullu S. Primary malignant melanoma of the middle ear mucosa: a case report. Kulak Burun Bogaz Ihtis Derg. 2006;16(2):83–6.
14. Whinney D, Kitchen N, Revesz T, Brookes G. Primary malignant melanoma of the cerebellopontine angle. Otol Neurotol. 2001;22(2):218–22.
15. Milbrath MM, Campbell BH, Madiedo G, Janjan NA. Malignant melanoma of the external auditory canal. Am J Clin Oncol. 1998;21(1):28–30.
16. Amando Garcia L, Suarez Nieto C, Madrigal Rubiales B, Garcia Garcia J. [External ear melanoma]. Acta Otorrinolaringol Esp. 2003;54(2):89–93.
17. Langman A, Yarington T, Patterson SD. Malignant melanoma of the external auditory canal. Otolaryngol Head Neck Surg. 1996;114(4):645–8.
18. Hynes B, Lubynski RA, Hynes B. Malignant melanoma of the external ear canal: a rare case. J Otolaryngol. 2004;33(6):401–3.
19. Banerjee AR, Meikle D, Dawes PJ, Deans JA. Malignant melanoma of the external auditory meatus. Clin Oncol (R Coll Radiol). 1993;5(4):255–6.
20. Kang S, Barnhill RL, Graeme-Cook F, Randolph G, Nadol JB, Sober AJ. Primary malignant melanoma of the external auditory canal: a case report with presentation as an aural polyp. Am J Otol. 1992;13(2):194–6.
21. Shih L, Crabtree JA. Carcinoma of the external auditory canal: an update. Laryngoscope. 1990;100(11):1215-1218.
22. Sambe S, Kobayashi K, Asakura K, Kataura A. [A case of malignant melanoma in the external auditory canal followed by systemic vasculitis]. Nippon Jibiinkoka Gakkai Kaiho. 1985;88(4):455–62.
23. Olariu B, Olariu D, Jianu S, Albastroiu F, Ciuchi V, Laky D. [Malignant melanoma of the external auditory canal treated by cryotherapy]. Rev Chir Oncol Radiol. 1984;29(4):299–311.
24. Urpegui Garcia A, Lahoz Zamarro T, Muniesa Soriano JA, et al. [Malignant melanoma of the middle ear, a rare site]. Acta Otorrinolaringol Esp. 1999;50(7):559–62.
25. Xenellis J, Mountricha A, Maragoudakis P, et al. A histological examination in the cases of initial diagnosis as chronic otitis media with a polypoid mass in the external ear canal. Auris Nasus Larynx. 2011;38(3):325–8.
26. Khan I, Mohamad S, Shakeel M, Jaramillo MJ. Aural metastasis from a nasal malignant melanoma: case report with literature review. J Laryngol Otol. 2011;125(12):1290–3.
27. Walther EK, Krick T. [Malignant melanoma of the temporal bone]. Laryngorhinootologie. 1993;72(1):48–50.
28. Hannan SA, Parikh A. Malignant melanoma of the external ear canal. Lancet. 2006;368(9548):1680.
29. Kazikdas KC, Onal K, Kuehnel TS, Ozturk T. An intradermal nevus of the external auditory meatus. Eur Arch Otorhinolaryngol. 2006;263(3):253–5.
30. EL MK Jr, Holmes WF, Harwick R. Primary melanoma of the middle ear. Laryngoscope. 1984;94(11 Pt 1):1459–60.
31. Sherman IW, Swift AC, Haqqani MT. Primary mucosal malignant melanoma of the middle ear. J Laryngol Otol. 1991;105(12):1061–4.
32. Banerjee A, Meikle D. Malignant melanoma of the middle ear. J Laryngol Otol. 1992;106(6):581.
33. Folz BJ, Niemann AM, Lippert BM, Hauschild A, Werner JA. [Mucous membrane melanomas of the upper aerodigestive tract. An analysis of 34 cases]. Laryngorhinootologie. 1997;76(5):289–94.
34. Oueslati Z, Touati S, Gritli S, et al. [Mucous malignant melanoma of the neck and face. Experience at the Salah Azaiz institute (Tunis)]. Rev Laryngol Otol Rhinol (Bord). 2001;122(4):237–40.
35. Uchida M, Matsunami T. Malignant amelanotic melanoma of the middle ear. Arch Otolaryngol Head Neck Surg. 2001;127(9):1126–8.
36. Luo H, Liang JJ, Jiang Y. [Primary malignant melanoma of the middle ear and mastoid: a case report]. Zhonghua Er Bi Yan Hou Tou Jing Wai Ke Za Zhi. 2008;43(11):865–6.
37. Curry JM, Kung BC, Willcox TO Jr. Malignant melanoma of the middle ear. Otolaryngol Head Neck Surg. 2007;136(5):856–7.
38. Tywonczuk-Szulc M, Kibilda B. Malignant melanoma of the auditory tube. Otolaryngol Pol. 2007;61(3):335–8.
39. Racic G, Kurtovic D, Roje Z, Tomic S, Dogas Z. Primary mucosal melanoma of the eustachian tube. Eur Arch Otorhinolaryngol. 2004;261(3):139–42.
40. Baek SJ, Song MH, Lim BJ, Lee WS. Mucosal melanoma arising in the eustachian tube. J Laryngol Otol. 2006;120(3):E17.
41. Lai CC, Tsay SH, Ho CY. Malignant melanoma of the eustachian tube. J Laryngol Otol. 2001;115(7):567–9.
42. Sakaki M, Shek TW, Hirokawa M, et al. Melanotic oncocytic metaplasia of the nasopharynx: a report of seven cases and review of the literature. Virchows Arch. 2004;444(4):345–9.
43. Piedra MP, Scheithauer BW, Driscoll CL, Link MJ. Primary melanocytic tumor of the cerebellopontine angle mimicking a vestibular schwannoma. Neurosurgery. 2006;59(1):E206.
44. Rodriguez-Zuniga, Milton Jose Max, Pablo Humberto Effio-Iman. Primary cerebellopontine angle melanoma: Case Report and Systematic Review. Polish Ann Med. 2017;24(2):268–75.
45. Kingdom TT, Lalwani AK, Pitts LH. Isolated metastatic melanoma of the cerebellopontine angle: case report. Neurosurgery. 1993;33(1):142–4.
46. Anderson TD, Weber RS, Guerry D, et al. Desmoplastic neurotropic melanoma of the head and neck: the role of radiation therapy. Head Neck. 2002;24(12):1068–71.
47. Beenken S, Byers R, Smith JL, Goepfert H, Shallenberger R. Desmoplastic melanoma. Histologic correlation with behavior and treatment. Arch Otolaryngol Head Neck Surg. 1989;115(3):374–9.
48. Pathak I, O'Brien CJ, Petersen-Schaeffer K, et al. Do nodal metastases from cutaneous melanoma of the head and neck follow a clinically predictable pattern? Head Neck. 2001;23(9):785–90.
49. O'Brien CJ, McNeil EB, McMahon JD, Pathak I, Lauer CS. Incidence of cervical node involvement in metastatic cutaneous malignancy involving the parotid gland. Head Neck. 2001;23(9):744–8.
50. Wick MR. Cutaneous melanoma: a current overview. Semin Diagn Pathol. 2016;33(4):225–41.
51. Amaral T, Sinnberg T, Meier F, et al. MAPK pathway in melanoma part II-secondary and adaptive resistance mechanisms to BRAF inhibition. Eur J Cancer. 2017;73:93–101.
52. Amann VC, Ramelyte E, Thurneysen S, et al. Developments in targeted therapy in melanoma. Eur J Surg Oncol. 2017;43(3):581–93.
53. Wagner JD, Park HM, Coleman JJ 3rd, Love C, Hayes JT. Cervical sentinel lymph node biopsy for melanomas of the head and neck and upper thorax. Arch Otolaryngol Head Neck Surg. 2000;126(3):313–21.

54. Carlson GW, Murray DR, Greenlee R, et al. Management of malignant melanoma of the head and neck using dynamic lymphoscintigraphy and gamma probe-guided sentinel lymph node biopsy. Arch Otolaryngol Head Neck Surg. 2000;126(3):433–7.
55. Wey PD, De La Cruz C, Goydos JS, Choi ML, Borah GL. Sentinel lymph node mapping in melanoma of the ear. Ann Plast Surg. 1998;40(5):506–9.
56. Balch CM, Gershenwald JE, S-J S, et al. Final version of 2009 AJCC melanoma staging and classification. J Clin Oncol. 2009;27(36):6199–206.
57. Lens M, Dawes M, Newton-Bishop J, Goodacre T. Tumour thickness as a predictor of occult lymph node metastases in patients with stage I and II melanoma undergoing sentinel lymph node biopsy. Br J Surg. 2002;89(10):1223–7.
58. Tardelli E, Mazzarri S, Rubello D, et al. Sentinel lymph node biopsy in cutaneous melanoma: standard and new technical procedures and clinical advances. A systematic review of the literature. Clin Nucl Med. 2016;41(12):e498–507.
59. Yang E, Linthicum FH Jr. Metastatic melanoma. Otol Neurotol. 2005;26(4):821–2.
60. Adler NR, Haydon A, McLean CA, Kelly JW, Mar VJ. Metastatic pathways in patients with cutaneous melanoma. Pigment Cell Melanoma Res. 2017;30(1):13–27.
61. Deroee AF, Joglekar S, Paparella MM. Malignant melanoma metastasis to temporal bone. Otol Neurotol. 2009;30(2):248–9.
62. Navarrete CM, Ruah CB, Schachern P, Paparella MM. Normal and metastatic melanin in the temporal bone. Am J Otolaryngol. 1995;16(1):33–9.
63. Kojima C, Iino Y, Nakamoto Y, Toriyama M. [Histopathological studies of temporal bones of patients with malignant melanoma]. Nippon Jibiinkoka Gakkai Kaiho. 1997;100(6):655–62.
64. Conley J, Juarbe C, Patow CA, Angel MF. Metastatic melanoma to the facial nerve. Plast Reconstr Surg. 1991;87(2):341–5.
65. Cohen JV, Tawbi H, Margolin KA, et al. Melanoma central nervous system metastases: current approaches, challenges, and opportunities. Pigment Cell Melanoma Res. 2016;29(6):627–42.
66. Arriaga MA, Lo WW, Brackmann DE. Metastatic melanoma to the cerebellopontine angle. Clinical and imaging characteristics. Arch Otolaryngol Head Neck Surg. 1995;121(9):1052–6.
67. Brackmann DE, Doherty JK. CPA melanoma: diagnosis and management. Otol Neurotol. 2007;28(4):529–37.
68. Delerue O, Destee A, Devos P. Bilateral metastases in the cerebellopontine angle. J Neurol Neurosurg Psychiatry. 1991;54(6):562.
69. Cervio A, Saadia D, Nogues M, Bas C, Coppola F. Metastatic melanoma within the internal auditory canal: a case report. Am J Otolaryngol. 1999;20(4):263–5.
70. Garcia Gonzalez LA, Redondo Ventura F. [Metastases in both internal auditive meatus of nasosinusal melanoma]. An Otorrinolaringol Ibero Am. 2005;32(6):537–44.
71. Jacob A, Brightman RP, Welling DB. Bilateral cerebellopontine angle metastatic melanoma: A case report. Ear Nose Throat J. 2007;86(7):388–90.
72. Yang AS, Bird P. Intracranial metastatic melanoma presenting with bilateral hearing loss. Otol Neurotol. 2009;30(2):243–4.
73. Fort M, Guet S, Husheng S, Calitchi E, Belkacemi Y. Role of radiation therapy in melanomas: systematic review and best practice in 2016. Crit Rev Oncol Hematol. 2016;99:362–75.
74. Ethun CG, Delman KA. The importance of surgical margins in melanoma. J Surg Oncol. 2016;113(3):339–45.
75. O'Brien CJ, Coates AS, Petersen-Schaefer K, et al. Experience with 998 cutaneous melanomas of the head and neck over 30 years. Am J Surg. 1991;162(4):310–4.
76. Bonnen MD, Ballo MT, Myers JN, et al. Elective radiotherapy provides regional control for patients with cutaneous melanoma of the head and neck. Cancer. 2004;100(2):383–9.
77. Agrawal S, Kane JM, Guadagnolo BA, Kraybill WG, Ballo MT. The benefits of adjuvant radiation therapy after therapeutic lymphadenectomy for clinically advanced, high-risk, lymph node-metastatic melanoma. Cancer. 2009;115(24):5836–44.
78. O'Brien CJ, Petersen-Schaefer K, Stevens GN, et al. Adjuvant radiotherapy following neck dissection and parotidectomy for metastatic malignant melanoma. Head Neck. 1997;19(7):589–94.
79. Ballo MT, Garden AS, Myers JN, et al. Melanoma metastatic to cervical lymph nodes: can radiotherapy replace formal dissection after local excision of nodal disease? Head Neck. 2005;27(8):718–21.
80. Chang DT, Amdur RJ, Morris CG, Mendenhall WM. Adjuvant radiotherapy for cutaneous melanoma: comparing hypofractionation to conventional fractionation. Int J Radiat Oncol Biol Phys. 2006;66(4):1051–5.
81. Filippi AR, Fava P, Badellino S, Astrua C, Ricardi U, Quaglino P. Radiotherapy and immune checkpoints inhibitors for advanced melanoma. Radiother Oncol. 2016;120(1):1–12.
82. Lens MB, Dawes M. Interferon alfa therapy for malignant melanoma: a systematic review of randomized controlled trials. J Clin Oncol. 2002;20(7):1818–25.
83. Eton O, Legha SS, Bedikian AY, et al. Sequential biochemotherapy versus chemotherapy for metastatic melanoma: results from a phase III randomized trial. J Clin Oncol. 2002;20(8):2045–52.
84. Xin Y, Huang Q, Zhang P, et al. Meta-analysis of the safety and efficacy of interferon combined with Dacarbazine versus Dacarbazine alone in cutaneous malignant melanoma. Medicine. 2016;95(16):e3406.
85. Pasquali S, Chiarion-Sileni V, Rossi CR, Mocellin S. Immune checkpoint inhibitors and targeted therapies for metastatic melanoma: a network meta-analysis. Cancer Treat Rev. 2017;54:34–42.
86. Amaral T, Sinnberg T, Meier F, et al. The mitogen-activated protein kinase pathway in melanoma part I— activation and primary resistance mechanisms to BRAF inhibition. Eur J Cancer. 2017;73:85–92.

Unusual Tumors of the Ear Canal

9

Paul W. Gidley

Abbreviations

ACC	Adenoid cystic carcinoma
CT	Computerized tomography
EAC	External auditory canal
ELST	Endolymphatic sac tumor
MEC	Mucoepidermoid carcinoma
MRI	Magnetic resonance imaging
PET/CT	Positron emission tomography/computerized tomography
PORT	Postoperative radiotherapy

Introduction

This chapter will describe benign and malignant tumors of the ear canal beyond squamous cell carcinoma, basal cell carcinoma, and melanoma. Adenoid cystic carcinoma is included in this chapter since it is thought to arise from ceruminous glands.

This chapter discusses the general anatomy of the ear canal, the nomenclature of ear canal tumors, and an in-depth analysis of the unusual tumors that occur within the ear canal.

The interested reader is directed to the Triological Society candidate's thesis by Hicks which is a classic monograph on clinical behavior of these tumors [1]. The histopathology of benign ceruminous tumors is described in detail by Thompson [2].

General Anatomy

The external canal has two parts: a lateral portion that has a cartilaginous framework and a medial bony portion. The cartilaginous portion of the canal comprises about one-third the length of the canal. The skin covering the cartilaginous canal is thin, measuring about 0.5–1 mm in thickness, firmly bound to perichondrium, with a thin subcutaneous tissue, while the skin of bony canal is about 0.2 mm thick, firmly bound to periosteum, and totally devoid of subcutaneous tissue.

Hair follicles and ceruminous glands are present in the cartilaginous canal, but they are not present in the bony canal [2]. The ear canal contains both sebaceous and modified sweat glands and ceruminous glands [3]. Sebaceous glands are abundant in the cartilaginous canal and open into the hair follicles of the canal. Ceruminous glands are modified apocrine glands [4]. As apocrine glands, ceruminous glands lose part of their cytoplasm with secretion. The ceruminous glands branch and drain into a duct which opens along with sebaceous gland ducts into the hair sacs found in the external auditory canal (EAC) [5]. The ceruminous glands are deep within the dermis and are usually located close to the cartilage of the canal.

Cerumen has a protective effect for the ear canal. The acidity of cerumen keeps the pH of the ear canal around 5.6–5.8. Additionally, as cerumen is waxy, it provides a waterproof coating for the ear canal skin [1]. Ceruminous glands do not have cholinergic or adrenergic innervation. The ear canal does not contain eccrine sweat glands [1]. Ceruminous glands, sebaceous glands, and hair follicles are located only in the membranous ear canal [6, 7].

The arterial supply to the ear canal is derived from branches of the posterior auricular, superficial temporal, and deep auricular arteries [1]. Venous blood drains by way of the maxillary and external jugular veins and the pterygoid plexus. The lymphatic drainage of the ear canal goes to nodes anterior, posterior, and inferior to the auricle. The inferior nodes drain to the intraparotid and jugulodigastric (Level 2) nodes. These jugulodigastric nodes also receive the lymph drainage from the external ear. The ear canal is supplied by the facial nerve for the superior part of the ear canal, the auriculotemporal nerve (mandibular division of trigeminal nerve) for the anterior portions of the meatus, the auricular branch of vagus nerve for the inferior portions of the canal, and the greater auricular nerve (C-3) for the posterior portions of the ear canal (Fig. 9.1).

P. W. Gidley, M.D., F.A.C.S.
Department of Head and Neck Surgery, The University of Texas M.D. Anderson Cancer Center, Houston, TX, USA
e-mail: pwgidley@mdanderson.org

P. W. Gidley, F. DeMonte (eds.), *Temporal Bone Cancer*, https://doi.org/10.1007/978-3-319-74539-8_9

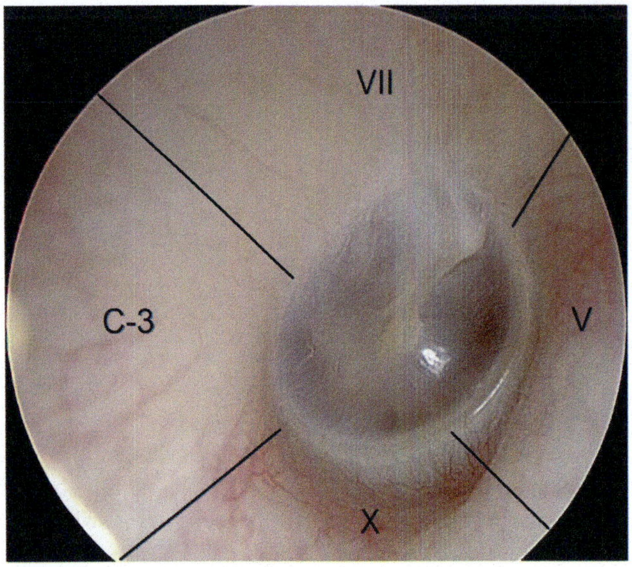

Fig. 9.1 Innervation of the ear canal

Table 9.1 Synonyms for ceruminous neoplasms of the external auditory canal (modified from Pallanch et al., Thompson et al.) [2, 9]

Adenocarcinoma of ceruminal type Adenoid cystic carcinoma Ceruminous adenocarcinoma Clear cell carcinoma Mucoepidermoid carcinoma	Adenoma ceruminalis Aural hydradenoma Ceruminoma (ceruminomata) Ceruminal adenoma Ceruminous adenoma Chondroid syringoma Cylindroma Cylindromatous deep hidroadenoma Cylindromatous lymphangioma Eccrine cylindroma Hidroadenoma Mixed tumor of skin Myoepithelioma Pleomorphic adenoma Syringocystadenoma papilliferum

Nomenclature

In 1894, Haug used the term ceruminoma to describe tumors of the external ear canal [8]. The nomenclature for ear canal tumors has been confusing ever since, given that the terms "ceruminoma" and "cylindroma" have been used to describe both benign and malignant tumors [2]. Many different terms have been used to describe and categorize these tumors (Table 9.1) [2, 9].

The rarity of these tumors, the use of the confusing term "ceruminoma," and the disagreement on the tissue of origin create the difficulties associated with studying these tumors [5]. Thus, the terms "ceruminoma" and "cylindroma" should be avoided [5, 7].

In 1972, Wetli suggested the pathologic organization of ear canal ceruminous gland tumors into four categories: (1) ceruminous adenoma, (2) pleomorphic adenoma, (3) adenoid cystic carcinoma, and (4) adenocarcinoma [10]. In 1991, the WHO rendered the term "ceruminoma" obsolete in favor of this nomenclature scheme [5]. Ceruminous adenocarcinoma is slightly more common than ceruminous adenomas [2].

Benign Ceruminous Tumors of the Ear Canal

The ceruminous glands of the ear canal produce wax and can give rise to benign tumors such as ceruminous adenoma, pleomorphic adenoma, and syringocystadenoma papilliferum or malignant tumors such as ceruminous adenocarcinoma, ceruminous adenoid cystic carcinoma, and ceruminous mucoepidermoid carcinoma [2, 4, 7]. Alternatively and theoretically, ectopic salivary gland tissue may give rise to tumors more commonly seen in the parotid gland, yet ectopic salivary gland tissue has never been found in the EAC.

Ceruminous gland tumors are difficult to diagnose due to their rare occurrence and the confusing nomenclature, classification, and tissue of origin [11]. Proper pathologic interpretation is necessary since treatment plans are distinctly different between managing a benign ear canal tumor versus a malignant tumor.

In 1951, Mark and Rothberg published the first case report of EAC adenoma [12]. Mills et al. reported a series of 32 ear canal lesions: 25 (78%) were squamous cell carcinomas, and the other 7 were various benign and malignant ceruminous neoplasms [5]. According to Thompson et al., benign ceruminous gland neoplasms comprise only 5.7% of all outer ear and ear canal tumors [2]. Only about 150 glandular tumors of the EAC have been reported worldwide [7, 11].

Thompson et al. reviewed the pathology from 41 ceruminous benign neoplasms diagnosed between 1970 and 2000 in the Armed Forces Institute of Pathology, and they identified another 32 cases in the English language literature from 1966 to 2004 [2]. In their series, ceruminous adenoma (n = 36) was the most common, followed by ceruminous pleomorphic adenoma (n = 4), and syringocystadenoma papilliferum (n = 1). The age range was 12–83 years. Men were slightly more affected than women; this finding is especially true for ceruminous pleomorphic adenomas. Left and right ears were equally affected. Tumors ranged in size from 0.5 to 2 cm in diameter, with a mean size of 1.2 cm. According to Diaz and Babu, frequencies are 88%, 10%, and 2% for ceruminous adenoma, ceruminous pleomorphic adenoma, and ceruminous syringocystadenoma papilliferum (SCAP), respectively [13].

Patients usually complain of a painless mass, ear canal blockage, hearing loss, and otalgia [7]. Alternatively, these tumors can occasionally mimic furunculosis [7, 14]. Symptom duration can be from 1 month up to 40 years, with a mean

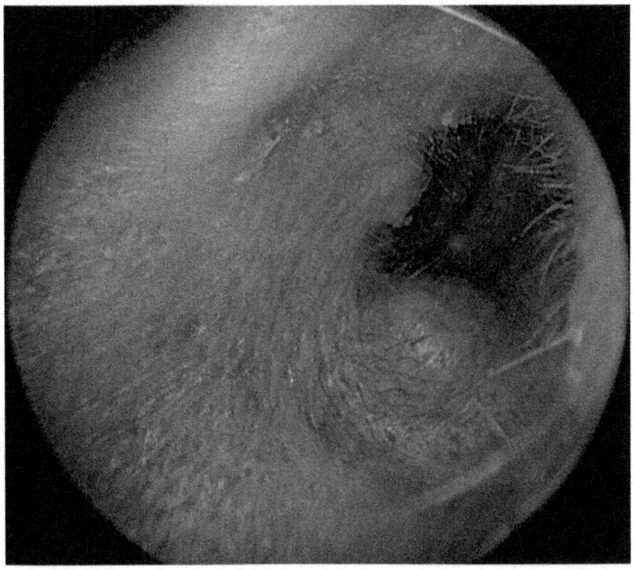

Fig. 9.2 Benign adenoma of the right ear canal

duration of 46 months [2]. On physical examination these tumors present as a smooth, soft, non-tender mass in the external auditory meatus (Fig. 9.2). However, one case has been described as an aural polyp associated with chronic otitis media [4]. Size ranges from 0.4 to 2 cm (mean 1.1 cm) in diameter [2]. The mean age at presentation is usually in the fifth decade, but a wide range from 5 to 85 years has been reported [2, 14].

Ceruminous Adenoma

Ceruminous adenoma is the most common benign tumor of the ear canal. These tumors become symptomatic when they obstruct the ear canal. For this reason, these tumors might be present for years prior to discovery [1]. They usually do not cause pain, unless obstruction of the canal precipitates otitis externa.

Benign adenomas are usually skin-covered, polypoid masses of various sizes in the ear canal. Hearing loss is secondary to obstruction. Otorrhea occurs only in the setting of canal obstruction and secondary otitis externa. Ceruminous adenoma has presented with clinical features suggesting furunculosis in the ear canal [7].

Pathologically, these tumors have glands with a two-layered structure analogous to ceruminous glands and a proliferation of myoepithelial cells. Histologically, these tumors have glands and small cysts lined by tubuloglandular proliferation of inner ceruminous cells surrounded by a spindled to cuboidal myoepithelial layer [2]. Cerumen pigment, CK7, and p63 are markers that help to distinguish this tumor from other tumors of the ear canal. The differential diagnosis includes ceruminous adenocarcinoma, meningioma, paraganglioma, and middle ear adenoma.

Treatment is wide local excision, removing the tumor in its entirety. Inadequate excision can lead to recurrence. If margins are clear and the pathology is conclusive, then no further treatment is needed. There is no role for radiotherapy.

Ceruminous Pleomorphic Adenoma

Ceruminous pleomorphic adenoma describes a mixed tumor with apocrine differentiation seen within the external auditory canal. There have been only about 35 cases reported in the world literature [1, 2, 4, 5, 15–27].

Typical symptoms are a slow-growing mass in the ear canal, sensation of blockage, or possible external otitis due to obstruction [1]. These tumors can be sessile or polypoid, smooth, mobile, and not adherent to underlying connective tissue. A very unusual case of lipomatous pleomorphic adenoma has been described [28].

CT and MRI are useful to document the extent of disease, to eliminate the parotid as the source of the tumor, and to identify any additional pathology medial to the tumor when it fully blocks the ear canal. On MRI, pleomorphic adenomas appear to have a well-defined margin and hypointensity on T1-weighted imaging and hyperintensity on T2-weighted imaging relative to the parotid gland; and these tumors enhance with contrast [19].

Complete excision is required, since inadequate excision leads to recurrence. When soft tissue margins are inadequate, the tumor capsule can be violated, and "seeding" of the tumor can occur [1]. Endaural incisions help to create enough exposure for complete tumor resection. Given the narrow confines of the bony canal, incomplete excision is frequent and usually leads to recurrence.

Adjuvant therapy is not necessary. Markou et al. [4] describe a case where a ceruminous pleomorphic adenoma presented as an aural polyp. The polyp arose from the posterior ear canal wall and extended into the middle ear. This tumor was removed with canal wall down mastoidectomy [4].

Histopathology shows a myxoid or pseudocartilaginous stroma with mucin or cuboidal cells. By definition, these tumors contain both epithelial and mesenchymal elements. There is pseudo-encapsulation.

Syringocystadenoma Papilliferum

Syringocystadenoma papilliferum (SCAP) is very rare cutaneous adnexal tumor of apocrine gland origin. These tumors usually arise on the scalp and face, usually in childhood or adolescence, and are often coexistent with congenital lesions such as nevus sebaceous [29]. Only 12 cases have been described that affect the ear canal [2, 13, 29–33]. A rare case report indicates this tumor can also occur on the pinna [34]. A unique case of ductal carcinoma arising from SCAP in the ear canal has been reported [13].

On MRI, SCAPs are reported to be intermediate signal intensity on T1- and T2-weighted imaging and slight enhancement on gadolinium enhanced T1-weighted images [30].

Malignant Ceruminous Tumors of the Ear Canal

Ceruminous Adenoid Cystic Carcinoma

Adenoid cystic carcinoma makes up about 20% of the malignant tumors of the ear canal; and it is the third most common malignancy of the ear canal behind squamous cell carcinoma and basal cell carcinoma (second most common in the series by Austin et al., 1994 [35], Yin et al., 2006 [36], and Chi et al. 2011 [37]; and fourth most common in the series by Madsen et al., 2008 [38]) [37, 39–45]. In the past, these tumors have been given the name "cylindroma," a very confusing term since it has been used to describe benign and malignant tumors [5, 11, 24, 46–49]. There are numerous case reports of ceruminous adenoid cystic carcinoma [1, 4, 5, 11, 24, 26, 27, 50–61].

Adenoid cystic carcinoma (ACC) makes up about 5–20% of the cancers of the EAC [60]. To date, there have only been a little over 100 cases reported in the English literature [62]. These tumors typically have an indolent course, and diagnosis is frequently delayed. This cancer is difficult to diagnose in an early stage because it is often subcutaneous or inconspicuous on a cursory examination of the ear canal (Fig. 9.3).

ACC typically occurs in the fifth or sixth decade of life. Dong et al. reported a mean age of 42 years (range 25–72 years) [63]. There have been conflicting reports about female predominance of disease [60]. Dong et al. reported a series of 22 patients, with 15 women and 7 men [63]. Liu et al. conducted an extensive review of the English literature and found a distinct female/male predominance of 57:36 cases or a ratio of 1.58 [62].

Ear pain is the most common symptom, perhaps related to perineural involvement. It is not unusual for there to be a history of otalgia for months or even years without a diagnosis until the lesion is finally found. Other symptoms are equally vague such as otorrhea, hearing loss, and bleeding. Dong et al. found that the mean duration of symptoms before diagnosis was 2 years (range 3 months to 30 years) [63]. They found that patients who suffered recurrence had a significantly longer duration of symptoms prior to diagnosis, 7.7 years versus 1.2 years. Every

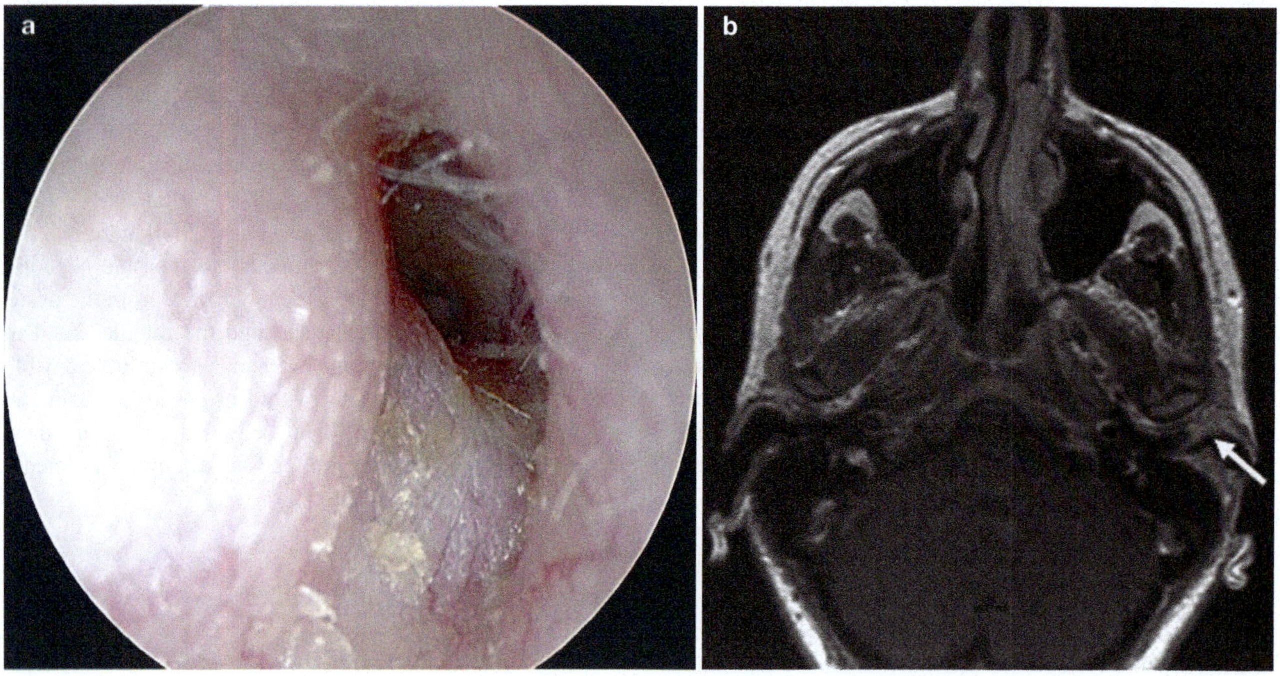

Fig. 9.3 Adenoid cystic carcinoma of left anterior ear canal in a 41-year-old woman. (**a**) Oto-endoscopic view, demonstrating the subcutaneous nature of these tumors. (**b**) Contrast-enhanced MRI showing non-specific thickening of the left ear canal (white arrow), the parotid gland is not involved

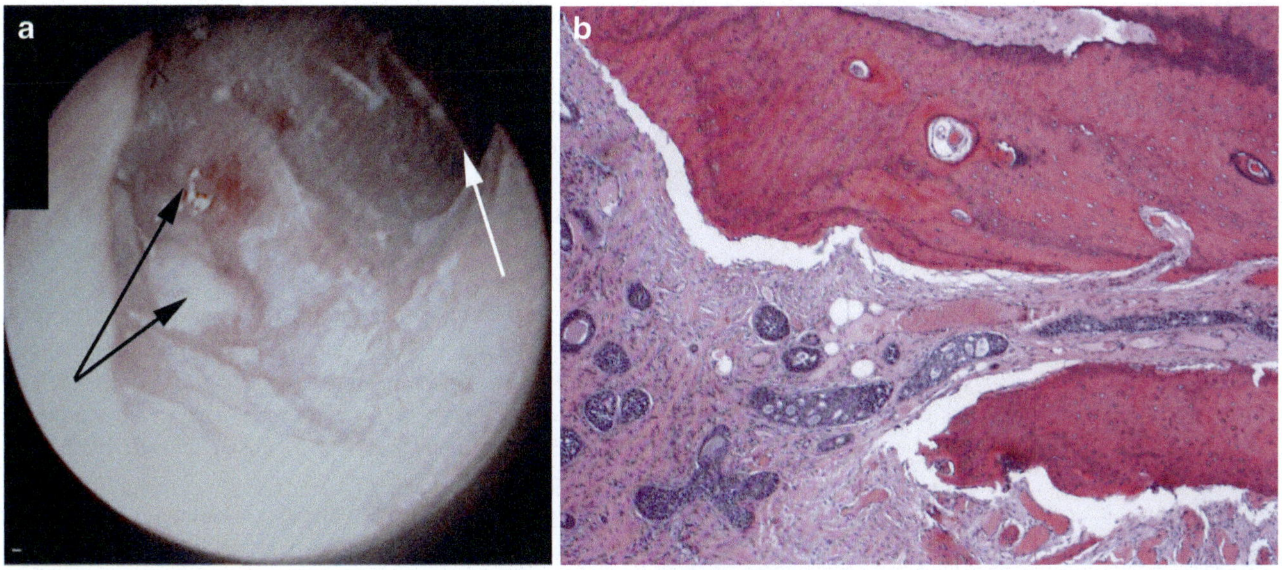

Fig. 9.4 Adenoid cystic carcinoma of the ear canal in a 60-year-old man treated with lateral temporal bone resection, parotidectomy, neck dissection, and temporalis flap for reconstruction. (**a**) Oto-endoscopic view of right ear canal (black arrows) and tympanic membrane (white arrow). (**b**) Histopathologic section showing bone invasion. Pathology report showed tubular and cribriform pattern with no perineural invasion. Bony invasion was identified, and he was treated with postoperative radiotherapy

patient who developed recurrence had had symptoms for more than 2 years [63].

These tumors are often subcutaneous and difficult to diagnosis until they become large enough to be easily seen (Fig. 9.4). Other symptoms, such as otorrhea, hearing loss, and pruritis, can also be found in relationship to these tumors. These relatively benign symptoms belie the pernicious nature of this malignancy.

Biopsy is the most important step in diagnosis. CT scan is important since it might show bony destruction from the tumor. These tumors tend to be locally aggressive, and lymph node metastases are rare. The Pittsburgh staging system has been applied to ACC of the EAC [60, 64]. The report by Gu et al. shows that the Pittsburgh staging system corresponded to survival [60].

Lateral temporal bone resection is required for tumors in the ear canal and has been shown to have better survival outcomes than local canal resection [60]. Tumors that have extended into the middle ear or mastoid will require subtotal temporal bone resection. Parotidectomy and lymph node dissection are more controversial, yet these procedures can be an important part of pathologic staging.

Postoperative radiotherapy (PORT) is indicated principally for cases with perineural spread. Other features which support the use of PORT include close or positive margins, lymphovascular invasion, high stage, soft tissue or bony invasion, solid histology, and lymph node involvement. Early-stage tumors with negative margins can simply be observed. Effective chemotherapy is lacking for adenoid cystic carcinoma.

Histopathologically, the cell of origin is most likely the ceruminous glands of the ear canal. The most common histologic subtype is the cribriform pattern (66%) followed by the tubular (27%) and solid patterns (7%) [62]. The literature is too limited to draw a conclusion about prognosis related to histologic pattern, but solid pattern is considered to have the worse prognosis based on clinical inference from salivary gland experience. The differential diagnosis includes basal cell carcinoma, mucoepidermoid carcinoma, and pleomorphic adenoma.

Perineural involvement is a frequent finding in adenoid cystic carcinoma and is estimated to be present in 80% of cases [62, 63]. Neural cell adhesion molecules have been identified in adenoid cystic carcinoma and might lead to the propensity for perineural spread [65]. The presence of perineural involvement significantly worsens prognosis [62]. Since ACC is notorious for perineural invasion, postoperative radiotherapy is usually required.

These tumors are locally aggressive. Invasion of adjacent soft tissue is reported in 59% and invasion into bone in 47%. Parotid gland invasion is reported in 24% [63]. Positive margins are a significant determinant of disease-free survival. Lymph node involvement is unusual. Lymphovascular invasion is rare, perhaps found in only 18% of cases [63]. Its presence indicates a higher chance of recurrence. These features of local invasion can make complete excision difficult.

Following adequate surgical excision and postoperative radiotherapy, most patients will not develop locoregional recurrence. Local recurrence happens in patients with inad-

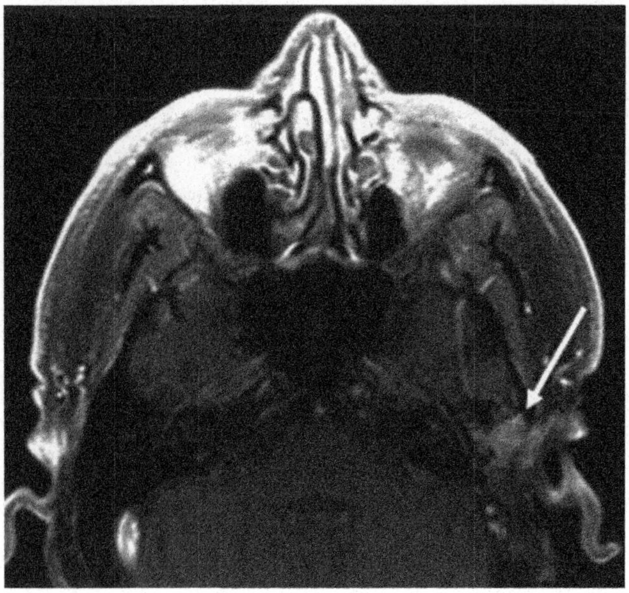

Fig. 9.5 Contrast-enhanced MRI of recurrent adenoid cystic carcinoma from the left ear canal (white arrow) in a 60-year-old man that presented with facial weakness

equate resection (Fig. 9.5). Recurrences typically occur within the first 2 years of therapy, although delayed local recurrences have been observed up to 5 years following adequate therapy.

Overall 5-year survival is around 70% [60]. These tumors often have the potential for late, distant metastatic spread. It is not uncommon for metastasis to appear 5–30 years later [1]. Dong et al. reported a mean time to recurrence of 8.1 years (median 8 years; range 1–15 years) [63]. A case of ceruminous adenoid cystic carcinoma that metastasized to the brain within 8 months of primary resection has been reported [55].

Ceruminous Adenocarcinoma

Ceruminous adenocarcinoma is the fourth most common cancer of the ear canal [37, 66]. In various large series of primary temporal bone cancers, adenocarcinoma may be listed as the third or fourth most common tumor seen [37, 41, 67]. In the series reported by Madsen et al., adenocarcinoma of the ear canal was the third most common cancer, but it accounted for only 6% of ear canal cancers [38]. Adenocarcinoma was the second most common temporal bone tumor and made up 12% of the patient cohort reported by Manolidis et al.; however, their series contained tumors of salivary gland origin [68].

Primary adenocarcinoma of the temporal bone is rare. McDonald et al. reported that fewer than 40 cases of primary ceruminous adenocarcinoma have been reported by 1995; and another dozen or so cases have been reported since then [1–5, 10, 11, 24, 26, 27, 54, 56, 66, 69–80].

While chronic ear infection has been linked to squamous cell carcinoma of the ear canal, no such correlation occurs with adenocarcinoma of the ear canal [81]. Symptoms of adenocarcinoma usually relate to ear canal blockage in the early stage [79]. Hearing loss, aural fullness, tinnitus, and deep pain are frequently reported symptoms with adenocarcinoma [81].

Physical examination can reveal a skin-covered tumor in the ear canal or might show an aural polyp [79]. Facial paralysis and bony erosion are commonly reported with adenocarcinoma [82]. Due to its vascular nature, ceruminous adenocarcinoma has also been confused clinically with paraganglioma [3].

Angiography will often disclose a vascular tumor, which can, at times, be mistaken for paraganglioma. CT scan can show bony erosion similar to paraganglioma [83]. CT scan is necessary to define the bony margins of the tumor. MRI is useful to characterize dural or brain involvement (Fig. 9.6). PET/CT is indicated in advanced stage disease to identify distant metastasis or to eliminate the ear canal lesion as a distant metastasis from another primary.

The differential diagnosis includes ceruminous adenoma, pleomorphic adenoma, ceruminous adenocarcinoma, eccrine cylindroma, syringocystadenoma papilliferum, adenoid cystic carcinoma, and metastatic adenocarcinoma [1, 2, 5, 24, 54]. The discernment of adenoma from adenocarcinoma can be difficult [5, 66, 84]. Mitotic hyperactivity, focal necrosis, stromal invasion, and desmoplastic stromal reaction are present in ceruminous adenocarcinoma and discriminate it from benign adenoma [66]. Additionally, ceruminous adenocarcinomas have features not found in adenomas, including soft tissue invasion, perineural invasion, irregular gland formation, pleomorphism, prominent nucleoli, increased and atypical mitotic figures, and tumor necrosis [2]. Low-grade tumors have irregular tubular or glandular structures. High-grade tumors have minimal to no apocrine differentiation and need to be distinguished from metastatic adenocarcinoma [66]. Unfortunately, the typical ceruminous adenocarcinoma demonstrates only a few of these features, blurring the lines between benign and malignant designation. Adenocarcinoma of the ear canal is an aggressive tumor.

In older literature, before 1990, endolymphatic sac tumors (ELST) were characterized as adenocarcinoma [85, 86]. ELST are papillary adenomas that arise from the endolymphatic sac. These tumors can grow to enormous size, infiltrating into bone and the cerebellopontine angle. ELST can be very vascular. CT and MRI are helpful to make the distinction between ELST and ear canal adenocarcinoma, since ELST arise along the posterior fossa and generally cause

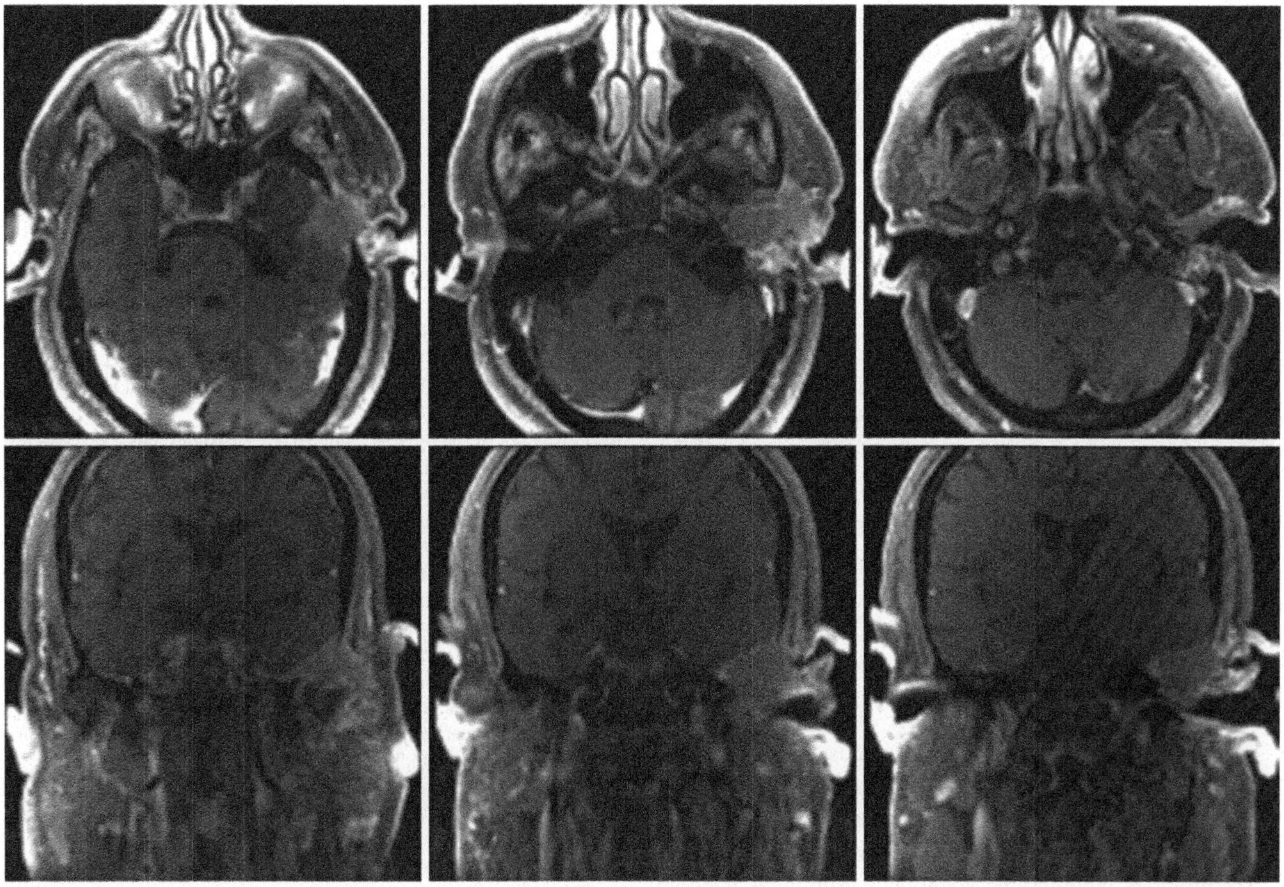

Fig. 9.6 High-grade ceruminous adenocarcinoma of the left ear canal in a 73-year-old man. He presented with a 2-year history of otorrhagia. His ear canal showed a skin-covered swelling that involves the entire anterior and superior ear canal. This swelling extended from the cartilaginous canal down to the level of the eardrum. Facial nerve function was normal. Contrast-enhanced MRI shows dural invasion. Subdural invasion but not brain invasion was found at operation. Final pathology report disclosed lymphovascular invasion with involved lymph nodes in the parotid and level IIB. Perineural invasion was not found

erosion of the labyrinth and therefore cause sensorineural hearing loss and vertigo as chief clinical sign.

Treatment of ceruminous adenocarcinoma is predicated on extent of disease. As with other temporal bone tumors, lateral temporal bone resection is indicated for tumors in the ear canal. Tumors that involve the middle ear or mastoid will require subtotal temporal bone resection. Parotidectomy and modified, selective neck dissection are recommended and necessary for proper staging [1, 5, 75, 79]. Extensive tumors that involve the temporomandibular joint, jugular foramen, or middle and posterior fossae will require combined resections that encompass these areas. Ceruminous adenocarcinoma has been described to invade the brain only in a few rare case reports [1, 71].

Lymph node metastasis is very rare in this condition. Distant metastasis to the liver and lung has been reported in high-grade adenocarcinoma from the middle ear [27].

Radiotherapy is indicated for patients with negative prognostic findings: high tumor grade, positive margins, lymph node metastases, perineural invasion, and bone invasion [69, 85]. Radiotherapy as a primary treatment has also been reported in some cases [76].

Recurrences are common with this tumor since it often present at a late stage [77]. Long-term recurrences, beyond 2 years, have been reported [77].

Ceruminous Mucoepidermoid Carcinoma of the EAC

Mucoepidermoid carcinoma (MEC) is the most common malignant tumor of the parotid gland. However, only eight cases of MEC of ceruminous gland origin and arising in the ear canal have been reported in the English literature [41, 87–93]. In the few reported cases, patient ages ranged from 29 to 62 (mean 49 years). These are locally invasive tumors with frequent lymph node metastases. Cases have been reported that are completely localized to the ear canal without lymph node metastasis [92].

Pathologically, these tumors demonstrate two cellular elements: squamous cells and mucous-secreting cells, with the presence of intermediate cells [92]. The proportions of these cellular elements allow grading: low, intermediate, and high. Low-grade tumors have a higher proportion of mucous cells. High-grade tumors have higher proportion of squamous cells.

The goal of surgical management is complete excision with negative margins. Usually, this requires lateral temporal bone resection. Lesser degrees of ear canal resection have been associated with recurrence [90, 93]. Given the potential for metastatic spread, parotidectomy and neck dissection are usually indicated. Postoperative radiotherapy is indicated for intermediate- and high-grade tumors. Postoperative radiotherapy is also indicated for positive lymph nodes, positive margins, and bony invasion. Postoperative radiotherapy with concurrent chemotherapy (carboplatin) has resulted in durable disease-free survival of 37 months in a single case. There are no reports with follow-up beyond 3 years.

Conclusion

This chapter discusses the diverse group of rare tumors that arise from the ceruminous glands of the external auditory canal. While previously described as "ceruminoma," this moniker has been replaced with more accurate, histopathologic descriptors: ceruminous adenoma, ceruminous pleomorphic adenoma, ceruminous adenoid cystic carcinoma, and ceruminous adenocarcinoma. Complete surgical excision is the main treatment modality for each of these tumors. Postoperative radiotherapy is indicated in malignant tumors that demonstrate perineural invasion, bony invasion, lymph node metastasis, or intermediate- to high-grade histology.

References

1. Hicks GW. Tumors arising from the glandular structures of the external auditory canal. Laryngoscope. 1983;93(3):326–40.
2. Thompson LD, Nelson BL, Barnes EL. Ceruminous adenomas: a clinicopathologic study of 41 cases with a review of the literature. Am J Surg Pathol. 2004;28(3):308–18.
3. Michel RG, Woodard BH, Shelburne JD, Bossen EH. Ceruminous gland adenocarcinoma: a light and electron microscopic study. Cancer. 1978;41(2):545–53.
4. Markou K, Karasmanis I, Vlachtsis K, Petridis D, Nikolaou A, Vital V. Primary pleomorphic adenoma of the external ear canal. Report of a case and literature review. Am J Otolaryngol. 2008;29(2):142–6.
5. Mills RG, Douglas-Jones T, Williams RG. 'Ceruminoma'—a defunct diagnosis. J Laryngol Otol. 1995;109(3):180–8.
6. El Demellawy D, Escott N, Salama S, Alowami S. Sebaceoma of the external ear canal: an unusual location. Case report and review of the literature. J Cutan Pathol. 2008;35(10):963–6.
7. Elsurer C, Senkal HA, Baydar DE, Sennaroglu L. Ceruminous adenoma mimicking furunculosis in the external auditory canal. Eur Arch Otorhinolaryngol. 2007;264(3):223–5.
8. Haug R. Beiträge zur Klinik und mikroskopischen Anatomie der Neubildungen des äusseren und mittleren Ohres. Eur Arch Otorhinolaryngol. 1894;36(3):170–206.
9. Pallanch JF, Weiland LH, McDonald TJ, Facer GW, Harner SG. Adenocarcinoma and adenoma of the middle ear. Laryngoscope. 1982;92(1):47-54.
10. Wetli CV, Pardo V, Millard M, Gerston K. Tumors of ceruminous glands. Cancer. 1972;29(5):1169–78.
11. Lassaletta L, Patron M, Oloriz J, Perez R, Gavilan J. Avoiding misdiagnosis in ceruminous gland tumours. Auris Nasus Larynx. 2003;30(3):287–90.
12. Mark I, Rothberg M. Mixed tumor of skin of external auditory canal. AMA Arch Otolaryngol. 1951;53(5):556–9.
13. Diaz RC, Babu SC. Ductal carcinoma arising from syringocystadenoma papilliferum in the external auditory canal. Otol Neurotol. 2007;28(6):873–4.
14. Giuseppe M, Serena B, Sandro B, Cristiano DN, Vincenzo S, Tommaso V, et al. Adenoma of the ceruminous gland (ceruminoma). Otol Neurotol. 2011;(2):32, e14–e35.
15. Tang X, Tamura Y, Tsutsumi Y. Mixed tumor of the external auditory canal. Pathol Int. 1994;44(1):80–3.
16. Lopez Campos D, Campos Banales ME, Lopez Aguado D. Primary pleomorphic adenoma (chondroid syringoma) of the external auditory canal. Case report and literature review. Acta Otorrinolaringol Esp. 2008;59(5):252–3.
17. Tsukahara K, Suzuki M, Tokashiki R, Motohashi R, Iwaya K. Pleomorphic adenoma of the external auditory canal complicated by hearing loss secondary to chronic otitis media. Auris Nasus Larynx. 2006;33(2):183–6.
18. Koyuncu M, Karagoz F, Kiliacarslan H. Pleomorphic adenoma of the external auditory canal. Eur Arch Otorhinolaryngol. 2005;262(12):969–71.
19. Masumura C, Horii A, Mishiro Y, Inohara H, Kitahara T, Takashima S, et al. Magnetic resonance imaging of pleomorphic adenoma arising from the external auditory canal. J Laryngol Otol. 2003;117(11):908–9.
20. Nardone M, Ferrara G, Nappi O, Di Maria D, Villari G. [Pleomorphic adenoma in unusual anatomic sites: case reports and review of literature]. Acta Otorhinolaryngol Ital. 2002;22(3):158–63.
21. Gerber C, Zimmer G, Linder T, Schuknecht B, Betts DR, Walter R. Primary pleomorphic adenoma of the external auditory canal diagnosed by fine needle aspiration cytology. A case report. Acta Cytol. 1999;43(3):489–91.
22. Baldus SE, Streppel M, Stennert E, Dienes HP. [Pleomorphic adenoma (mixed tumor) of the external auditory canal. Differential diagnosis of the tumors of the ceruminal glands]. Pathologe. 1999;20(2):125–9.
23. Haraguchi H, Hentona H, Tanaka H, Komatuzaki A. Pleomorphic adenoma of the external auditory canal: a case report and review of the literature. J Laryngol Otol. 1996;110(1):52–6.
24. Mansour P, George MK, Pahor AL. Ceruminous gland tumours: a reappraisal. J Laryngol Otol. 1992;106(8):727–32.
25. Suzuki K, Baba S, Miyamoto N. Pleomorphic adenoma of the external auditory canal in Japan, with a case report. Auris Nasus Larynx. 1991;18(3):271–9.
26. Lahoz Zamarro MT, Valero Ruiz J, Royo Lopez J, Yus Gotor C, Camara F. [Mixed tumor of the external auditory canal]. Acta Otorrinolaringol Esp. 1990;41(1):53–6.
27. Dehner LP, Chen KT. Primary tumors of the external and middle ear. Benign and malignant glandular neoplasms. Arch Otolaryngol. 1980;106(1):13–9.
28. Kuwabara H, Haginomori S, Takamaki A, Ito K, Takenaka H, Kurisu Y, et al. Lipomatous pleomorphic adenoma of the ceruminous gland. Pathol Int. 2006;56(1):51–3.
29. Presutti L, Alicandri-Ciufelli M, Mattioli F, Marchioni D, Costantini M. A case of syryngocystadenoma papilliferum (SCAP) involving middle ear, presenting with otomastoiditis and cerebral abscess. Auris Nasus Larynx. 2008;35(3):401–3.

30. Kamakura T, Horii A, Mishiro Y, Takashima S, Kubo T. Magnetic resonance imaging of syringocystadenoma papilliferum of the external auditory canal. Auris Nasus Larynx. 2006;33(1):53–6.
31. Muller R, Theissig F. [Syringocystadenoma papilliferum of the outer ear canal]. Laryngorhinootologie. 1995;74(1):43–5.
32. Lee CK, Jang KT, Cho YS. Tubular apocrine adenoma with syringocystadenoma papilliferum arising from the external auditory canal. J Laryngol Otol. 2005;119(12):1004–6.
33. Marioni G, Brescia G, Staffieri C, Poletti A, Staffieri A. Syringocystoadenoma papilliferum of the external ear canal: an immunohistochemical study. Acta Otolaryngol. 2004;124(6):761–2.
34. Bakshi J, Parida PK. Syringocystadenoma papilliferum: report of first case on the pinna. J Laryngol Otol. 2006;120(12):e45.
35. Austin JR, Stewart KL, Fawzi N. Squamous cell carcinoma of the external auditory canal. Therapeutic prognosis based on a proposed staging system. Arch Otolaryngol Head Neck Surg. 1994;120(11):1228–32.
36. Yin M, Ishikawa K, Honda K, Arakawa T, Harabuchi Y, Nagabashi T, et al. Analysis of 95 cases of squamous cell carcinoma of the external and middle ear. Auris Nasus Larynx. 2006;33(3):251–7.
37. Chi FL, Gu FM, Dai CF, Chen B, Li HW. Survival outcomes in surgical treatment of 72 cases of squamous cell carcinoma of the temporal bone. Otol Neurotol. 2011;32(4):665–9.
38. Madsen AR, Gundgaard MG, Hoff CM, Maare C, Holmboe P, Knap M, et al. Cancer of the external auditory canal and middle ear in Denmark from 1992 to 2001. Head Neck. 2008;30(10):1332–8.
39. Nyrop M, Grontved A. Cancer of the external auditory canal. Arch Otolaryngol Head Neck Surg. 2002;128(7):834–7.
40. Breau RL, Gardner EK, Dornhoffer JL. Cancer of the external auditory canal and temporal bone. Curr Oncol Rep. 2002;4(1):76–80.
41. Kollert M, Draf W, Minovi A, Hofmann E, Bockmuhl U. [Carcinoma of the external auditory canal and middle ear: therapeutic strategy and follow up]. Laryngorhinootologie. 2004;83(12):818–23.
42. Dornhoffer JL, Gardner W, Breau RL. Malignancy of the temporal bone: a review of 32 cases at the university of Arkansas for medical sciences. Skull Base. 2001;11(Suppl 2):54–5.
43. Conley J, Schuller DE. Malignancies of the ear. Laryngoscope. 1976;86(8):1147–63.
44. Shih L, Crabtree JA. Carcinoma of the external auditory canal: an update. Laryngoscope. 1990;100(11):1215–8.
45. Pensak ML, Gleich LL, Gluckman JL, Shumrick KA. Temporal bone carcinoma: contemporary perspectives in the skull base surgical era. Laryngoscope. 1996;106(10):1234–7.
46. Pulec JL, Parkhill EM, Devine KD. Adenoid cystic carcinoma (cylindroma) of the external auditory canal. Trans Am Acad Ophthalmol Otolaryngol. 1963;67:673–94.
47. Lo JS, Snow SN, Mohs FE. Cylindroma treated by Mohs micrographic surgery. J Dermatol Surg Oncol. 1991;17(11):871–4.
48. Volter C, Baier G, Schwager K, Muller JG, Rose C. [Cylindrocarcinoma in a patient with Brooke-Spiegler syndrome]. Laryngorhinootologie. 2002;81(3):243–6.
49. Mashkevich G, Undavia S, Iacob C, Arigo J, Linstrom C. Malignant cylindroma of the external auditory canal. Otol Neurotol. 2006;27(1):97–101.
50. Cankar V, Crowley H. Tumors of ceruminous glands: a clinicopathological study of 7 cases. Cancer. 1964;17:67–75.
51. Ahmed GM, Nath DK. Ceruminous gland tumour (a case report). J Laryngol Otol. 1988;102(4):346–9.
52. Ito K, Ito T, Tsukuda M, Kanisawa M. An immunohistochemical study of adenoid cystic carcinoma of the external auditory canal. Eur Arch Otorhinolaryngol. 1993;250(4):240–4.
53. Fernandez Perez A, Fernandez-Nogueras Jimenez F, Moreno Leon J, Fernandez Sanchez A. [Cystic adenoidal carcinoma of the external ear]. Acta Otorrinolaringol Esp. 1994;45(2):111–3.
54. Fenniche S, Haouet S, Mdimagh H, Chatti S, Maamouri M, Kchir N, et al. [Tumors of the ceruminous glands]. Ann Pathol. 1995;15(2):147–9.
55. Conlin PA, Mira JL, Graham SC, Kaye KS, Cordero J. Ceruminous gland adenoid cystic carcinoma with contralateral metastasis to the brain. Arch Pathol Lab Med. 2002;126(1):87–9.
56. Durko T, Danilewicz M, Pajor A. [Glandular neoplasms of the external auditory canal—clinical and morphologic observations]. Otolaryngol Pol. 2003;57(1):51–7.
57. Garbyal RS, Kumar M, Bohra A. Adenoid cystic carcinoma of ceruminous gland: a case report. Indian J Pathol Microbiol. 2006;49(4):587–9.
58. Crestani S, Vellin JF, Nohra O, Gabrillargues J, Kemeny JL, Gilain L, et al. [Adenoid cystic carcinoma of the external auditory canal]. Ann Otolaryngol Chir Cervicofac. 2007;124(6):314–7.
59. Ouaz K, Robier A, Lescanne E, Bobillier C, Moriniere S, Bakhos D. Cancer of the external auditory canal. Eur Ann Otorhinolaryngol Head Neck Dis. 2013;130(4):175–82.
60. FM G, Chi FL, Dai CF, Chen B, Li HW. Surgical outcomes of 43 cases with adenoid cystic carcinoma of the external auditory canal. Am J Otolaryngol. 2013;34(5):394–8.
61. Zhen S, Fu T, Qi J, Wen J. [Adenoid cystic carcinoma of external auditory canal: 8 cases report]. Lin Chung Er Bi Yan Hou Tou Jing Wai Ke Za Zhi. 2015;29(4):343–5.
62. Liu SC, Kang BH, Nieh S, Chang JL, Wang CH. Adenoid cystic carcinoma of the external auditory canal. J Chin Med Assoc. 2012;75(6):296–300.
63. Dong F, Gidley PW, Ho T, Luna MA, Ginsberg LE, Sturgis EM. Adenoid cystic carcinoma of the external auditory canal. Laryngoscope. 2008;118(9):1591–6.
64. Chang CH, Shu MT, Lee JC, Leu YS, Chen YC, Lee KS. Treatments and outcomes of malignant tumors of external auditory canal. Am J Otolaryngol. 2009;30(1):44–8.
65. Shang J, Sheng L, Wang K, Shui Y, Wei Q. Expression of neural cell adhesion molecule in salivary adenoid cystic carcinoma and its correlation with perineural invasion. Oncol Rep. 2007;18(6):1413–6.
66. Yang CY, Shu MT, Chen BF. Ceruminous adenocarcinoma. Otol Neurotol. 2010;31(6):1011–2.
67. Moore MG, Deschler DG, McKenna MJ, Varvares MA, Lin DT. Management outcomes following lateral temporal bone resection for ear and temporal bone malignancies. Otolaryngol Head Neck Surg. 2007;137(6):893–8.
68. Manolidis S, Pappas D Jr, Von Doersten P, Jackson CG, Glasscock ME 3rd. Temporal bone and lateral skull base malignancy: experience and results with 81 patients. Am J Otol. 1998;19(6 Suppl):S1–15.
69. McDonald M, Brophy BP, Raymond W. Intracranial invasion from a primary adenocarcinoma arising in the middle and external ear. Aust N Z J Surg. 1995;65(6):454–6.
70. Hageman ME, Becker AE. Intracranial invasion of a ceruminous gland tumor. A follow-up of 12 years. Arch Otolaryngol. 1974;100(5):395–7.
71. Saito R, Kodaki K, Shiobara R, Toya S, Kanzaki J. Ceruminoma with intracranial invasion—case report. Neurol Med Chir (Tokyo). 1990;30(13):1034–7.
72. Urbiola Marcilla E. [Ceruminous adenocarcinoma: report of a case]. Rev Med Univ Navarra. 1990;34(3):135–7.
73. Miani C, Russolo M, Silvestri F. [Glandular tumors of the middle ear: a case of primary ceruminous adenoma]. Acta Otorhinolaryngol Ital. 1990;10(3):295–301.
74. Contreras A, Marzo M, Orts M, Mallea I, Morant A, Martinez E, et al. [Adenocarcinoma of the ceruminous glands: report of three cases]. Acta Otorrinolaringol Esp. 1994;45(1):49–51.
75. Soon SL, Bullock M, Prince ME. Ceruminous adenocarcinoma: a rare tumour of the external auditory canal. J Otolaryngol. 2001;30(6):373–7.
76. Shimatani Y, Kodani K, Mishima K, Ametani M, Ogawa T, Shabana M. [Evaluation of the results of radiotherapy for carcinoma involving the external auditory canal or middle ear]. Nippon Igaku Hoshasen Gakkai Zasshi. 2002;62(13):739–43.
77. Tzagaroulakis A, Pasxalidis J, Papadimitriou N, Boussiotou A, Nikolopoulos T, Korres S, et al. [Recurrent ceruminous adenocar-

cinoma of the external auditory canal]. ORL J Otorhinolaryngol Relat Spec. 2003;65(5):300–2.
78. Amonkar GP, Amonkar PP, Rege JD. Bilateral axillary apocrine nevi—a case report. Indian J Pathol Microbiol. 2005;48(1):22–3.
79. Kim CW, Rho YS, Cho SJ, Lee CH, Bae WJ. A case of ceruminous adenocarcinoma of the external auditory canal presenting as an aural polyp. Am J Otolaryngol. 2008;29(3):205–8.
80. Selcuk A, Ensari S, Cetin MA, Sak SD, Dere H. Ceruminous gland carcinoma of the external auditory canal presenting as chronic otitis media. B-ENT. 2007;3(4):195–9.
81. Carroll WR, Niparko JK, Zappia JJ, McClatchey KD. Primary adenocarcinoma of the temporal bone. A case with 40-year follow-up. Arch Otolaryngol Head Neck Surg. 1991;117(4):439–41.
82. Dadas B, Alkan S, Turgut S, Basak T. Primary papillary adenocarcinoma confined to the middle ear and mastoid. Eur Arch Otorhinolaryngol. 2001;258(2):93–5.
83. Goebel JA, Smith PG, Kemink JL, Graham MD. Primary adenocarcinoma of the temporal bone mimicking paragangliomas: radiographic and clinical recognition. Otolaryngol Head Neck Surg. 1987;96(3):231–8.
84. D'Haene N, Saal I, Louryan S, Choufani G, Hassid S, Remmelink M, et al. [External auditory meatus adenocarcinoma]. Rev Med Brux. 2004;25(2):103–6.
85. Glasscock ME 3rd, McKennan KX, Levine SC, Jackson CG. Primary adenocarcinoma of the middle ear and temporal bone. Arch Otolaryngol Head Neck Surg. 1987;113(8):822–4.
86. Li JC, Brackmann DE, Lo WW, Carberry JN, House JW. Reclassification of aggressive adenomatous mastoid neoplasms as endolymphatic sac tumors. Laryngoscope. 1993;103(12):1342–8.
87. Pulec JL. Glandular tumors of the external auditory canal. Laryngoscope. 1977;87(10):1601–12.
88. Kinney SE, Wood BG. Malignancies of the external ear canal and temporal bone: surgical techniques and results. Laryngoscope. 1987;97(2):158–64.
89. Magliulo G, Fusconi M, Pulice G. Mucoepidermoid carcinoma of the external auditory canal: case report. Am J Otolaryngol. 2003;24(4):274–7.
90. Bared A, Dave SP, Garcia M, Angeli SI. Mucoepidermoid carcinoma of the external auditory canal (EAC). Acta Otolaryngol. 2007;127(3):280–4.
91. Chung JH, Lee SH, Park CW, Tae K. Mucoepidermoid carcinoma in the external auditory canal: a case report. Cancer Res Treat. 2012;44(4):275–8.
92. Magliulo G, Ciniglio Appiani M, Colicchio MG, Soldo P, Gioia CR. Mucoepidermoid carcinoma of the external auditory canal. Otol Neurotol. 2012;33(3):e21–2.
93. Mourad WF, KS H, Shourbaji RA, Harrison LB. Trimodality approach for ceruminous mucoepidermoid carcinoma of the external auditory canal. J Laryngol Otol. 2013;127(2):203–6.

Unusual Tumors of the Middle Ear

10

Paul W. Gidley

Introduction

Middle ear tumors are more uncommon than ear canal tumors. Often, these tumors present as conductive hearing loss or as chronic otitis media. This chapter reviews the tumors that occur in the middle ear, excepting squamous cell carcinoma.

Gurgel et al. performed a SEER database search of middle ear carcinomas from 1973 to 2004 and identified 215 middle ear carcinomas [1]. The mean age was 60.7 years. Squamous cell carcinoma (62.8%) was the most frequent tumor type followed by adenocarcinoma (18.2%) and other carcinomas (13.0%). The 5-year survival rate was 36.4%, with squamous cell carcinoma having a much worse prognosis than adenocarcinoma. They found that surgery and radiotherapy had the highest survival rate.

Clinically, these tumors present as conductive hearing loss or chronic otitis media. Physical examination might reveal a retrotympanic mass. For middle ear tumors, exploratory middle ear biopsy is often required to make the diagnosis [2]. The pathologic nomenclature has evolved over time, and middle ear adenomatous neoplasms, neuroendocrine adenomatous middle ear neoplasm, and carcinoid tumors are grouped under the same heading. These tumors have relatively benign behavior, but occasionally metastatic disease can occur. Middle ear adenocarcinomas are a rare, potentially metastatic, and fatal tumor. Inverting papilloma, Schneiderian papilloma, and Schneiderian carcinoma are considered as a spectrum of a single clinical entity. These tumors have extensive invasion, which makes complete surgical excision difficult; and recurrence is relatively common.

The treatment for these rare tumors is complete surgical excision. Recurrence is related to incomplete excision. Radiotherapy has a smaller and less defined role for these unusual middle ear tumors than for squamous cell carcinoma.

P. W. Gidley, M.D., F.A.C.S.
Department of Head and Neck Surgery, The University of Texas M.D. Anderson Cancer Center, Houston, TX, USA
e-mail: pwgidley@mdanderson.org

Middle Ear Adenomatous Neoplasms, Neuroendocrine Adenomatous Middle Ear Neoplasm, and Carcinoid Tumors

Middle ear adenomatous neoplasms (MEAN) encompass a spectrum of diagnoses including carcinoid tumor, middle ear carcinoid, neuroendocrine middle ear tumor, middle ear adenoma, adenomatous tumors of the middle ear, adenocarcinoids, and amphicrine tumors [3]. These tumors are grouped together since they share a common phenotypic and immunopositivity of epithelial and endocrine markers [4].

Neuroendocrine adenomas of the middle ears (NAME) are rare benign tumors that have both neuroendocrine and epithelial properties. These tumors were first described by Derlacki in 1976 [5]. About 100 of these tumors have been reported in the literature; and they account for about 2% of middle ear tumors [6].

Neuroendocrine carcinoma is a very rare tumor of the middle ear. Their incidence is estimated to be 1:40,000 through 1:200,000 persons per year [3]. Carcinoid tumor and middle ear adenoma are probably the same clinical entity [7]. Carcinoid tumors of the middle ear are classified as a low-grade, well-differentiated neuroendocrine carcinoma. In a recent review of the literature, Ramsey et al. identified only 46 cases published in the English literature [8]. While the traditional nomenclature seems to indicate a benign pathology, this tumor has the potential for metastatic spread.

Initially only case series of primary adenomatous neoplasm or low-grade adenocarcinomas of the middle ear and temporal bone were described [9, 10]. Eden et al. described four cases of primary adenomatous neoplasm of the middle ear, and three of these tumors were found behind an intact tympanic membrane and confined to the middle ear without inner ear erosion [10]. These three tumors filled the middle ear but did not erode the ossicles. These tumors were described as reddish-brown and easily removed from the middle ear.

Goebel et al. reported three primary adenomatous middle ear tumors that present with symptoms confused for glomus

P. W. Gidley, F. DeMonte (eds.), *Temporal Bone Cancer*, https://doi.org/10.1007/978-3-319-74539-8_10

jugulare [11]. The radiographic imaging, including arteriography showing highly vascular tumors, presented in the article is most likely consistent with endolymphatic sac tumor (ELST). Glasscock et al. described four patients with low-grade adenocarcinoma of the middle ear and temporal bone. Their patients presented with vertigo and hearing loss. Two tumors seemed to arise in the middle ear and two arose from the posterior surface of the temporal bone between the sigmoid sinus and the internal auditory canal. These latter tumors were probably ELST.

Clinical Presentation

Average age at presentation is 43 years (range 16–72 years) [8]. Left and right ears are equally affected. Male to female ratio is 1.4:1.

Symptoms

Hearing loss is the most common presenting symptom [8]. Aural fullness and tinnitus are the second most common symptoms [12]. Facial paralysis and lymph node metastasis have been reported with neuroendocrine carcinoma [13].

Physical Findings

Most tumors produce conductive hearing loss and an opaque eardrum (Fig. 10.1). The middle ear mass can cause the TM to bulge outwardly. Alternatively, the middle ear mass can extend into the ear canal and obscure the view of the TM. Facial paralysis has been reported, and it is due primarily to nerve compression and not nerve invasion [7]. These findings often prompt intervention such as myringotomy with or without tube, permitting diagnosis, or CT scan followed by middle ear exploration for biopsy.

Nine cases of carcinoid tumor in the ear canal have been reported [8, 14, 15]. The MDACC series includes two patients with carcinoid tumor of the ear canal that presented as a polyp (Fig. 10.2). As pictured, this patient had a large right lower lung lobe carcinoid tumor, raising the possibility that the ear canal lesion was a metastasis from this lung primary tumor.

Diagnostic Imaging

CT is the preferred method of evaluating these middle ear tumors. This method gives excellent bony detail and helps to identify the extent of disease, especially if the mastoid and middle ear remain partially aerated. CT is also a reasonable choice for assessing for possible metastatic disease into the neck and parotid gland. While MRI cannot demonstrate the bony anatomy of the middle ear, these carcinoid tumors of the middle ear do enhance with gadolinium (Fig. 10.1d) [16].

PET/CT is reasonable to assess for metastatic disease or to rule out other carcinoid tumors. Octreotide scanning has been useful in localizing gastrointestinal tumors, and it has a reported sensitivity of 89%. However, octreotide scan has been reported in just one case for middle ear carcinoid tumor [17].

Pathology

Grossly, these tumors are reddish-brown to pale yellow in color. Occasionally these tumors can be seen through an intact tympanic membrane [12]; however, for most patients, the diagnosis is made through middle ear exploration and biopsy.

Pathologically, the tumors are described as arranged in cords, nests, and rosette-like patterns. The cells have small, uniform nuclei with finely stippled chromatin. The cytoplasm varies from clear to eosinophilic. Immunohistochemical analysis is positive for keratin, vimentin, chromogranin, and neuron-specific enolase [12, 18, 19]. Electron microscopy shows dense core, intracytoplasmic granules.

Batsakis and El-Naggar [20] divided adenomatous tumors of the middle ear into two groups: mixed and papillary. Mixed tumors are the more common entity and include pathologic patterns described as acinar, solid, trabecular, cribriform, or carcinoid-like. Mixed tumors are more prominent in men, and papillary tumors are more common in women. These tumors are always confined to the middle ear and mastoid, commonly misdiagnosed as chronic otitis media, and rarely demonstrate an involvement of the otic capsule or the facial nerve. Conversely, papillary tumors always extend to the petrous apex, frequently involve the middle and posterior fossa, and usually involve the facial nerve.

As a group, carcinoid tumors are relatively common tumors of the lung and gastrointestinal tract. These tumors arise from the enterochromaffin-Kulchitsky cells of the GI tract. These cells are part of the amine precursor uptake and decarboxylation (APUD) system. These cells can synthesize, store, and secrete many chemical messengers (serotonin and norepinephrine) and neuropeptides (adrenocorticotropic hormone, calcitonin, and antidiurectic hormone). These hormones are responsible for carcinoid syndrome. Carcinoid syndrome consists of diarrhea, cardiovascular symptoms, and flushing. Only one case of middle ear carcinoid tumor has been associated with carcinoid syndrome [21].

Murphy et al. first described neuroendocrine differentiation of a middle ear tumor in 1980 [22]. The neural crest cells have been postulated as the origin of these tumors in the middle ear [19].

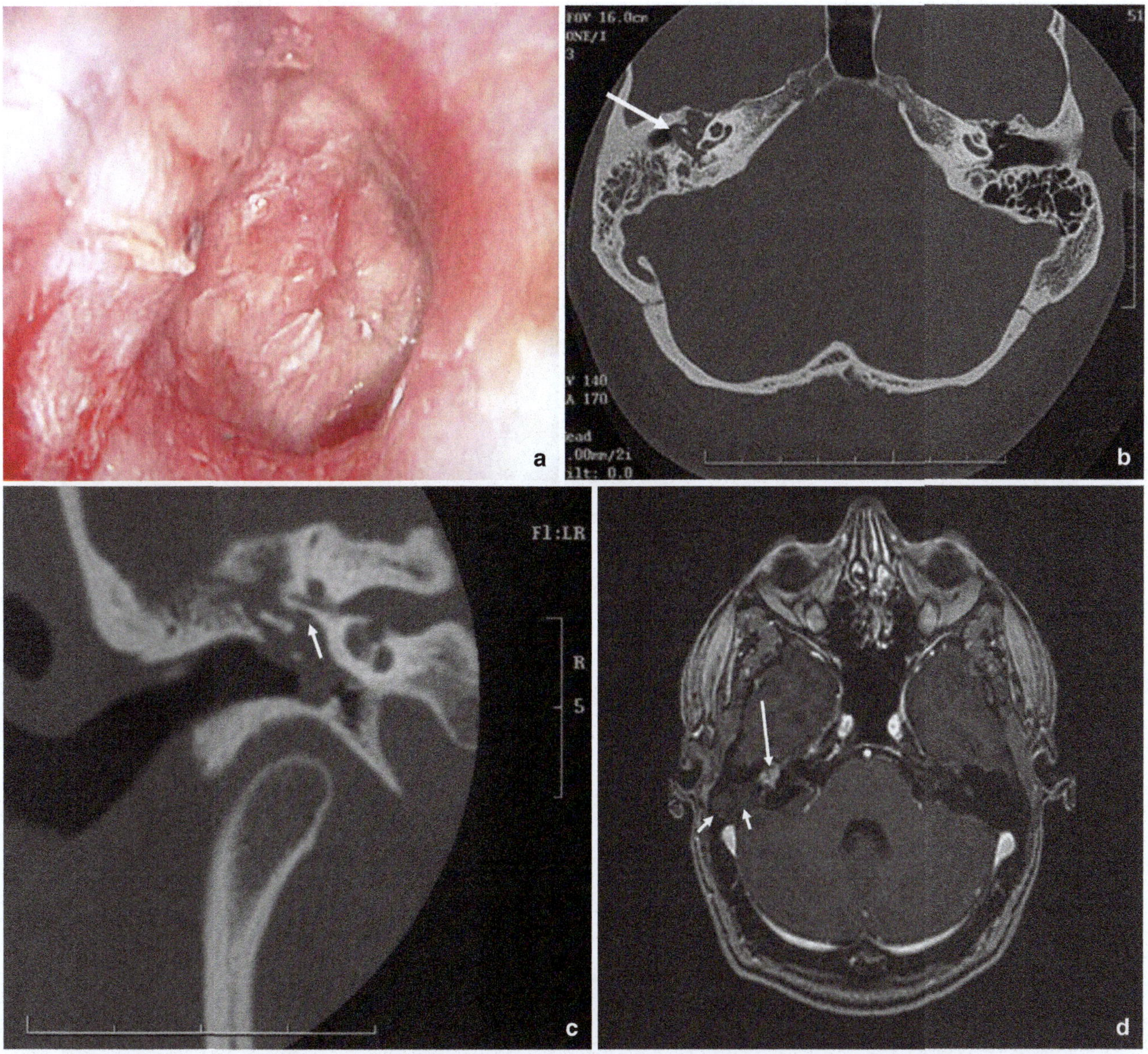

Fig. 10.1 Carcinoid tumor of the right middle ear, presenting as conductive hearing loss and a middle ear mass. (**a**) Oto-endoscopic view. (**b**) Non-contrast axial CT showing the ossicles engulfed by tumor (arrow) and opacified mastoid air cells due to obstruction. (**c**) Non-contrast coronal CT, showing an intact tympanic facial nerve canal (small arrow). (**d**) Contrast-enhanced T1 MRI, showing the enhancing tumor (long arrow) versus the non-enhancing mastoid fluid (short arrows). This tumor was resected via a canal wall up tympanomastoidectomy. The incus was removed due to tumor involvement. No recurrent tumor was identified in an ossiculoplasty performed 6 months later. He has been followed with serial imaging and has remained free of disease for more than 10 years

Treatment

Treatment is complete surgical excision, usually with tympanomastoidectomy. CT imaging is required to know the extent of disease and for treatment planning. Tumors that are limited to the middle ear and mastoid can usually be excised through a canal wall up modified radical mastoidectomy with a facial recess approach. This gives adequate exposure to the tumor, allowing complete excision.

The tumors usually surround and envelope the ossicular chain. Dividing the incudostapedial joint or removal of the incus is necessary to remove tumor around the stapes. The tumor is usually easily removed from the stapes. Care must be exercised when removing disease along the facial nerve, since these tumors can erode bone and expose the facial nerve. Direct facial nerve invasion has also been described [8].

Reconstruction is performed as one would for cholesteatoma. Planned, second-look middle ear exploration is performed 6–12 months later to evaluate and remove any recurrent disease and to refine ossiculoplasty [3].

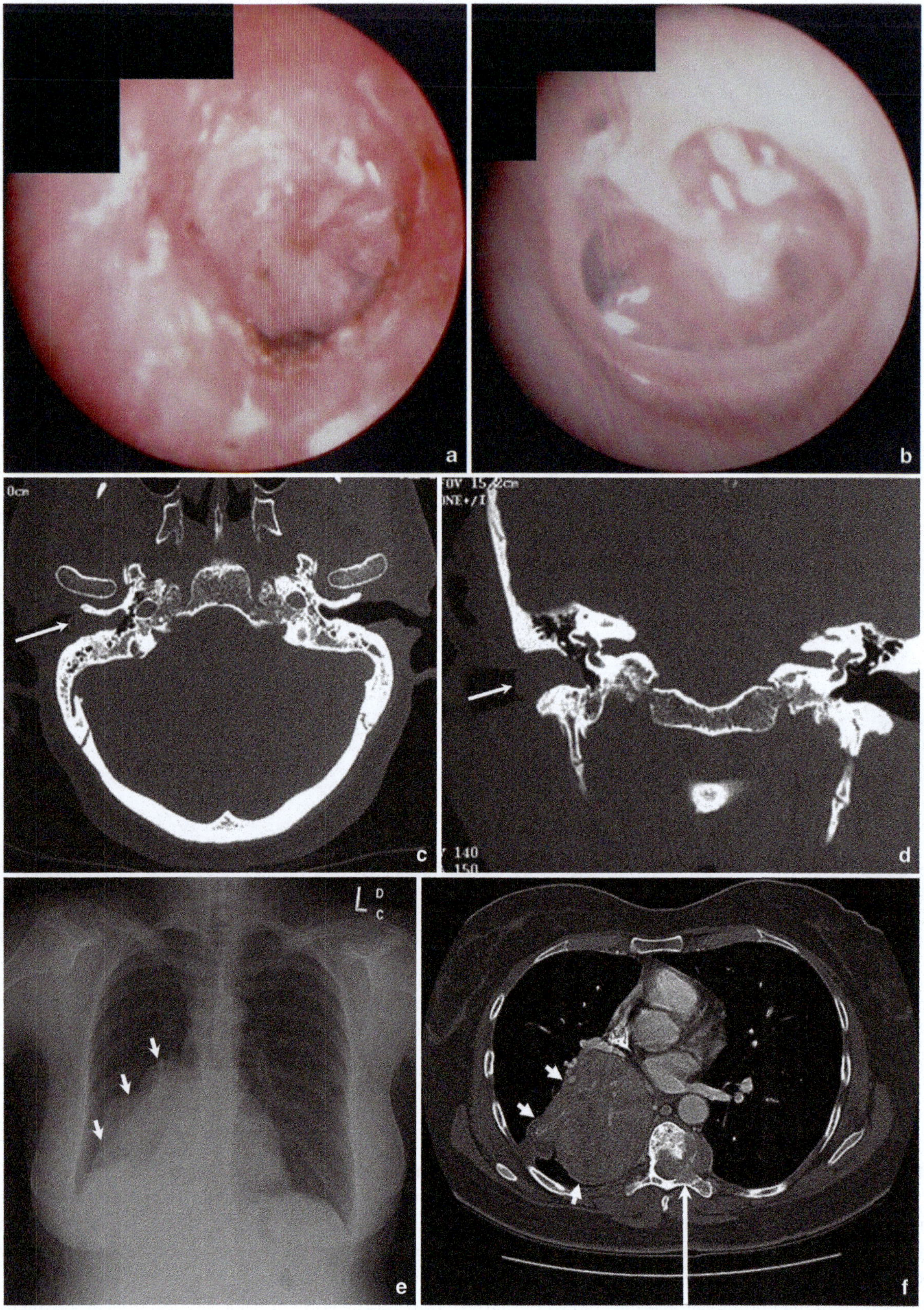

Fig. 10.2 Neuroendocrine carcinoma in a 46-year-old woman that presented as a polyp in the right ear canal. The polyp was removed by the referring physician. Oto-endoscopic photograph of (**a**) right ear after polyp removal and (**b**) left ear, which shows an atelectatic left TM with incudostapedial joint erosion. Non-contrast CT scan axial (**c**) and coronal (**d**) of the temporal bone showing the polyp filling the right ear canal (white arrow). The middle ear is aerated bilaterally. (**e**) Chest X-ray shows large right lower lobe mass (short white arrows). (**f**) Chest CT shows this large mass (short white arrows), which extended into the spinal canal at T9 (long white arrow). Biopsy of this mass revealed carcinoid tumor. Liver metastases were also identified at presentation

In his review of the literature, Ramsay et al. identified that radical mastoidectomy is the most common procedure performed to remove this tumor [8]. They report that ossicular involvement was found in 72% of cases, mastoid involvement in 20%, and Eustachian tube involvement in 9%.

Marchioni et al. have described their experience using a transcanal endoscopic approach for benign middle ear neoplasms, including carcinoid tumors [23].

For more aggressive tumor, especially tumors that have eroded into the ear canal or are recurrent, lateral temporal bone resection has been used. Tumors that extend into the labyrinth can be safely excised through a subtotal temporal bone resection.

Tumors can involve the facial nerve, requiring facial nerve exploration and repair [8].

Disease that has spread into the parotid and neck is excised with parotidectomy and neck dissection; however, there is no evidence to support performing these procedures as a prophylactic measure for the clinically negative sites.

Disease that extends intracranially is excised using frozen section to guide the extent of resection, followed by dural repair and microvascular free flap (Fig. 10.3).

Adjuvant Therapy

There is little to no evidence regarding the use of radiotherapy for carcinoid tumors. Tumors that exhibit aggressive behavior, such as bony erosion, or multiple recurrences have been treated with postoperative radiotherapy. Ramsey et al. identified only five patients who had been treated with radiotherapy; doses ranged from 45 to 60 Gy [8].

While chemotherapy is a part of treatment for pulmonary and gastrointestinal carcinoid tumors, there is no evidence of the use of chemotherapy for middle ear neuroendocrine carcinoma.

Recurrence

Recurrence occurs in almost 20% of cases, due to less than complete resection (Fig. 10.4). In their review of the literature, Ramsey et al. found a local recurrence rate of 22% [8]. Local recurrence rates were higher in patients who underwent tympanotomy (recurrence rate = 29%) than those who were treated with radical mastoidectomy (10%); however, this difference was not statistically significant.

Patients must be followed for several years to detect recurrence. The average interval for recurrence is around 13 years [8].

While laryngeal carcinoids are known to metastasize, this metastatic spread is much less common with temporal bone carcinoids [18]. Ramsey et al. identified four patients (9%) who developed regional metastases. Regional metastases were to cervical lymph nodes in one patient and to intraparotid lymph nodes in three patients [8]. Pellini et al. describe a case of metastatic temporal bone carcinoid tumor with 29 of 51 lymph nodes positive for tumor (see also Fig. 10.3f) [18].

Middle Ear Adenocarcinoma

Middle ear adenocarcinoma is very rare, with less than 80 cases reported in the literature [24–26]. It must be differentiated from middle ear adenoma [27, 28].

These tumors present as chronic otitis media [24]. Middle ear adenocarcinoma often presents as a retrotympanic mass [10]. In the case of middle ear adenocarcinoma, physical examination might reveal a vascular middle ear tumor, which can be easily mistaken for paraganglioma. It is important to differentiate adenocarcinoma of the middle ear from a metastatic lesion, since metastatic colon adenocarcinoma to the middle ear has been described [29].

CT and MRI are crucial to define the limits of the tumor (Fig. 10.5). These tumors can be invasive and extend into the middle fossa and temporal lobe [30].

Complete excision with negative margins is the goal of surgical treatment [31, 32]. Low-grade adenocarcinoma of the middle ear can often be excised through a tympanomastoidectomy [10]. For tumors that are limited to the ear canal, lateral temporal bone resection is indicated. For tumor that involves the middle ear, subtotal temporal bone resection is indicated [2]. Facial nerve involvement is frequently reported in middle ear adenocarcinoma. Facial nerve grafting is indicated where possible.

Intracranial invasion from primary (ceruminous) adenocarcinoma of the middle ear and ear canal has been described [31]. Only a very few patients with middle ear adenocarcinoma have been described to invade intracranially [30].

Inverting Papilloma, Schneiderian Papilloma, and Schneiderian Carcinoma

Inverting papilloma (IP), also known as Schneiderian papilloma, is a benign but locally aggressive tumor that usually arises from the ectodermally derived sinonasal tract, especially from the lateral nasal wall [33, 34]. The natural history of inverting papilloma has three key features: tendency to recur after excision, multicentricity, and potential for malignant transformation [34]. Pathologically, sinonasal IP is identical to middle ear IP.

Three theories have been proposed to explain the development of these tumors: (1) extension from the sinonasal tract, (2) ectopic Schneiderian mucosa in the middle ear, or (3)

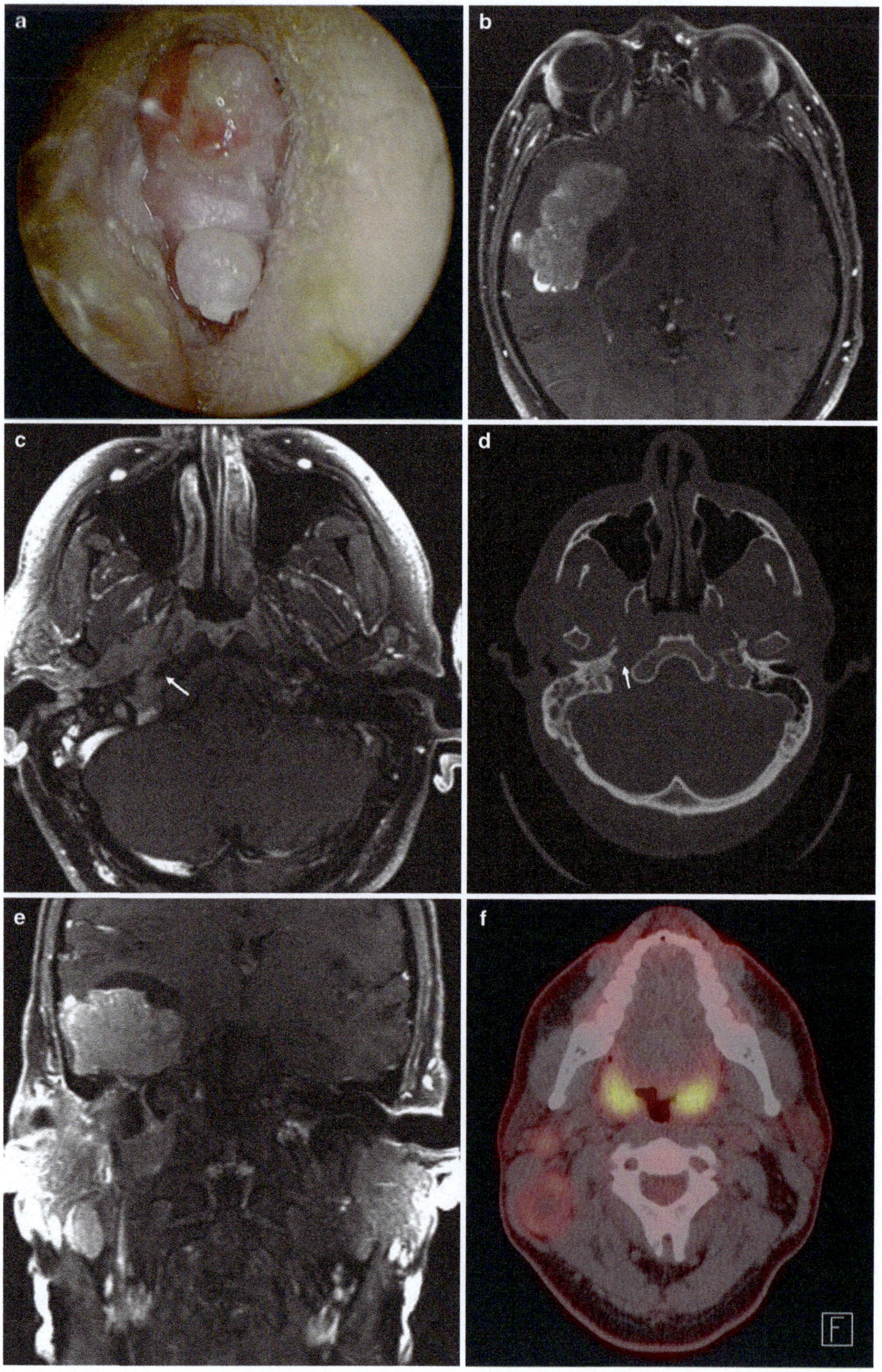

Fig. 10.3 Neuroendocrine carcinoma of the right temporal bone with metastases to the right neck. (**a**) Oto-endoscopic view of right ear canal mass. (**b**) Contrast-enhanced T1 axial MRI showing intracranial portion of tumor. (**c**) Contrast-enhanced T1 axial MRI showing disease around carotid artery (arrow). (**d**) Axial CT scan at same level as Fig. 10.3c, showing bony destruction at carotid canal (arrow). (**e**) Contrast-enhanced T1 coronal MRI, showing both the intracranial and the subtemporal portions of this tumor. (**f**) Axial PET/CT showing metastatic disease in the right neck

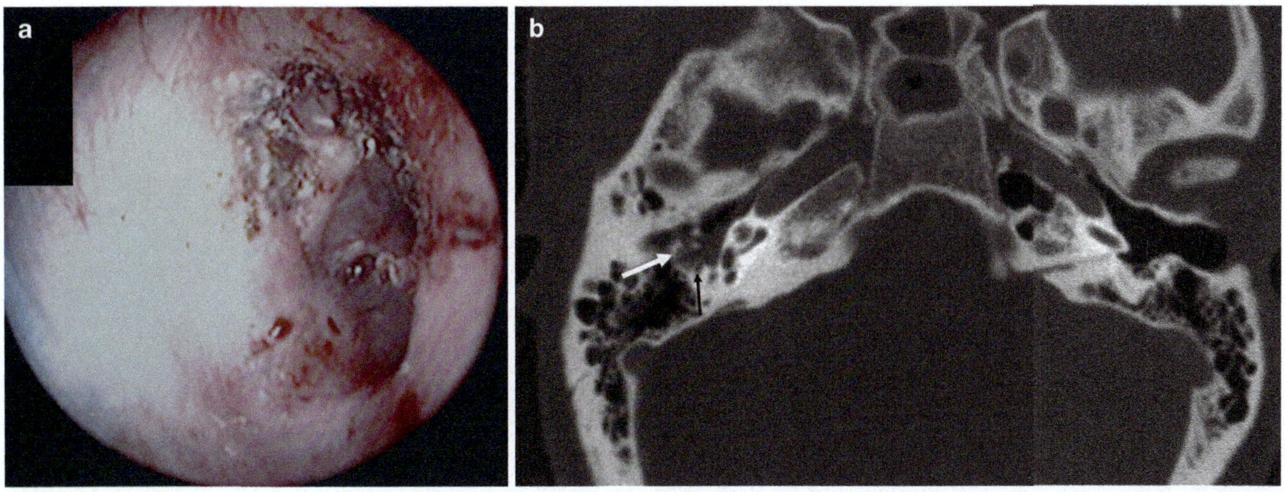

Fig. 10.4 Recurrent carcinoid tumor in a 29-year-old woman treated with a tympanoplasty elsewhere 4 years earlier. (**a**) Oto-endoscopic view, showing tumor bulging the posterior tympanic membrane. (**b**) Axial CT showing bony erosion at the fossa incudis (white arrow). The facial canal is indicated by the black arrow. She was treated with lateral temporal bone resection. Final pathology report indicated bony erosion; therefore, postoperative radiotherapy was administered. She has been disease free for 6 years

seeding of tumor cells from surgical resection of sinonasal IP. Extension from the sinonasal tract is the most widely cited [35–38]. The second theory proposes that IP arises from multicentric or ectopic Schneiderian mucosa in the middle ear [39]. Shen et al. demonstrate a case, which seems to support this theory [34]. Lastly, surgical excision of a sinonasal IP theoretically could seed tumor cells into the middle ear through the Eustachian tube [40].

Primary Schneiderian papillomas are middle ear tumors that are diagnosed without any prior sinonasal disease. These cases tend to have a prior history of chronic otitis media, which leads to myringotomy and biopsy for diagnosis [41]. Secondary Schneiderian papillomas develop in the middle ear following or synchronously with sinonasal disease.

Stone et al. reported the first case of inverting papilloma of the middle ear and mastoid [35]. This patient had a prior history of inverting papilloma in the right lateral nasal wall and maxillary sinus. Later this patient was found to have extensive inverting papilloma in the middle ear and mastoid with erosion of the horizontal canal, tegmen, and posterior fossa plate.

In a systematic review, Carlson et al. identified 32 cases of inverting papilloma affecting the temporal bone [42]. The median age at diagnosis was 54 years (range 19–81 years); and 56% were men. Fifty-nine percent (59%) were associated with sinonasal disease, and 41% were isolated to the temporal bone. There have been three cases of bilateral temporal bone inverting papilloma [39, 43, 44] and two cases of middle ear involvement with malignant transformation [43, 45]. Malignant transformation has been reported more commonly with secondary Schneiderian papillomas than with primary papillomas [43].

Patients with primary temporal bone Schneiderian papillomas tended to be younger, tended to be female, and tended to have less intracranial spread when compared to secondary temporal bone Schneiderian papillomas [42].

Schneiderian papillomas are associated with human papilloma virus (HPV) infections, and HPV positivity is associated with poor outcomes but not necessarily a clear association with malignancy [33, 36, 42, 46]. However, the rate of HPV positivity for primary temporal bone Schneiderian papillomas is only about 20–30% compared to 76% for sinonasal Schneiderian papillomas [33, 42].

Progesterone has been implicated as possible influence on the growth of inverting papilloma of the temporal bone [47]. Progesterone receptors have been identified in two of three cases reported by Shen et al. [34] Air pollution has been linked to Schneiderian papillomas in the nose [48]. Lastly, outdoor and industrial occupations (construction, textile, printing, paper making, and electronics) have been implicated as a significant risk factor for inverting papillomas [49].

The most common symptoms of Schneiderian papillomas of the middle ear are conductive hearing loss and otorrhea. The most common physical finding was tumor bursting through the tympanic membrane in 53% of reported cases. Facial paralysis has been reported in six cases; and all of these cases were associated with either severe dysplasia or invasive carcinoma. Temporal bone CT shows nonspecific opacification of the middle ear and mastoid. These tumors enhance with gadolinium. (Fig. 10.6).

The clinical differential diagnosis includes paraganglioma, papilloma, carcinoid tumor, squamous cell carcinoma, adenocarcinoma, and sarcoma. Diagnosis depends on biopsy, which can usually be performed through a transcanal approach.

Definitive treatment for IP requires complete surgical excision. Surgeons have reported using radical mastoidectomy with obliteration [41], Fisch type A [50], and Fisch type C

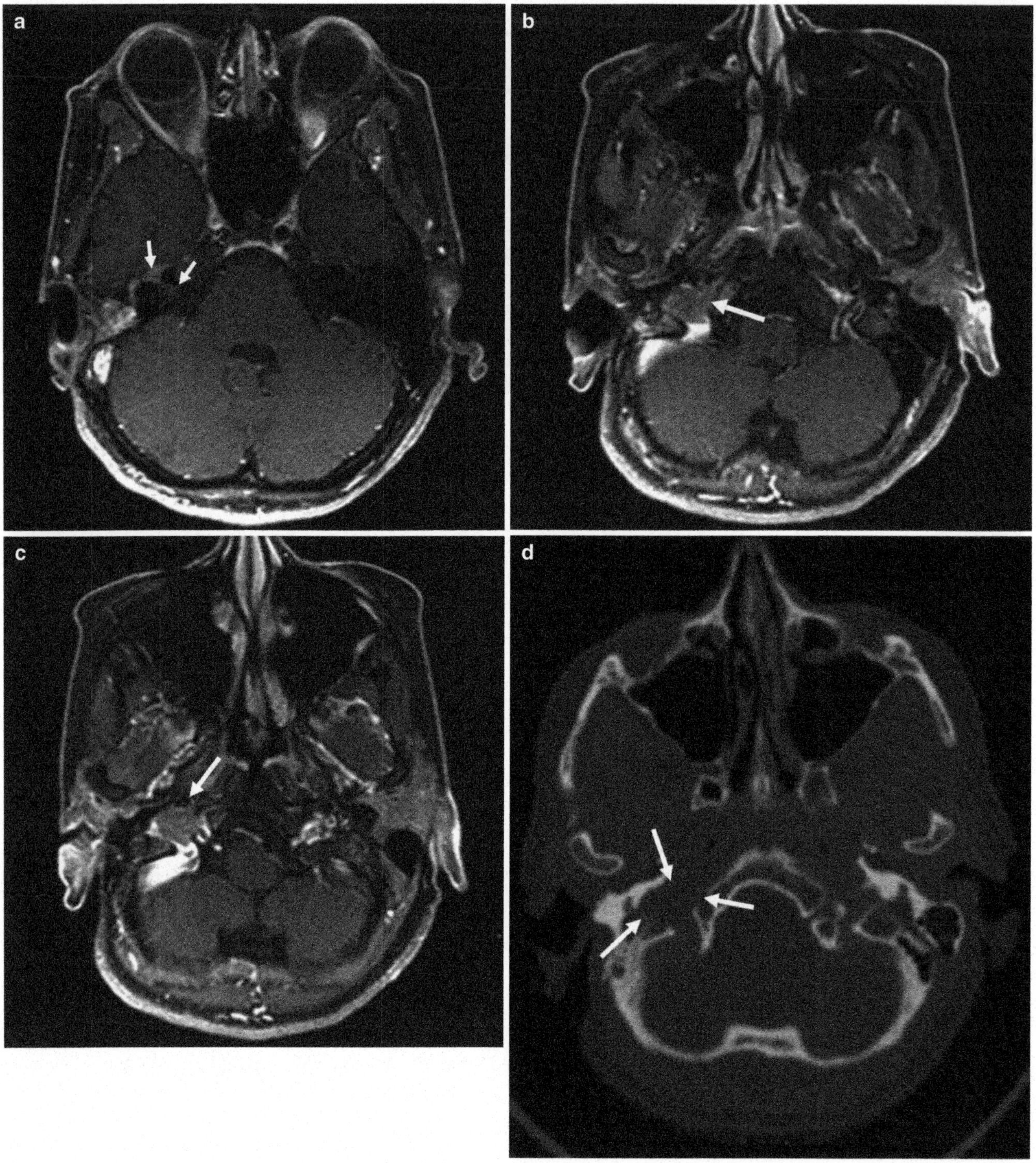

Fig. 10.5 Adenocarcinoma of middle ear. This 58-year-old woman presented with recurrent adenocarcinoma of the middle ear after canal wall down tympanomastoidectomy performed elsewhere 2 years previously. She developed episodic dizziness and lower cranial nerve dysfunction. Axial contrast-enhanced T1 MRI showing (**a**) enhancement of facial nerve and internal auditory canal (arrows), (**b**) tumor filling jugular bulb (arrow) and obstructing sigmoid sinus, and (**c**) tumor abutting carotid artery (arrow). (**d**) Axial CT showing bony destruction at level of jugular foramen (arrows). A subtotal temporal bone resection with jugular foramen resection was used to remove this tumor. She was treated with postoperative radiotherapy and had good locoregional control of her disease. She died of liver metastases 3 years later

[36] approaches to resect disease adequately. However, many cases have extensive disease with bony erosion and adherence to the underlying dura [45, 51]. Carotid artery and internal auditory canal involvement have also been reported [36, 43, 45, 50, 52]. A high level of surgical suspicion must be maintained around the carotid artery since erosive bony involvement around the carotid can lead to the artery being dehiscent and biopsy of tissue here can lead to catastrophic

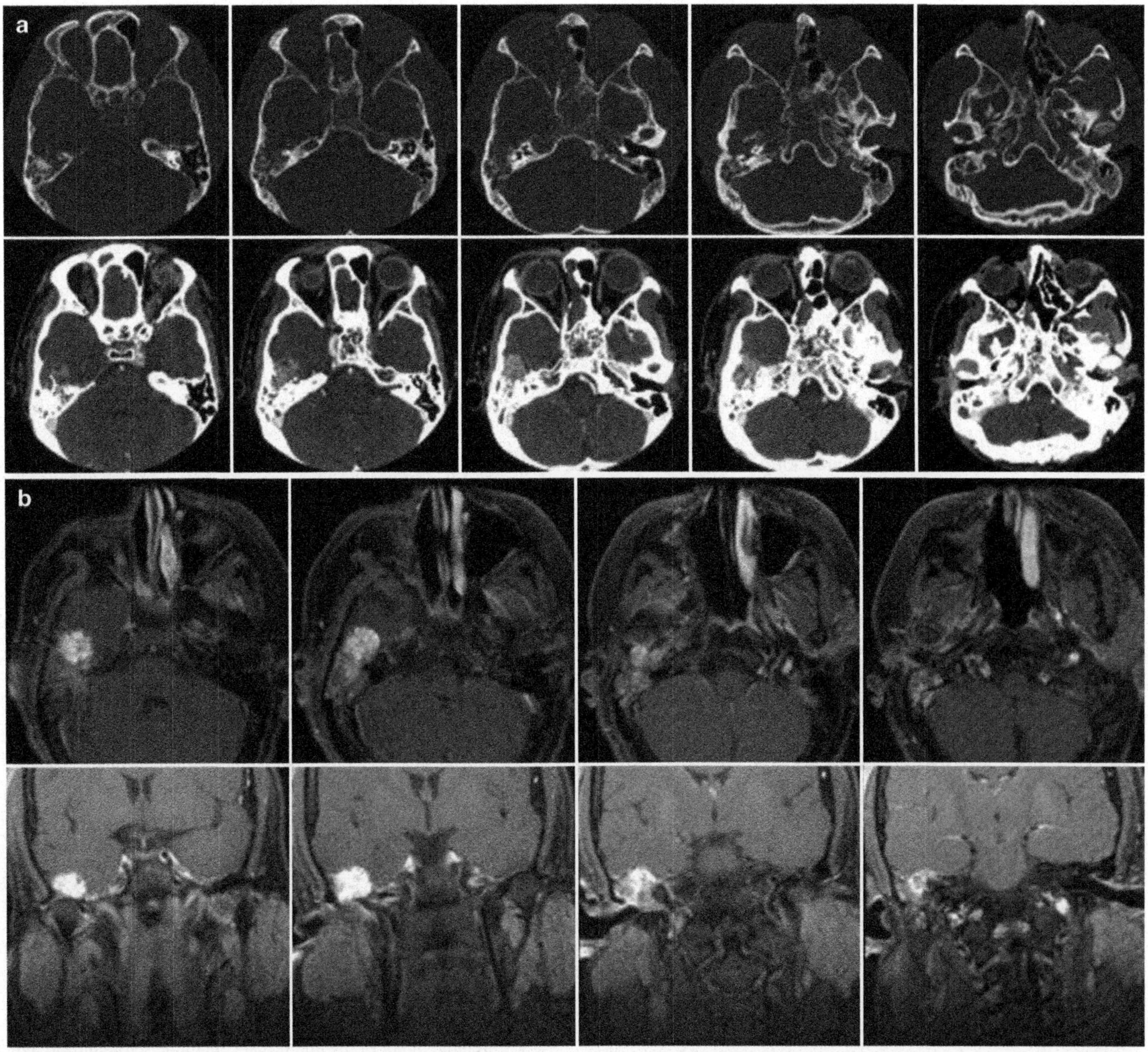

Fig. 10.6 Secondary Schneiderian carcinoma of the right middle ear and temporal bone in a 19-year-old man. He originally presented with sinonasal Schneiderian carcinoma at age 13, which was treated with surgery and radiotherapy. (**a**) Contrast-enhanced CT, bone windows in upper pane and soft tissue windows in lower pane. (**b**) Contrast-enhanced MRI, axial images in upper pane and coronal images in lower pane

hemorrhage. Due to the thin nature of the tegmen, intracranial involvement has been reported in 20 cases, a much higher incidence than for sinonasal inverting papilloma [45].

Radiotherapy for sinonasal inverting papilloma has been implicated in malignant transformation. For temporal bone inverting papilloma, radiotherapy is reserved for cases with proven malignant transformation; and it has also been used in cases of nonmalignant inverting papilloma, which could not be completely resected [43, 45]. Radiotherapy has been used in less than 40% of reported cases.

The recurrence rate after surgical resection remains high (30–60%), which is much higher than the reported recurrence rate for sinonasal inverting papilloma (10–17%) [33, 42, 43]. The recurrence rate between primary and secondary tumors is roughly equivalent (50% compared to 60%, respectively) [34]. Recurrences have been documented to occur from 6 months to 15 years following initial treatment, with most occurring within the first 2 years of diagnosis.

Schneiderian papillomas can transform into Schneiderian carcinoma. The rate of malignant transformation is higher for temporal bone Schneiderian papillomas (40% malignant transformation) than for sinonasal Schneiderian papillomas (5–13%) [33, 43]. Fewer than 20 cases of primary temporal bone Schneiderian carcinoma have been described; roughly another 15 cases of secondary temporal bone Schneiderian carcinoma involvement have been reported. The recurrence rate of Schneiderian carcinoma (69%) is much higher than in those cases without malignant transformation (36%) [34]. Schneiderian carcinoma has a slight female predominance (55%).

Lymphoepithelial-Like Carcinoma

Lymphoepithelial-like carcinomas (LELCs) are tumors that are histologically similar to nasopharyngeal carcinoma, but these tumors arise in areas of the head and neck different from the nasopharynx. The most common sites are the salivary glands, especially the parotid, sinonasal tract, and larynx; but LELCs have been described arising in the middle ear and temporal bone [53]. There have only been six cases of LELC in the middle ear reported in the literature. All of these tumors were associated with Epstein-Barr virus (EBV) infection. Four of six patients were from Guangdong province of China.

Clinically, these patients have hearing loss, aural fullness, pain, and cranial nerve palsies. All of these patients had a history of long-standing otitis media. Otoscopy showed polypoid granulation tissue-like mass in the middle ear extending to the ear canal. None of these patients had disease in the nasopharynx.

Surgery with postoperative radiotherapy has been used and appears to be appropriate therapy for these tumors.

Aggressive Papillary Tumor of the Middle Ear

Papillary tumors that arise within the middle ear without involvement of the endolymphatic sac have been described. Tysome et al. described a 68-year-old woman with a tumor filling the middle ear and no evidence of petrous temporal bone involvement [54]. Muller et al. also described an "endolymphatic sac tumor" confined to the middle ear, which clinically mimicked a glomus tympanicum tumor [55]. Further literature search found additional three cases [2, 30, 56].

These tumors tend to grow along pathways of least resistance and fill the middle ear and mastoid [57].

A mouse model was serendipitously discovered while creating a mouse model for mutant EGFR-driven lung cancer [58]. These mice developed head tilt at median age 25 weeks, and MRI showed bilateral tympanic cavity tumors. These tumors originated from epithelial cells in the tympanic cavity. Mutant EGFR was expressed by immunohistochemical studies. Trial of tyrosine kinase inhibitors, afatinib and cetuximab, was found to reduce tumor volume by 67% and normalized head tilt and gait.

Conclusion

Middle ear cancers are rare. These tumors usually present as conductive hearing loss or chronic otitis media. Transcanal biopsy is necessary for definitive diagnosis, since imaging findings are nonspecific. Complete surgical excision is required for adequate treatment. Radiotherapy is reserved for tumors that show aggressive pathologic behavior or for recurrence.

References

1. Gurgel RK, Karnell LH, Hansen MR. Middle ear cancer: a population-based study. Laryngoscope. 2009;119(10):1913–7.
2. Dadas B, Alkan S, Turgut S, Basak T. Primary papillary adenocarcinoma confined to the middle ear and mastoid. Eur Arch Otorhinolaryngol. 2001;258(2):93–5.
3. Duderstadt M, Forster C, Welkoborsky HJ, Ostertag H. Adenomatous tumors of the middle ear and temporal bone: clinical, morphological and tumor biological characteristics of challenging neoplastic lesions. Eur Arch Otorhinolaryngol. 2012;269(3):823–31.
4. Bell D, El-Naggar AK, Gidley PW. Middle ear adenomatous neuroendocrine tumors: a 25-year experience at MD Anderson Cancer Center. Virchows Arch. 2017;471(5):667–72.
5. Derlacki EL, Barney PL. Adenomatous tumors of the middle ear and mastoid. Laryngoscope. 1976;86(8):1123–35.
6. Almuhanna K. Neuroendocrine adenoma of the middle ear with the history of otitis media and carcinoma of the cheek: a case report. BMC Res Notes. 2014;7:532.
7. Torske KR, Thompson LD. Adenoma versus carcinoid tumor of the middle ear: a study of 48 cases and review of the literature. Mod Pathol. 2002;15(5):543–55.
8. Ramsey MJ, Nadol JB Jr, Pilch BZ, McKenna MJ. Carcinoid tumor of the middle ear: clinical features, recurrences, and metastases. Laryngoscope. 2005;115(9):1660–6.
9. Gulya AJ, Glasscock ME, Pensak ML. Primary adenocarcinoma of the temporal bone with posterior fossa extension: case report. Laryngoscope. 1986;96(6):675-7.
10. Eden AR, Pincus RL, Parisier SC, Som PM. Primary adenomatous neoplasm of the middle ear. Laryngoscope. 1984;94(1):63–7.
11. Goebel JA, Smith PG, Kemink JL, Graham MD. Primary adenocarcinoma of the temporal bone mimicking paragangliomas: radiographic and clinical recognition. Otolaryngol Head Neck Surg. 1987; 96(3):231–8.
12. Chan KC, CM W, Huang SF. Carcinoid tumor of the middle ear: a case report. Am J Otolaryngol. 2005;26(1):57–9.
13. Ouaz K, Robier A, Lescanne E, Bobillier C, Moriniere S, Bakhos D. Cancer of the external auditory canal. Eur Ann Otorhinolaryngol Head Neck Dis. 2013;130(4):175–82.
14. Ferri E, Cavaleri S, Ianniello F, Longo L. [Primitive carcinoid tumor of the middle ear: a case report and review of literature]. Acta Otorhinolaryngol Ital. 1999;19(2):91–6.
15. Hosoda S, Tateno H, Inoue HK, Isojima G, Kondo S, Konishi T. Carcinoid tumor of the middle ear containing serotonin and multiple peptide hormones. A case report and review of the pathology literature. Acta Pathol Jpn. 1992;42(8):614–20.
16. Phelps PD, Lloyd GA. Magnetic resonance with gadolinium DTPA for the investigation of temporal bone tumours. Clin Otolaryngol Allied Sci. 1989;14(3):251–62.
17. Nikanne E, Kantola O, Parviainen T. Carcinoid tumor of middle ear. Acta Otolaryngol. 2002;119(11):1081–4.
18. Pellini R, Ruggieri M, Pichi B, Covello R, Danesi G, Spriano G. A case of cervical metastases from temporal bone carcinoid. Head Neck. 2005;27(7):644–7.
19. Bold EL, Wanamaker JR, Hughes GB, Rhee CK, Sebek BA, Kinney SE. Adenomatous lesions of the temporal bone immunohistochemical analysis and theories of histogenesis. Am J Otol. 1995;16(2):146–52.
20. Batsakis JG. El-Naggar AK. Papillary neoplasms (Heffner's tumors) of the endolymphatic sac. Ann Otol Rhinol Laryngol. 1993;102(8 Pt 1):648–51.
21. Latif M, Madders D, Barton R, Shaw P. Carcinoid tumour of the middle ear associated with systemic symptoms. J Laryngol Otol. 1987;101(05):480–6.
22. Murphy GF, Pilch ZB, Dickersin GR, Goodman ML, Nadol JB. Carcinoid tumor of the middle ear. Am J Clin Pathol. 1980; 73(6):816–23.

23. Marchioni D, Alicandri-Ciufelli M, Gioacchini FM, Bonali M, Presutti L. Transcanal endoscopic treatment of benign middle ear neoplasms. Eur Arch Otorhinolaryngol. 2013;270(12): 2997–3004.
24. Morita M, Mori N, Takashima H, Miki H, Sakai SI. Primary poorly differentiated adenocarcinoma of the middle ear. Auris Nasus Larynx. 1994;21(1):59–63.
25. Carroll WR, Niparko JK, Zappia JJ, McClatchey KD. Primary adenocarcinoma of the temporal bone. A case with 40-year follow-up. Arch Otolaryngol Head Neck Surg. 1991;117(4):439–41.
26. Glasscock ME 3rd, McKennan KX, Levine SC, Jackson CG. Primary adenocarcinoma of the middle ear and temporal bone. Arch Otolaryngol Head Neck Surg. 1987;113(8):822–4.
27. Devaney KO, Boschman CR, Willard SC, Ferlito A, Rinaldo A. Tumours of the external ear and temporal bone. Lancet Oncol. 2005;6(6):411–20.
28. Thompson LD, Nelson BL, Barnes EL. Ceruminous adenomas: a clinicopathologic study of 41 cases with a review of the literature. Am J Surg Pathol. 2004;28(3):308–18.
29. Merrick Y. Metastatic colon adenocarcinoma of the middle ear. Arch Otorhinolaryngol. 1983;238(2):103–5.
30. Paulus W, Romstock J, Weidenbecher M, Huk WJ, Fahlbusch R. Middle ear adenocarcinoma with intracranial extension. Case report. J Neurosurg. 1999;90(3):555–8.
31. McDonald M, Brophy BP, Raymond W. Intracranial invasion from a primary adenocarcinoma arising in the middle and external ear. Aust N Z J Surg. 1995;65(6):454–6.
32. Mansour P, George MK, Pahor AL. Ceruminous gland tumours: a reappraisal. J Laryngol Otol. 1992;106(8):727–32.
33. van der Putten L, Bloemena E, Merkus P, Hensen EF. Schneiderian papilloma of the temporal bone. BMJ Case Rep. 2013;2013
34. Shen J, Baik F, Mafee MF, Peterson M, Nguyen QT. Inverting papilloma of the temporal bone: case report and meta-analysis of risk factors. Otol Neurotol. 2011;32(7):1124–33.
35. Stone DM, Berktold RE, Ranganathan C, Wiet RJ. Inverted papilloma of the middle ear and mastoid. Otolaryngol Head Neck Surg. 1987;97(4):416–8.
36. Jones ME, Wackym PA, Said-Al Naief N, Brandwein M, Shaari CM, Som PM, et al. Clinical and molecular pathology of aggressive schneiderian papilloma involving the temporal bone. Head Neck. 1998;20(1):83–8.
37. Chhetri D, Gajjar N, Bhuta S, Andrews J. Pathology forum. Quiz case 2. Schneiderian-type papilloma of the middle ear. Arch Otolaryngol Head Neck Surg. 2001;127:79,80–2.
38. Liu ZW, Walden A, Lee CA. Sinonasal inverted papilloma involving the temporal bone via the eustachian tube: case report. J Laryngol Otol. 2013;127(3):318–20.
39. Altug T, Sunar O, Bilgin H. [Inverted papilloma. Apropos of a multicentric case]. Rev Laryngol Otol Rhinol (Bord). 1989;110(3): 299–301.
40. Miller PJ, Jacobs J, Roland JT, Cooper J, Mizrachi HH. Intracranial inverting papilloma. Head Neck. 1996;18(5):450–4.
41. Pou AM, Vrabec JT. Inverting papilloma of the temporal bone. Laryngoscope. 2002;112(1):140–2.
42. Carlson ML, Sweeney AD, Modest MC, Van Gompel JJ, Haynes DS, Neff BA. Inverting papilloma of the temporal bone: report of four new cases and systematic review of the literature. Laryngoscope. 2015;125(11):2576–83.
43. Uchida M, Fujita T, Okamoto K, Ueda M, Ushijima C, Dejima K. [A case of Schneiderian middle-ear and sinonasal papilloma with intracranial complications]. Nihon Jibiinkoka Gakkai Kaiho. 2011;114(9):768–73.
44. Uchida M, Fujita T, Okamoto K, Ueda M, Ushijima C, Dejima K. A case of Schneiderian middle-ear and sinonasal papilloma with intracranial complications. Nihon Jibiinkoka Gakkai Kaiho. 2011;114(9):768–73.
45. Dingle I, Stachiw N, Bartlett A, Lambert P. Bilateral inverted papilloma of the middle ear with intracranial involvement and malignant transformation: first reported case. Laryngoscope. 2012;122(7):1615–9.
46. Marioni G, Altavilla G, Busatto G, Blandamura S, De Filippis C, Staffieri A. Detection of human papillomavirus in temporal bone inverted papilloma by polymerase chain reaction. Acta Otolaryngol. 2003;123(3):367–71.
47. Blandamura S, Marioni G, de Filippis C, Giacomelli L, Segato P, Staffieri A. Temporal bone and sinonasal inverted papilloma: the same pathological entity? Arch Otolaryngol Head Neck Surg. 2003;129(5):553–6.
48. Calderon-Garciduenas L, Delgado R, Calderon-Garciduenas A, Meneses A, Ruiz LM, De La Garza J, et al. Malignant neoplasms of the nasal cavity and paranasal sinuses: a series of 256 patients in Mexico City and Monterrey. Is air pollution the missing link? Otolaryngol Head Neck Surg. 2000;122(4):499–508.
49. Sham CL, Lee DL, Cv H, Tong MC. A case-control study of the risk factors associated with sinonasal inverted papilloma. Am J Rhinol Allergy. 2010;24(1):e37–40.
50. Zhou H, Chen Z, Li H, Xing G. Primary temporal inverted papilloma with premalignant change. J Laryngol Otol. 2011;125(2):206–9.
51. Wassef S, Battra P, Barnett S. Skull base inverted papilloma: a comprehensive review. ISRN Surg. 2012;2012:175903.
52. Acevedo-Henao CM, Talagas M, Marianowski R, Pradier O. Recurrent inverted papilloma with intracranial and temporal fossa involvement: a case report and review of the literature. Cancer Radiother. 2010;14(3):202–5.
53. Wenig BM. Lymphoepithelial-like carcinomas of the head and neck. Semin Diagn Pathol. 2015;32(1):74–86.
54. Tysome JR, Harcourt J, Patel MC, Sandison A, Michaels L. Aggressive papillary tumor of the middle ear: a true entity or an endolymphatic sac neoplasm? Ear Nose Throat J. 2008;87(7): 378–81.
55. Muller M, Zammit-Maempel I, Hill J, Wilkins B. An unusual middle-ear mass. J Laryngol Otol. 2010;124(1):108–10.
56. Schick B, Kronsbein H, Kahle G, Prescher A, Draf W. Papillary tumor of the temporal bone. Skull Base. 2001;11(1):25–33.
57. Levin RJ, Feghali JG, Morganstern N, Llena J, Bradley MK. Aggressive papillary tumors of the temporal bone: an immunohistochemical analysis in tissue culture. Laryngoscope. 1996;106(2 Pt 1):144–7.
58. Kawabata S, Hollander MC, Munasinghe JP, Brinster LR, Mercado-Matos JR, Li J, et al. Epidermal growth factor receptor as a novel molecular target for aggressive papillary tumors in the middle ear and temporal bone. Oncotarget. 2015;6(13):11357–68.

Unusual Tumors of the Temporal Bone

11

Paul W. Gidley

Introduction

This chapter discusses rare cancers of the temporal bone beyond squamous cell carcinoma. These tumors have unique clinical characteristics and natural histories. The diagnosis and management of each tumor type are discussed in detail. This chapter does not discuss benign tumors of the temporal bone, such as paragangliomas or meningiomas.

Endolymphatic Sac Tumor

Endolymphatic sac tumors (ELSTs) are benign tumors that arise from the endolymphatic sac and produce sensorineural hearing loss and vestibulopathy. ELSTs are characteristically highly vascular and locally aggressive with infiltration of the temporal bone. Several different terms have been used to describe this tumor, including primary adenocarcinoma of the middle ear of papillary type, papillary adenoma tumor (PAT), PAT of the temporal bone, or low-grade adenocarcinoma of the temporal bone [1].

Embryologically, the endolymphatic sac is derived from neuroectoderm. Anatomically, the endolymphatic sac is located on the posterior surface of the temporal bone, between the posterior semicircular canal and sigmoid sinus. This structure is thought to regulate the fluid volume and ionic balance of the inner ear. The endolymphatic sac connects to the common crus of the bony labyrinth through the endolymphatic duct. The endolymphatic sac has two layers, which are continuous with the posterior fossa dura, and between these layers is a rugose lining [2].

The first case reported was probably by Brandt in 1921 who described a destructive tumor of the temporal bone that histologically resembled renal cell carcinoma [3]. However, the first definitive report of ELST was by Hassard et al. (1984) who described a tumor of the endolymphatic sac discovered during endolymphatic sac decompression for Meniere's disease [4]. Gaffey et al. (1988) noted the association of biologically aggressive growth with papillary histology and proposed the term aggressive papillary middle ear tumor [5]. Heffner (1989) characterized the pathologic findings of aggressive papillary tumors of the temporal bone and opined the endolymphatic sac as the origin [6]. Li et al. (1993) proposed that these invasive papillary tumors of the temporal bone be classified as ELST [7]. Batsakis and El-Naggar (1993) described in detail the pathologic features associated with ELST [8].

von Hippel-Lindau Syndrome

These tumors are associated with von Hippel-Lindau disease (VHL). The first patient with VHL was described by Eugen von Hippel as a tumor of the petrous bone [9]. ELST can be the initial presentation of VHL in approximately 30% of patients [10]. VHL is an autosomal dominant syndrome associated with mutation of the *VHL* gene on the short arm of chromosome 3 (3p25–p26) [11–13]. The *VHL* gene acts as a tumor suppressor, and it was first identified in 1993 by Latif et al. [11] These tumorigeneses follow along the two-hit hypothesis of Knudson [14] Mutation of the von Hippel-Lindau tumor suppressor gene has also been identified in sporadic ELST [12].

The incidence of VHL is approximately 1 case/39,000 people per year. VHL comprises the association of multiple tumor types including ELST, CNS and retinal hemangioblastomas, pheochromocytomas, renal cysts and carcinomas, cystadenomas of the reproductive adnexal organs, and pancreatic cysts and neuroendocrine tumors [15–19].

ELST occurs in 4–16% of patients with VHL [1, 10, 18, 20, 21]. Bilateral ELST has been found in patients with VHL [22–25]. The *VHL* germline mutation is present in approximately 39% of ELST [10]. Since ELST can be the initial presentation of VHL, VHL genetic testing is recommended for patients with ELST.

P. W. Gidley, M.D., F.A.C.S.
Department of Head and Neck Surgery, The University of Texas M.D. Anderson Cancer Center, Houston, TX, USA
e-mail: pwgidley@mdanderson.org

P. W. Gidley, F. DeMonte (eds.), *Temporal Bone Cancer*, https://doi.org/10.1007/978-3-319-74539-8_11

VHL Surveillance

Given that hearing loss is a common outcome from ELSTs and that hearing can be preserved with removal of small tumors, surveillance in VHL is necessary to identify tumors at an early stage [26]. Surveillance begins in infancy for children with a family history of VHL or a known genetic defect. Newborn hearing screening and annual eye/retinal examinations are important in early childhood. Hearing assessment and eye examinations continue throughout childhood to adulthood. Audiograms are performed whenever VHL patients complain of hearing loss, tinnitus, vertigo, or aural fullness.

MRIs are performed in children with hearing loss, tinnitus, vertigo, or repeated ear infections. By age 16, MRI of the brain and spinal cord is recommended every 2–3 years to rule out both ELST and hemangioblastomas [27].

Abdominal ultrasound and plasma-free metanephrines are used to identify pheochromocytomas.

Epidemiology

These tumors are rare. By 2004, Bambakidis had identified 149 cases of ELSTs in both VHL and non-VHL patients [28]. Their retrospective review identified 103 patients with sporadic ELST. There were 55 men and 48 women, with an age range of 15–77 (mean 52.5 years). They identified 46 VHL patients with ELST. There were 15 men and 31 women, with an age range of 7–63 years (mean 31.3 years). Bilateral hearing loss was found in 1% of sporadic cases and 28% of syndromic cases. Facial weakness was found in 38% of syndromic cases versus 49% in sporadic cases.

There have been at least another 150 cases reported since then. The youngest patient ever reported with ELST was 4 years old [29].

An international database of endolymphatic sac tumors identified 93 patients with ELST [10]. From this international ELST registry, the average age of diagnosis was 31 years (range 6–78 years) [10]. Twenty-five had sporadic ELST, and 68 patients had VHL-associated (syndromic) ELST. The mean age is slightly older in sporadic ELSTs (40 years) compared to VHL-associated tumors (30 years, $p = 0.002$). In this registry, there were 52 women to 41 men. Sporadic tumors tended to occur more commonly in men than women (60% versus 40%), while syndromic tumors tended to occur more frequently in women than men (63% versus 32%). Bilateral tumors were found in 19% and only occurred in VHL patients. Asymptomatic tumors were found only in syndromic patients, perhaps due to heightened vigilance.

Patient Features

These histologically benign tumors show aggressive growth clinically. These tumors originate on the posterior surface of the temporal bone as extradural growths. They grow anteriorly and laterally into the labyrinth and middle ear, posteriorly and medially into the cerebellopontine angle and cerebellum, inferiorly into the jugular bulb, and superiorly and anteriorly along the petrous apex to the carotid canal. ELST that grows into the sphenoid sinus has been reported [30]. They erode through the temporal bone into the middle ear, and they can produce deficits in cranial nerves V-XI [31].

Clinically these tumors present with gradual hearing loss, vertigo, tinnitus, or facial paralysis [30]. Sensorineural hearing loss (SNHL) is the most common complaint, in approximately 95–100% of patients [10, 28, 32]. SNHL tends to develop in young adulthood, with an average age of onset of 22 years [20].

This hearing loss can be sudden (43%) or progressive (43%) [10, 33]. SNHL can be mild to profound. Tumors that erode into the otic capsule are associated with profound hearing loss [33]. In tumors without otic capsule erosion, intralabyrinthine hemorrhage is associated with sudden hearing loss. Butman et al. described a cohort of 38 patients with ELST and VHL [33]. Large tumors with otic capsule erosion had profound SNHL. In patients without otic capsule invasion, SNHL developed in 82%, either suddenly or gradually. Intralabyrinthine hemorrhage was identified in 79% of the ears with sudden hearing loss but occurred in none of the patients with gradual or normal hearing.

Tinnitus is found nearly as often, in 92% of patients [10]. Vertigo and disequilibrium are found in about 62% [19–21]. The combination of SNHL, vertigo, and tinnitus can mimic Meniere's disease [4, 34–36]. Autopsy findings in a patient with VHL and symptoms of Meniere's disease identified endolymphatic hydrops and a microscopic ELST [19]. Butman et al. reported that 54% of VHL patients with ELST had the triad of hearing loss, tinnitus, and vertigo [33].

Interestingly, tumor size does not correlate with SNHL or vestibular symptoms [33]. In fact, audiovestibular symptoms occur frequently in tumors 2–3 mm in size. These small tumors can be associated with intralabyrinthine hemorrhage and sudden hearing loss. This observation is supported by autopsy findings in a VHL patient with sudden hearing loss who had a microscopic ELST with hemosiderin in the inner ear [19]. Therefore, the mechanisms of hearing loss in ELST can be from direct otic capsule erosion, intralabyrinthine hemorrhage, or endolymphatic hydrops.

Since these tumors are slow growing and their symptoms can be vague, diagnosis can be delayed by more than 8 years following symptom onset [37].

Facial weakness and paralysis have been reported in patients with ELST, but this occurs much less frequently than hearing loss, vertigo, or tinnitus [32, 36–38]. CN X palsy has also been reported [38].

Occasionally these tumors erode into the middle ear and ear canal (Fig. 11.1).

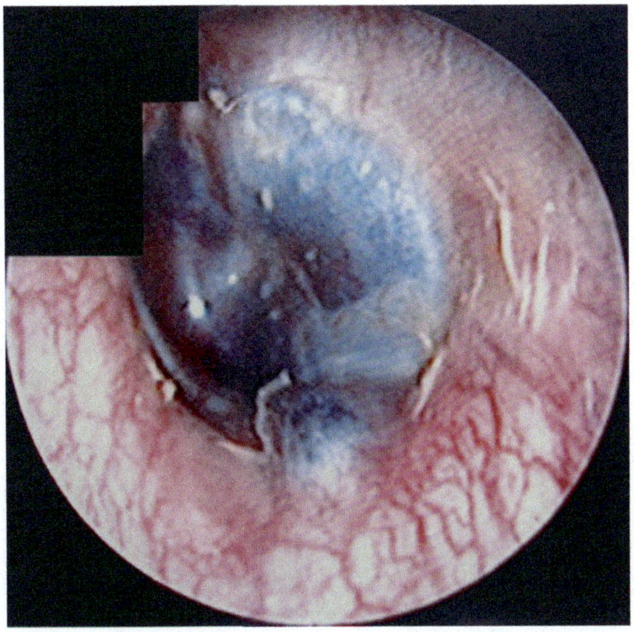

Fig. 11.1 Oto-endoscopic view of ELST involving the middle ear and mastoid. This tumor produced hemorrhagic middle ear secretions very similar to cholesterol granuloma

Audiovestibular Evaluation

Audiogram is an essential test to measure hearing function in these patients. The incidence of hearing loss varies from 70 to 95%, depending on the cohort size. Patients with sporadic ELST tend to present with hearing loss [37], whereas patients with VHL can have ELST identified before hearing loss.

Videonystagmography (VNG) is worthwhile to perform in patients with a complaint of vertigo. In patients with sporadic ELST, VNG usually demonstrates absent caloric response on the tumor side; and patients with syndromic ELST usually have vestibular hypofunction [37].

Diagnostic Imaging

ELSTs occur on the posterior surface of the temporal bone at the location of the endolymphatic sac. The endolymphatic sac is retrolabyrinthine in position and located between the internal auditory canal and sigmoid sinus (Fig. 11.2). With time and growth, these tumors erode surrounding the bone. These tumors are highly vascular, and they show avid contrast enhancement. CT scan is helpful to define the bone anatomy and the changes associated with tumor growth. ELSTs are isodense with gray matter on unenhanced CT scan. With contrast, CT shows a vascular, enhancing, and destructive lesion of the posterior surface of the temporal bone. CT demonstrates (1) aggressive soft tissue mass; (2) stippled, reticular, or speculate areas of calcification within

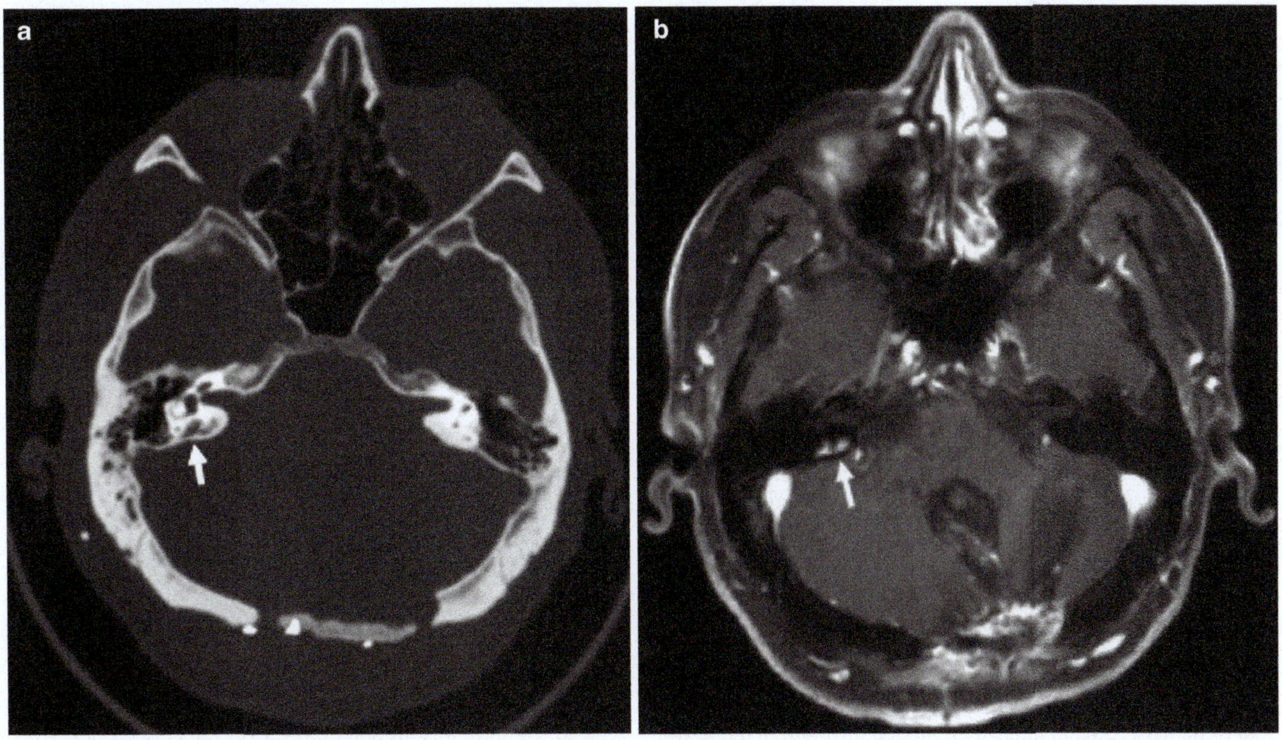

Fig. 11.2 Asymptomatic ELST in a 37-year-old man with VHL syndrome. (**a**) Axial imaging: upper panel, bone window CT; lower panel, contrast enhanced T1 MRI. (**b**) Coronal imaging: upper paenl, bone window CT; lower panel, contrast enhanced T1 MRI. (**c**) Audiogram showing symmetric high-frequency sensorineural hearing loss

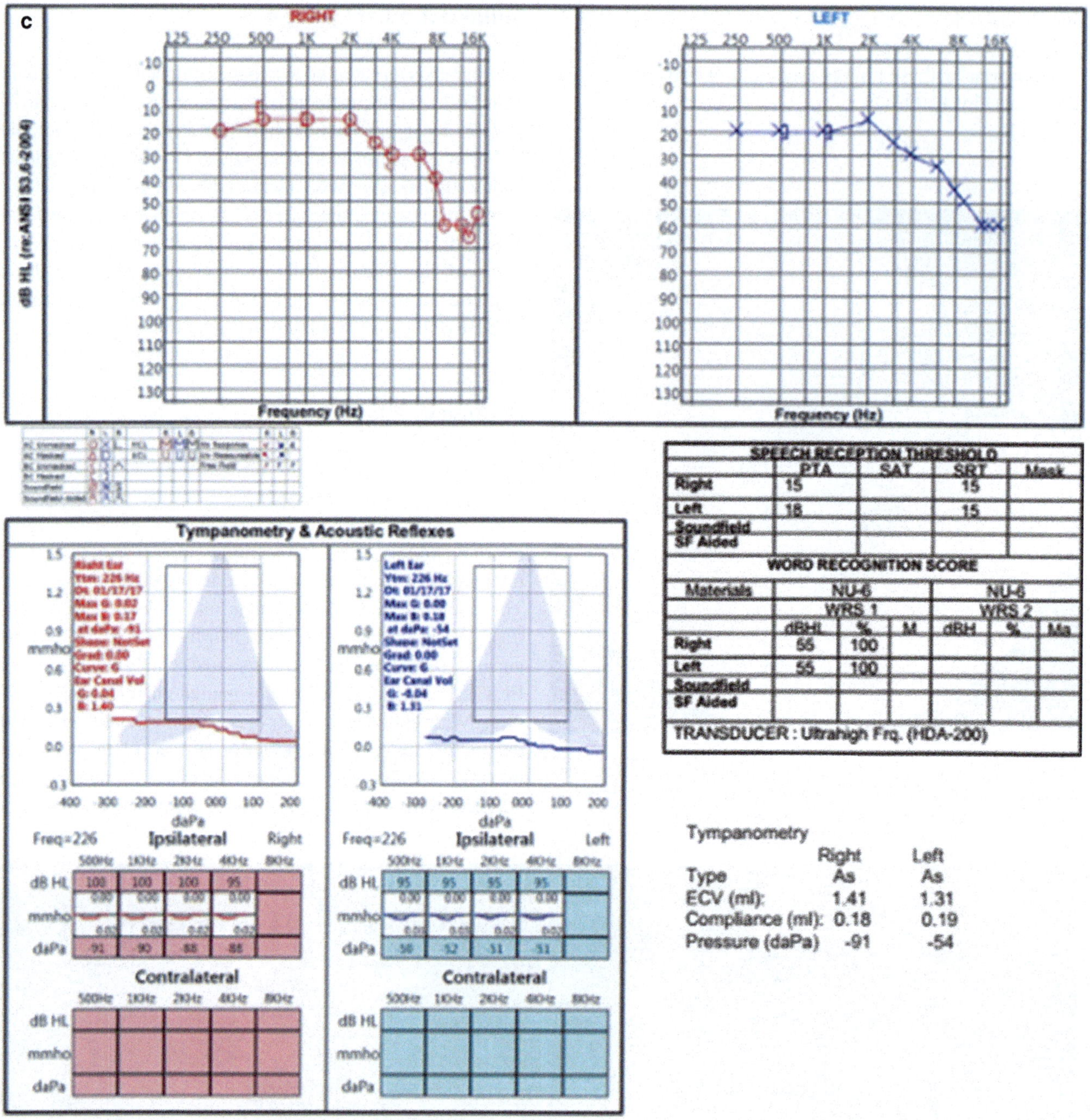

Fig. 11.2 (continued)

the tumor; and (3) a rim of calcification along the posterior margin of the tumor [36, 38, 39].

ELST has a heterogeneous appearance on unenhanced T1 MRI sequences, with areas of hyperintensity suggesting intratumoral hemorrhage and cholesterol granuloma formation [39, 40]. Isointense areas on pre-contrast T1 correspond to enhancing areas on post-contrast T1 imaging. Tumors less than 3 cm have a circumferential rim of increased signal intensity located at the periphery of the tumor, and larger tumors have multiple foci of increased signal intensity scattered throughout the lesion [41]. MRI demonstrates a heterogeneous tumor that enhances brightly with contrast and displays hyperintense signal on T2.

ELSTs can be mistaken for paragangliomas based on imaging characteristics. Paragangliomas are more common that ELSTs, but they demonstrate similar vascular, enhancing, and destructive patterns on imaging. The location of tumor growth is perhaps the best defining feature that separates these two tumor types. Other tumors in the differential include ceruminous gland adenocarcinoma, choroid plexus papillomas, meningioma, metastatic carcinoma, and chordoma [37, 38, 42].

Radiographically undetectable ELST has been described [19, 26, 34, 43]. Kim et al. describe a series of three VHL patients with audiovestibular symptoms prior to radiologic evidence of ELST. Binderup et al. describe a patient in whom a tumor was not found until almost 17 years following symptom onset [43]. This patient developed low-frequency SNHL prior to sudden profound hearing loss. His tumor, however, was not radiologically present until 4 months after the onset of deafness.

Intralabyrinthine hemorrhage associated with sudden hearing loss can be the first sign of ELST [33, 44]. Intralabyrinthine hemorrhage is defined on MR as abnormal isolated intralabyrinthine increased signal on pre-contrast T1-weighted images. Intralabyrinthine hemorrhage has also been identified in a patient with sudden hearing loss whose tumor was otherwise not visible on MRI or CT but was found on surgical exploration [33].

Angiography is often performed for these tumors to define the vascular anatomy. These tumors usually have blood supply from (1) the inferior tympanic artery, a branch of the ascending pharyngeal artery; (2) stylomastoid artery, a branch of the occipital or posterior auricular artery; (3) intrapetrous branch of the carotid artery; (4) anterior and posterior cerebellar arteries; and (5) petrous branch of the middle meningeal artery [38, 41, 45]. Embolization is performed for larger tumors to minimize blood loss.

Staging System for ELST

Bambakidis et al. proposed a staging system for ELSTs [28]. Their staging system uses "Grade," but "Stage" is used here to emphasize size of the tumor and to avoid confusion about tumor grade. Stage I tumors are confined to the temporal bone, middle ear, and/or external auditory canal. Stage II tumors extend into the posterior fossa. Stage III tumors involve the posterior and middle cranial fossae. Stage IV tumors extend to the clivus or sphenoid wing. Stage IV tumors are thought to make up only 2–4% of ELSTs.

Schipper et al. classified these tumors into three types: type A is locally confined without erosion of the temporal bone nor infiltration of the subarachnoid space; type B has bony infiltration of the labyrinth and clinical hearing loss; type C has infiltration of the sigmoid sinus and jugular vein [46].

Wait and Watch

Surveillance programs for VHL patients are likely to identify asymptomatic ELSTs. For these patients with normal hearing, observation with annual MRI and audiogram might be a reasonable option, since these tumors are typically slow growing [37]. Alternatively, the risk of observation is that sudden hearing loss from intralabyrinthine hemorrhage could occur, even without tumor growth. If observation is pursued, there must be clear understanding and agreement on what development would trigger intervention. Since progressive or sudden hearing loss is common in patients with ELST, small tumors with normal hearing should proceed to surgical resection [19]. In patients with bilateral tumors, the decision to observe versus offer treatment is especially thorny. If the goal is to preserve hearing, offering surgery to a patient with a small tumor might permit hearing preservation and complete tumor removal [26].

Alternatively, in patients who have lost hearing, the decision for surgery is based on prevention of further neurologic damage.

Surgery

Treatment is complete surgical excision. Identification of ELSTs when they are small and before hearing loss occurs is optimal. Surgical resection of small tumors can alleviate vestibular symptoms and preserve hearing [26, 36, 47, 48]. For the patient with VHL, who might develop visual loss and gait impairment, preserving hearing is a vital goal to maintain overall quality of life.

Megerian et al. describe three different surgical approaches for hearing preservation in patients with small ELST and good hearing: transmastoid, retrolabyrinthine-transdural, and retrosigmoid approaches [47]. In their description, the transmastoid approach was possible in one case because the tumor could be peeled off the inner layer of the endolymphatic sac, so that the dura was not violated. The disadvantage of this approach is that unless the mastoid is thoroughly aerated, it can be difficult to have enough access to the endolymphatic sac. In the retrolabyrinthine approach, the sigmoid sinus, posterior semicircular canal, facial canal, and jugular bulb were skeletonized; and the dura was sharply incised circumferential to the tumor. A fat graft was used to repair the dural defect. The retrosigmoid approach was used for a tumor that protruded slightly into the vestibule from the posterior aspect of the labyrinth. The tumor was seen through the posterior fossa dura. The dura was incised circumferentially, and the tumor was gently elevated off the bone and out of the vestibule. The common crus was drilled away to remove remnants of tumor, and the inner ear was sealed with Gelfoam and Surgicel. The disadvantage of this approach is that it can be difficult to delineate the posterior semicircular canal and endolymphatic duct from the posterior fossa, and it can be associated with a slightly higher CSF leak rate due to exposure of mastoid air cells.

Kim et al. describe in detail the retrolabyrinthine posterior petrosectomy approach for small ELST with intact hearing [26]. "Small" denotes no otic capsule invasion. In this approach, they emphasize the removal of the endolymphatic sac and involved duct, and they opine that this helps to minimize the chance for recurrence. They reported stable hearing and resolution of vertigo in all five patients.

Larger tumors generally destroy the labyrinth and present with profound hearing loss. The translabyrinthine, transcochlear, or transjugular approaches are required for larger tumors. Timmer et al. reported subtotal resection in three out of five patients with sporadic ELST [37].

The facial nerve is preserved in patients with normal facial function, even if the nerve is engulfed in tumor. In this circumstance, the tumor can generally be separated from the nerve (Fig. 11.3). Kupferman et al. described a 4-year-old boy who presented with serous otitis media, profound SNHL, and facial paralysis from ELST [29]. The facial nerve was transposed anteriorly and preserved; his final facial nerve function was House-Brackmann II. Rodrigues et al. found that tumor infiltration was present in patients with preoperative facial paralysis [48].

Intraoperatively, these tumors can be surrounded by air cells filled with hemosiderin-laden tissue and areas of old hemorrhage similar to cholesterol granuloma.

Radiotherapy for ELST

Radiotherapy has been used only for a few patients, usually in the postoperative period after subtotal excision or for recurrent tumors [17, 38, 49, 50]. Timmer et al. describe a 78-year-old patient who underwent primary radiotherapy (total dose 60 Gy) for an ELST [37]. The intracerebellar portion of this patient's tumor shrunk, but the intrapetrous portion did not change. These changes remained stable until the patient's death about 4 years later.

Stereotactic radiosurgery (SRS) has been used in only a few cases as a primary treatment modality [51–53]. SRS led to tumor shrinkage in one case and no change in two cases [51, 53]. SRS has been used for isolated intracranial recurrences with some success [32, 53]. In the MD Anderson series, we encountered one patient who was treated with SRS for an ELST. He presented to our center 12 years later with a massive tumor (Fig. 11.4). After two subtotal resections, he underwent IMRT with a total dose of 50.4 Gy; and his tumor has decreased slightly in size over 4 years.

Recurrence

Incomplete tumor excision leads to persistent growth and recurrence. Since these tumors are benign, care should be exercised to preserve as much normal function as possible. Tumor around the carotid artery can be particularly difficult to resect with normal margins and can lead to tumor recurrence. Revision surgery can be performed, but it runs the risk of facial paralysis. Multiply recurrent tumors might increase the risk of metastasis although only a few cases of metastatic ELST have been reported [54]. Radiotherapy has been used to control local disease following surgical excision [38].

Giant-Cell Tumor

Giant-cell tumors (GCTs) are histologically benign but locally aggressive tumors [55]. Because of the local destructive nature and the potential for metastatic spread, these tumors are often included in case series of temporal bone malignancies [56]. The overall incidence is estimated at 1 case/1 million population/year [57]. They occur more commonly in the epiphyses of long bone, but they can occur within the cranium particularly within the temporal bone, sphenoid, and ethmoid [58]. Only 1–2% of GCT is found in the craniofacial region [58, 59]. The proclivity of GCT to occur in the temporal and sphenoid bones might relate to their endochondral ossification rather than intramembranous ossification for other bones of the craniofacial region [58, 60]. Temporal bone and sphenoid are the site for 94% of GCT in the craniofacial region [60]. GCT has been reported to involve the jugular foramen, and thus they can mimic paraganglioma with respect to anatomic location, cranial nerve deficits, and vascularity [61]. GCTs can also occur at two different locations in the same patient, without the earmarks of metastatic disease [62].

Etiology

The etiology is unclear, and the most likely pathogenesis involves reactive hyperplasia secondary to inflammation [63]. In 2002, the World Health Organization classified these tumors as benign synovium lesions with four subtypes: bone, soft tissue, synovial, and tendon sheath [63].

Epidemiology

GCTs occur in the fourth through sixth decade of life, and the incidence is slightly higher in women than men [58, 64, 65]. GCTs have been reported in children as young as 2 years of age [57, 66, 67].

These tumors can arise from the temporomandibular joint, and up to one-third of these tumors invade intracranially. There have only been about 100 cases of temporal bone GCT reported in the English literature in the last 40 or 50 years [60, 68]. The earliest report of GCT in the temporal bone was by Doderlein in 1913 [67]. Zhang et al. published in English the largest, single institutional series of 18 patients with GCT

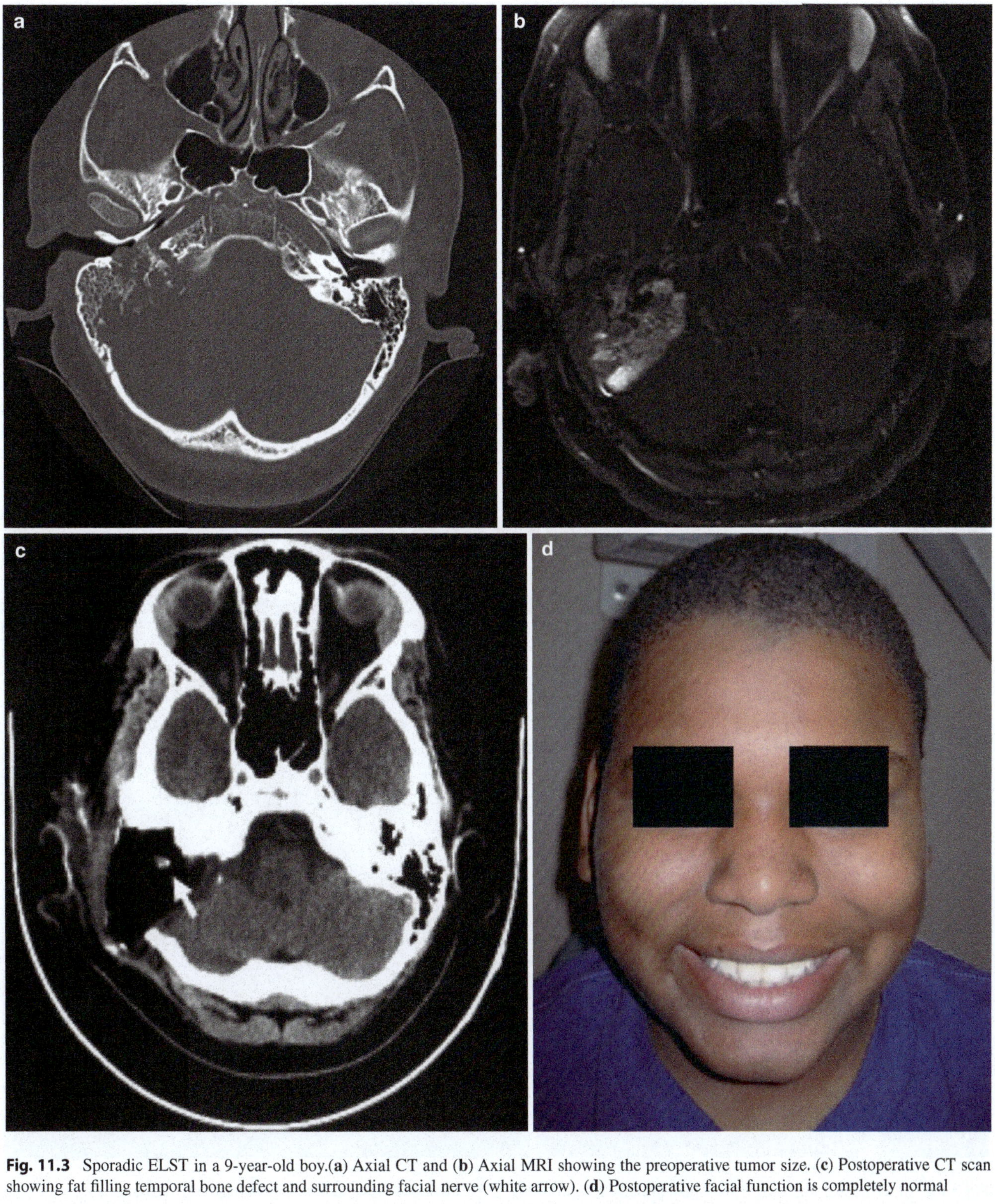

Fig. 11.3 Sporadic ELST in a 9-year-old boy.(**a**) Axial CT and (**b**) Axial MRI showing the preoperative tumor size. (**c**) Postoperative CT scan showing fat filling temporal bone defect and surrounding facial nerve (white arrow). (**d**) Postoperative facial function is completely normal

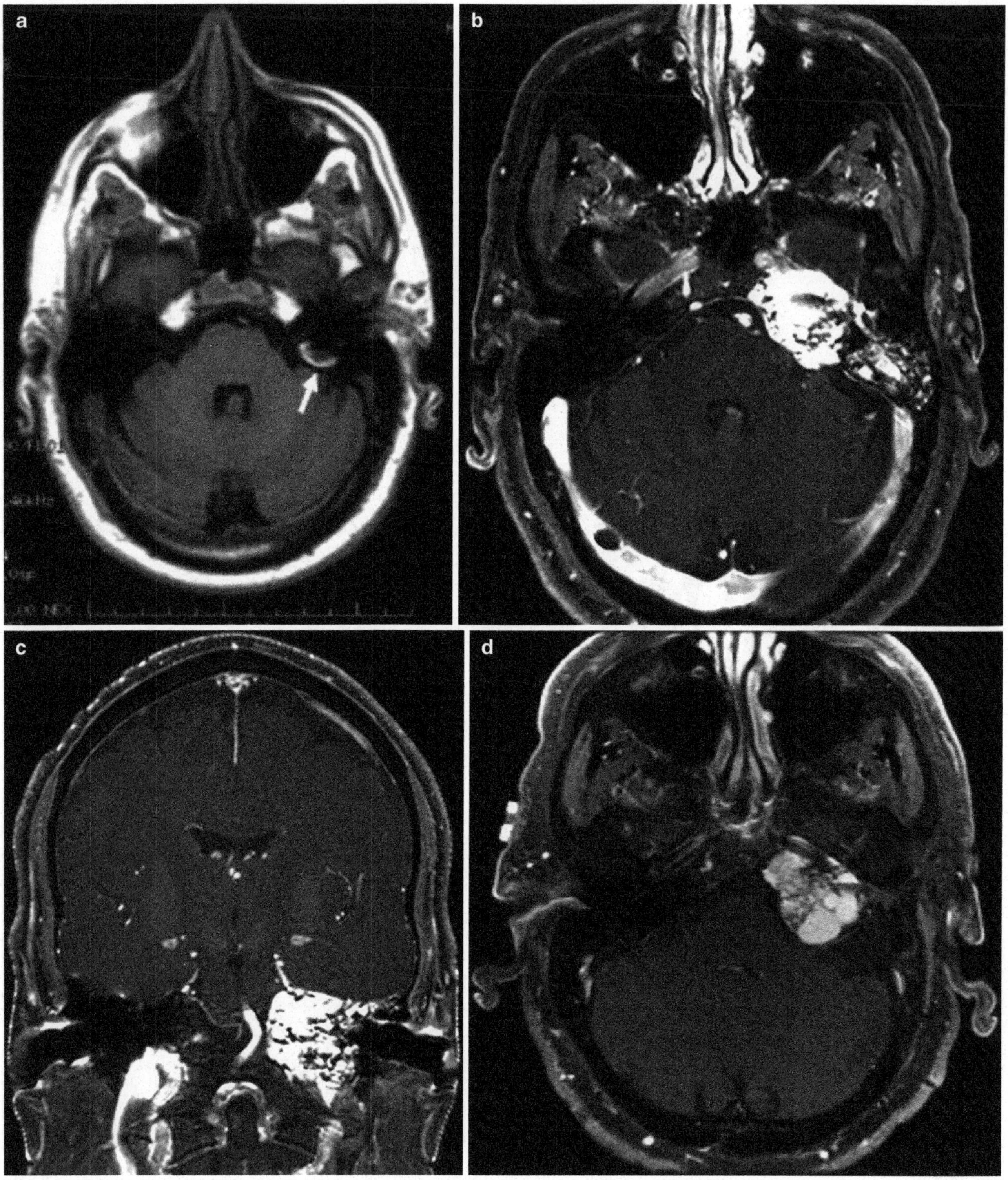

Fig. 11.4 ELST treated with SRS. This patient presented to our center 12 years after SRS. (**a**) Axial contrast-enhanced MRI of tumor (white arrow) prior to SRS. Note the rim enhancement of early-stage ELST. Tumor at presentation to our center (**b**) axial and (**c**) coronal MRI. This tumor was resected via a transcochlear approach with preservation of the facial nerve. (**d**) Axial MRI 1 year after first resection. An additional resection was performed via the same approach with preservation of the facial nerve and carotid artery. One year later he underwent IMRT for residual tumor. (**e**) Axial MRI prior to IMRT. (**f**) Axial MRI 6 years after presentation and 4 years after IMRT, showing tumor shrinkage. He continues to have normal facial function

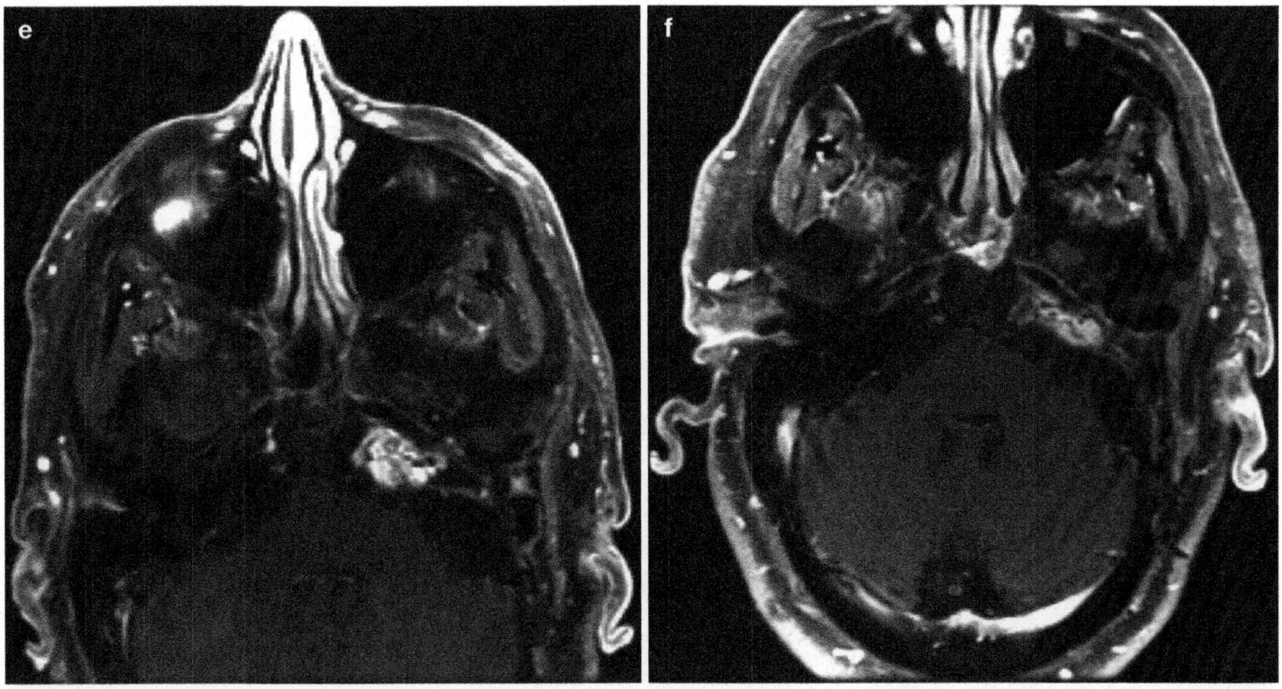

Fig. 11.4 (continued)

of the skull over an 18-year period [60]. Cui et al. reported a series of 23 patients at a single institution in China [69]. Malignant GST has been described with metastases to the lymph nodes and lung [68, 70].

Clinical Presentation

Principal symptoms are headache, hearing loss, tinnitus, swelling, and trismus. Tumor growth can lead to facial paralysis [60]. Symptoms may be present for many years prior to diagnosis [68]. In unusual cases, GCT can lead to Garcin syndrome, which is progressive, unilateral weakness in at least 7 of the 12 cranial nerves associated with osteoclastic involvement of the skull base [71].

GCTs can involve the middle ear, temporomandibular joint, squamous portion of the temporal bone, mastoid, middle cranial fossa, and greater wing of sphenoid [72]. This anatomic diversity means that these tumors tend to invade into the external ear canal and produce conductive hearing loss or invade into the Eustachian tube and produce chronic serous otitis media (Fig. 11.5).

Diagnostic Imaging

The combination of CT and MRI usually correctly identifies these tumors. CT shows soft tissue mass with bony erosion or expansion [73]. The bony margins are scalloped with cyst formation. About 40% of GCTs have a "soap bubble appearance" [74]. MRI shows the mass with low signal intensity on T1 imaging, and extremely low T2 imaging, reflecting hemosiderin deposition from prior hemorrhage [75]. The extremely low T2-imaging feature is considered highly indicative of GCT [60]. These tumors enhance with contrast on MR. These tumors show active uptake of F18-FDG on PET/CT [68]. Digital subtraction angiography can show an abundant blood supply [60].

The differential diagnosis includes giant cell reparative granuloma (GCRG), chondroblastoma, chondrosarcoma, osteoblastoma, osteolytic metastasis, synovial chondromatosis, synovial sarcoma, and synovial hemangioma [58, 60, 68]. GCRGs are difficult to distinguish histologically from GCT, except that GCRGs typically arise from the mandible, usually have a preceding history of trauma, and typically arise in the second decade of life and by the presence of osseous metaplasia in GCRG [60, 74, 76]. GCRG is radiographically indistinguishable from GCT [76].

Pathology

Histologically, these tumors are made up of three different cell types: osteoclast-like multinucleated giant cells, round mononuclear cells resembling monocytes, and spindle-shaped, fibroblast-like stromal cells [66]. The collection of multinucleated osteoclasts led to the older, European term of osteoclastoma [57, 77, 78]. Tissue specimens also contain foam cells, siderophages, and inflammatory cells [68]. Multinucleated giant cells stain positive for CD68 and CD45, clusterin, and vimentin [60, 79]. Mononuclear cells are positive for CD68. Tumors may be focally positive with S100.

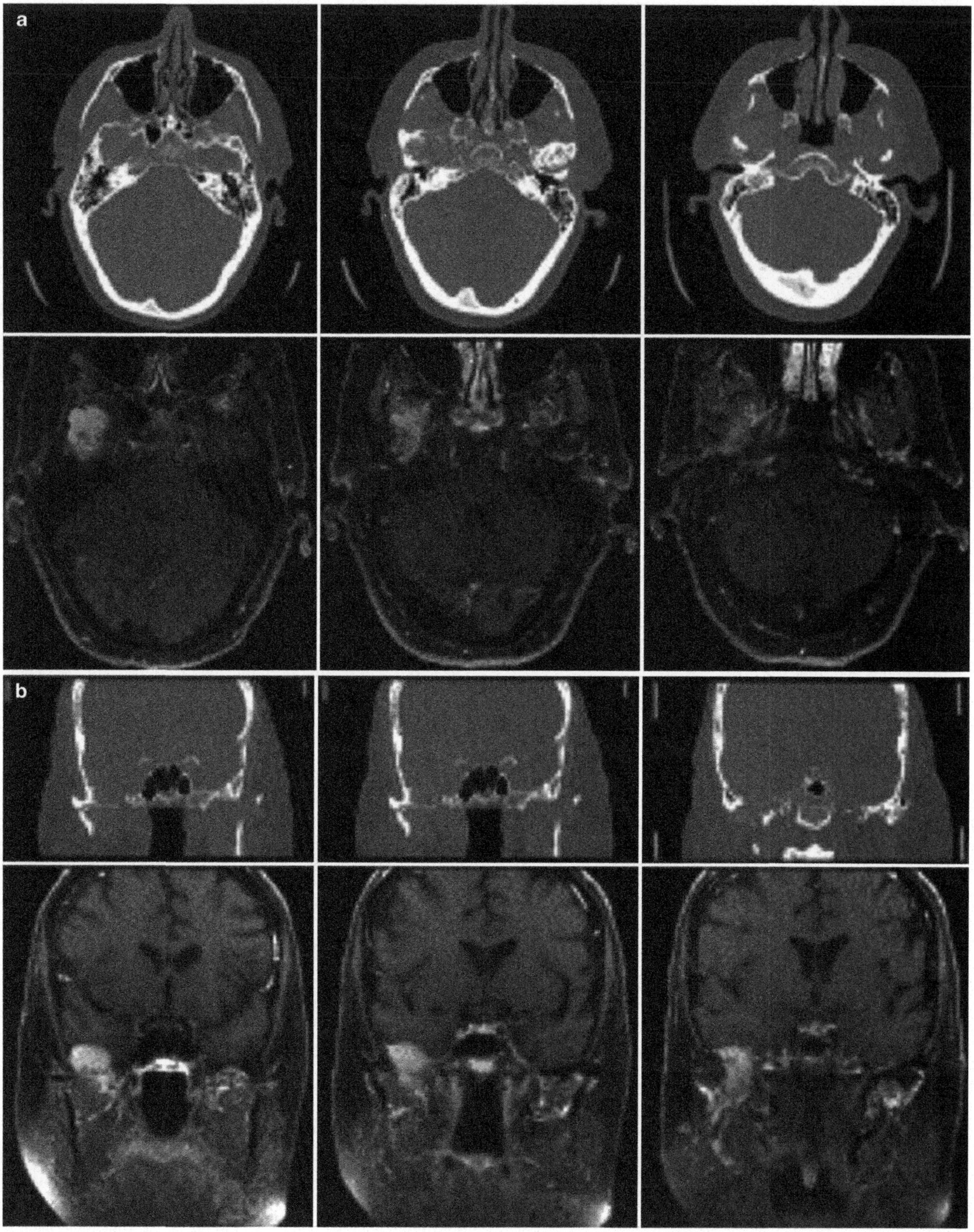

Fig. 11.5 Giant-cell tumor of right temporomandibular joint involving the right middle ear and middle fossa. (**a**) Axial imaging: upper panel, bone window CT; lower panel, contrast enhanced T1 MRI. (**b**) Coronal imaging: upper paenl, bone window CT; lower panel, contrast enhanced T1 MRI

Treatment

Surgical excision is the main treatment modality. Complete removal is the goal, but it is difficult to achieve in the temporal bone given the proximity of vital structures. The infratemporal approaches (ITF-A, -B, and -D) and middle cranial fossa approaches have been described to remove these tumors [62, 68]. Approaches to remove this tumor and preserve hearing have also been described [80].

Radiotherapy is an adjuvant to surgical resection or as an alternative to surgery in cases that are otherwise unresectable [65]. Radiation therapy can be considered when vital structures are involved and to prevent recurrences. Radiotherapy does improve local control rates in patients with positive margins [65]. It is also indicated in patients in whom aggressive surgical therapy would result in significant functional morbidity. Doses range from 25 to 65 Gy (median 46 Gy), with the typical dosage being 45 Gy [65]. Specific dose recommendations are lacking, however, due to small sample sizes in the radiotherapy literature. The benefit of radiotherapy must be weighed against the potential risks of malignant transformation and osteoradionecrosis [64, 65, 81].

Chemotherapy has been used for tumors that recur despite aggressive surgery and radiotherapy [81]. In the past, chemotherapy as used for sarcomas has been used for GCT. This protocol consists of methotrexate, Adriamycin, and cyclophosphamide. Interferon alpha-2a has been used as a salvage therapy; however, this form of therapy is not recommended when gross disease is causing significant morbidity since treatment response is delayed [65]. Denosumab, a monoclonal antibody against RANK ligand, has been shown to be promising for treatment of GCT of long bones [70]. There has not been a study demonstrating its effectiveness for craniofacial GCT [60].

Recurrence and Survival

Recurrences can occur in one-third to one-half of patients, and complete surgical excision with negative margins is required to minimize the chance of recurrence [58, 68]. Zhang et al. performed a systematic review of the English language literature and identified 76 cases of skull base GCT in addition to their own 18 cases. They performed an analysis of overall survival (OS) and event-free survival (EFS) for this cohort of patients. Event-free survival is significantly better in patients who had gross total resection versus patients who had subtotal resection (STR). Patients who had subtotal resection with postoperative radiotherapy did better than patients who had STR and no radiotherapy [60].

Hemangiopericytoma

Hemangiopericytomas (HPCs), now classified as solitary fibrous tumors, are frequently located in the lower extremities, pelvis (SFT), and retroperitoneum [82]. They make up about 3% of soft tissue sarcomas [83]. Between 15 and 30% of HPCs occur within the head and neck, most of which are in the soft tissues of the scalp, face, neck, nasal cavities, and paranasal sinuses [82, 84, 85]. HPCs make up about 1% of intracranial tumors [86]. One-third of cases are multicentric, usually within the same anatomic location [87]. These tumors usually present in the fifth and sixth decade [82, 87]. Only 5–10% of tumors occur in childhood [87]. These tumors are typically slow growing and painless. A case with 30-year history of hemangiopericytoma has been described [83].

Epidemiology

SFT/HPC involving the temporal bone tumors is rare; perhaps only 15 cases have been reported [85, 88–94]. HPCs in proximity to the jugular foramen can be frequently confused with paragangliomas [95]. HPC of the cerebellopontine angle may also be confused with acoustic neuroma (Fig. 11.6) [96]. These tumors often present as large, late-stage tumors that involve the middle fossa floor, external auditory canal, and zygoma [97].

Pathology

HPC was first described by Stout and Murray in 1942 [98]. These tumors arise from the pericytoma cells of Zimmerman, which are smooth muscle cells arranged around the blood vessels and are separated from endothelial cells by the basement membrane [83]. As such, these tumors have a mesenchymal origin. Tumor vessels demonstrate an unusual pattern of arrangement similar to stag horns and antlers.

Originally classified as atypical meningioma, the designation was changed in 1993 by WHO, to recognize HPC as a separate pathologic entity given its malignancy and its non-meningothelial origin [86]. Currently these tumors are classified as solitary fibrous tumors and are associated with the NAB2-STAT6 gene fusion arising from recurrent intrachromosomal rearrangements on chromosome 12q [99]. HPC can produce insulin-like growth factors, which stimulate neoplastic proliferation and can produce a clinical picture of hypoglycemia [82].

Pathologic features associated with malignancy include size greater than 5 cm, four or more mitotic figures per ten

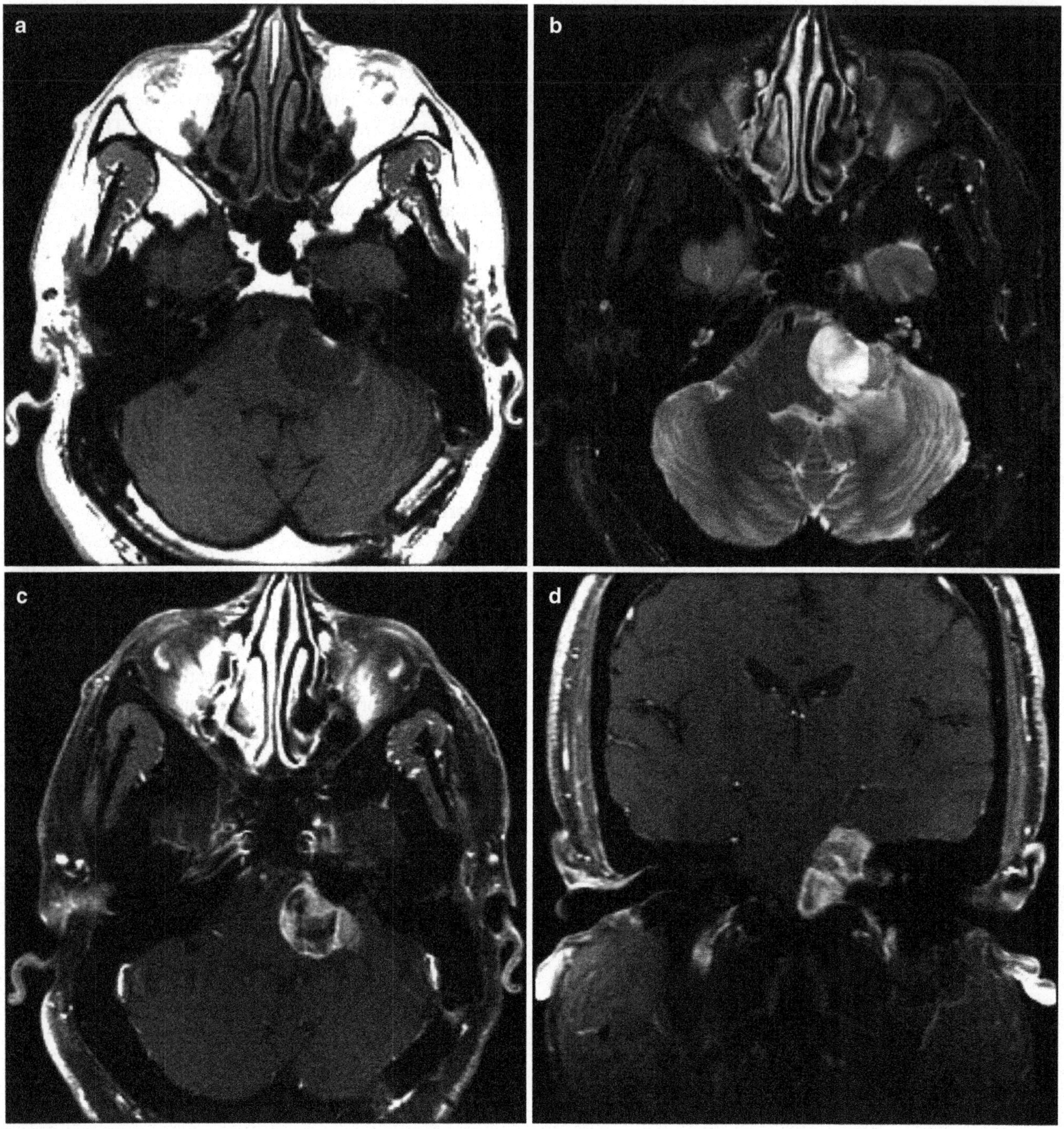

Fig. 11.6 Hemangiopericytoma of the left cerebellopontine angle. He presented with complete left-sided hearing loss and facial weakness. MRI images at the level of the internal auditory canal: non-contrast axial (**a**) T1 and (**b**) T2; contrast-enhanced T1 (**c**) axial and (**d**) coronal

high-power fields, high degree of cellularity, pleomorphic cells, hemorrhage, and necrosis [82]. Immunohistochemistry shows positive vimentin reaction, and most tumors express CD34 and CD99. These tumors are negative for S-100, actin, and desmin [84]. The pathologic differential diagnosis includes fibrous histiocytoma, synovial sarcoma, mesenchymal chondrosarcoma, and atypical meningiomas [82].

Diagnostic Imaging

There are no pathognomonic features on radiography. Radiographs show a well-circumscribed soft tissue mass that displaces neighboring structures [82]. CT shows these tumors as having heterogeneous enhancement with focal areas of necrosis; a nodular, well-defined border; and minimal surrounding edema [85, 100]. On MRI, these tumors are isointense to the brain on T1- and T2-weighted imaging and enhance intensely with contrast, although a fraction of tumors will show areas of necrosis and cystic changes [93, 100]. A "dural tail" is seen in less than 10% of cases [100]. Angiography reveals a vascular tumor with arterial dilation and diffuse capillary blush or opacification on the arterial phase and dilatation of draining vessels on the venous phase [82]. Preoperative embolization is indicated to try to minimize intraoperative blood loss.

Treatment

Treatment is primarily surgical, and complete surgical resection is required to avoid recurrence [89, 101]. However, obtaining negative margins in the temporal bone is difficult, since en bloc resection is associated with high morbidity rates. Tumor location, dural sinus involvement, dense vascularity, and neural involvement often limit the extent of resection [102]. Preoperative embolization is essential given the rich blood supply associated with these tumors [85].

Radiotherapy has been recommended for high-grade lesions and for incomplete resection. Radiotherapy achieves local tumor control in 80%, but patients are still at risks for distant disease [83]. These tumors are considered radiosensitive with doses greater than 50 Gy; however, radiotherapy is not indicated as primary treatment due to recurrences even after doses greater than 70 Gy [84].

The ability of stereotactic radiosurgery (SRS) to deliver a high dose while minimizing radiation effects to surrounding tissues is an advantage in this patient population; and the role of SRS has been reviewed in a meta-analysis [103]. The recommended marginal dose should be higher than 14 Gy. Tumor control with Gamma Knife radiosurgery ranges from 46 to 93% depending on the length of follow-up, where longer follow-up is associated with a lower control rate.

Recurrence and Survival

In the intracranial hemangiopericytoma literature, only a subtotal resection can be achieved in about two-thirds of patients with skull base involvement and/or dural sinus involvement [102]. Recurrence is more common with tumors larger than 6 cm or when dural sinuses are involved; and local recurrence rates range from 26 to 80% (Fig. 11.7) [103]. In this population, postoperative radiotherapy is recommended and has been shown to improve overall survival and local recurrence rates [102, 103]. The recurrence rate has been shown to decrease from 88% with surgery alone to 12.5% with surgery and postoperative radiotherapy [104].

Metastasis occurs in 10–60% of cases considering all primary tumor locations. The most frequent sites for metastases are the lung, liver, and bone (Fig. 11.8); and local recurrence usually precedes distant metastasis [82, 90]. The median time to systemic metastasis is about 80 months [103]. Lymph node involvement is rare. Prolonged follow-up is required since recurrences grow slowly and may not produce symptoms for 10 years or more [85]. Recurrences have been reported decades after original diagnosis [83, 89]. High-grade tumors have a 10-year survival of 29% [(83)]

Extrapolating from the intracranial HPC literature, local control, disease-free survival, and overall survival are greater when patients receive radiotherapy postoperatively [100, 101, 105, 106]. Guthrie et al. showed that progression-free survival is improved with postoperative radiotherapy, increasing from 29 months in the surgery-alone group to 74 months in the adjuvant radiotherapy group [107]. Sonabend et al. examined the Surveillance, Epidemiology, and End Results (SEER) database for hemangiopericytoma and found that an overall survival benefit was gained when gross total resection was accomplished combined with postoperative radiotherapy [102].

Conclusion

This chapter has described three tumor types that occur within the temporal bone: endolymphatic sac tumors, giant-cell tumors, and hemangiopericytoma or solitary fibrous tumors. These tumors can present at advanced stage and produce significant bony destructions. Diagnostic imaging is essential to define extent of disease and to narrow the differential diagnosis. Surgical excision is the mainstay of therapy; however, the location of tumor near vital structures often impairs complete resection. Radiotherapy has been used in the postoperative setting to control local disease.

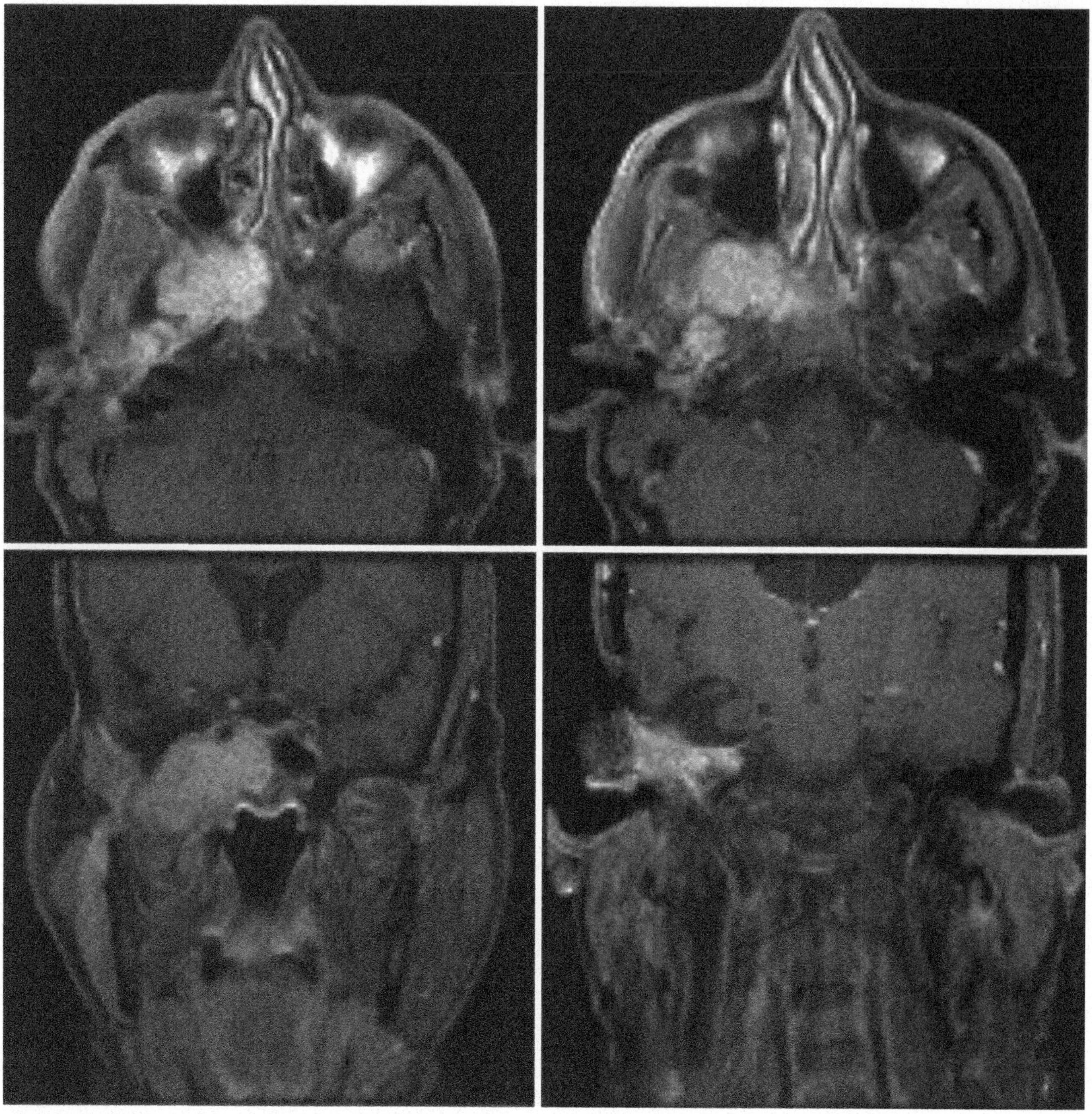

Fig. 11.7 Recurrent hemangiopericytoma of the right temporal bone and infratemporal fossa. Contrast-enhanced T1 MRI. Upper panes are axial images; lower panes are coronal images

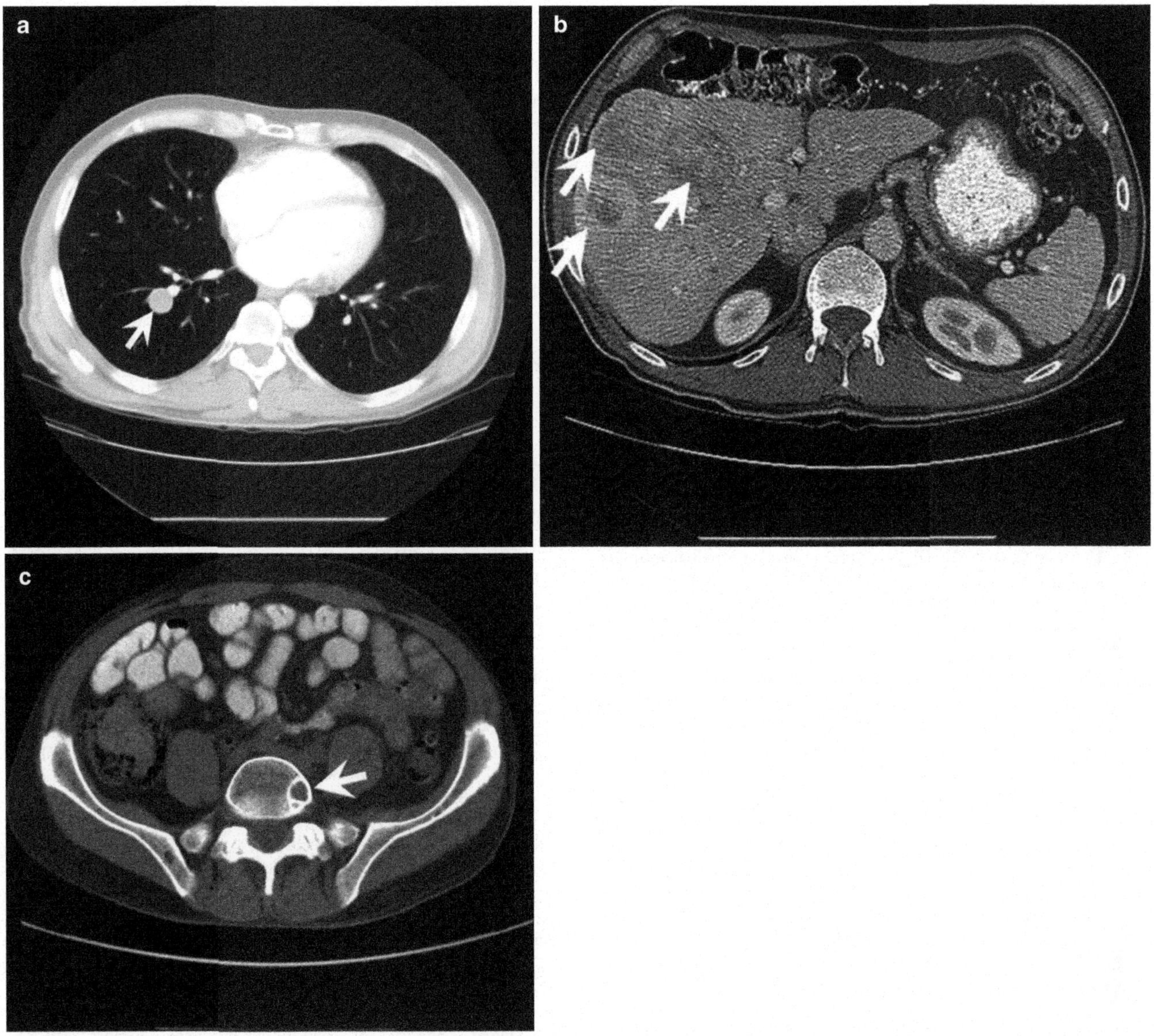

Fig. 11.8 CT showing (**a**) lung, (**b**) liver, and (**c**) bone metastases (white arrows) from the same patient presented in Fig. 11.7

References

1. Duderstadt M, Forster C, Welkoborsky HJ, Ostertag H. Adenomatous tumors of the middle ear and temporal bone: clinical, morphological and tumor biological characteristics of challenging neoplastic lesions. Eur Arch Otorhinolaryngol. 2012;269(3):823–31.
2. Kempermann G, Neumann H, Volk B. Endolymphatic sac tumours. Histopathology. 1998;33(1):2–10.
3. Brandt R. Zur Frage der Angiomatosis retinae. Graefes Arch Clin Exp Ophthalmol. 1921;106(1):127–65.
4. Hassard A, Boudreau S, Cron C. Adenoma of the endolymphatic sac. J Otolaryngol. 1984;13(4):213.
5. Gaffey MJ, Mills SE, Fechner RE, Intemann SR, Wick MR. Aggressive papillary middle-ear tumor: a clinicopathologic entity distinct from middle-ear adenoma. Am J Surg Pathol. 1988;12(10):790–4.
6. Heffner DK. Low-grade adenocarcinoma of probable endolymphatic sac origin a clinicopathologic study of 20 cases. Cancer. 1989;64(11):2292–302.
7. Li JC, Brackmann DE, Lo WW, Carberry JN, House JW. Reclassification of aggressive adenomatous mastoid neoplasms as endolymphatic sac tumors. Laryngoscope. 1993;103(12):1342–8.
8. Batsakis JG, El-Naggar AK. Papillary neoplasms (Heffner's tumors) of the endolymphatic sac. Ann Otol Rhinol Laryngol. 1993;102(8 Pt 1):648–51.
9. von Hippel E. Vorstellung eines Patienten mit einer sehr ungewohnlichen Netzhaut. Wiesbaden: XXIV Verstellung der ophthalmologischen Gesellschaft. JF Bergman; 1896.
10. Bausch B, Wellner U, Peyre M, Boedeker CC, Hes FJ, Anglani M, et al. Characterization of endolymphatic sac tumors and von Hippel-Lindau disease in the International Endolymphatic Sac Tumor Registry. Head Neck. 2016;38(Suppl 1):E673–9. https://doi.org/10.1002/hed.24067.

11. Latif F, Tory K, Gnarra J, Yao M, Duh F-M, Orcutt ML, et al. Identification of the von Hippel-Lindau disease tumor suppressor gene. Science. 1993;260:1317.
12. Hamazaki S, Yoshida M, Yao M, Nagashima Y, Taguchi K, Nakashima H, et al. Mutation of von Hippel-Lindau tumor suppressor gene in a sporadic endolymphatic sac tumor. Hum Pathol. 2001;32(11):1272–6.
13. Kawahara N, Kume H, Ueki K, Mishima K, Sasaki T, Kirino T. VHL gene inactivation in an endolymphatic sac tumor associated with von Hippel-Lindau disease. Neurology. 1999;53(1):208–10.
14. Knudson AG. Mutation and cancer: statistical study of retinoblastoma. Proc Natl Acad Sci. 1971;68(4):820–3.
15. Lonser RR, Glenn GM, Walther M, Chew EY, Libutti SK, Linehan WM, et al. von Hippel-Lindau disease. Lancet. 2003;361(9374):2059–67.
16. Gaffey MJ, Mills SE, Boyd JC. Aggressive papillary tumor of middle ear/temporal bone and adnexal papillary cystadenoma. Manifestations of von Hippel-Lindau disease. Am J Surg Pathol. 1994;18(12):1254–60.
17. Kunzel J, Agaimy A, Hornung J, Lell M, Ganslandt O, Semrau S, et al. Sporadic endolymphatic sac tumor—a diagnostic and therapeutic challenge. Int J Clin Exp Pathol. 2014;7(5):2641–6.
18. Poulsen MLM, Gimsing S, Kosteljanetz M, Møller HU, Brandt CA, Thomsen C, et al. Von Hippel-Lindau disease: surveillance strategy for endolymphatic sac tumors. Genet Med. 2011;13(12):1032–41.
19. Lonser RR, Kim HJ, Butman JA, Vortmeyer AO, Choo DI, Oldfield EH. Tumors of the endolymphatic sac in von Hippel-Lindau disease. N Engl J Med. 2004;350(24):2481–6.
20. Manski TJ, Heffner DK, Glenn GM, Patronas NJ, Pikus AT, Katz D, et al. Endolymphatic sac tumors. A source of morbid hearing loss in von Hippel-Lindau disease. JAMA. 1997;277(18):1461–6.
21. Choo D, Shotland L, Mastroianni M, Glenn G, Cv W, Linehan WM, et al. Endolymphatic sac tumors in von Hippel—Lindau disease. J Neurosurg. 2004;100(3):480–7.
22. Eby TL, Makek MS, Fisch U. Adenomas of the temporal bone. Ann Otol Rhinol Laryngol. 1988;97(6 Pt 1):605–12.
23. Megerian CA, McKenna MJ, Nuss RC, Maniglia AJ, Ojemann RG, Pilch BZ, et al. Endolymphatic sac tumors: histopathologic confirmation, clinical characterization, and implication in von Hippel-Lindau disease. Laryngoscope. 1995;105(8 Pt 1):801–8.
24. Poe DS, Tarlov EC, Thomas CB, Kveton JF. Aggressive papillary tumors of temporal bone. Otolaryngol Head Neck Surg. 1993;108(1):80–6.
25. Noel FL, Benecke JE Jr, Carberry JN, House JW, Patterson M. Adenomas of the mastoid and middle ear. Otolaryngol Head Neck Surg. 1991;104(1):133–4.
26. Kim HJ, Butman JA, Brewer C, Zalewski C, Vortmeyer AO, Glenn G, et al. Tumors of the endolymphatic sac in patients with von Hippel-Lindau disease: implications for their natural history, diagnosis, and treatment. J Neurosurg. 2005;102(3):503–12.
27. Alliance V. Suggested surveillance 2017. https://vhl.org/wp-content/uploads/2016/05/Surveillance-guidelines.pdf.
28. Bambakidis NC, Megerian CA, Ratcheson RA. Differential grading of endolymphatic sac tumor extension by virtue of von Hippel-Lindau disease status. Otol Neurotol. 2004;25(5):773–81.
29. Kupferman ME, Bigelow DC, Carpentieri DF, Bilaniuk LT, Kazahaya K. Endolymphatic sac tumor in a 4-year-old boy. Otol Neurotol. 2004;25(5):782–6.
30. Bambakidis NC, Rodrigue T, Megerian CA, Ratcheson RA. Endolymphatic sac tumor metastatic to the spine. Case report. J Neurosurg Spine. 2005;3(1):68–70.
31. Reijneveld J, Hanlo P, Groenewoud G, Jansen G, van Overbeeke K, Tulleken C. Endolymphatic sac tumor: a case report and review of the literature. Surg Neurol. 1997;48(4):368–73.
32. Carlson ML, Thom JJ, Driscoll CL, Haynes DS, Neff BA, Link MJ, et al. Management of primary and recurrent endolymphatic sac tumors. Otol Neurotol. 2013;34(5):939–43.
33. Butman JA, Kim HJ, Baggenstos M, Ammerman JM, Dambrosia J, Patsalides A, et al. Mechanisms of morbid hearing loss associated with tumors of the endolymphatic sac in von Hippel-Lindau disease. JAMA. 2007;298(1):41–8.
34. Lee KJ, Kirsch CF, Lai C, Ishiyama A. Endolymphatic sac tumor presenting with Ménière's disease. Otolaryngol Head Neck Surg. 2010;142(6):915–6.
35. Ong YK, Chee NW, Hwang PY, Goh J. Endolymphatic sac tumour: a rare cause of recurrent vertigo. Singapore Med J. 2006;47(7):627–30.
36. Hansen MR, Luxford WM. Surgical outcomes in patients with endolymphatic sac tumors. Laryngoscope. 2004;114(8):1470–4.
37. Timmer FC, Neeskens LJ, Van De Hoogen FJ, Slootweg PJ, Dunnebier EA, Pauw BH, et al. Endolymphatic sac tumors: clinical outcome and management in a series of 9 cases. Otol Neurotol. 2011;32(4):680–5.
38. Poletti AM, Dubey SP, Barbo R, Pericotti S, Fiamengo B, Colombo G, et al. Sporadic endolymphatic sac tumor: its clinical, radiological, and histological features, management, and follow-up. Head Neck. 2013;35(7):1043–7.
39. Patel NP, Wiggins RH 3rd, Shelton C. The radiologic diagnosis of endolymphatic sac tumors. Laryngoscope. 2006;116(1):40–6.
40. Ho VT, Rao VM, Doan HT, Mikaelian DO. Low-grade adenocarcinoma of probable endolymphatic sac origin: CT and MR appearance. AJNR Am J Neuroradiol. 1996;17(1):168–70.
41. Mukherji SK, Albernaz VS, Lo WW, Gaffey MJ, Megerian CA, Feghali JG, et al. Papillary endolymphatic sac tumors: CT, MR imaging, and angiographic findings in 20 patients. Radiology. 1997;202(3):801–8.
42. Al-Anazi AR, Holliday W, Sheikh B, Gentili F. Extraosseous endolymphatic sac low-grade adenocarcinoma mimicking posterior fossa meningioma. J Neurosurg. 2001;95(5):893–6.
43. Binderup ML, Gimsing S, Kosteljanetz M, Thomsen C, Bisgaard ML. von Hippel-Lindau disease: deafness due to a non-MRI-visible endolymphatic sac tumor despite targeted screening. Int J Audiol. 2013;52(11):771–5.
44. Eze N, Huber A, Schuknecht B. De novo development and progression of endolymphatic sac tumour in von Hippel-Lindau disease: an observational study and literature review. J Neurol Surg B Skull Base. 2013;74(5):259–65.
45. Lo WW, Applegate LJ, Carberry JN, Solti-Bohman LG, House JW, Brackmann DE, et al. Endolymphatic sac tumors: radiologic appearance. Radiology. 1993;189(1):199–204.
46. Schipper J, Maier W, Rosahl S, Berlis A, Laszig R. Tumour staged surgery of endolymphatic sac tumors (ELST). Laryngorhinootologie. 2004;83(8):493–500.
47. Megerian CA, Haynes DS, Poe DS, Choo DI, Keriakas TJ, Glasscock Iii ME. Hearing preservation surgery for small endolymphatic sac tumors in patients with von Hippel-Lindau syndrome. Otol Neurotol. 2002;23(3):378–87.
48. Rodrigues S, Fagan P, Turner J. Endolymphatic sac tumors: a review of the St. Vincent's hospital experience. Otol Neurotol. 2004;25(4):599–603.
49. SJ Y, Chen YD, Gao F, Qiu XG, Chang H. Endolymphatic sac papillary tumor: a case report. Chin Med J (Engl). 2011;124(22):3828–9.
50. Gupta R, Vaidhyswaran AN, Murali V, Kameswaran M. Endolymphatic sac papillary carcinoma treated with surgery and post-operative intensity-modulated radiotherapy: a rare case report. J Cancer Res Ther. 2010;6(4):540–2.
51. Balasubramaniam S, Deshpande RB, Misra BK. Gamma knife radiosurgery in jugular foramen endolymphatic sac adenocarcinoma. J Clin Neurosci. 2009;16(5):710–1.
52. Virk JS, Randhawa PS, Saeed SR. Endolymphatic sac tumour: case report and literature review. J Laryngol Otol. 2013;127(4):408–10.
53. Ferreira MA, Feiz-Erfan I, Zabramski JM, Spetzler RF, Coons SW, Preul MC. Endolymphatic sac tumor: unique features of two cases and review of the literature. Acta Neurochir. 2002;144(10):1047–53.

54. Guha D, Menard C, Evans W, Gentili F, Zadeh G. Flap reconstruction and hyperbaric oxygen therapy in the management of temporal bone osteoradionecrosis in an endolymphatic sac tumor: case report. Skull Base Rep. 2011;1(2):125–8.
55. Byun JH, Park KB, Ko JS, Ahn SK. Giant cell tumor of Infratemporal fossa and mandibular condyle: a case report. J Int Adv Otol. 2015;11(1):88–91.
56. Kinney SE, Wood BG. Malignancies of the external ear canal and temporal bone: surgical techniques and results. Laryngoscope. 1987;97(2):158-64.
57. Germano A, Caruso G, Caffo M, Galatioto S, Belvedere M, Cardia E. Temporal osteoclastoma: an exceptional lesion in infancy. Childs Nerv Syst. 1998;14(4–5):213–7.
58. Akyigit A, Karlidag T, Sakallioglu O, Polat C, Keles E. Giant cell tumor of bone involving the temporomandibular joint and temporal bone. J Craniofac Surg. 2014;25(4):1397–9.
59. ZH L, Yao ZW. Giant cell tumour of the posterior cranial fossa: a case report. Br J Radiol. 2011;84(1007):e206–9.
60. Zhang Z, Xu J, Yao Y, Chu S, Cheng H, Chen D, et al. Giant cell tumors of the skull: a series of 18 cases and review of the literature. J Neurooncol. 2013;115(3):437–44.
61. Rosenbloom JS, Storper IS, Aviv JE, Hacein-Bey L, Bruce JN. Giant cell tumors of the jugular foramen. Am J Otolaryngol. 1999;20(3):176–9.
62. Roberts DS, Faquin WC, Deschler DG. Temporal bone giant cell tumour: report of a second primary giant cell tumour of the temporal bone and infratemporal fossa. B-ENT. 2011;7(4):301–3.
63. Ong HS, Zhang CP, YQ W, Ji T. Update on the surgical management of temporomandibular joint-centered tendon sheath giant cell tumor with intradural extension: introducing a cost-effective method in using temporal bone for skull base reconstruction in preventing brain hernia. J Craniofac Surg. 2014;25(5):1769–72.
64. Wang Y, Honda K, Suzuki S, Ishikawa K. Giant cell tumor at the lateral skull base. Am J Otolaryngol. 2006;27(1):64–7.
65. Caudell JJ, Ballo MT, Zagars GK, Lewis VO, Weber KL, Lin PP, et al. Radiotherapy in the management of giant cell tumor of bone. Int J Radiat Oncol Biol Phys. 2003;57(1):158–65.
66. Elder JB, Berry C, Gonzalez-Gomez I, Kreger MD, McComb JG. Giant cell tumor of the skull in pediatric patients. Report of two cases. J Neurosurg. 2007;107(1 Suppl):69–74.
67. Dinning TA. Osteoclastoma of the petrous temporal bone; report of a case benefited by deep x-ray therapy. Aust N Z J Surg. 1953;22(4):253–7.
68. Pina S, Fernandez M, Maya S, Garcia RA, Noor A, Pawha PS, et al. Recurrent temporal bone tenosynovial giant cell tumor with chondroid metaplasia: the use of imaging to assess recurrence. Neuroradiol J. 2014;27(1):97–101.
69. Cui Y, Zong XY, Hao SY, Zhang YZ. Microsurgical treatment of giant cell tumor of skull. Zhonghua Yi Xue Za Zhi. 2010;90(23):1622–4.
70. Liu J, Yang H, Sun R, Yang Z, Zhu Z. Retrospective analysis of patients with rare-site and metastatic giant cell tumor. Chin J Cancer Res. 2013;25(5):585–92.
71. Bibas-Bonet H, Fauze RA, Lavado MG, Paez RO, Nieman J. Garcin syndrome resulting from a giant cell tumor of the skull base in a child. Pediatr Neurol. 2003;28(5):392–5.
72. Prasad SC, Piccirillo E, Nuseir A, Sequino G, De Donato G, Paties CT, et al. Giant cell tumors of the skull base: case series and current concepts. Audiol Neurootol. 2014;19(1):12–21.
73. Lee HJ, Lum C. Giant-cell tumor of the skull base. Neuroradiology. 1999;41(4):305–7.
74. Jain S, Sam A, Yohannan DI, Kumar S, Joshi D, Kumar A. Giant cell tumor of the temporal bone—an unusual presentation. Clin Neurol Neurosurg. 2013;115(5):646–8.
75. Tang JY, Wang CK, Su YC, Yang SF, Huang MY, Huang CJ. MRI appearance of giant cell tumor of the lateral skull base: a case report. Clin Imaging. 2003;27(1):27–30.
76. Borges BB, Fornazieri MA, Bezerra AP, Martins LA, Pinna Fde R, Voegels RL. Giant cell bone lesions in the craniofacial region: a diagnostic and therapeutic challenge. Int Forum Allergy Rhinol. 2012;2(6):501–6.
77. Ashamallah RS. Osteoclastoma of the petrous temporal bone. J Laryngol Otol. 1978;92(10):905–9.
78. Buter JJ, Chilla R. Giant cell tumor of the temporal bone (osteoclastoma). Eur Arch Otorhinolaryngol. 1997;254(6):298–300.
79. Fisher M, Biddinger P, Folpe AL, McKinnon B. Chondroid tenosynovial giant cell tumor of the temporal bone. Otol Neurotol. 2013;34(6):e49–50.
80. Takata Y, Hidaka H, Ishida K, Kobayashi T. Giant cell reparative granuloma of the temporal bone successfully resected with preservation of hearing. J Laryngol Otol. 2013;127(7):716–20.
81. Lee MY, Lee EJ. Giant cell tumor of the petrous temporal bone with direct invasion into the middle ear. J Craniofac Surg. 2006;17(4):797–800.
82. Guerrissi JO, Miranda MG, Olivier R. Giant hemangiopericytoma of mandible: a propos of a case: a variant of the surgical technique for protection of the articular fosse. J Craniofac Surg. 2006;17(3):523–7.
83. Brucoli M, Giarda M, Valente G, Benech A. Hemangiopericytoma of the infratemporal fossa: progression toward malignancy in a 30-year history. J Craniofac Surg. 2005;16(6):1146–50.
84. Bianchi B, Poli T, Bertolini F, Sesenna E. Malignant hemangiopericytoma of the infratemporal fossa: report of a case. J Oral Maxillofac Surg. 2002;60(3):309–12.
85. Birzgalis AR, Ramsden RT, Lye RH, Richardson PL. Haemangiopericytoma of the temporal bone. J Laryngol Otol. 1990;104(12):998–1003.
86. Shi ZP, Lin YS, Lin CK, Chen HC, Wang CH. Multiple metastatic progression of meningeal hemangiopericytoma initially diagnosed as atypical meningioma with temporal bone invasion. Otolaryngol Head Neck Surg. 2009;140(2):278–80.
87. Hornoy P, Sonigo P, Fallet-Bianco C, Largiliere P, Teillac D, Gomes H, et al. Fetal hemangiopericytoma with an associated cerebral anomaly. Ultrasound Obstet Gynecol. 2005;26(1):81–5.
88. Tewfik TL, Finlayson M, Attia EL. Hemangiopericytoma of the temporal bone. J Otolaryngol. 1981;10(1):72–7.
89. Schick B, Brors D, Draf W. Experiences with hemangiopericytoma in cranial base surgery. Laryngorhinootologie. 1998;77(5):256–63.
90. Cross DL, Mixon C. Temporal bone hemangiopericytoma. Otolaryngol Head Neck Surg. 1996;114(4):631.
91. Magliulo G, Terranova G, Cordeschi S. Hemangiopericytoma and temporal bone. An Otorrinolaringol Ibero Am. 1999;26(1):67–74.
92. Megerian CA, McKenna MJ, Nadol JB Jr. Non-paraganglioma jugular foramen lesions masquerading as glomus jugulare tumors. Am J Otol. 1995;16(1):94–8.
93. Chin LS, Rabb CH, Hinton DR, Apuzzo ML. Hemangiopericytoma of the temporal bone presenting as a retroauricular mass. Neurosurgery. 1993;33(4):728–31; discussion 31–2.
94. Chlangani D, Saxena R, Popli S, Bharadwaj T. Hemangiopericytoma of the postauricular region. J Laryngol Otol. 1970;84:457–61.
95. Weber AL, McKenna MJ. Radiologic evaluation of the jugular foramen. Anatomy, vascular variants, anomalies, and tumors. Neuroimaging Clin N Am. 1994;4(3):579–98.
96. Tashjian VS, Khanlou N, Vinters HV, Canalis RF, Becker DP. Hemangiopericytoma of the cerebellopontine angle: a case report and review of the literature. Surg Neurol. 2009;72(3):290–5.
97. Sade B, Budur K, Lee DK, Franco K, Lee JH. Major depression with psychosis after resection of a giant middle fossa hemangiopericytoma. Surg Neurol. 2006;65(3):290–2; discussion 2.
98. Stout AP, Murray MR. Hemangiopericytoma: a vascular tumor featuring Zimmermann's pericytes. Ann Surg. 1942;116(1):26.
99. Thway K, Ng W, Noujaim J, Jones RL, Fisher C. The current status of solitary fibrous tumor: diagnostic features, variants, and genetics. Int J Surg Pathol. 2016;24(4):281–92.

100. Zhou JL, Liu JL, Zhang J, Zhang M. Thirty-nine cases of intracranial hemangiopericytoma and anaplastic hemangiopericytoma: a retrospective review of MRI features and pathological findings. Eur J Radiol. 2012;81(11):3504–10.
101. Rutkowski MJ, Jian BJ, Bloch O, Chen C, Sughrue ME, Tihan T, et al. Intracranial hemangiopericytoma. Cancer. 2012;118(6):1628–36.
102. Sonabend AM, Zacharia BE, Goldstein H, Bruce SS, Hershman D, Neugut AI, et al. The role for adjuvant radiotherapy in the treatment of hemangiopericytoma: a surveillance, epidemiology, and end results analysis: clinical article. J Neurosurg. 2014;120(2):300–8.
103. Spina A, Boari N, Gagliardi F, Donofrio CA, Franzin A, Mortini P. The current role of gamma knife radiosurgery in the management of intracranial haemangiopericytoma. Acta Neurochir. 2016;158(4):635–42.
104. Dufour H, Métellus P, Fuentes S, Murracciole X, Régis J, Figarella-Branger D, et al. Meningeal hemangiopericytoma: a retrospective study of 21 patients with special review of postoperative external radiotherapy. Neurosurgery. 2001;48(4):756–63.
105. Soyuer S, Chang EL, Selek U, McCutcheon IE, Maor MH. Intracranial meningeal hemangiopericytoma: the role of radiotherapy. Cancer. 2004;100(7):1491–7.
106. Melone AG, D'Elia A, Santoro F, Salvati M, Delfini R, Cantore G, et al. Intracranial hemangiopericytoma—our experience in 30 years: a series of 43 cases and review of the literature. World Neurosurg. 2014;81(3):556–62.
107. Guthrie BL, Ebersold MJ, Scheithauer BW, Shaw EG. Meningeal hemangiopericytoma: histopathological features, treatment, and long-term follow-up of 44 cases. Neurosurgery. 1989;25(4):514–22.

Hematologic Malignancies Affecting the Temporal Bone

12

Paul W. Gidley, Nathan Fowler, and Marc-Elie Nader

Abbreviations

ABVD	Adriamycin, bleomycin, vinblastine, and dacarbazine
ALL	Acute lymphocytic leukemia
AML	Acute myeloid leukemia
APL	Acute promyelocytic leukemia
ATRA	All-*trans* retinoic acid
CLL	Chronic lymphocytic leukemia
CML	Chronic myeloid leukemia
CNS	Central nervous system
CSF	Cerebrospinal fluid
CT	Computerized tomography
DLBCL	Diffuse large B-cell lymphoma
EAC	External auditory canal
EMP	Extramedullary plasmacytoma
HIV	Human immunodeficiency virus
HL	Hodgkin's lymphoma
Hyper-CVAD	Cyclophosphamide, mesna, doxorubicin, vincristine, dexamethasone
IAC	Internal auditory canal
IT	Intrathecal
LDH	Lactate dehydrogenase
MD	Myeloproliferative disorder
MDS	Myelodysplastic syndrome
MM	Multiple myeloma
MRI	Magnetic resonance imaging
MS	Myeloid sarcoma
NHL	Non-Hodgkin's lymphoma
PET/CT	Positron emission tomography/computerized tomography
PLB	Primary lymphoma of bone
SPB	Solitary plasmacytoma of bone

P. W. Gidley, M.D., F.A.C.S. (✉) · N. Fowler, M.D.
M.-E. Nader, M.D., M.Sc.
Department of Head and Neck Surgery, The University of Texas M.D. Anderson Cancer Center, Houston, TX, USA
e-mail: pwgidley@mdanderson.org; nfowler@mdanderson.org; mnader@mdanderson.org

Introduction

Hematologic malignancies are broadly divided into lymphoma, leukemia, and myeloma. Although most presentations involve the bone marrow, peripheral blood, and occasionally the spleen, the temporal bone can occasionally be affected as a primary site or as part of a systemic presentation. Diffuse large B-cell lymphoma is the most common subtype of lymphoma and can present with involvement of the ear canal and temporal bone. Leukemias, both acute and chronic, have also been known to involve the temporal bone. Leukemic infiltration of the marrow and periosteum primarily involves the petrous apex, and it can extend to involve the inner ear, middle ear, and facial nerve. Tumorous accumulation of acute leukemia can involve the air spaces of the temporal bone, and it is often referred to as myeloid sarcoma. Presenting symptoms are very similar to acute otitis media. Plasma cell disorders such as myeloma and plasmacytoma have also been described within the temporal bone with various presentations. This chapter will describe the manifestations and clinical course of hematologic malignancies involving the ear and temporal bone.

Lymphoma

Lymphoma is a highly heterogeneous disease which is typically divided into Non-Hodgkin's lymphoma (NHL) and Hodgkin's lymphomas (HL), which make up approximately 90% and 10% of new cases, respectively [1]. Both subtypes can be further subclassified and have a widely variable presentation and clinical course. While some patients can present with slowly growing, painless adenopathy in the head and neck, others present with rapidly growing disease, pain, and classic "B" symptoms such as night sweats, fevers, and/or weight loss. Indolent lymphomas such as follicular and

P. W. Gidley, F. DeMonte (eds.), *Temporal Bone Cancer*, https://doi.org/10.1007/978-3-319-74539-8_12

marginal zone lymphoma have mean overall survival ranging from 10–20 years. Typical therapy in indolent lymphoma is associated with high overall response rates but frequent relapses. In contrast, aggressive lymphomas such as diffuse large B-cell and classical Hodgkin's lymphoma follow a rapidly progressive clinical course, but these diseases are associated with cure following frontline therapy in over 60% of patients.

Hodgkin's Lymphoma

The incidence of HL has remained stable over the last two decades and is more frequent in men than in women [2]. It has a bimodal distribution which peaks in young adults and in patients over 60 years of age.

HL is divided into two main types: nodular lymphocyte predominant HL, with an indolent clinical course, and classical HL. Classic Hodgkin's disease is further subdivided into the following four subtypes: nodular sclerosis, mixed cellularity, lymphocyte-depleted, and unclassifiable.

Although HL typically presents as painless lymphadenopathy, more than 56% of patients have a mediastinal mass and can present with dyspnea, cough, or superior vena cava obstruction [2]. Only 5–8% of HL have bone marrow involvement. Histologic diagnosis of HL is based on the identification of the multinucleated large Reed-Sternberg cells surrounded by an inflammatory infiltrate. Staging of HL is based on the modified Ann Arbor system.

Patients presenting with early stage disease (Stage I–IIA) have an excellent overall survival exceeding 90% with radiotherapy and combination chemotherapy such as adriamycin, bleomycin, vinblastine, and dacarbazine (ABVD) [2]. Advanced disease has excellent long-term outcomes with progression free survival of 70% and overall survival of 82–90%.

Although Hodgkin's disease rarely affects the ear canal, middle ear, or temporal bone, several cases have been reported in the literature. Maithrea et al. reported a case of Hodgkin's disease affecting the middle ear and ear canal that presented with facial paresis [3]. Staging workup did not reveal any other site of disease. This patient was treated with ABVD chemotherapy, and his facial nerve function returned to normal.

Liu et al. also reported a case of primary HL in the left temporal bone associated with an intracranial abscess [4]. This 49-year-old woman presented with a 5-month history of a painful mass in the left mastoid region. She did not have any hearing loss, tinnitus, or dizziness. MRI showed a heterogeneous enhancing lesion of the left temporal bone. At mastoidectomy, necrotic tissue was filling the air cell spaces, and an epidural abscess was found. Pathology confirmed a CD30+ lymphocyte rich classic HL.

Non-Hodgkin's Lymphoma

Non-Hodgkin's lymphoma (NHL) accounts for nearly 90% of all newly diagnosed lymphomas. The incidence of NHL in the population has been rising steadily for decades and affects about 73,000 patients in the USA in 2016 [1]. In children, lymphoma remains the third most diagnosed malignancy.

Like HL, classic symptoms of NHL include painless lymphadenopathy as well as systemic symptoms including fevers, night sweats, weight loss, and fatigue. NHL can involve any organ and, hence, can be associated with a wide range of clinical presentations. Diagnosis requires lymph node biopsy. Initial workup includes careful history and physical, bone marrow biopsy, lactate dehydrogenase (LDH), and imaging studies.

About 85–90% of NHL are derived from B cells, while the remaining lymphomas are derived from T cell or NK cells [1]. Diffuse large B-cell lymphoma (DLBCL) is the most common subtype of NHL. Virtually all cases of HIV-associated NHL are of B-cell origin, and approximately half of these cases are extranodal [5].

Peripheral T-cell lymphomas commonly involve the skin as well as various extranodal sites. Common subtypes include mycosis fungoides, cutaneous anaplastic large T-cell lymphoma, and peripheral T-cell lymphoma not otherwise specified (NOS).

Approximately 25% of all cases of extranodal NHL occur in the head and neck, which represents the second most common site of extranodal involvement (6, 7). While Waldeyer's ring is the most common site for lymphoma to develop in the head and neck, the temporal bone can occasionally be a primary site for lymphoma. Most primary temporal bone lymphomas are NHL [4].

Improvements in conventional treatment, such as the addition of rituximab to combination chemotherapy for NHL, have resulted in improved outcomes for patients with localized and systemic disease [8]. Although historical studies have demonstrated the potential for cure with localized radiotherapy in early stage disease, modern combined approaches incorporating systemic chemotherapy have improved relapse rates [1].

HIV, organ transplantation, obesity and autoimmune disorders, such as rheumatoid arthritis, Sjogren's syndrome, and systemic lupus erythematosus (SLE), are risk factors for NHL [1]. Extranodal NK-T-cell lymphoma and Burkitt's lymphoma are also strongly associated with Epstein-Barr virus infection [1].

Burkitt's lymphoma is highly aggressive with cell doubling time of 24–48 h [9–11]. Burkitt's lymphoma is associated with the chromosomal translocation activating the c-MYC oncogene. Burkitt's lymphoma is the most common childhood cancer where malaria is holoendemic [10].

In non-endemic areas, the incidence of Burkitt's lymphoma is very high in immunosuppressed patients, especially when associated with HIV infection.

Cutaneous T-cell lymphoma, also known as mycosis fungoides, is primarily a malignancy of T-helper (CD4+) cells [12]. While T-cell lymphoma often presents with cutaneous involvement, it only rarely involves the outer ear. The disease is associated with three clinical stages: patch, plaque, and tumor stages. Each stage can progress over several years and, if left untreated, can eventually become bulky with large dome-shaped cutaneous nodules evident. Presentation at this stage is often associated with visceral involvement, and prognosis is poor.

External Ear

Both B-cell and T-cell lymphoma can involve the external ear. The incidence of T-cell involvement might be slightly higher in primary cases, potentially due to mycosis fungoides involving of the external ear. Both children and adults have been reported with primary lymphoma of the outer ear. Strahan and Calcaterra (1971) reported the first case of ear involvement, along with face, oropharynx, and external auditory canal (EAC), from T-cell lymphoma [13].

Lymphoma of the outer ear typically presents with redness and swelling and can be easily mistaken for perichondritis, especially if there is a history of prior ear trauma or a cartilage-piercing earring (Fig. 12.1). Given the indolent nature of some lymphomas, patients can have symptoms for many years prior to diagnosis [14]. Several cases of NHL presenting only an external ear swelling have been reported, involving children as young as 8 months of age and adults [12, 14–23]. Similar to systemic presentations, most adults are in the fifth or sixth decade of life at presentation.

Mantle cell lymphoma is an uncommon and aggressive form of NHL [17]. The disease has a propensity to involve the gastrointestinal tract and has only rarely been reported to involve the outer ear (Fig. 12.2) [17].

Involvement of the skin of the outer ear can be seen in patients with localized or systemic mycosis fungoides and can present as a plaque or ulcerated tumor (Fig. 12.3). Several cases of mycosis fungoides involving the outer ear have been reported [13, 24–28].

Diagnosis depends on adequate biopsy, and tissue must be sent for histological examination by an experienced hematopathologist. Treatment depends on the extent of disease as well as the subtype of lymphoma and varies from chemotherapy alone, radiotherapy alone, and combined modality approaches. Small studies have reported patients with isolated, single-site disease treated with radiotherapy alone [14, 20, 21]; most patients will receive additional systemic chemotherapy. Rarely intrathecal chemotherapy prophylaxis is used to minimize future central nervous system involvement [18, 23]. Adjuvant radiotherapy has also been reported in a few cases [22].

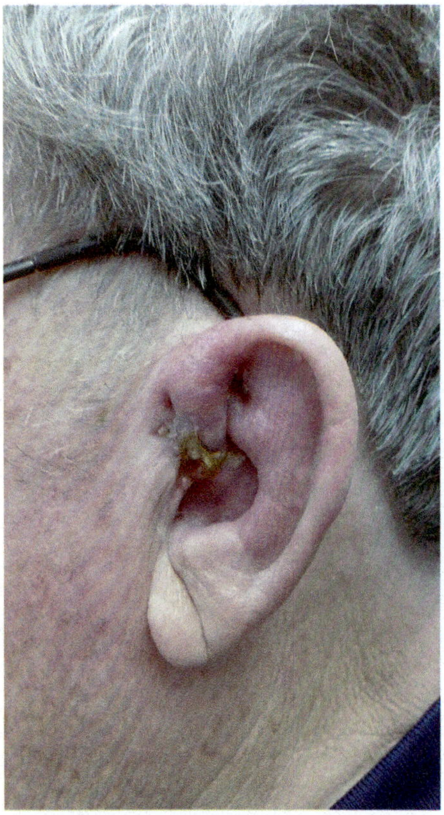

Fig. 12.1 The outer ear as a primary site of NHL

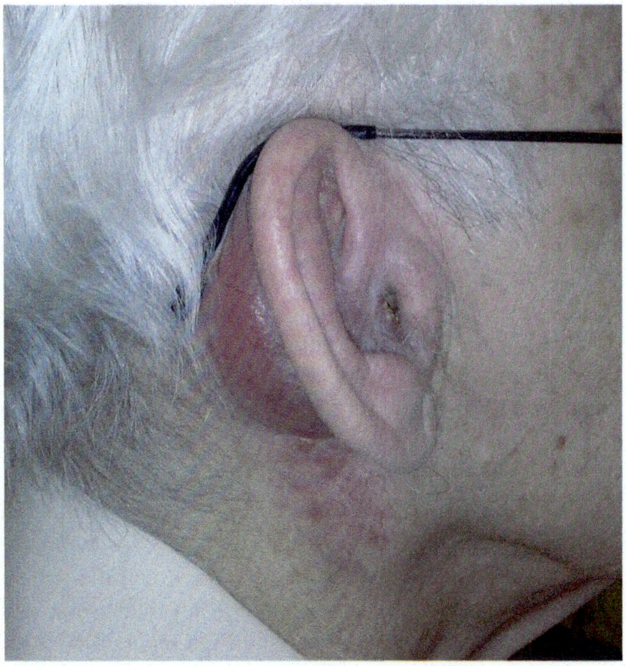

Fig. 12.2 Recurrent mantle cell lymphoma involving the outer ear

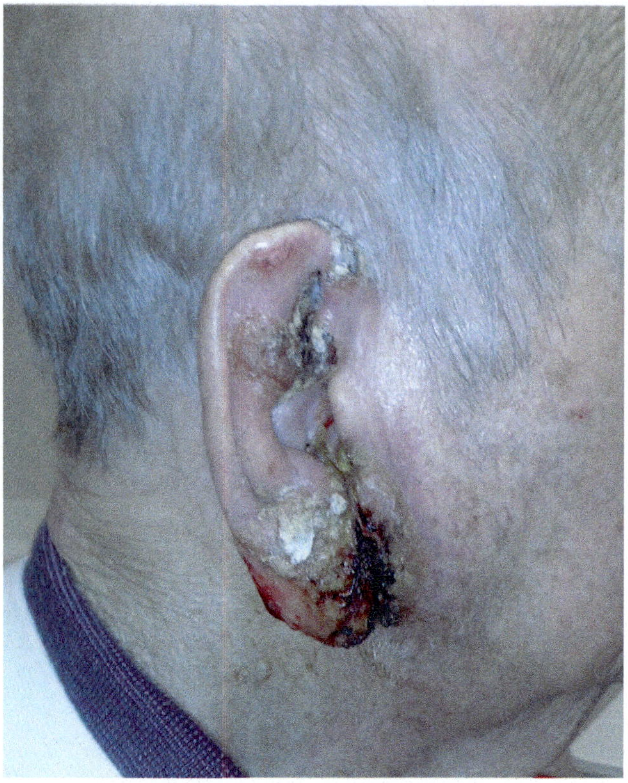

Fig. 12.3 Mycosis fungoides of the outer ear

External Ear Canal

Primary lymphoma of the ear canal is extremely rare, with less than a dozen cases reported [6, 7, 29–35]. Both B-cell and T-cell lymphomas have been reported. These patients, generally, are older and many are in the eighth or ninth decade of life [7, 30]. Most patients have been women.

Patients generally present with symptoms of otitis externa, such as otalgia and otorrhea, and hearing loss. Physical examination shows a reddish, raised bulge in the ear canal. This swelling may or may not involve the tympanic membrane (Fig. 12.4). An unusual case presented with a cauliflower-like growth in both ear canals [34]. Bilateral ear canal lymphoma has been reported [36].

CT examination shows a soft tissue mass, usually without bone destruction. Open biopsy is required for diagnosis, but frequently the diagnosis can be missed if the tissue is not sent for immediate immunologic staining and flow cytometry.

These patients are generally treated with systemic chemotherapy and radiotherapy. Isolated cases have been reported with lateral temporal bone resection as well as systemic chemotherapy; in this case the tumor recurred and the patient received salvage high dose chemotherapy with stem cell transplantation [31]. Kieserman and Finn reported NHL of the EAC in an HIV+ patient; this lymphoma extended into

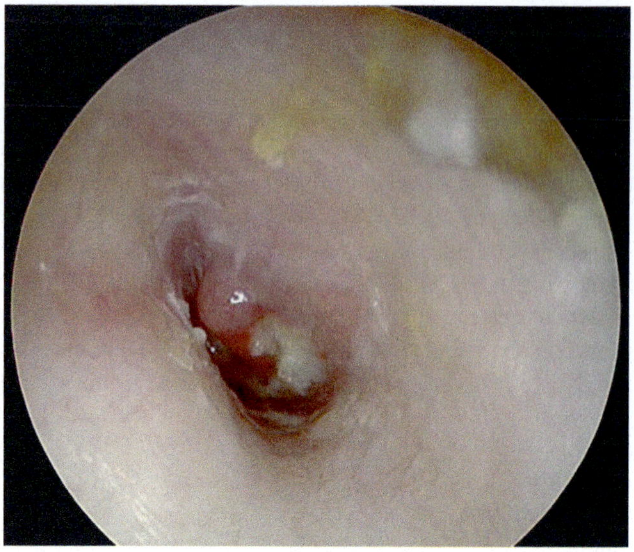

Fig. 12.4 Mycosis fungoides of the ear canal and tympanic membrane

the nasopharynx and was treated with radiotherapy 46 Gy [35].

Middle Ear

In patients with systemic lymphoma, serous otitis media is a common occurrence. Many patients will have evidence of lymphoma in the middle ear effusion. Okura and Kaga reported their experience with middle ear effusions in patients with lymphoma, observing evidence of lymphoma in the middle ear effusion in 5 of 16 ears [37].

Fewer than 30 cases of primary lymphoma of the middle ear have been reported [30, 38, 39]. Both children and adults have been reported with primary lymphoma of the middle ear. Cases generally present as otitis media that does not resolve with antibiotic therapy. Physical examination can reveal a reddish mass from the superior two-thirds of the tympanic membrane and extending into the external auditory canal [40]. Facial weakness and pain are also frequently reported [3, 40–42]. Cerebral venous thrombosis has been reported in one case of NHL involving the middle ear [39].

Middle ear exploration with or without mastoidectomy is performed for biopsy (Fig. 12.5), and an amorphous mass of pale fleshy tissue has been described filling the entire middle ear space [42]. Despite the clinical presentation of facial paresis, the fallopian canal may be intact [42].

The majority of reported lymphoma cases of the middle ear have been classified as DLCBL and are treated with systemic chemotherapy. CNS prophylaxis is added to the chemotherapy regimen in children.

Temporal Bone

The temporal bone is frequently involved secondarily by lymphoma. As mentioned previously, middle ear effusions in lymphoma patients often contain lymphoma cells. Several temporal bone histopathologic studies have demonstrated lymphoma in almost half of the temporal bones of lymphoma patients that were studied, indicating the systemic nature of the disease [43–45].

However, primary lymphoma of the temporal bone is very rare [4, 9, 36, 46–51]. In a series of 287 patients with NHL, Conley et al. found only one case of the temporal bone as the primary site [52].

Primary lymphoma of the temporal bone has been broadly classified together with primary lymphoma of the bone (PLB) [36]. PLB accounts for only 1–2% of lymphoma and 3–5% of extranodal lymphoma [53]. Diffuse large B-cell lymphoma accounts for 75–80% of cases and is associated with statistically longer survival after diagnosis when compared to other pathologic types [53, 54].

The original diagnostic criteria for PLB were put forth by Coley (1950): (1) a primary focus in a single bone on admission, (2) unequivocal histologic proof of lymphoma in a bone lesion, and (3) only regional metastases present on admission or if the onset of symptoms of the primary tumor preceded the appearance of the metastasis by 6 months [55]. The World Health Organization uses two criteria: (1) a single skeletal site, with or without regional lymph node involvement, and (2) multiple bones are involved, but there is no visceral or lymph node involvement [56].

In a retrospective analysis of adult patients with skeletal PLB, Lewis et al. found that the median age was 45 years (range 23–76 years) and that men outnumbered women, 2:1 [53]. The most common sites of involvement are the femur, pelvis, humerus, tibia, and radius.

In a literature review, Ogawa et al. identified 18 cases of PLB of the temporal bone and middle ear in patients ranging from 2–81 years [36]. In their review, the most common symptoms included otalgia, hearing loss, and aural fullness. Three of the 18 patients presented with facial palsy. A soft tissue mass was found in the EAC in 5 of 18 patients. Ten out of 12 cases were B-cell type.

Systemic symptoms, such as fever or night sweats, are usually absent in primary temporal bone lymphoma. In examining all sites of PLB, Beal et al. found that such B symptoms were present in only 15% of patients [54].

Conductive hearing loss is more common than sensorineural hearing loss, since the otic capsule is resistant to tumor invasion. Sensorineural hearing loss is usually related to auditory nerve invasion. However, lymphoma of the skull base can be associated with multiple cranial nerve deficits [47, 48].

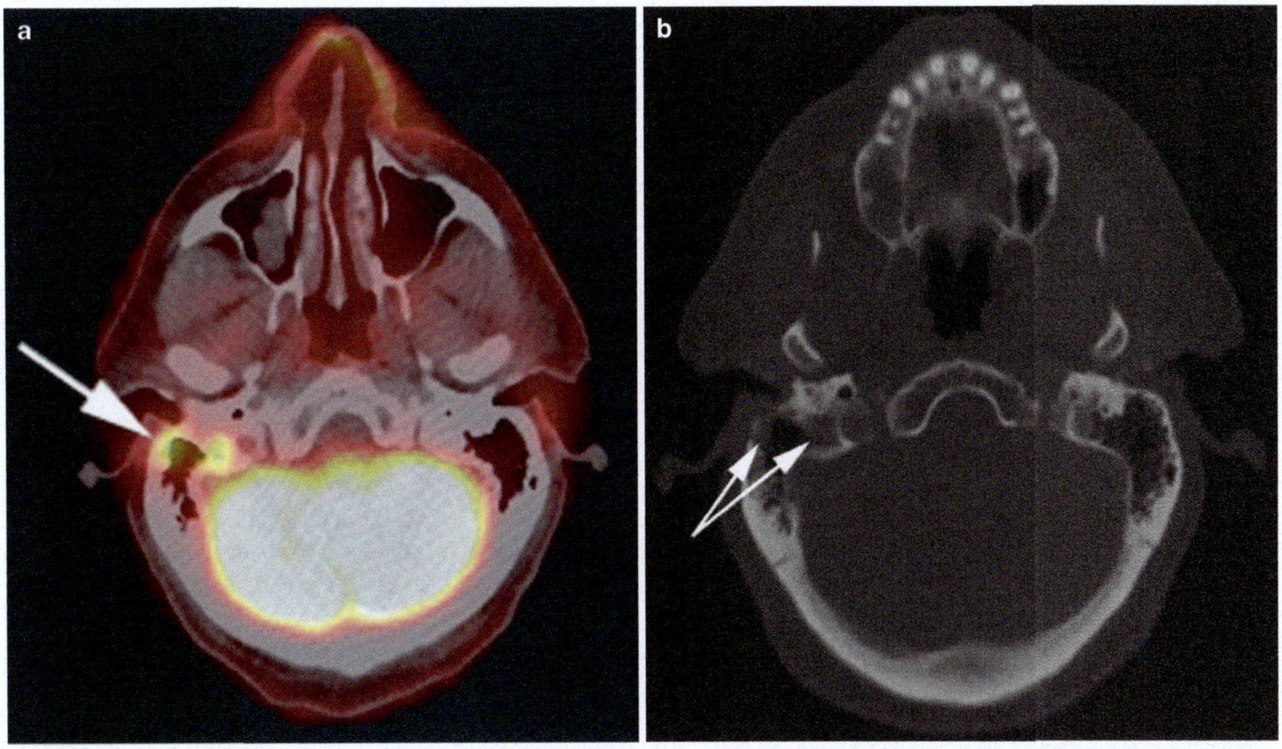

Fig. 12.5 NHL of the mastoid. (**a**) PET/CT showing FDG-avid uptake in the right mastoid. (**b**) Non-contrast axial CT scan. (**c**) Audiogram. Bony erosion and a reddish, cellular soft tissue mass were found in the mastoid

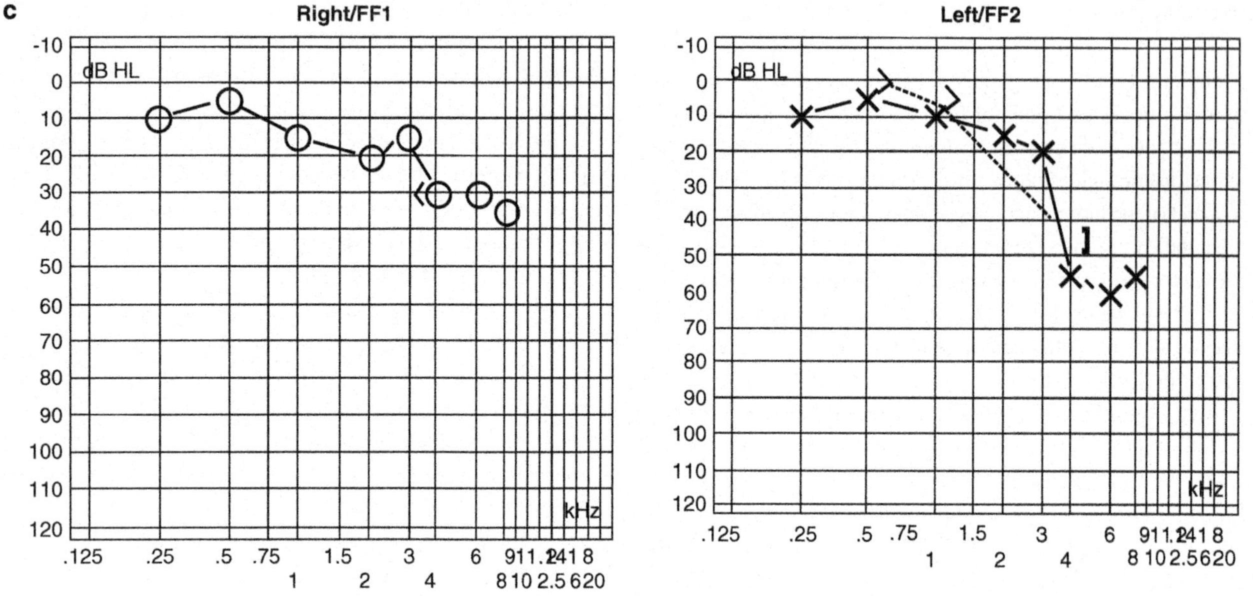

	Right
AC	
BC	
FF	
IP	

	Left
AC	
BC	70
FF	
IP	

SRT PTA Right:- PTA Left:-

Transducer	Test type	Intensity	Masking	Aided	ISF440 List
Left	HL	10			Spondee A
Right	HL	15			Spondee B

WR PTA Right:- PTA Left:-

Transducer	WR	Intensity	Masking	Score	Aided	ISF440 List
Left	WR1	55		100		NU-6 LIST 1A
Right	WR1	55		100		NU-6 LIST 2A

Fig. 12.5 (continued)

When temporal bone lymphoma is classified as a primary bone lymphoma, favorable prognostic factors include age younger than 40 years, the use of combined modality therapy (chemoradiation), an absence of B symptoms (fever, night sweats, and weight loss), normal lactate dehydrogenase levels, and female gender.

CT and MRI are useful for the diagnosis of PLB. CT can show patchy destruction of the mastoid and temporal bone [50] or extensive soft tissue density in the middle ear and mastoid [57]. PET imaging is useful for staging and might be preferable for assessment of remission. Treatment usually requires radiotherapy and chemotherapy [36, 46, 49, 51, 54] versus chemotherapy alone [50, 57]. Overall 5-year survival is 60–90% [36, 54]. However, some tumors are fulminant in nature, and rapid decline and death can occur despite aggressive treatment [51].

Leukemia of the Temporal Bone

Otolaryngologists commonly see leukemia patients for head and neck infections [58, 59]. Very rarely is the ear canal and temporal bone a site for primary leukemia. However, the systemic manifestations of the leukemia can involve the temporal bone, especially the petrous apex.

Leukemia has long been known to affect hearing. Deafness in leukemia was first described by Donné in 1844 [60]. Politzer (1884) is the first to describe leukemic temporal bone changes, including degeneration of the membranous labyrinth and osteoneogenesis in the cochlea [61]. Several authors from the late nineteenth century and early twentieth century have also described leukemic infiltration in the temporal bones, facial nerve, and middle and inner ears [62]. Druss, in 1945, clarified the otologic complications secondary to leukemia through a study of the medical records of 148 patients with leukemia [63].

Otologic signs and symptoms, such as hearing loss, otorrhea, otalgia, vertigo, and otorrhagia, occur in 32–69% of leukemia patients [64–66]. Hearing loss is the most common otologic complaint in patients with leukemia [64, 67, 68]. Sudden sensorineural hearing loss can occur with either acute or chronic leukemias [69]. Signs of leukemic infiltration in the ear and temporal bone include red or thickened tympanic membrane, hemotympanum, exudates in the middle ear, acute otitis media, mastoiditis, conductive or sensorineural hearing loss, dizziness, vertigo, or facial paralysis [62].

Acute Leukemias

Acute leukemias are broadly divided into cells of lymphoid origin (e.g., acute lymphocytic leukemia) and cells of myeloid origin (acute myeloid leukemia). Acute lymphoblastic leukemia (ALL) is a heterogeneous group of lymphoid disorders that arise from a monoclonal proliferation and expansion of immature lymphoid cells in the marrow, blood, and other organs [70]. Acute lymphoblastic leukemia is the most common malignancy in childhood, accounting for 25% of all pediatric cancers and 75% of all pediatric leukemia [71]. The incidence is 1.5 cases per 100,000 population. About 6000 cases of acute lymphoblastic leukemia are diagnosed in the USA every year [72].

Conventional treatment for ALL follows the schedule of induction chemotherapy with CNS prophylaxis, followed by consolidation and intensification, followed by maintenance therapy [70]. Induction and consolidation use hyper-CVAD (cyclophosphamide, mesna, doxorubicin, vincristine, dexamethasone) with CNS prophylaxis of intrathecal methotrexate and cytarabine. Maintenance therapy consists of 6-mercaptopurine, methotrexate, prednisone, and vincristine.

Acute myeloid leukemia (AML) occurs at any age but is most common in the fifth and sixth decades; it accounts for only 15% of childhood leukemias [73]. Men and women are equally affected. About 25% of patients present with infection. Petechiae and other signs of bleeding are common. Lymphadenopathy is uncommon.

Management of AML is initially aimed at stabilizing the platelet count and treating presenting infections. Chemotherapy is rapidly introduced in two stages: induction therapy followed by consolidation therapy. Bone marrow transplantation can follow consolidation therapy [74]. CNS prophylaxis is generally not required in adult AML, since the incidence of CNS leukemia is less than 2% and since induction chemotherapy includes the CNS penetrating agent, cytarabine.

Chronic Leukemias

Indolent leukemias derived from mature white cells are termed chronic leukemias [75]. Chronic leukemias are divided based on immunostaining as either B-cell or T-cell derived. B-cell leukemias are four times more common than T-cell leukemias in Western countries. T-cell leukemias frequently present with skin involvement, and patients with skin lesions in the head and neck may present first to otolaryngologists. Cutaneous lesions in B-cell chronic lymphocytic leukemia (CLL) are common but usually occur late in the course of disease [76].

Ninety-five percent (95%) of patients with chronic myelogenous leukemia (CML) will demonstrate the presence of the Philadelphia chromosome (translocation t(9;22)(q34;q11)).

External Ear

Similar to lymphoma, cutaneous manifestations of chronic lymphocytic leukemia on the outer ear have been described. CLL has the highest incidence of cutaneous manifestations of all the leukemias [62]. Several case reports have described CLL affecting the outer ear and presenting as nodules on the helix, swelling of the ear lobes, or cauliflower ear [76–83].

Skin manifestations of leukemia vary from nodules, papules, infiltrations, plaques, ulcerations, or exfoliative erythroderma [62]. External ear swelling in the earlobes or helix has been described in patients with CLL [62, 76, 77]. These nodules are typically firm, erythematous or violaceous, and painless. These skin manifestations of CLL have been treated with localized radiotherapy [62] and ultraviolet B phototherapy [77].

Ear Canal

Several authors have reported extramedullary relapse of acute promyelocytic leukemia (APL) in the external auditory canal following treatment with all-*trans* retinoic acid (ATRA) [68, 84–87]. APL is a subtype of AML characterized by severe hemorrhage, translocation t(15;17), and response to ATRA. A unique feature of APL is extramedullary relapse following treatment with ATRA. ATRA has been shown to cause APL cells to express intercellular adhesion molecule-1(ICAM-1), leukocyte function-associated antigen-1, and other adhesion molecules [84]. Relapse of APL in the ear canal can have a good response to arsenic trioxide (As_2O_3), perhaps because arsenic accumulates in skin, hair, and nails. Au et al. describe two patients with external canal relapse of APL [87]. Breccia et al. describe seven patients with relapse of APL in the ear canal or mastoid [68]. Leukemic infiltration of the ear canal associated with AML relapse has been treated with radiotherapy [88].

Middle Ear

Hemorrhage, inflammatory changes, and leukemic infiltration associated with the disease can occur in the middle ear, inner ear, and cranial nerve VII and VIII. Serous otitis media is frequently seen in patients with leukemia or lymphoma especially following prolonged hospitalization, such as after bone marrow transplantation. Thrombocytopenia can lead to tympanic membrane or middle ear hemorrhage (Fig. 12.6).

Okura and Kaga studied the middle ear effusions in 8 of 35 ears of patients with leukemia. Floating tumor cells were found in four of eight ears and tumor infiltration around the Eustachian tube in three ears [37].

Primary leukemia can involve any site of bone marrow, including the skull base (Fig. 12.7). Extramedullary spread of leukemia usually heralds bone marrow relapse [89]. Relapsed leukemia has presented as acute otitis media [90, 91], otitis externa [92], facial palsy [93, 94], or cholesteatoma [89]. These cases are treated with standard re-induction chemotherapy followed by local radiation therapy.

Leukemic Infiltration

As occurs with metastatic solid tumors, the petrous apex is the most common site for leukemias to involve the temporal bone [95]. Kelemen opined that leukemia in the temporal bone evolved through the sequence of hemorrhage, leukemic infiltration, organization to connective tissue, suppuration, formation of new bone, and lastly degeneration into cholesterol granuloma [96]. From the petrous apex, tumor cells permeate the submucosal vasculature and ultimately are carried into the tubotympanic cavity [66]. Leukemia infiltration can involve the mucosa of the middle ear and mastoid, facial nerve, and the skin of the external auditory canal [65, 97, 98].

Leukemic infiltration of the temporal bone arises through either hematogenous spread or through the CSF [66], and it has been identified in as many as 36% of temporal bones [64, 65, 97]. In leukemic patients who develop hearing loss, the classic finding is leukemic infiltration of the petrous apex followed by hemorrhage in the inner ear (Fig. 12.8) [67, 99]. Hemorrhage in the inner ear can result in either sudden hearing loss or disequilibrium [100]. While leukemic infiltration is most commonly seen with acute leukemia, sudden and bilateral hearing loss due to labyrinthine hemorrhage has been identified in chronic leukemia as well [98, 99].

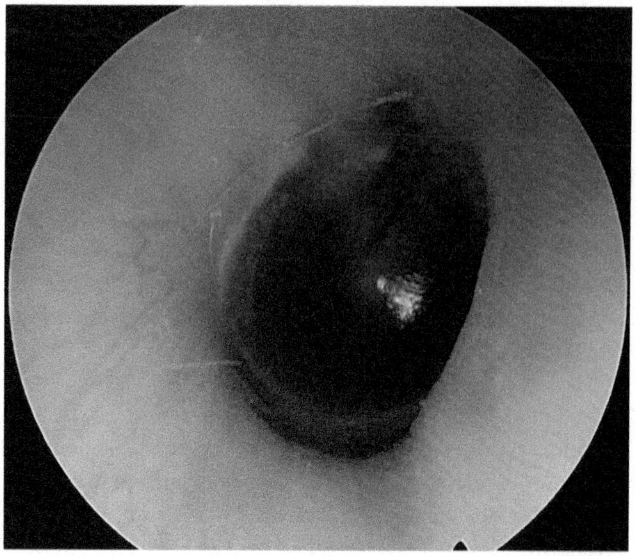

Fig. 12.6 Hemotympanum due to thrombocytopenia in a leukemia patient

Paparella et al. studied 45 temporal bones from 25 patients with various types of leukemia [65]. They identified three general categories of pathologic findings among these temporal bones: leukemic infiltration, hemorrhage, and infection. They found leukemic infiltration of the mucoperiosteum of the middle ear in 36%. This infiltration can involve the ossicles and the tendons of the intratympanic muscles. The tympanic membrane was infiltrated in 24% of patients. Ear canal infiltration was found in 12%. Leukemic infiltration of the bone marrow spaces of the petrous apex was found in every patient. Leukemic infiltration of the internal auditory canal (IAC) was found in 44%. The perineurium and endoneurium of CNs VII and VIII were infiltrated [65]. In their series, only one patient had hemorrhage in the inner ear. They found evidence of acute infection in only 16% of patients; all four patients had acute leukemia [65].

Terao et al. described the histopathologic temporal bone findings in 13 patients with acute lymphocytic leukemia [66]. Nine of these patients had otologic complaints including hearing loss, otalgia, otorrhea, and vertigo. Hemorrhage was a common finding in the middle ear, cochlea and vestibule. Leukemic infiltration was observed in the petrous apex, middle ear, vestibule, and internal auditory canal. Floating tumor cells were found in the middle ear effusions in three patients. Inflammatory changes were found in the cochlea and vestibule. Ossicular destruction, tympanic membrane perforation, and granulation tissue were observed in four patients.

Sando and Egami described a 78-year-old woman with a history of CLL who developed sudden hearing loss in the

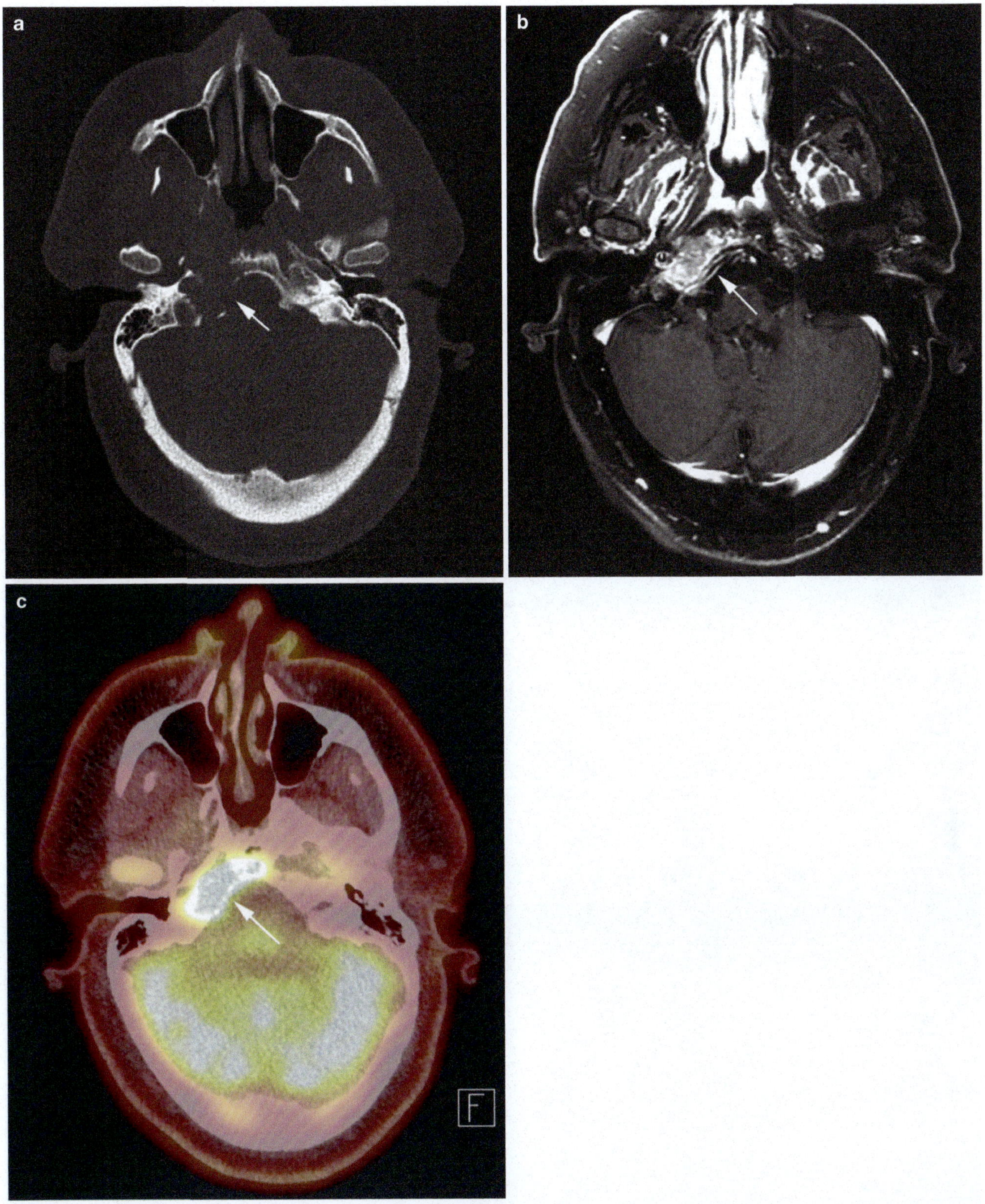

Fig. 12.7 Acute B-cell lymphoblastic leukemia involving the base of skull. The diagnosis was made by sternal bone marrow biopsy. (**a**) CT bone windows, showing erosion of the occipital condyle (arrow). (**b**) MRI T1 contrast. (**c**) PET/CT

right ear following transfusion [100]. She died 6 months later, and an autopsy showed extensive leukemic infiltration into the spleen, liver, lungs, and vascular spaces. Temporal bone pathologic evaluation showed leukemic hemorrhage in the perilymphatic and endolymphatic spaces in the cochlea and vestibular system. The authors attributed the sudden hearing loss to hemorrhage in the cochlea [100].

Smith et al. describe a case of a 62-year-old man with bilateral hearing loss, bilateral primary horizontal and vertical nystagmus, left facial paresis, absent jaw jerk, and absent gag reflex from Philadelphia chromosome negative CML [101]. His tumor did not respond to cytosine arabinoside, hydroxyurea, and busulfan. He did not recover hearing. He died 8 months after diagnosis. Postmortem examination showed normal auditory nerves. The vestibular nerves were atrophic with loss of vestibular ganglion cells in the IAC. The cochleae had been obliterated by myxoid fibrous tissue. Spiral ganglion cells were absent in the middle and apical regions, and the organ of Corti was atrophic with hydrops. The horizontal canals were occluded by fibrous material.

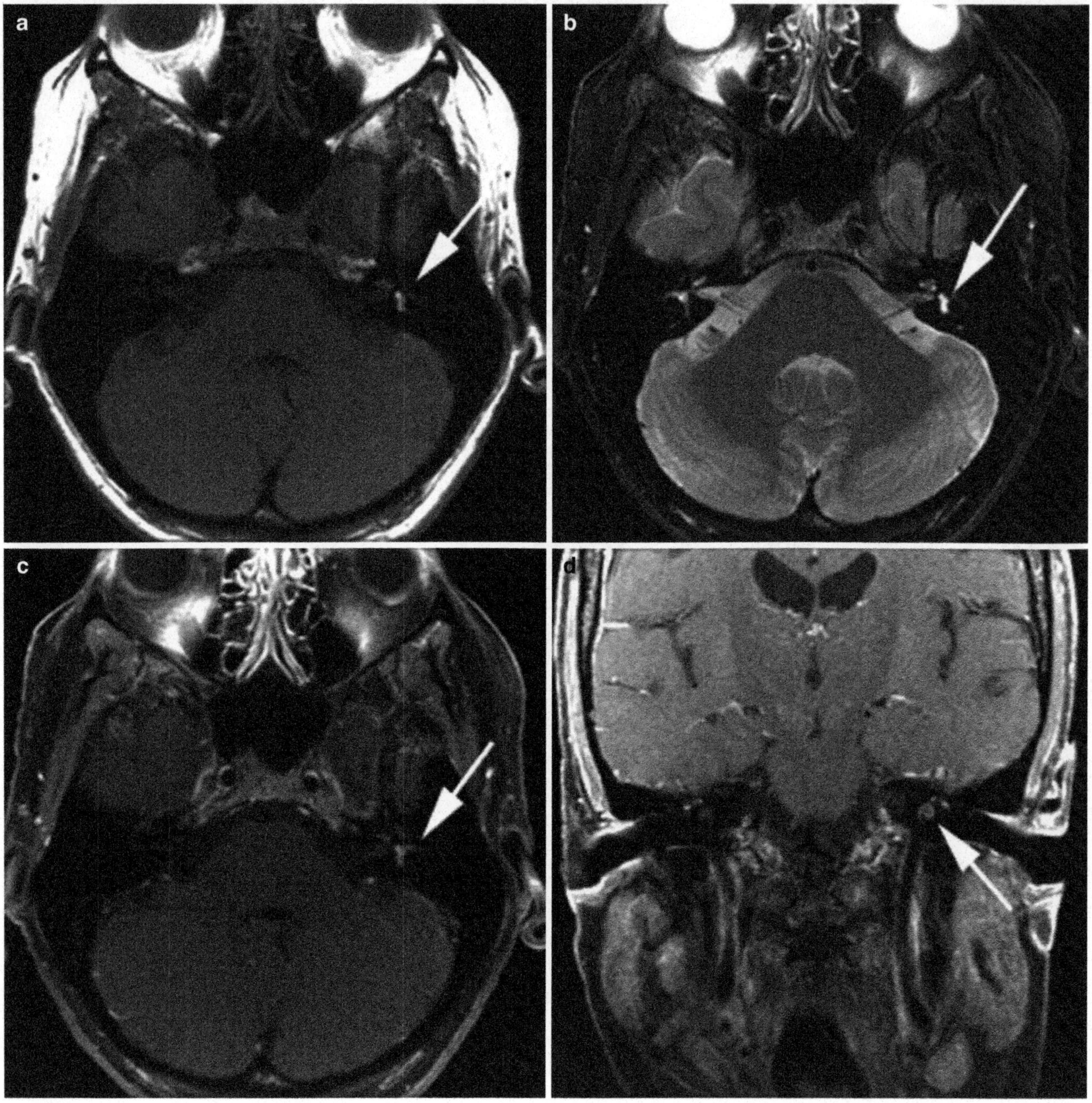

Fig. 12.8 Intralabyrinthine hemorrhage in a patient with APL. Sudden onset hearing loss and dizziness were the presenting symptoms of this patient's leukemia. MRI shows hyperintense signal within the left inner ear. (**a**) Non-contrast T1, (**b**) non-contrast T2, (**c**) contrast T1 axial, (**d**) contrast T1 coronal, (**e**) audiogram demonstrating profound hearing loss in the left ear

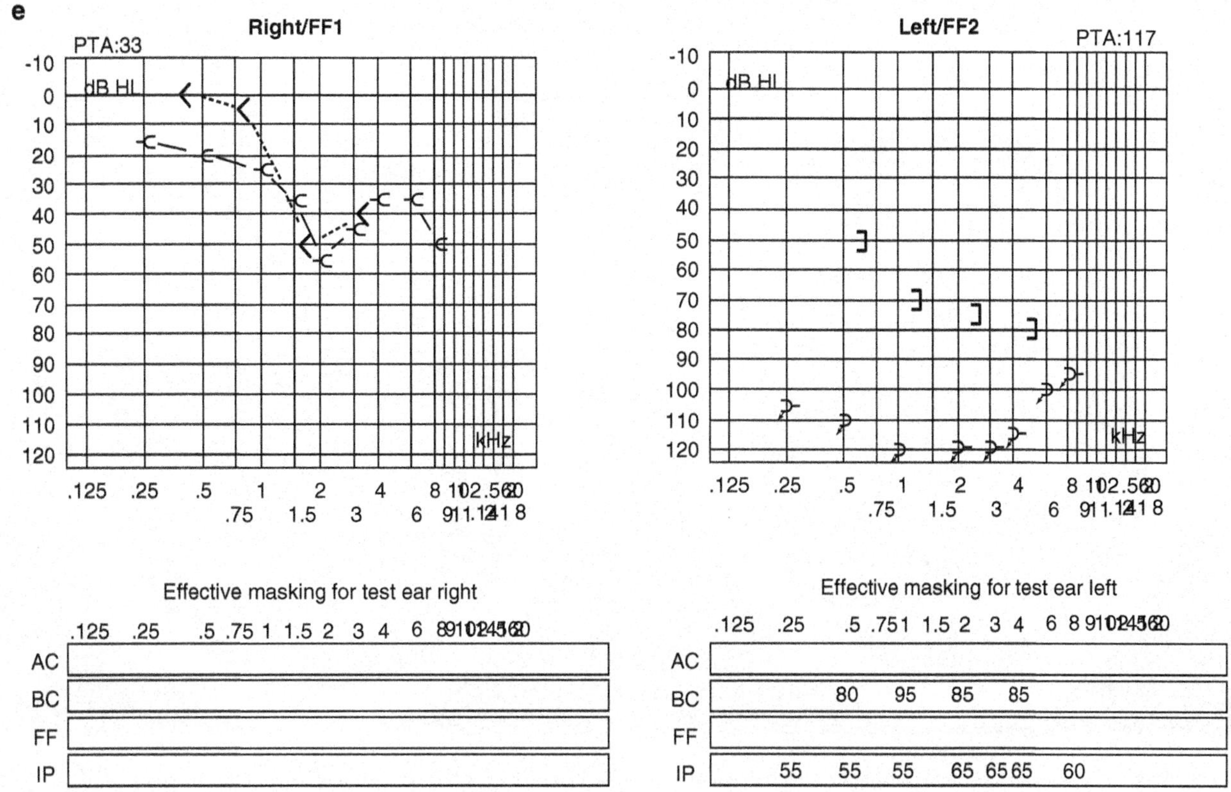

SRT PTA Right: 33.3 PTA Left: 116.7					
Transducer	Test type	Intensity	Masking	Aided | Binaural	ISF440 List
Insert Right	HL	25	--		Spondee A
Insert Left	HL	NR	50		Spondee A

WR PTA Right: 33.3 PTA Left: 116.7						
Transducer	WR	Intensity	Masking	Score	Aided | Binaural	ISF440 List
Insert Right	WR1	65		96		NU-6 LIST 1A
Insert Left	WR1	NR	50			NU-6 LIST 2A

Fig. 12.8 (continued)

The maculae of the saccule and utricle were absent. While these findings can occur with labyrinthitis, there was no evidence of infection. Hyperviscosity and hemorrhage were also excluded as a cause. Leukemic infiltration was suspected as the cause, and leukemic cells theorized as absent due to response from therapy [101].

Cranial Nerve and CNS Involvement

Cranial nerve findings in leukemia patients usually indicate leptomeningeal disease; MRI and CSF studies are important to evaluate for this possibility (Fig. 12.9). CNS leukemia is

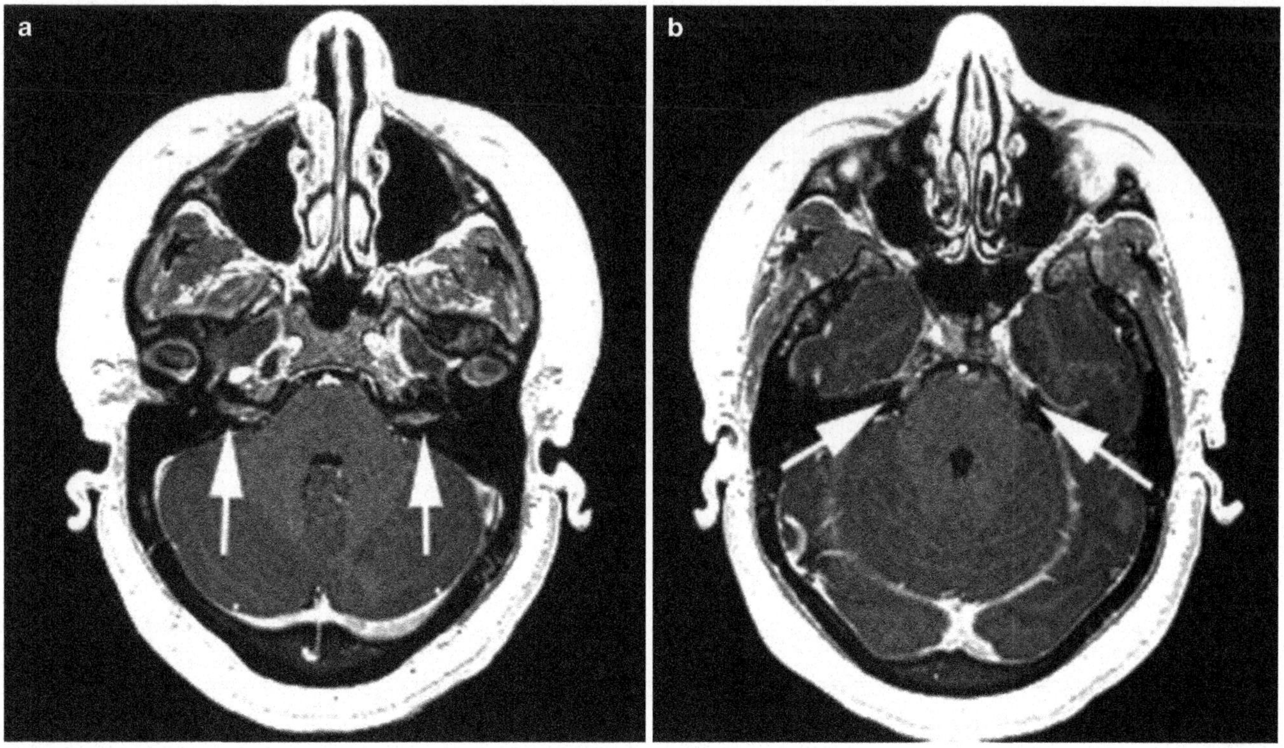

Fig. 12.9 Acute lymphocytic leukemia causing leptomeningeal disease in facial nerve (**a**, white arrows) and trigeminal nerves (**b**, white arrows) on contrast-enhanced MRI. Audiogram was normal

diagnosed by (1) the demonstration of blast cell in CSF, (2) CT or MRI findings of leptomeningeal spread, and (3) new onset of neurologic deficits in the setting of presenting or relapsed leukemia that cannot otherwise be explained by another cause [102]. Eighty-five percent of patients will have abnormal CSF studies [66].

CNS involvement occurs in <5% of patients with acute myeloid leukemia, compared with 25–50% of patients with lymphoid leukemia [102]. Since CNS relapse has such a poor prognosis, upfront intrathecal (IT) therapy is often included in the primary treatment of leukemia as a prophylactic measure. When gross disease is present in the CNS, tumor cells can block the normal flow of CSF and minimize the effectiveness of IT therapy.

CSF leukemic infiltration occurs along the perineurium of the nerves in the internal auditory canal and is conducted along the cochlear and vestibular nerves into the cochlea, vestibule, and semicircular canals [66]. The facial nerve is the most common cranial nerve affected [103], although nearly one-third of patients will have more than one cranial nerve affected. Sklansky et al. reported that the incidence of facial paralysis was 2.8% in patients with acute nonlymphocytic leukemia and 13.3% of patients with ALL [104].

In their paper, Paryani et al. examined 52 children with ALL or NHL and CNS disease [103]. Twenty (38%) of these children had cranial nerve paresis or palsy; and the nerve deficit usually developed over 24 to 48 hours. The combination of intrathecal chemotherapy and radiotherapy was most effective for restoring function and controlling disease.

In the setting of AML, facial paralysis is most likely related to recurrence of disease [105, 106]. Bilateral facial paralysis has been reported as a sign of recurrent AML [105]. Rhee et al. reported a case of an 11-year-old boy who developed direct leukemic infiltration of the facial nerve and parotid gland 5 years after remission of ALL [71]. Only a few case reports show facial palsy as a presenting sign of childhood AML [73].

Klausen et al. reported a case of a 60-year-old woman with CLL who developed complete facial paralysis associated with tumor protruding through the TM, and she was treated with radiotherapy [107].

Aikawa and Ohtani examined the temporal bones of a 32-year-old man with AML who died of CNS leukemia [108]. He had aural fullness for 4 months and dizziness for 1 month before he succumbed to his disease. Leukemic cells were found in the CSF. On postmortem examination, leukemic cells had infiltrated the scala tympani of the basal turn of the cochlea, the saccule, the posterior semicircular canal, and the vestibulocochlear nerves. Leukemic infiltration was identified in the external auditory canal, the tympanic membrane, the middle ear mucosa, and the bone marrow of the temporal bone [108].

Treatment

Treatment is based upon the subtype of leukemia and usually involves chemotherapy with or without stem cell transplant. Radiotherapy to the skull base, whole brain, or craniospinal axis has been used in adult patients with cranial nerve manifestations of leptomeningeal disease from leukemia [102]. Radiotherapy may be potentially advantageous as treatment is not affected by tumor cells blocking the flow of CSF, as is the case with IT therapy. Walker et al. analyzed 163 adults with CNS leukemia (41% AML, 41% ALL, and 17% CLL or CML) [102]. The mean survival time was 3.8 months after radiotherapy. Facial nerve deficit was present in 28%, followed closely by optic nerve deficits. Resolution of deficit was seen in 15%, improvement in 54%, and stable disease in 15%, and progressive findings in 17%. Patients who had isolated CNS involvement (i.e., negative bone marrow disease) benefitted the most from radiotherapy.

Myeloid Sarcoma

Chloroma, granulocytic sarcoma, and myeloid sarcoma are synonyms used to describe one or more tumor masses consisting of immature myeloid cells at an extramedullary site [109]. The term chloroma was coined by King in 1853 [110] and applies to the greenish color these tumors can exhibit due to the myeloperoxidase enzyme. Myeloid sarcoma (MS) is the preferred term and can herald or occur currently with AML, myeloproliferative disorder (MD), myelodysplastic syndrome (MDS), or the blastic phase of chronic myelogenous leukemia [109, 111].

Myeloid sarcoma is seen in 3–8% of all patients with AML [111]. MS can be the presenting sign of AML M2 subtype and is associated with the t(8; 21) cytogenic abnormality. MS in patients with a history of leukemia indicates recurrence and an imminent downturn in clinical course. These tumors can often be misdiagnosed as lymphoblastic lymphoma, Burkitt's lymphoma, or DLBCL.

The symptoms of MS of the temporal bone are nonspecific: hearing loss, vertigo, facial palsy, tinnitus, aural fullness, and otalgia [88, 112]. MS can mimic otomastoiditis and otitis externa [111, 113, 114].

Facial palsy has been described due to MS in several case reports. Kaufman et al. describe a case of facial paralysis in a 2-year-old boy as the presenting sign of granulocytic sarcoma [115]. Levy et al. described a 3-year-old boy who presented with left otitis media, left facial paralysis, left abducens, and ataxia due to MS of the petrous portion of the temporal bone [116].

Chapman and Johnson described a 35-year-old man with recurrent AML presenting with right otorrhea, fever, otalgia, and right facial paralysis due to mastoid chloroma [117]. His physical examination showed an edematous right ear canal and the TM could not be seen. Biopsy of the mastoid showed AML. CSF studies showed high WBC in the spinal fluid. He was treated with intrathecal methotrexate and cytosine arabinoside followed by whole brain radiation.

MS involving the cerebellopontine angle has been described and can present with sudden sensorineural hearing loss, facial paralysis, and lower cranial nerve dysfunction [88, 118]. In this setting, resection is performed to treat brainstem compression and hydrocephalus. Murakami et al. reported a case of myeloid sarcoma involving the temporal bone and presenting with intracranial hemorrhage [112]. This tumor rebled 8 days after hemorrhage evacuation, and the patient died 4 days later.

When MS affects bone, CT typically demonstrates a lytic lesion. On MRI, MS has signal intensity similar to bone marrow, and the lesion enhances with contrast [111]. Based on imaging alone, MS cannot be distinguished from lymphoma, meningioma, or pseudotumor. Biopsy is required for final diagnosis, although the clinical context usually suggests the diagnosis.

The role of surgery is biopsy only. MS are generally sensitive to radiation therapy [115]. Overall survival for MS is short, with chemotherapy giving survival time on average of 7 months.

Plasmacytoma of the Temporal Bone

Plasma cell tumors are a monoclonal proliferation of immunoglobulin-secreting plasma cells of hematopoietic origin [119, 120]. Multiple myeloma (MM) is the disseminated form of the malignant plasma cell disorder, and it generally produces multiple lytic bone lesions, monoclonal antibodies in the serum and urine, and pathologic fractures [119]. Plasmacytomas are classified into two types: solitary plasmacytoma of the bone (SPB) and extramedullary plasmacytoma (EMP) [120]. Plasmacytomas primarily affect middle-aged and older adults; the average age of patients with EMP is 45 years and that of SPB is 51 years. About 70% of plasmacytomas occur in men. SPB usually involves the axial skeleton, especially the vertebrae. In the temporal bone, solitary plasmacytomas arise from the petrous portion of the temporal bone due to its rich bone marrow. EMP occurs in the upper airway and mandible. Diagnosis of solitary osseous plasmacytoma is made in the absence of clinical, radiologic, or pathologic evidence of disseminated disease.

Several case reports of plasmacytoma in the temporal bone are found in the literature [119, 121–137]. Chiang et al. (1998) reviewed the English literature and found 11 cases of plasmacytoma of the temporal bone; 4 cases of EMP and 7 cases of SPB [133]. Symptoms include unilateral conductive hearing loss, tinnitus, aural pressure, otorrhea, and pain. Often, the clinical picture can suggest acute otitis media. Hearing loss, facial paralysis, and lower cranial nerve deficits have also been reported and indicate that the diagnosis is more than inflammatory middle ear disease.

On CT these lesions are associated with bone loss and soft tissue density. On MRI, these tumors are isointense on T1 imaging and isointense to hyperintense on T2 imaging. These tumors show mild to marked enhancement with contrast (Fig. 12.10).

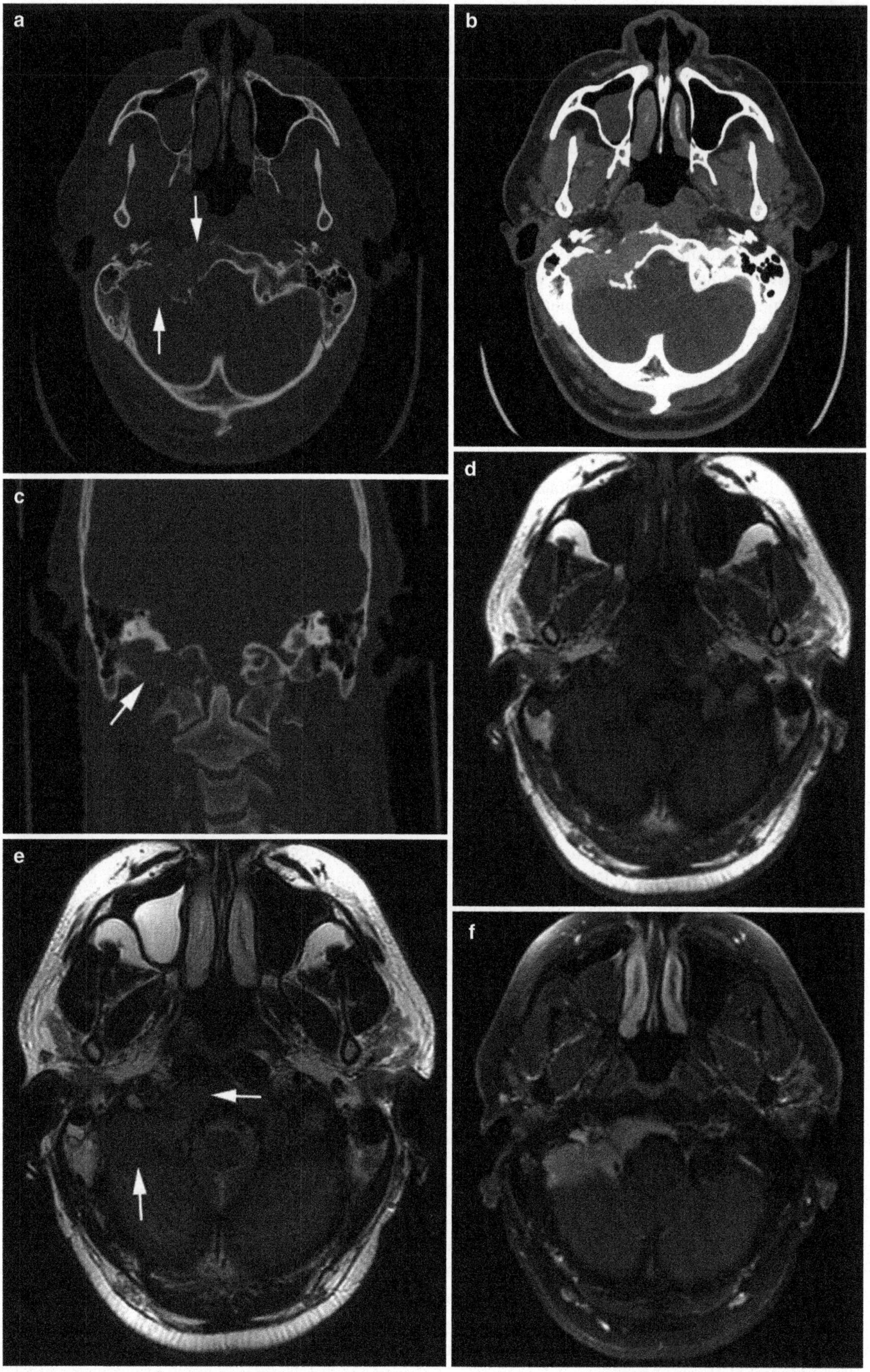

Fig. 12.10 Plasmacytoma of the right temporal bone that presented with headache. This patient had normal hearing and no evidence of disease in the middle ear. Contrast-enhanced axial CT scan bone windows (**a**), showing erosion of the right skull base (arrows), and (**b**) soft tissue windows. (**c**) Coronal CT scan, showing erosion of the skull base (arrow). MRI images showing (**d**) T1 and (**e**) T2 non-contrast images and (**f**) contrast-enhanced T1

Diagnosis depends on biopsy, usually requiring mastoidectomy. The differential should include plasma cell granuloma, lymphoma, paragangliomas, and hemangiopericytoma.

Solitary plasmacytoma of the bone has been treated with radiotherapy only or with combined chemotherapy and radiotherapy. A few case reports indicate surgical treatment for isolated disease [119, 131]. SPB is believed to be a precursor to multiple myeloma, and long-term follow-up is indicated. Within 3 to 5 years, about 50% of patients will develop multiple myeloma. The average survival of SPB is 86 to 114 months [133].

Conclusion

Hematologic malignancies can involve the ear and temporal bone rarely as the primary site of involvement or as a manifestation of systemic disease. The signs and symptoms are vague and can be mistaken for common ear disorders such as perichondritis, otitis externa, otitis media, and mastoiditis. Associated symptoms such as fever, night sweats, and weight loss should suggest a systemic illness. Persistent cytopenias also suggest potential marrow involvement by lymphoma or leukemia, and monoclonal gammopathy might suggest an occult plasma cell malignancy. Diagnostic tests and imaging are required to help refine the differential diagnosis. Definitive diagnosis is based on tissue biopsy with hematopathologic interpretation, Biopsy of disease in the ear canal, middle ear, or mastoid is required when findings are isolated to the temporal bone. Treatment is dependent on an accurate diagnosis.

References

1. Armitage JO, Gascoyne RD, Lunning MA, Cavalli F. Non-Hodgkin lymphoma. Lancet. 2017;390(10091):298–310.
2. Townsend W, Linch D. Hodgkin's lymphoma in adults. Lancet. 2012;380(9844):836–47.
3. Maithrea N, Periyathamby S, Mohamad I. Primary Hodgkin's lymphoma of the middle ear: a rare cause of facial nerve palsy. Egypt J Ear Nose Throat Allied Sci. 2017;18(1):67–9.
4. Liu Y, Chen Q, Si Y, Zhang ZG. Hodgkin's lymphoma of the temporal bone accompanied by intracranial abscess. Otol Neurotol. 2014;35(2):e95–6.
5. Biggar RJ, Rabkin CS. The epidemiology of AIDS-related neoplasms. Hematol Oncol Clin North Am. 1996;10(5):997–1010.
6. Khaw B, Sivalingam S, Pathamanathan SS, Tan TS, Naicker M. Simultaneous non-Hodgkin lymphoma of the external auditory canal and thyroid gland: a case report. Ear Nose Throat J. 2014;93(12):508–11.
7. Hersh SP, Harrison WG, Hersh DJ. Primary B cell lymphoma of the external auditory canal. Ear Nose Throat J. 2006;85(9):597–9.
8. Coiffier B, Lepage E, Brière J, Herbrecht R, Tilly H, Bouabdallah R, et al. CHOP chemotherapy plus rituximab compared with CHOP alone in elderly patients with diffuse large-B-cell lymphoma. N Engl J Med. 2002;346(4):235–42.
9. Vigier S, Nicollas R, Roman S, Barlogis V, Coulibaly B, Triglia JM. Burkitt's leukemia presenting as atypical acute mastoiditis in a 7-month-old child. Arch Pediatr. 2013;20(12):1317–20.
10. Molyneux EM, Rochford R, Griffin B, Newton R, Jackson G, Menon G, et al. Burkitt's lymphoma. Lancet. 2012;379(9822):1234–44.
11. Oyetunji NM, Ladapo AA. Burkitt's lymphoma of the mastoid temporal bone. J Laryngol Otol. 1981;95(10):1063–7.
12. Baumgartner BJ, Eusterman V, Myers J, Massengill P. Initial report of a cutaneous T-cell lymphoma appearing on the auricular helix. Ear Nose Throat J. 2000;79(5):391–4. 6
13. Strahan RW, Calcaterra TC. Otolaryngologic aspects of mycosis fungoides: a case report. Laryngoscope. 1971;81(12):1912–6.
14. Darvay A, Russell-Jones R, Acland KM, Lampert I, Chu AC. Systemic B-cell lymphoma presenting as an isolated lesion on the ear. Clin Exp Dermatol. 2001;26(2):166–9.
15. Levin RJ, Henick DH, Cohen AF. Human immunodeficiency virus-associated non-Hodgkin's lymphoma presenting as an auricular perichondritis. Otolaryngol Head Neck Surg. 1995;112(3):493–5.
16. Clayton AS, McCollough M, Barekman CL. Primary cutaneous B-cell lymphoma. Cutis. 1998;62(2):69–72.
17. Moody BR, Bartlett NL, George DW, Price CR, Breer WA, Rothschild Y, et al. Cyclin D1 as an aid in the diagnosis of mantle cell lymphoma in skin biopsies: a case report. Am J Dermatopathol. 2001;23(5):470–6.
18. Lewis WB, Patel U, Roberts JK, Palis J, Teot L. Angiocentric T-cell lymphoma of the temporal bone. Otolaryngol Head Neck Surg. 2002;126(1):85–6.
19. Zanation AM, Ebert CS Jr, Coffey CS, Dubin MG, Rose AS. Precursor B-cell lymphoblastic lymphoma presenting as an isolated external ear swelling in a two-year-old child. Int J Pediatr Otorhinolaryngol. 2005;69(5):695–9.
20. Fika Z, Karkos PD, Badran K, Williams RE. Primary cutaneous aggressive epidermotropic CD8 positive cytotoxic T-cell lymphoma of the ear. J Laryngol Otol. 2007;121(5):503–5.
21. Bittencourt AL, Rothers S, Boente P, Santos R. Primary cutaneous eosinophil-rich anaplastic large cell lymphoma: report of an unusual case and literature review. J Cutan Med Surg. 2008;12(2):88–92.
22. Greve J, Bas M, Schipper J, Hoffmann TK. Primary cutane manifestation of a precursor-B-lymphoblastic lymphoma in the external ear. Laryngorhinootologie. 2008;87(10):728–30.
23. Indudharan R, Arni T, Myint KK, Jackson N. Lymphoblastic lymphoma/leukaemia presenting as perichondritis of the pinna. J Laryngol Otol. 1998;112(6):592–4.
24. Fenwick JD. Mycosis fungoides involving the external auditory meatus. J Laryngol Otol. 1975;89(11):1155–9.
25. Brennan JA. The head and neck manifestations of mycosis fungoides. Laryngoscope. 1995;105(5):478–80.
26. Chuang TY, WP S, Muller SA. Incidence of cutaneous T cell lymphoma and other rare skin cancers in a defined population. J Am Acad Dermatol. 1990;23(2 Pt 1):254–6.
27. Molina Utrilla R, Lao Luque J, Perello Scherdel E, Companyo Hermo C, Casamitjana Claramunt F. Otomycosis. Case reports of 18 months in the general University Hospital of the Valle de Hebron in Barcelona. An Otorrinolaringol Ibero Am. 1994;21(3):255–63.
28. Zackheim HS, Lebo CF, Wasserstein P, McNutt NS, Epstein EH, Meyler S, et al. Mycosis fungoides of the mastoid, middle ear, and CNS: literature review of mycosis fungoides of the CNS. Arch Dermatol. 1983;119(4):311–8.
29. Maiche AG, Teerenhovi L, Isokangas O. Diffuse centrocytic malignant lymphoma with unusual sites—report on two cases with possible etiological factors. Acta Oncol. 1991;30(6):767–8.
30. Merkus P, Copper MP, Van Oers MH, Schouwenburg PF. Lymphoma in the ear. ORL J Otorhinolaryngol Relat Spec. 2000;62(5):274–7.
31. Fish BM, Huda R, Dundas SA, Lesser TH. B-cell lymphoma of the external auditory meatus. J Laryngol Otol. 2002;116(1):39–41.
32. Gonzalez Delgado A, Argudo Marco F, Sanchez Martinez N, Sprekelsen Gasso C. T cell non-Hodgkin's lymphoma of the external auditory canal. Acta Otorrinolaringol Esp. 2008;59(4):200–1.
33. Bruschini L, De Vito A, Fortunato S, Pelosini M, Cervetti G, Petrini M, et al. A case of primary non-Hodgkin's lymphoma of the external auditory canal. Case Rep Otolaryngol. 2013;2013:138397.

34. Shuto J, Ueyama T, Suzuki M, Mogi G. Primary lymphoma of bilateral external auditory canals. Am J Otolaryngol. 2002;23(1): 49–52.
35. Kieserman SP, Finn DG. Non-Hodgkin's lymphoma of the external auditory canal in an HIV-positive patient. J Laryngol Otol. 1995;109(8):751–4.
36. Ogawa S, Tawara I, Ueno S, Kimura M, Miyazaki K, Nishikawa H, et al. De novo CD5-positive diffuse large B-cell lymphoma of the temporal bone presenting with an external auditory canal tumor. Intern Med. 2006;45(11):733–7.
37. Okura SI, Kaga K. Temporal bone pathology of leukemia and malignant lymphoma with middle ear effusion. Auris Nasus Larynx. 1994;21(1):1–7.
38. Roberts JM, Fastenberg J, Redd E, Foyt D. Primary diffuse large B-cell lymphoma presenting as chronic otomastoiditis. J Otol Rhinol. 2017;71:951–9.
39. Saito A, Jia W, Sasaki T, Mizukami H, Sasaki A, Shinkawa H, et al. B-cell malignant lymphoma presenting as otitis media and mastoiditis associated with sinus thrombosis. Case Rep Neurol. 2014;6(2):161–5.
40. Schmedes GW, Rizk HG, Lambert PR. Middle ear mass with facial weakness. JAMA Otolaryngol Head Neck Surg. 2015;141(1):89–90.
41. Kanzaki S, Saito H, Mori T, Shimasaki N, Mukai M, Ogawa K. Thirteen-month-old boy with malignant lymphoma having symptoms mimicking acute otitis media and mastoiditis with facial palsy. ORL J Otorhinolaryngol Relat Spec. 2011;73(5):266–70.
42. Lang EE, Walsh RM, Leader M. Primary middle-ear lymphoma in a child. J Laryngol Otol. 2003;117(3):205–7.
43. Paparella MM, El-Fiky FM. Ear involvement in malignant lymphoma. Ann Otol Rhinol Laryngol. 1972;81(3):352–63.
44. Kobayashi K, Igarashi M, McBride RA, Saito R, Kataura A. Temporal bone pathology of metastatic T-cell lymphoma. Acta Otolaryngol Suppl. 1988;447:113–9.
45. Okamura H, Ohtani I, Nakamura N, Abe M, Wakasa H. Four cases of metastatic lymphoma into the temporal bone. Auris Nasus Larynx. 1992;19(1):29–35.
46. Tucci DL, Lambert PR, Innes DJ Jr. Primary lymphoma of the temporal bone. Arch Otolaryngol Head Neck Surg. 1992;118(1):83–5.
47. Jiang ZY, Saadia-Redleaf MI. Primary lymphoma of the temporal bone presenting as XIIth cranial nerve weakness. Ear Nose Throat J. 2011;90(3):125–7.
48. Sritharan N, Moghadam A, Choroomi S, Stone H. Primary non-Hodgkin lymphoma of the petrous temporal bone. Otol Neurotol. 2012;33(2):e11–2.
49. Cakmak O, Kutluk T, Akyol MU, Ruacan S. Angiocentric lymphoma involving the temporal bone in a child. Eur Arch Otorhinolaryngol. 1999;256(5):262–5.
50. Koral K, Curran JG, Thompson A. Primary non-Hodgkin's lymphoma of the temporal bone. CT findings. Clin Imaging. 2003;27(6):386–8.
51. Danino J, Joachims HZ, Ben-Arieh Y, Hefer T. Weyl-Ben-Arush M. T cell lymphoma of the ear presenting as mastoiditis. J Laryngol Otol. 1997;111(9):852–4.
52. Conley SF, Staszak C, Clamon GH, Maves MD. Non-hodgkin's lymphoma of the head and neck: the university of iowa experience. Laryngoscope. 1987;97(3):291-300.
53. Lewis VO, Primus G, Anastasi J, Doherty D, Montag AG, Peabody TD, et al. Oncologic outcomes of primary lymphoma of bone in adults. Clin Orthop Relat Res. 2003;415:90–7.
54. Beal K, Allen L, Yahalom J. Primary bone lymphoma: treatment results and prognostic factors with long-term follow-up of 82 patients. Cancer. 2006;106(12):2652–6.
55. Coley BL, Higinbotham NL, Groesbeck HP. Primary reticulum-cell sarcoma of bone: summary of 37 cases 1. Radiology. 1950;55(5):641–58.
56. Unni K, Hogendoorn P, editors. Malignant lymphoma. World Health Organization classification of tumours pathology and genetics of tumours of soft tissue and bone. Lyon: IARC; 2002. p. 306–8.
57. Liu Y-L, Tung C-L, Yang Y-L, Lin D-T, Lin K-H, Liao HL. Precursor B-cell lymphoblastic lymphoma of the ear in a 7-year-old child. J Clin Oncol. 2012;30(21):e184–e7.
58. Kontoyiannis DP, Chagua MR, Ramirez I, Prieto V. Locally invasive auricular aspergillosis after ear piercing in a neutropenic patient with leukemia. Am J Hematol. 2003;73(4):296–7.
59. Borner D, Marsch WC, Fischer M. Necrotizing otitis externa caused by Stenotrophomonas maltophilia. Hautarzt. 2003;54(11):1080–2.
60. Donné A. Cours de microscopie complémentaire des études médicales: anatomie microscopique et physiologie des fluides de l'économie. Paris: J.-B. Baillière; 1844.
61. Politzer A. Pathologische Veranderungen im Labyrinthe bei leukamischer Taubheit. Cong Int Otol. 1885;3:139.
62. Gotay V. Unusual otologic manifestation of chronic lymphocytic leukemia. Laryngoscope. 1976;86(12):1856–63.
63. Druss JG. Aural manifestations of leukemia. Arch Otolaryngol. 42:267–74.
64. Shanbrom E, Finch SC. The auditory manifestations of leukemia. Yale J Biol Med. 1958;31:144–56.
65. Paparella MM, Berlinger NT, Oda M, el-Fiky F. Otological manifestations of leukemia. Laryngoscope. 1973;83(9):1510–26.
66. Terao K, Cureoglu S, Schachern PA, Paparella MM, Morita N, Nomiya S, et al. Pathologic correlations of otologic symptoms in acute lymphocytic leukemia. Am J Otolaryngol. 2011;32(1):13–8.
67. Schuknecht HF, Igarashi M, Chasin WD. Inner ear hemorrhage in leukemia. A case report. Laryngoscope. 1965;75:662–8.
68. Breccia M, Petti MC, Testi AM, Specchia G, Ferrara F, Diverio D, et al. Ear involvement in acute promyelocytic leukemia at relapse: a disease-associated 'sanctuary'? Leukemia. 2002;16(6):1127–30.
69. Chae SW, Cho JH, Lee JH, Kang HJ, Hwang SJ. Sudden hearing loss in chronic myelogenous leukaemia implicating the hyperviscosity syndrome. J Laryngol Otol. 2002;116(04):291–3.
70. Jabbour E, Borthakur G, Buesos-Ramos C, Kantarjian H, Faderl S. Acute lymphoblastic Leukemia. In: Kantarjian H, Wolff R, Koller C, editors. MD Anderson manual of medical oncology. New York: McGraw-Hill; 2006. p. 3–17.
71. Rhee D, Myssiorek D, Zahtz G, Diamond A, Paley C, Shende A. Recurrent attacks of facial nerve palsy as the presenting sign of leukemic relapse. Laryngoscope. 2002;112(2):235–7.
72. Inaba H, Greaves M, Mullighan CG. Acute lymphoblastic leukaemia. Lancet. 2013;381(9881):1943–55.
73. Takhenchangbam DS, Laishram RS, Thoudem TS, Sunita A, Imchen LT. Proptosis and facial palsy as an unusual clinical presentation of acute myeloid leukemia. Iran J Cancer Prev. 2013;6(1):52–4.
74. Wiernik PH. Diagnosis and treatment of adult acute myeloid leukemia other than acute promyelocytic leukemia. In: Wiernik PH, Goldman JM, Dutcher JP, Kyle RA, editors. Neoplastic diseases of the blood. 5th ed. New York: Springer; 2013. p. 375–401.
75. Adelson RT, Samy RN, Lindberg G. T-cell prolymphocytic leukemia presenting as an ear canal mass. Otol Neurotol. 2004;25(6):1006–8.
76. Kindem S, Traves V, Requena C, Alcalá R, Llombart B, Serra-Guillén C, et al. Bilateral cauliflower ear as the presenting sign of B-cell chronic lymphocytic leukemia. J Cutan Pathol. 2014;41(2):73–7.
77. Porter WM, Sidwell RU, Catovsky D, Bunker CB. Cutaneous presentation of chronic lymphatic leukaemia and response to ultraviolet B phototherapy. Br J Dermatol. 2001;144(5):1092–4.
78. Kim PS, Sheth PB. Asymptomatic cauliflower ears in a 73-year-old man. Diagnosis: leukemia cutis in the setting of indolent

B-cell chronic lymphocytic leukemia (B-CLL). Arch Dermatol. 2011;147(12):1443–8.
79. Morales-Avellaneda T, Gonzalez-Ramirez AI, Rodriguez-Alfonso B, Mucientes-Rasilla J, Garcia-Berrocal JR, De Diego B. Clinical-scintigraphy discordance in a case of malignant external otitis. Rev Esp Med Nucl Imagen Mol. 2012;31(5):267–9.
80. Vester K, Treudler R, Paasch U, Becker C, Liebmann A, Simon JC, et al. Specific bilateral ear infiltration as an early manifestation of chronic lymphocytic leukaemia. Eur J Dermatol. 2012;22(2):265–6.
81. Koletsa T, Patsatsi A, Kostopoulos I, Georgiou E, Sotiriadis D. Ear lobe involvement in chronic lymphocytic leukemia. J Dtsch Dermatol Ges. 2013;11(1):80–2.
82. Kleijwegt FS, van Krimpen C, Faber LM. An elderly man with swelling and discolouration of the right earlobe. Neth J Med. 2015;73(5):253. 6-7
83. Raufi A, Alsharedi M, Khelfa Y, Griswold DC, Lebowicz Y. Leukemia cutis in a patient with chronic lymphocytic leukemia presenting as bilateral helical nodules. SAGE Open Med Case Rep. 2016;4:2050313x16683624.
84. Marchetti M, Falanga A, Giovanelli S, Oldani E, Barbui T. All-trans-Retinoic Acid Increases Adhesion To Endothelium Of The Human Promyelocytic Leukaemia Cell Line NB4. Br J Haematol. 1996;93(2):360–6.
85. Tobita T, Shinjyo K, Yanagi M, Takeshita A, Ohnishi K, Ohno R. Relapse in the external auditory canal of acute promyelocytic leukemia after treatment with all-trans retinoic acid. Intern Med. 1997;36(7):484–6.
86. Yagita M, Onishi R, Yamagata N, Shimazaki C, Kudoh H, Kobayashi M, et al. Extramedullary relapse in the external auditory canal in a patient with acute promyelocytic leukemia treated with all-trans retinoic acid and autologous peripheral blood stem cell transplantation. Rinsho Ketsueki. 1998;39(9):709–15.
87. WY A, Chan GC, Chim CS, Shek TW, Ooi GC, Ho WK, et al. Unusual sites of involvement by hematologic malignancies. Case 3. External auditory canal tumor: a rare chloroma in acute promyelocytic leukemia with a complete response to arsenic trioxide. J Clin Oncol. 2001;19(19):3993–5.
88. Gokcan MK, Batikhan H, Calguner M, Tataragasi AI. Unilateral hearing loss as a presenting manifestation of granulocytic sarcoma (chloroma). Otol Neurotol. 2006;27(1):106–9.
89. Effat KG, Naguib AW. Simultaneous leukaemic infiltrate and cholesteatoma in the same temporal bone. J Laryngol Otol. 1998;112(9):867–9.
90. Khan AA, Nazir S, Ahmed A. Relapse of acute myeloid leukemia presenting as acute otitis media. QJM. 2010;103(7):533–4.
91. Millot F, Klossek JM, Brizard F, Brizard A, Vandermarq P, Babin P, et al. Recurrence of childhood acute lymphoblastic leukemia presenting as a tumor of the middle ear: a case report. J Pediatr Hematol Oncol. 1997;19(4):351–3.
92. Sharma S, Banerjee A. Acute otitis externa—an unusual presentation of relapse of acute lymphoblastic leukaemia. Indian J Pathol Microbiol. 1986;29(3):215–7.
93. Almadori G, Del Ninno M, Cadoni G, Di Mario A, Ottaviani F. Facial nerve paralysis in acute otomastoiditis as presenting symptom of FAB M2, T8; 21 leukemic relapse. Case report and review of the literature. Int J Pediatr Otorhinolaryngol. 1996;36(1):45–52.
94. Wuillemin WA, Vischer MW, Tobler A, Fey MF. Relapse of acute myeloblastic leukaemia presenting as temporal bone chloroma with facial nerve paralysis. Ann Oncol. 1993;4(4):339–40.
95. Gloria-Cruz TI, Schachern PA, Paparella MM, Adams GL, Fulton SE. Metastases to temporal bones from primary nonsystemic malignant neoplasms. Arch Otolaryngol Head Neck Surg. 2000;126(2):209–14.
96. Kelemen G. Aural pathohistology in leukemia. ORL J Otorhinolaryngol Relat Spec. 1975;37(6):321–32.
97. Zechner G, Altmann F. The temporal bone in leukemia. Histological studies. Ann Otol Rhinol Laryngol. 1969;78(2):375–87.
98. Naraev BG, Linthicum FH Jr. Rapid hearing loss in chronic lymphocytic leukemia. Otol Neurotol. 2006;27(3):445–6.
99. Taljebini M, Linthicum FH Jr. Hearing loss in chronic lymphocytic leukemia. Otol Neurotol. 2007;28(2):282–3.
100. Sando I, Egami T. Inner ear hemorrhage and endolymphatic hydrops in a leukemic patient with sudden hearing loss. Ann Otol Rhinol Laryngol. 1977;86(4):518–24.
101. Smith N, Bain B, Michaels L, Craven E. Atypical Ph negative chronic myeloid leukaemia presenting as sudden profound deafness. J Clin Pathol. 1991;44(12):1033–4.
102. Walker GV, Shihadeh F, Kantarjian H, Allen P, Rondon G, Kebriaei P, et al. Comprehensive craniospinal radiation for controlling central nervous system leukemia. Int J Radiat Oncol Biol Phys. 2014;90(5):1119–25.
103. Paryani SB, Donaldson SS, Amylon MD, Link M. Cranial nerve involvement in children with leukemia and lymphoma. J Clin Oncol. 1983;1(9):542–5.
104. Sklansky BD, Jafek BW, Wiernik PH. Otolaryngologic manifestations of acute leukemia. Laryngoscope. 1974;84(2):210–30.
105. Leite da Silveira P, Goncalves Silva V, Rizzato Paschoal J, Nizam Pfeilsticker L. Bilateral peripheral facial palsy and mastoid infiltration as symptoms of relapsed acute myeloid leukemia. Eur Ann Otorhinolaryngol Head Neck Dis. 2015;132(1):41–3.
106. Juhn YJ, Inoue S. Facial nerve palsy as an early manifestation of relapse in T-cell acute lymphoblastic leukemia. Ear Nose Throat J. 1996;75(3):157–60.
107. Klausen OG, Lind O, Mella O. Facial nerve paralysis caused by tumor-forming chronic lymphatic leukemia: a case report. J Otolaryngol. 1990;19(1):76–8.
108. Aikawa T, Ohtani I. Temporal bone findings in central nervous system leukemia. Am J Otolaryngol. 1991;12(6):320–5.
109. Pileri S, Ascani S, Cox M, Campidelli C, Bacci F, Piccioli M, et al. Myeloid sarcoma: clinico-pathologic, phenotypic and cytogenetic analysis of 92 adult patients. Leukemia. 2007;21(2):340–50.
110. King A. A case of chloroma. Monthly J Med. 1853;17(97):b1.
111. Lee B, Fatterpekar GM, Kim W, Som PM. Granulocytic sarcoma of the temporal bone. AJNR Am J Neuroradiol. 2002;23(9):1497–9.
112. Murakami M, Uno T, Nakaguchi H, Yamada SM, Hoya K, Yamazaki K, et al. Isolated recurrence of intracranial and temporal bone myeloid sarcoma—case report. Neurol Med Chir (Tokyo). 2011;51(12):850–4.
113. Chang K-H, Kim D-K, Jun B-C, Park Y-S. Temporal bone myeloid sarcoma. Clin Exp Otorhinolaryngol. 2009;2(4):198–202.
114. Sugimoto Y, Nishii K, Sakakura M, Araki H, Usui E, Lorenzo VF, et al. Acute myeloid leukemia with t(8;21)(q22;q22) manifesting as granulocytic sarcomas in the rhinopharynx and external acoustic meatus at relapse after high-dose cytarabine: case report and review of the literature. Hematol J. 2004;5(1):84–9.
115. Kaufman BA, Jones L, Zutter MM, Park TS. Megakaryoblastic leukemia presenting as a temporal bone granulocytic sarcoma. Case report. J Neurosurg. 1993;79(1):128–31.
116. Levy R, Shvero J, Sandbank J. Granulocytic sarcoma (chloroma) of the temporal bone. Int J Pediatr Otorhinolaryngol. 1989;18(2):163–9.
117. Chapman P, Johnson SA. Mastoid chloroma as relapse in acute myeloid leukaemia. J Laryngol Otol. 1980;94(12):1423–7.
118. Kao SC, Yuh WT, Sato Y, Barloon TJ. Intracranial granulocytic sarcoma (chloroma): MR findings. J Comput Assist Tomogr. 1987;11(6):938–41.

119. Jun HJ, Choi J, Kim KM, Chae SW. Multiple myeloma with isolated plasmacytoma in temporal bone. Otol Neurotol. 2013;34(7):107–8.
120. Lorsbach RB. Update on the diagnosis and classification of the plasma cell neoplasms. Surg Pathol Clin. 2010;3(4):1061–89.
121. Abemayor E, Canalis RF, Greenberg P, Wortham DG, Rowland JP, Sun NC. Plasma cell tumors of the head and neck. J Otolaryngol. 1988;17(7):376–81.
122. Rowland PH, Valentine BA, Stebbins KE, Smith CA. Cutaneous plasmacytomas with amyloid in six dogs. Vet Pathol. 1991; 28(2):125–30.
123. Sato M, Kanai N, Yamamoto S, Take H, Kuyama J, Shiraki T, et al. Giant plasmacytoma of the skull which appeared in the clinical course of multiple myeloma—a case report. No To Shinkei. 1993;45(8):753–7.
124. Wax MK, Yun KJ, Omar RA. Extramedullary plasmacytomas of the head and neck. Otolaryngol Head Neck Surg. 1993;109(5):877–85.
125. George JC, Caldemeyer KS, Kreipke DL, Chalian AA, Moran CC. Solitary plasmacytoma of the mastoid bone presenting as coalescent mastoiditis. Arch Otolaryngol Head Neck Surg. 1994;120(12):1393–4.
126. Panosian MS, Roberts JK. Plasmacytoma of the middle ear and mastoid. Am J Otol. 1994;15(2):264–7.
127. Weber AL, McKenna MJ. Radiologic evaluation of the jugular foramen. Anatomy, vascular variants, anomalies, and tumors. Neuroimaging Clin N Am. 1994;4(3):579–98.
128. Megerian CA, McKenna MJ, Nadol JB Jr. Non-paraganglioma jugular foramen lesions masquerading as glomus jugulare tumors. Am J Otol. 1995;16(1):94–8.
129. Janicki PT, Adams JS, JT ME Jr. Plasma cell granuloma of the temporal bone. Am J Otol. 1996;17(1):123–6.
130. Mantyla R, Kinnunen J, Bohling T. Intracranial plasmacytoma: a case report. Neuroradiology. 1996;38(7):646–9.
131. Matsuda M, Nakazawa T, Kizuki H, Matsumura K, Nakasu S, Handa J. Solitary plasmacytoma of the skull vault—case report. Neurol Med Chir (Tokyo). 1996;36(6):388–92.
132. Dazert S, Baier G, Aletsee C, Hagen R. Extramedullary plasmacytoma—manifestation in petrous bone. Laryngorhinootologie. 1997;76(9):559–61.
133. Chiang SK, Canalis RF, Ishiyama A, Eversole LR, Becker DP. Plasmacytoma of the temporal bone. Am J Otolaryngol. 1998;19(4):267–73.
134. Yetiser S, Talas D, Akkaya A, Deveci S. Plasmacytoma of the temporal bone: management with a combination of surgery and radiotherapy. Acta Otolaryngol. 2001;121(8):915–8.
135. Ruenes R, Palacios E. Plasmacytoma of the petrous temporal bone. Ear Nose Throat J. 2003;82(9):672.
136. Jayagopal S, Berry MG, Ross G, Armour A, Howcroft AJ. A case of squamous cell carcinoma associated with plasmacytoma. Br J Plast Surg. 2004;57(2):172–3.
137. Wang X, Wu P, Ge R. Clinical characteristics of solitary plasmacytoma of temporal bone. Lin Chung Er Bi Yan Hou Tou Jing Wai Ke Za Zhi. 2012;26(10):477–80.

Sarcomas of the Temporal Bone

13

Jamie A. Ku, Paul W. Gidley, and Erich M. Sturgis

Introduction

Sarcomas are rare malignancies, comprising of less than 1% of all cancers in the United States [1]. They represent a heterogeneous group of tumors of mesenchymal origin with a wide array of clinical behavior. While more than 70 histologic types have been identified, sarcomas can be broadly categorized into two types: soft-tissue sarcoma and bone sarcoma. Sarcomas are further classified based on the tissue of origin, histologic subtype and grade, anatomic subsite, and clinicopathologic and genetic features [2]. For instance, sarcoma can arise from cells of adipose, muscle, vascular, stromal, nerve sheath, cartilage, or bony tissues. While classifying sarcomas based on the tissue of origin is helpful in developing a standardized nomenclature for both clinical and research applications, understanding the histologic grades and genetic modifications is essential in determining the overall prognosis as well as the effective treatment stratification for each patient. The *World Health Organization (WHO) Classification of Tumours of Soft Tissue and Bone* provides diagnostic criteria based on morphologic, immunohistochemical, and genetic/molecular data, and the latest fourth edition, published in February 2013, now includes categories based on biological behavior and aggressiveness (benign vs. locally aggressive, or rarely metastasizing intermediate types vs. malignant) [3].

In adults, the majority of soft-tissue sarcomas arise in an extremity, followed by the trunk and the retroperitoneum. Only about 10% of sarcomas originate in the head and neck region [4]. In contrast, in the pediatric population, up to 35% of all sarcomas manifest in the head and neck region [5]. Additionally, while only 1% of all primary head and neck malignancies in adults are sarcomas, approximately 14% of all pediatric head and neck malignancies are sarcomas, with rhabdomyosarcoma being the most common subtype [6]. A large Surveillance, Epidemiology, and End Results (SEER) database analysis of 11,481 adult patients and 1,244 pediatric patients with head and neck sarcomas found that the most common subsites were the skin and soft tissues (63%), followed by the bones of the skull and face (11%) [7]. In a review of approximately 2,000 adult patients with sarcoma of the head and neck evaluated at The University of Texas MD Anderson Cancer Center between 1970 and 2013, the most frequent anatomic subsites included the scalp and face (30%), followed by the sinonasal cavity/anterior skull base (23%). Upper aerodigestive tract and parotid/neck regions each accounted for 19%. Sarcomas arising from the ear or lateral/posterior skull base were quite rare, at only 8% (Fig. 13.1a). In the pediatric and adolescent cohort of 396 patients, the sinonasal cavity and anterior skull base accounted for 28% of cases, while the ear and the lateral or posterior skull base was the site of origin in 9% of this patient population [8] (Fig. 13.1b).

Malignant neoplasms involving the temporal bone are exceedingly rare, with an annual incidence estimated at between 1 and 6 per million [9, 10]. The majority of these are either direct extensions from advanced periauricular skin cancer or parotid salivary gland malignancies rather than primary ear canal and middle ear cancers [11, 12]. The most common primary sites for metastatic disease to the temporal bone are the breast, lung, and prostate [13]. In terms of histologic diagnoses, tumors of epithelial origin, including squamous cell carcinoma and basal cell carcinoma, occur

J. A. Ku, M.D. (✉)
Cleveland Clinic Head and Neck Institute, Cleveland, OH, USA

P. W. Gidley, M.D., F.A.C.S.
Department of Head and Neck Surgery, The University of Texas M.D. Anderson Cancer Center, Houston, TX, USA
e-mail: pwgidley@mdanderson.org

E. M. Sturgis, M.D., M.P.H.
Department of Head and Neck Surgery, The University of Texas M.D. Anderson Cancer Center, Houston, TX, USA

Department of Epidemiology, The University of Texas M.D. Anderson Cancer Center, Houston, TX, USA

Christopher and Susan Damico Chair in Viral Associated Malignancies, The University of Texas M.D. Anderson Cancer Center, Houston, TX, USA
e-mail: esturgis@mdanderson.org

P. W. Gidley, F. DeMonte (eds.), *Temporal Bone Cancer*, https://doi.org/10.1007/978-3-319-74539-8_13

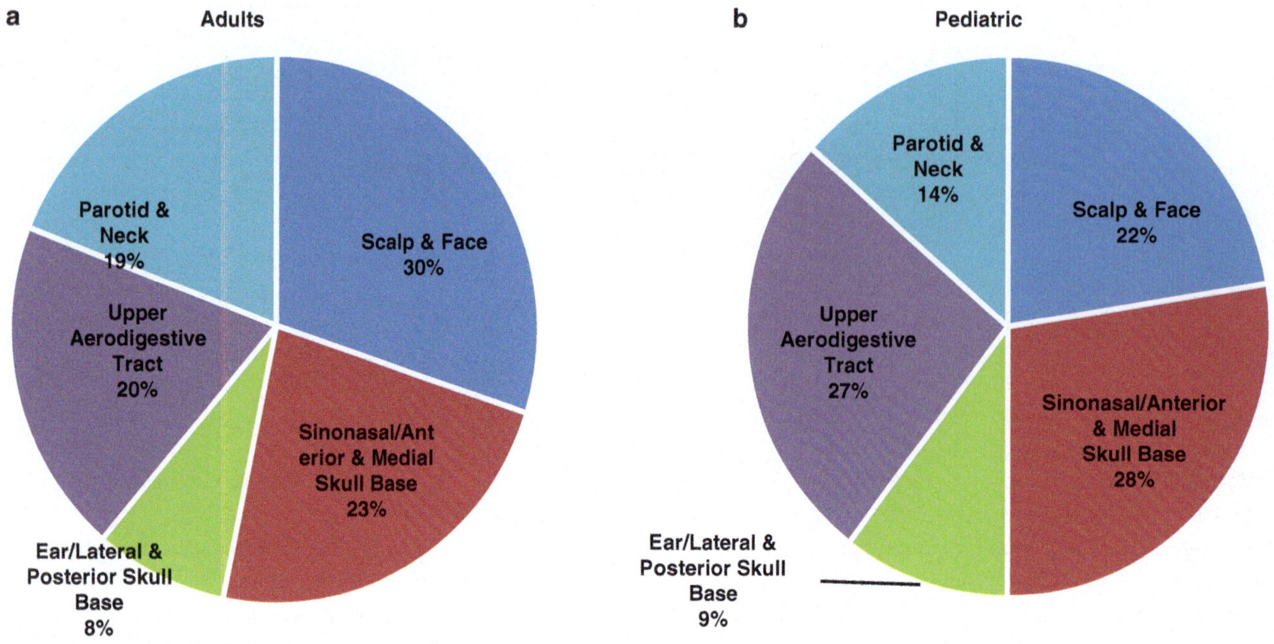

Fig. 13.1 Subsite distribution of sarcomas of the head and neck region presenting to the University of Texas MD Anderson Cancer Center 1970–2013 (**a**) adult cohort and (**b**) pediatric cohort

most frequently, followed by salivary origin [11]. Sarcomas occur much less frequently, comprising about 6–8% of all temporal bone tumors in two large series of patients with malignant temporal bone tumors treated at two high-volume comprehensive cancer centers [10, 14]. Because of their rarity, temporal bone sarcomas are only described in the literature as case reports or as part of a larger series of patients with temporal bone malignancies or sarcomas of the head and neck. The most frequently described types of sarcomas of the temporal bone are Ewing's sarcoma, rhabdomyosarcoma, and chondrosarcoma. There also have been case series and reports of more rare types, such as synovial sarcoma, osteosarcoma, angiosarcoma, leiomyosarcoma, and liposarcoma [15–25].

Radiation-associated sarcoma is a rare but devastating long-term complication of irradiation of the temporal bone [26] (Fig. 13.2). Patients receiving radiotherapy for tumors of the nasopharynx, oropharynx, the skull base, the parotid gland, and the periauricular region are at risk of developing radiation-associated malignancies (RAM). The latency between the completion of radiotherapy and the development of RAM can range from 3 to 30 years [27, 28]. The two most common types of RAM are sarcoma and squamous cell carcinomas [28–30]. The exact mechanism of radiation-associated sarcomas is not well characterized, although mutations in the *p53* gene have been implicated [31]. In a retrospective review of 13 patients presenting to the University of Texas MD Anderson Cancer Center from 1999 to 2012 with RAM of the temporal bone, the authors found that radiation-associated sarcomas were also more likely to present with disease extending beyond the external auditory canal, have positive surgical margins, and have disease recurrence compared to radiation-associated carcinomas [28]. Ultimately, patients with a diagnosis of sarcoma had a significantly worse disease-specific survival compared to patients with a diagnosis of carcinoma (33.3% vs. 90.0% 3-year disease-specific survival) [28]. A heightened concern, therefore, is imperative in any patients with a history of irradiation for head and neck cancer presenting with symptoms of otorrhea, otalgia, hearing loss, and facial nerve weakness or paralysis, and if a mass is present and confirmed by cross-sectional imaging, biopsy is mandated.

Management

Patient Evaluation

Table 13.1 illustrates the common presenting signs and symptoms of patients with temporal bone sarcoma. Many of the symptoms can mimic chronic otitis media or otitis externa. Thus, patients presenting with severe and refractory ear infection should undergo further evaluation and work-up. Facial palsy is an ominous presenting symptom and should raise the suspicion for an aggressive malignant process. Trismus and pain with eating may indicate involvement of the temporomandibular joint and or muscles of mastication. Vertigo may be a sign of inner ear or labyrinth invasion. Finally, with dural and intracranial invasion, patients may present with headaches, cerebral spinal fluid leak, or meningitis.

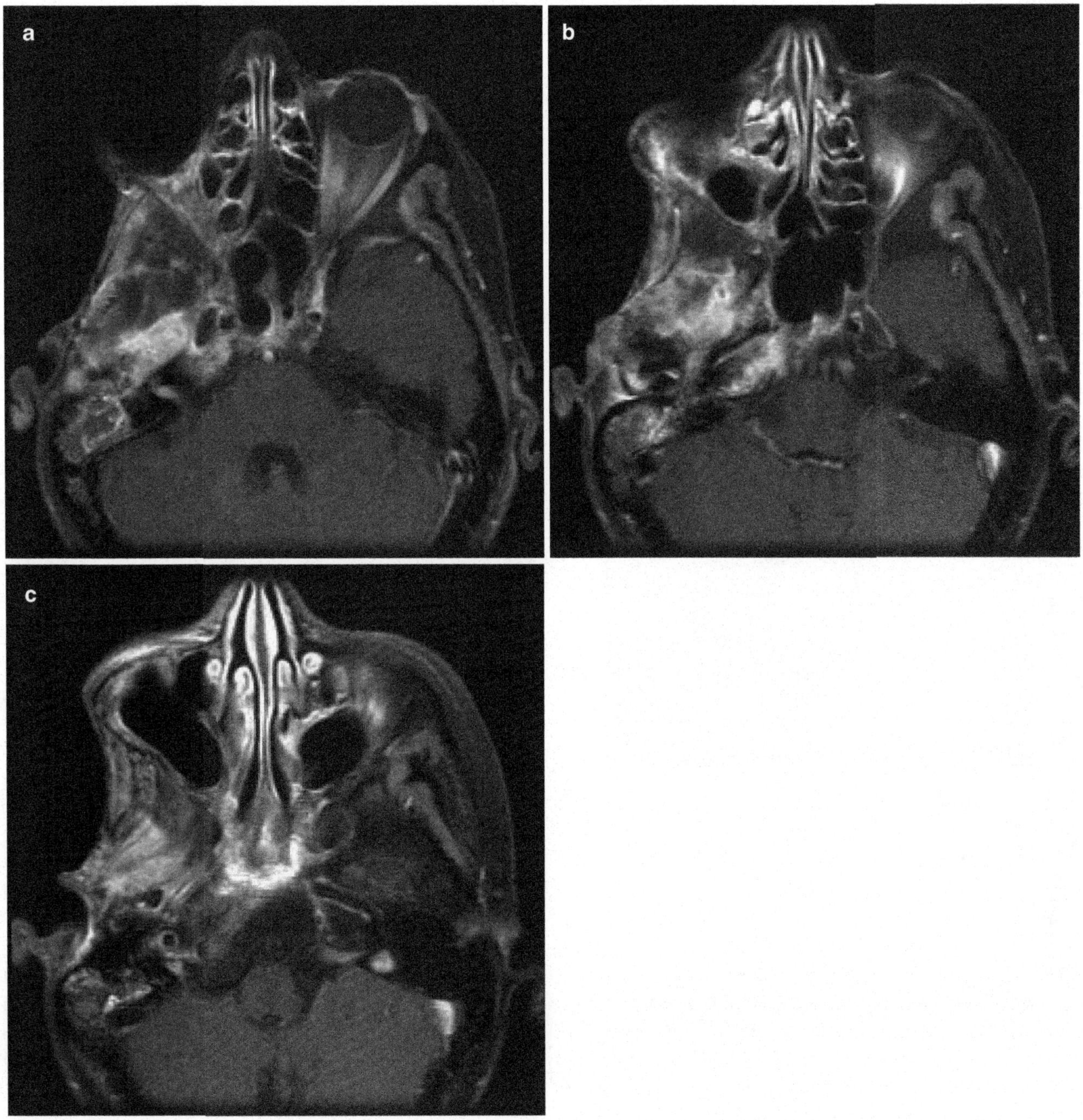

Fig. 13.2 High-grade spindle cell sarcoma of the right temporal bone 7 years after surgery and radiotherapy for an adenoid cystic carcinoma of the right lacrimal gland. Contrast-enhanced T1 images (**a**–**c**)

A detailed history and complete head and neck examination, including a full cranial nerve assessment, is performed. Assessment of neurologic function may reveal various cranial nerve palsies, depending on the extension of the tumor out of the temporal bone into other anatomic spaces. These deficits include diplopia with the involvement of the petrous apex; multiple ophthalmic abnormalities such as visual loss, diplopia, proptosis, and chemosis with extension into the orbital apex; ophthalmic abnormalities with the addition of trigeminal paresthesia with further involvement of the cavernous sinus; and isolated numbness in the distribution of the mandibular branch of the trigeminal nerve with the involvement of the infratemporal fossa. In addition, physical examination should include a close inspection of the external ear, external auditory canal, tympanic membrane, periauricular skin, parotid gland, and cervical lymph nodes. Binocular micro-otoscopy may reveal a soft-tissue mass that may be amenable to a biopsy if located in an easily accessible location (Fig. 13.3).

An audiogram is obtained to document any hearing loss, whether sensorineural, conductive, or mixed. Once a

Table 13.1 List of common presenting symptoms and physical findings in patients with temporal bone sarcoma

Otalgia	Aural polyp
Otorrhea	Lymphadenopathy
Hearing loss	Parotid or retroauricular mass
Tinnitus/vertigo	Facial paralysis
Facial nerve weakness	Cranial nerve 3, 4, 6 palsies
Diplopia/visual disturbances	Trigeminal paresthesia
Periauricular mass	
Trismus	
Headaches	

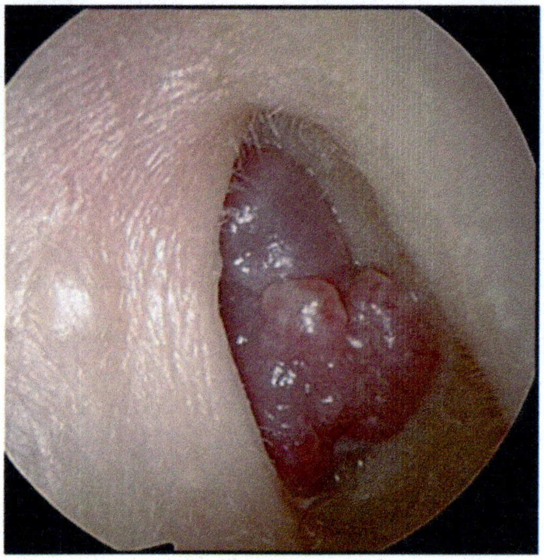

Fig. 13.3 Leiomyosarcoma filling the right external auditory canal (from the Department of Head and Neck Surgery, MD Anderson Cancer Center; with permission)

temporal bone process is suspected, the next step in diagnosis is radiologic imaging, with high-resolution fine-cut computed tomography (CT) and magnetic resonance imaging (MRI) being complementary in portraying bony vs. soft-tissue tumor characteristics as well as tumor extension. While CT provides superior detail of bony structures and can identify early cortical erosions, MRI provides better soft-tissue resolution, especially if suspecting dural, orbital, bone marrow, or perineural involvement. The lung is the most likely site for distant metastatic disease from most head and neck sarcomas, and additional investigation, such as CT chest or fluorodeoxyglucose-positron emission tomography imaging, may be warranted to rule out distant metastasis.

Staging

The Seventh Edition American Joint Committee on Cancer (AJCC) staging system for soft-tissue sarcoma is the most widely used staging system that relies upon tumor size and depth of invasion, histologic grading, and the presence of regional or distant metastatic disease (Table 13.2) [32]. Because the Seventh Edition AJCC staging system is not site-specific and does not take into account the critical anatomic considerations specific to the head and neck, the validity and applicability of this staging system to head and neck sarcomas have been questioned in the past. An analysis of 319 patients with head and neck sarcoma at Memorial Sloan-Kettering Cancer Center was performed to determine the validity of the AJCC staging system in the head and neck and concluded that oncologic outcomes of head and neck sarcoma patients can be accurately predicted using the Seventh Edition AJCC staging system [33], though improvements are needed. Currently, there is no staging system that has been approved for temporal bone sarcoma by the AJCC. However, the Eighth Edition AJCC system, which is scheduled to be published in 2017, will have separate T-categories for head and neck sarcomas as well as updates to the grading system, but new stage groupings for head and neck sarcomas are yet to be determined (Table 13.2) [34].

Treatment

Because of the rarity of temporal bone sarcomas, it is often necessary to infer best practice from the recommended treatment in the management of the specific type of sarcoma from other parts of the body. Surgery has traditionally been the cornerstone of treatment for head and neck sarcomas. With data collected from several cooperative groups indicating improved patient outcomes, multimodality treatment has now become the standard of care. These updated treatment protocols now include radiation and multidrug chemotherapy, either as neoadjuvant, adjuvant, or as primary therapy. Therefore, treatment of sarcoma, in general, requires input from multidisciplinary team members, including medical oncology, radiation oncology, head and neck surgery, neurootology, neurosurgery, pathology, and reconstructive surgery teams.

Examples of Temporal Bone Sarcomas

Based on the case reports and case series in the literature, the most frequently described types of sarcomas of the temporal bone are rhabdomyosarcoma, Ewing's sarcoma, osteosarcoma, chondrosarcoma, and leiomyosarcoma.

Rhabdomyosarcoma

Rhabdomyosarcomas (RMS) are highly malignant tumors arising from undifferentiated skeletal muscle. This is the

Table 13.2 AJCC staging system for soft-tissue sarcomas

Seventh edition		Eighth edition (specific to head and neck)	
T-categories		*T-categories*	
Tx	Primary tumor cannot be assessed	Tx	Primary tumor cannot be assessed
T1	<5 cm in greatest dimension (a, superficial; b, deep)	T1	≤2 cm in greatest dimension
T2	≥5 cm in greatest dimension (a, superficial; b, deep)	T2	>2 and ≤4 cm in greatest dimension
		T3	>4 cm in greatest dimension
		T4	Invasion of adjoining structures (a, orbit, skull base, dura, central compartment viscera, facial skeleton, or pterygoid muscles; b, brain, carotid artery encasement, prevertebral muscles, or central nervous system via perineural spread)
N-categories		*N-categories*	
N0	No regional lymph node metastases	N0	No regional lymph node metastases
N1	Regional lymph node metastases	N1	Regional lymph node metastases
M-categories		*M-categories*	
M0	No distant metastases	M0	No distant metastases
M1	Distant metastases	M1	Distant metastases
Grade-categories		*Grade-categories*	
Gx	Grade cannot be assessed	Gx	Grade cannot be assessed
G1	Total differentiation, mitotic count, and necrosis score of 2 or 3	G1	Total differentiation, mitotic count, and necrosis score of 2 or 3
G2	Total differentiation, mitotic count, and necrosis score of 4 or 5	G2	Total differentiation, mitotic count, and necrosis score of 4 or 5
G3	Total differentiation, mitotic count, and necrosis score of 6 or higher	G3	Total differentiation, mitotic count, and necrosis score of 6 or higher
Stage groupings		*Stage groupings*	
IA	T1a-b, Gx or G1, N0, M0	As yet to be defined	
IB	T2a-b, Gx or G1, N0, M0	As yet to be defined	
IIA	T1a-b, G2-3, N0, M0	As yet to be defined	
IIB	T2a-b, G2, N0, M0	As yet to be defined	
III	T2a-b, G3, N0, M0	As yet to be defined	
	Any T, any G, N1, M0	As yet to be defined	
IV	Any T, any G, any N, M1	As yet to be defined	

most common soft-tissue sarcoma in the pediatric population, accounting for over 60% of all soft-tissue sarcoma in this population. RMS of childhood have been associated with multiple syndromes, including Beckwith-Wiedemann syndrome, Costello syndrome, Li-Fraumeni syndrome, Noonan syndrome, and neurofibromatosis [35]. RMS of the head and neck region in children are divided into three subsites: orbital, parameningeal (which includes the temporal bone), and nonorbital nonparameningeal. The current WHO classification includes four histologic subgroups: embryonal, alveolar, spindle cell/sclerosing, and pleomorphic, with the first two being the most frequent subgroups. Of these various subclassifications, the orbital and embryonal subtypes have the best prognosis. Parameningeal cases have worse outcome, likely reflecting the challenges of achieving negative surgical margins [36, 37]. While the temporal bone is considered a parameningeal site, the majority of temporal bone RMS is the embryonal histology [38].

While approximately 30% of all pediatric RMS occur in the head and neck, the temporal bone is an uncommon site of origin (Fig.13.4), occurring in only 4–10% of cases [36, 38, 39]. In a large Surveillance, Epidemiology, and End Results (SEER) study analyzing 558 patients with head and neck RMS from 1973 to 2007, parameningeal RMS accounted for 44%, of which 4% arose from the middle ear [36]. The staging system for RMS, established by the Soft-Tissue Sarcoma Committee of the Children's Oncology Group (COG-STS), utilizes (1) tumor stage at the time of the diagnosis based on clinical and radiologic features, (2) completeness of surgical resection and the degree of residual disease based on surgical histopathology, and (3) tumor histology, stage, and group to classify into low-, intermediate-, and high-risk categories [40, 41]. The 5-year survival rate of RMS of the temporal bone and the middle ear has improved significantly from 0 to 41% due to the efforts of multiple cooperative groups, such as the Intergroup Rhabdomyosarcoma Study (IRS) Group and the COG-STS Group, and the advancement in new radiation and chemotherapeutic regimens [42, 43]. The most recent studies have demonstrated an overall 5-year disease-free survival ranging from 66% to 80% in pediatric patients with RMS of the ear and temporal bone [38, 39].

Ewing's Sarcoma

Ewing's sarcoma is a small round blue cell tumor affecting bone and soft tissue. The molecular genetic translocation t(11:22)(q24; q12) is pathognomonic for the diagnosis of Ewing's sarcoma [44, 45]. This translocation in the EWSR1 and ETS genes results in a fusion protein that act as a transcription factor for ETS target genes. Ewing's sarcoma occurs more frequently in the pediatric population, and it is the second most common bony malignancy in children, after

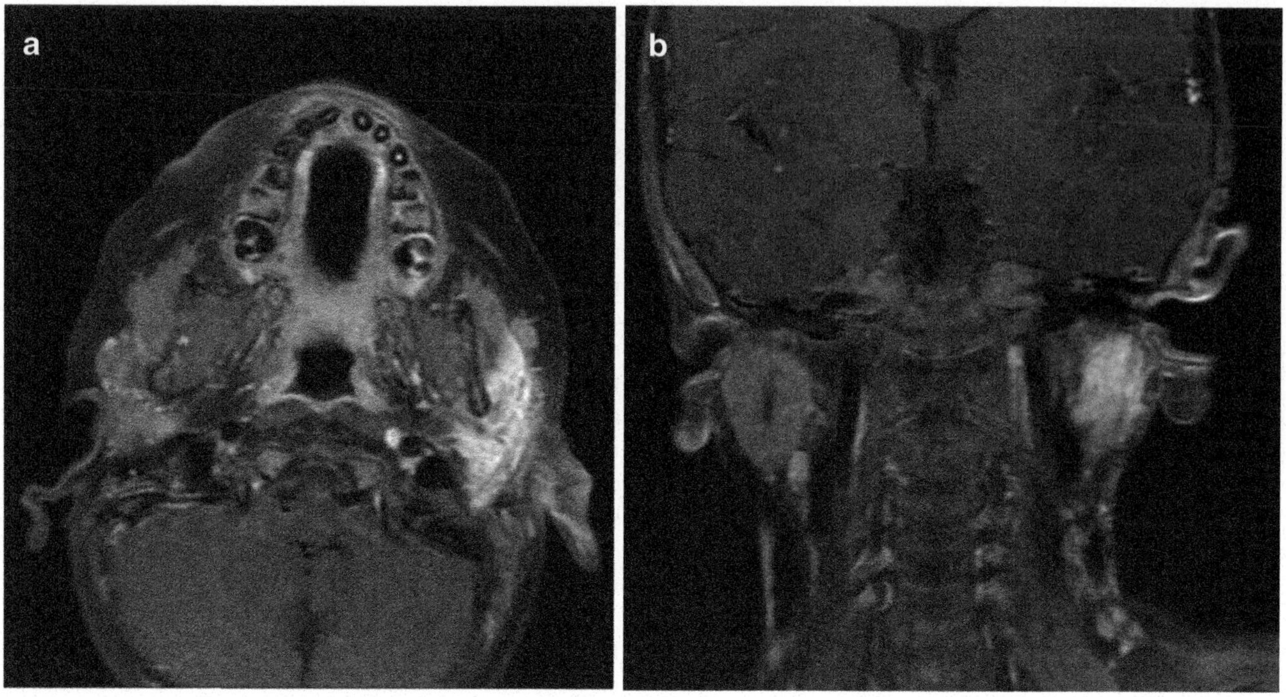

Fig.13.4 Rhabdomyosarcoma involving the left temporal bone in a 3-year-old girl. Contrast-enhanced MRI, axial (**a**) and coronal (**b**)

osteosarcoma [46]. It typically involves the long bones, pelvis, and ribs [46]. Although it can originate at extraosseous soft-tissue sites, Ewing's sarcoma is less common in the head and neck region, accounting for only 4–9% of all cases [47, 48]. Ewing's sarcoma of the head and neck usually involves the mandible, skull (including the temporal bone), and the maxilla.

There have only been a few case reports of Ewing's sarcoma presenting in the ear canal or the temporal bone [49–56] (Fig.13.5). In one study describing a 40-year single-institutional experience of Ewing's sarcoma of the head and neck, only 1 out of 9 patients with head and neck Ewing's sarcoma presented in the temporal bone [57]. Patients usually present with a rapidly enlarging and painful mass in the head and neck. Due to the expansile nature of the mass that can lead to increased intracranial pressure, patients can present with headache, nausea, vomiting, papilledema, as well as lower cranial nerve palsy. In CT imaging, radiologic findings of bone expansion and remodeling associated with a soft-tissue mass may mimic an intracranial neoplasm, fibrous dysplasia, or neurofibromatosis [58] (Fig.13.5). Similar to RMS, Ewing's sarcoma responds best to multimodality therapy. A subgroup analysis within the Intergroup Rhabdomyosarcoma Study Group has found that optimal treatment of Ewing's sarcoma is surgical excision, followed by a chemotherapy regimen of vincristine, actinomycin D, and cyclophosphamide (VAC) with adjuvant radiotherapy reserved for residual gross or microscopic disease, though most oncologists typically might start with neoadjuvant chemotherapy [59, 60]. For patients with large tumors or tumors in locations that are not amenable to surgical excision, concomitant chemoradiation is most frequently utilized [47, 60]. The 3-year and 5-year overall survival are 80–87% and 53%, respectively [47, 48, 60].

Osteosarcoma

Osteosarcoma is a malignant tumor of mesenchymal origin with cells producing immature osteoid. It is the most common primary sarcoma of the bone in children and young adults. Osteosarcoma has a bimodal age distribution with an adolescent presentation in the second decade of life and a second peak in the eighth decade of life [61]. The incidence in osteosarcoma in the 0–24-year-old group is approximately four per million [62]. The most frequently affected anatomic location is the metaphyseal portion of the long bones, such as the femur [61]. The true etiology of osteosarcoma remains unknown but appears to be multifactorial. This includes both genetic and environmental factors, with ionizing radiation being the most common associated environmental factor. There is also an association with hereditary retinoblastoma and Li-Fraumeni syndromes, likely due to genetic mutations resulting in inactivation of the retinoblastoma or p53 pathways [63, 64]. In the elderly population, genetic changes associated with Paget's disease have been linked to the increased risk of developing secondary osteosarcomas [65].

Osteosarcoma of the head and neck represents about 5–15% of all sarcomas in this region [7, 8]. Osteosarcoma of the head and neck exhibits a clinical behavior and natural history that are distinct from those of osteosarcoma of other anatomic sites. Unlike osteosarcoma of the long bone, head and neck osteosarcomas usually affect patients in their third or fourth decades of life [66–68]. Additionally, while osteosarcomas of non-head and neck sites have a high distant metastatic rate of 80% [61], osteosarcoma of the head and neck have a much lower rate of distant metastases, at around 7–21%, most commonly to the lung and bone [69–71]. Finally, it is more challenging to obtain a negative margin in head and neck osteosarcomas, making it difficult to obtain local control of the disease. A typical presentation of head

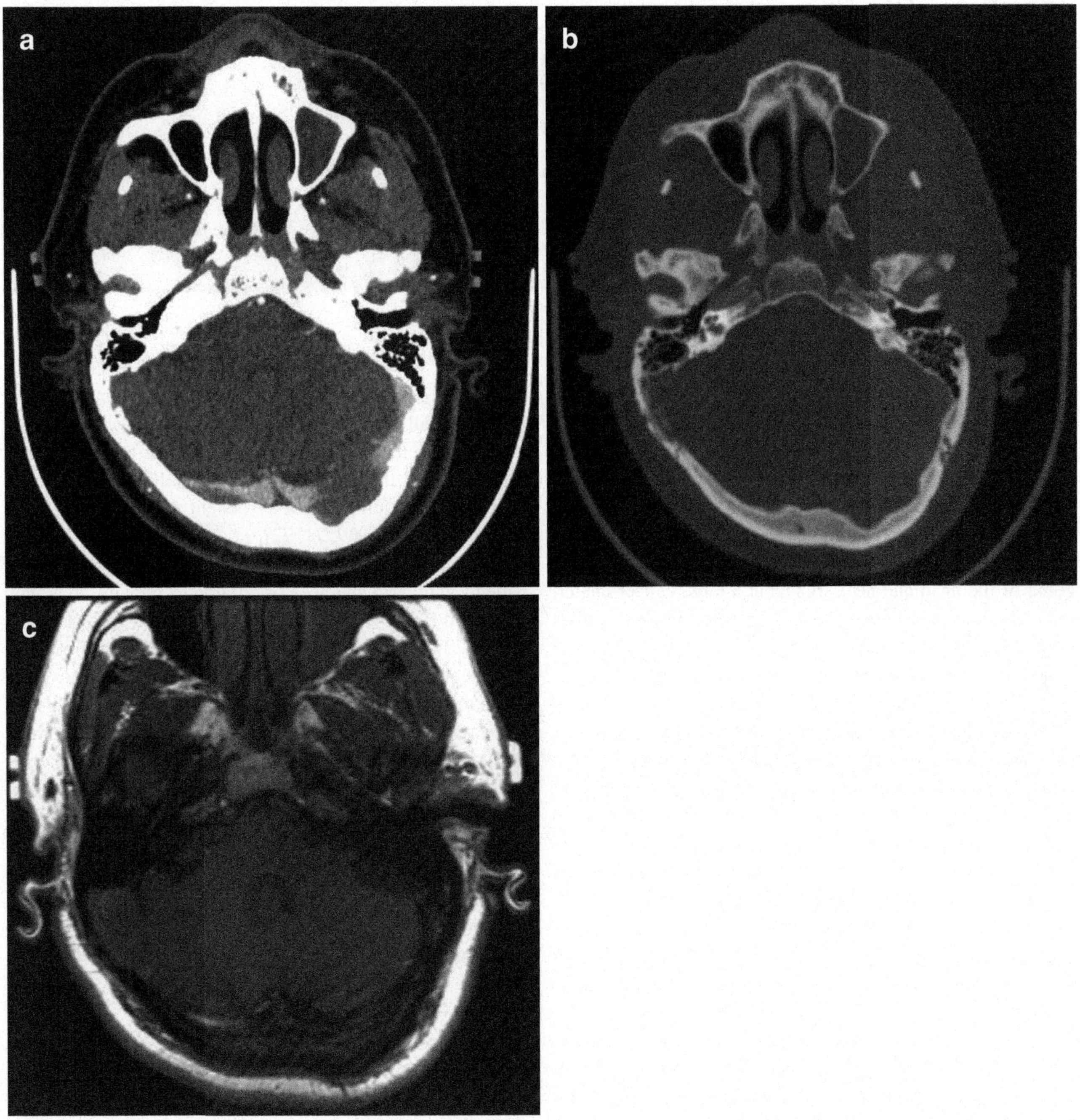

Fig. 13.5 A 43-year-old man with Ewing's sarcoma metastasis to the right temporal bone and occipital bone. The tumor has obstructed the transverse and sigmoid sinuses. CT soft tissue (**a**) and bone (**b**) windows. MRI noncontrast (**c**) T1 and (**d**) T2, and (**e**) contrast-enhanced T1

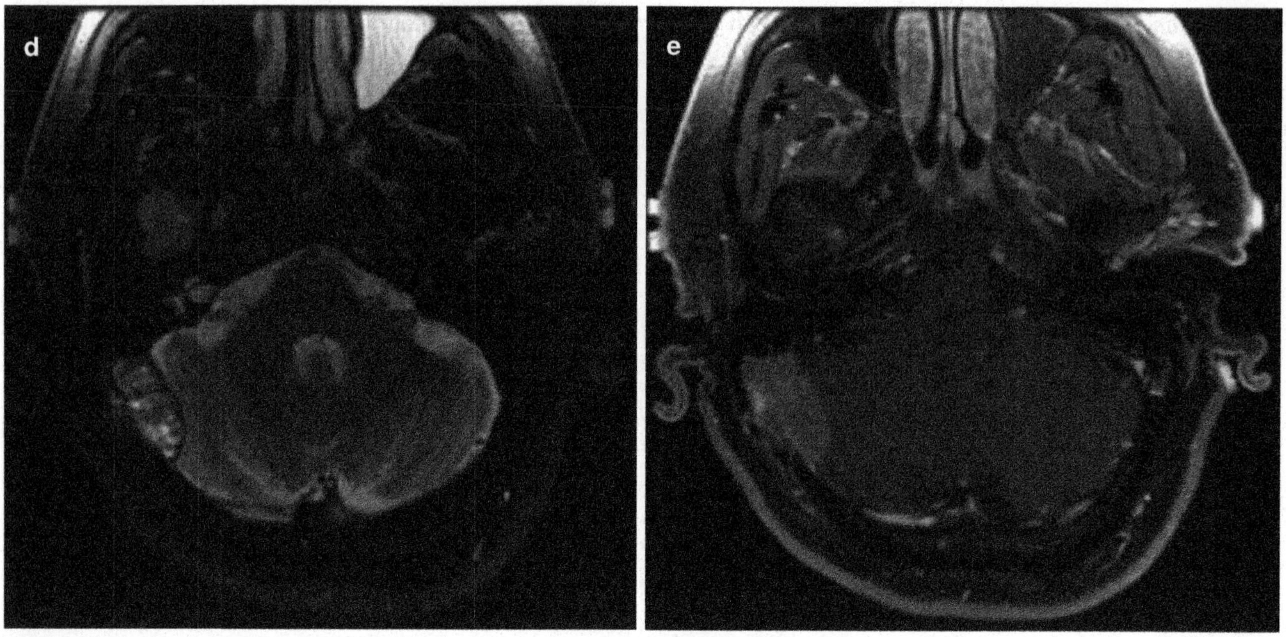

Fig. 13.5 (continued)

and neck osteosarcoma includes swelling and pain in the affected bone [72]. This usually involves dental pain and loose teeth, since the majority of tumors involve the mandibular and maxillary bones [66, 68, 71, 72]. Osteosarcomas of the temporal bone are extremely rare, with only a handful of case reports in the literature [19, 20, 73–77]. In one of the largest, retrospective series of 127 patients with osteosarcoma of the head and neck treated at a large cancer center, only 2% were of the temporal bone (Figs.13.6 and 13.7) [71]. Many of the reported cases of temporal bone osteosarcoma were in association with previous radiation treatment to the head and neck, typically for nasopharyngeal cancer.

The primary management of osteosarcoma is total surgical eradication of the tumor with negative margins. Since the regional metastatic rate is rare, elective surgical treatment of the cervical lymph nodes is unnecessary [66]. There is no consensus on treatment regimens incorporating chemotherapy and radiotherapy, but many studies have investigated the role of these agents in both neoadjuvant and adjuvant settings. Adjuvant radiation has been utilized in the setting of high-grade tumors, large primary lesions, close or positive margins, or inoperability. Multiple retrospective studies have demonstrated improvement in local control and overall survival in patients with head and neck osteosarcoma with positive resection margins when treated with adjuvant radiation [69, 71]. The exact role of systemic chemotherapy in the management of head and neck osteosarcoma remains to be established. A systematic review of 201 patients with craniofacial osteosarcoma published in 1997 found improvement in the overall and disease-free survival rates when chemotherapy was employed in either neoadjuvant or adjuvant settings [78]. On the contrary, there are multiple retrospective series demonstrating a lack of benefit with the addition of chemotherapy [66–69, 71, 72].

Regardless of the treatment regimen, the overall survival of patients with head and neck osteosarcoma remains poor, with an overall 5-year survival rate ranging from 55 to 70% [7, 66, 69, 71, 72]. This is in contrast to an overall survival of 70–90% in patients with osteosarcoma of other anatomic sites [61]. Local recurrence is the most common reason for poor survival in patients with osteosarcoma of the head and neck [68]. Surgical margin status remains the only significant prognostic factor in osteosarcoma [66, 68, 69, 71, 72, 79]. Origin of the osteosarcoma in the head and neck region directly affects prognosis, presumably due to the inverse relationship between the critical neurovascular anatomy and a chance for complete resection [72]. Thus, osteosarcomas originating from the mandible and maxilla have improved survival compared to those in extragnathic locations [66–69].

Chondrosarcoma

Chondrosarcoma is a cartilage-forming malignant tumor originating from cartilaginous cells that produce chondroid matrix [80]. It is the second most common primary malignancy

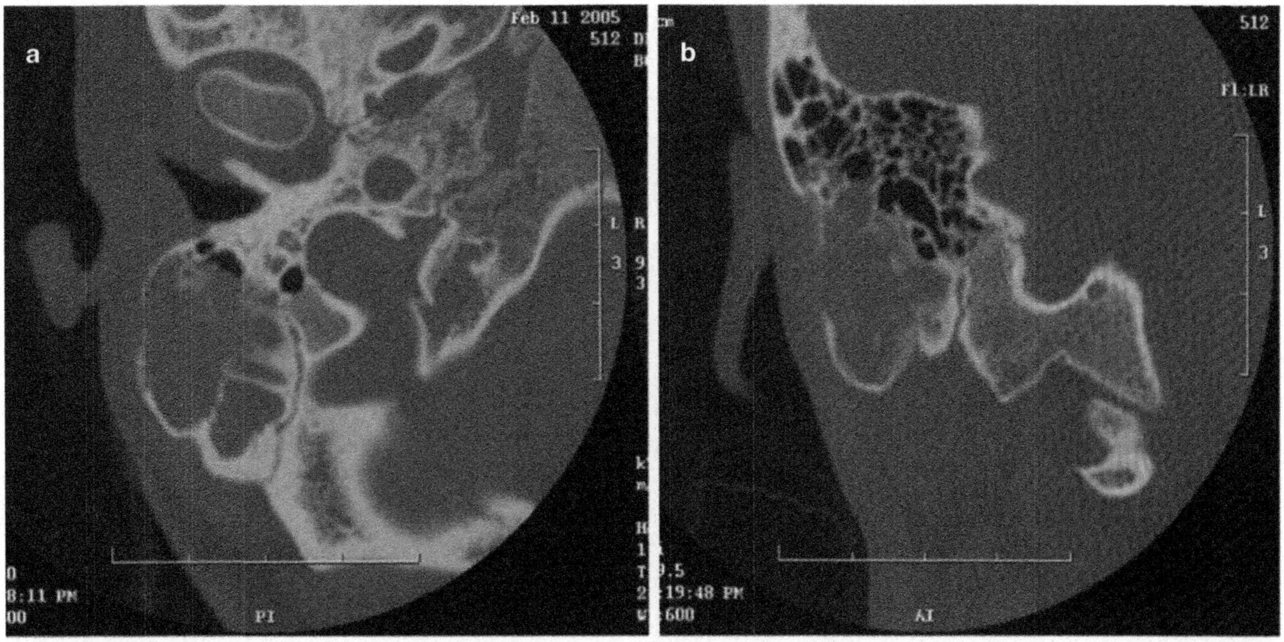

Fig.13.6 Noncontrast CT (**a**) axial and (**b**) coronal of osteosarcoma of the right mastoid in a 26-year-old woman

of the bone, with osteosarcoma being the most common [81]. Rarely, chondrosarcomas can develop in the soft tissue, presumably from cartilaginous differentiation of primitive mesenchymal cells. Primary chondrosarcoma arises from cartilage, bone, or soft tissue, while secondary chondrosarcoma arises from a malignant transformation of a benign cartilaginous tumor, such as osteochondroma. Maffucci syndrome and Ollier disease are syndromes associated with chondrosarcomas arising from malignant degeneration of benign enchondromas [82]. There are five variants of chondrosarcoma—conventional, clear cell, mesenchymal, periosteal, and dedifferentiated [80].

About 5–10% of chondrosarcoma present in the head and neck region [83] and about 5–10% of head and neck sarcomas are chondrosarcoma [84, 85]. The majority of the head and neck chondrosarcomas are located in the bones or joints of the skull and the skull base, including the sinonasal tract and the mandible [86, 87]. The remaining occurs in laryngotracheal subsites as well as other head and neck soft-tissue sites [86, 87]. Within the skull, there is a predilection for the clivus and petrous portion of the temporal bone [88, 89] (Fig.13.8). Temporal bone chondrosarcomas usually arise in the region of the foramen lacerum, where sphenopetrosal, petro-occipital, and sphenooccipital synchondroses converge [90]. Because a variety of inflammatory and neoplastic processes occur at the petrous apex, anatomic imaging with high-resolution CT and MRI is critical in the differential diagnosis of these lesions [91, 92].

In general, chondrosarcomas are locally invasive tumors that rarely metastasize. They are felt to be resistant to chemotherapy or radiation. Thus, surgical excision with negative margins remains the only curative treatment paradigm. Local recurrence still remains a concern, even in low-grade lesions [85, 87]. Therefore, for tumors with positive margins and high-grade lesions, adjuvant radiation therapy may be warranted. Incidences of regional nodal metastases and distant metastases are each <10% [87]. In a large, population-based analysis of 682 patients with chondrosarcoma of the head and neck using the SEER database, chondrosarcomas of the head and neck had significantly higher 10-year disease-specific survival and overall survival than non-head and neck chondrosarcomas [86]. Overall 5-year survival rate is reported to be 54–78% [84, 87]. This may be attributed to the finding that the vast majority of chondrosarcomas of the head and neck are well or moderately differentiated [86, 87]. They also tend to present at an earlier stage when compared to non-head and neck chondrosarcomas [86, 87].

Leiomyosarcoma

Leiomyosarcoma is thought to be derived from smooth muscle in the cutaneous or subcutaneous layer [93] or from pluripotent, undifferentiated mesenchymal cells. Being that it is

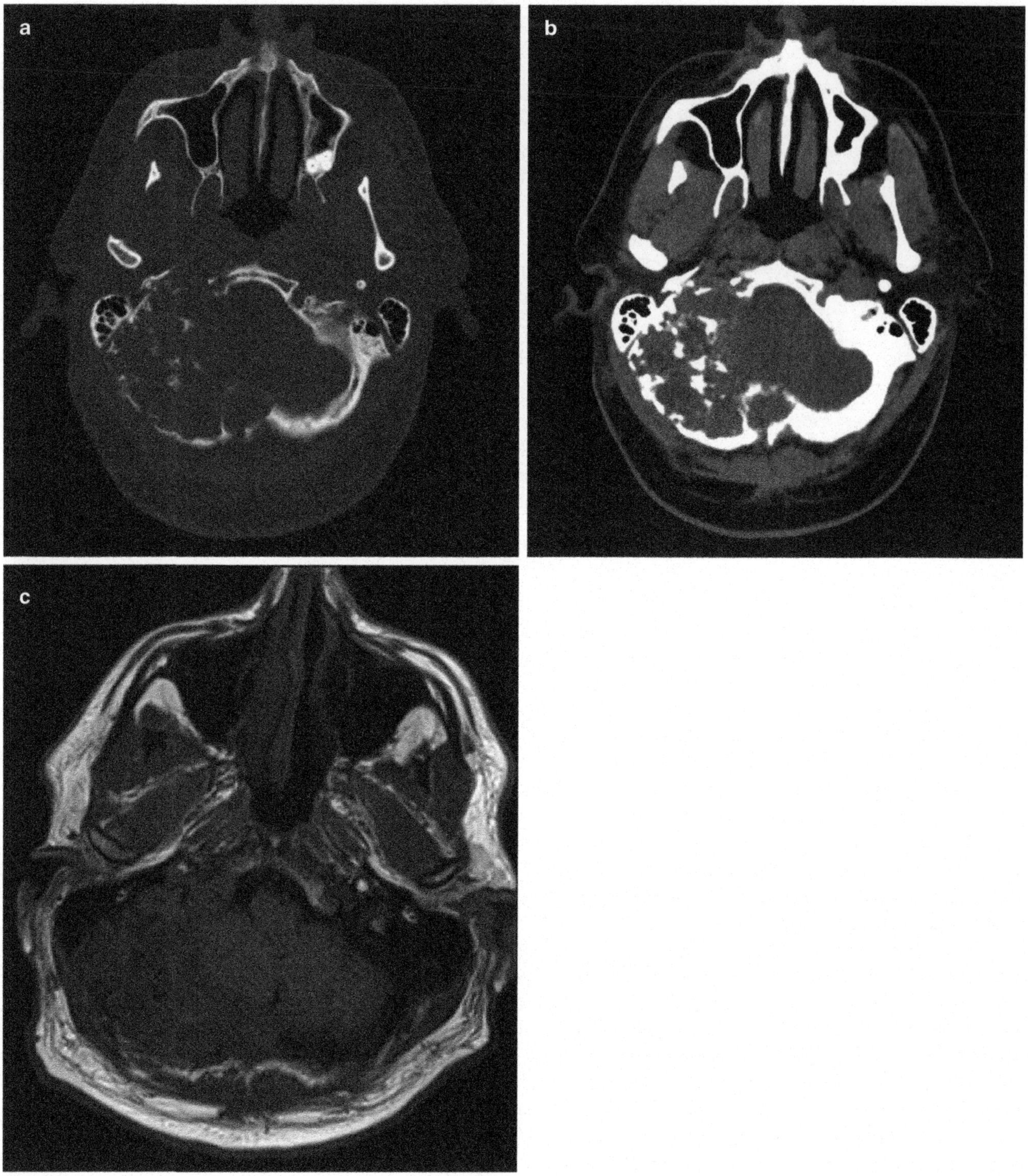

Fig. 13.7 Osteosarcoma in a 53-year-old man. Axial CT (**a**) bone window and (**b**) soft-tissue window. Axial noncontrast MRI (**c**) T1 and (**d**) T2, and (**e**) contrast-enhanced T1

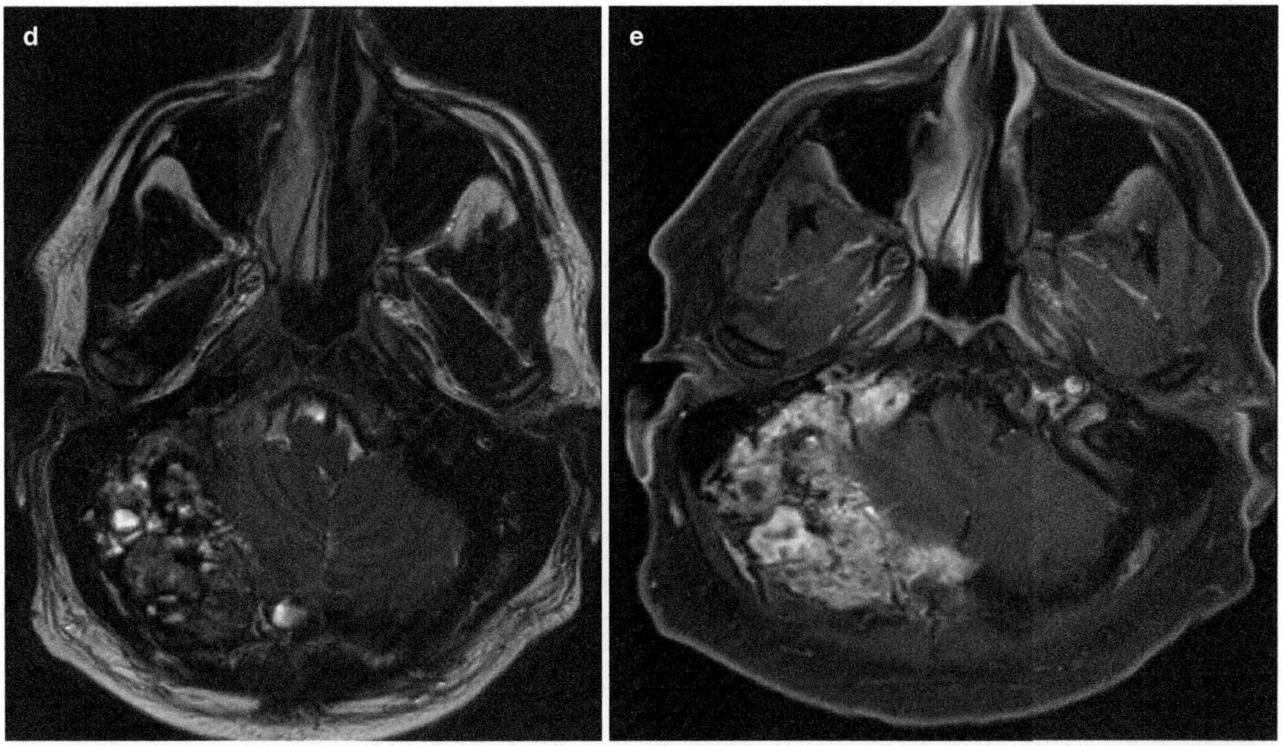

Fig. 13.7 (continued)

one of the less common soft-tissue sarcomas to originate in the head and neck region, a possible primary tumor in a pelvic or abdominal site resulting in a metastatic lesion in the head and neck should be considered and ruled out [94–101]. Within the head and neck region, the skin and the deep soft tissue of the face and neck represent the most frequent location of leiomyosarcoma [96, 102]. It generally affects patients in their fifth decade of life or later [96, 103, 104]. Leiomyosarcoma of the temporal bone and the external auditory canal is exceedingly rare, with only six case reports in the literature [24, 25, 105–108] (Fig.13.9).

The primary treatment modality for leiomyosarcoma is complete surgical resection. Without adequate resection with negative margins, the rate of local recurrence is high. Although the rate of regional metastases is extremely low [96, 103, 109], distant metastasis is more common, affecting 20–45% of patients [103, 110]. Although the effectiveness of adjuvant therapy in leiomyosarcoma has not been elucidated, adjuvant chemotherapy and radiation therapy may be indicated in high-grade tumors, those with close or positive margins, and those with metastatic disease. Accurate estimates of overall survival are difficult to assess due to the rarity of these sarcomas in the head and neck, but the larger series report an OS rate between 60% and 100% [95, 96, 104]. However, a worse prognosis has been demonstrated for high-grade leiomyosarcoma, with OS as low as 53–60% [95, 104]. Additionally, patients with cutaneous leiomyosarcoma have improved outcome when compared to those with noncutaneous leiomyosarcoma [104].

Summary

Temporal bone sarcoma is a rare entity originating from various types of mesenchymal cells. The most frequently described types of sarcomas of the temporal bone are Ewing's sarcoma, rhabdomyosarcoma, and chondrosarcoma. Presenting symptoms can mimic chronic otitis media or otitis externa, and thus, index of suspicion should be high in patients presenting with severe and refractory ear infection, especially in the setting of a history of prior irradiation to the head and neck region. Surgical resection with negative margins remains the cornerstone of treatment for temporal bone sarcomas, with a clear role of radiation and chemotherapy for high-grade tumors and those with close or positive margins, either as neoadjuvant or adjuvant therapy depending on the specific type of sarcoma. Treatment goals should include achieving local disease control while minimizing distant metastasis. Evaluation and management of patients with temporal bone sarcoma require a multidisciplinary team of experienced clinicians and surgeons to achieve the best outcome.

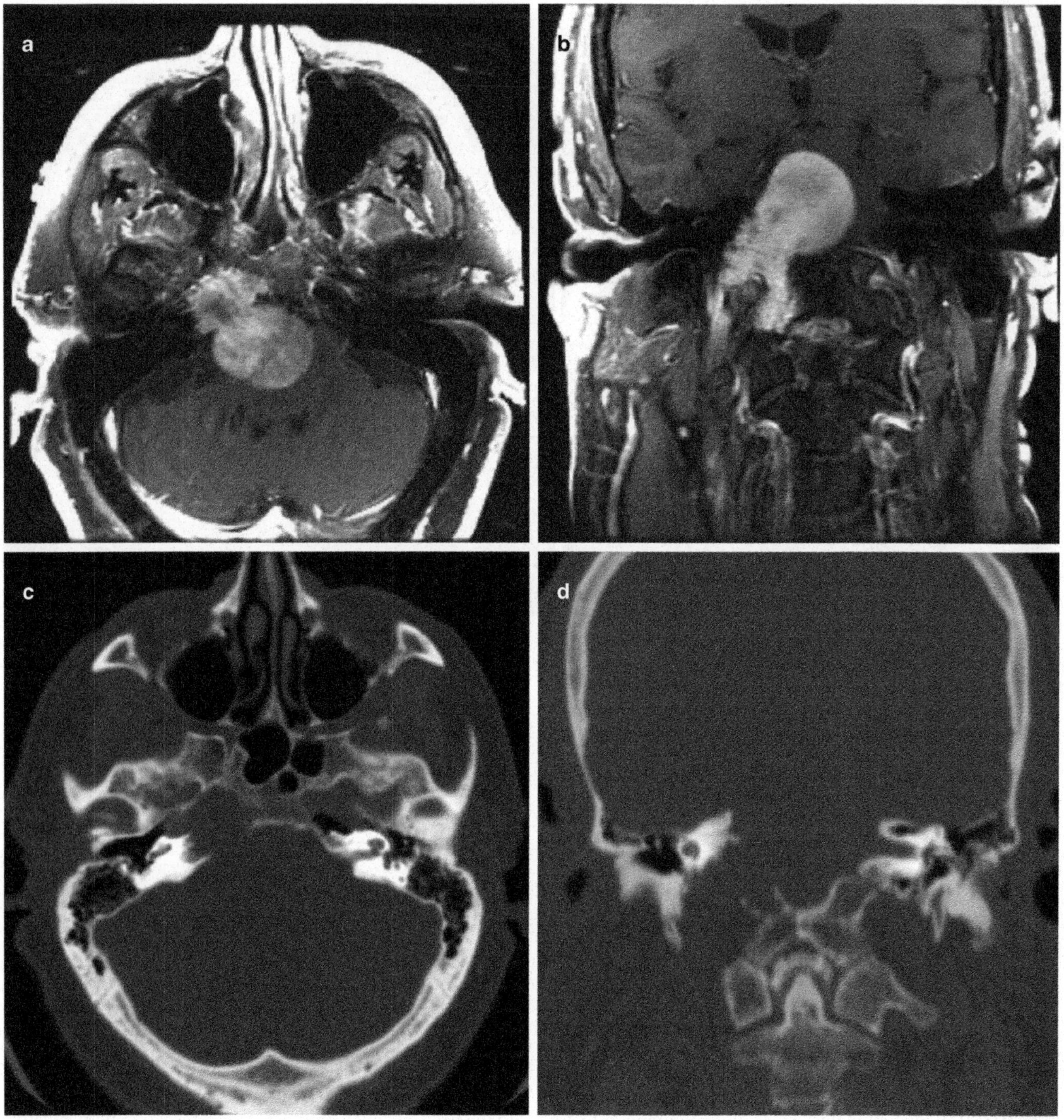

Fig. 13.8 MRI and CT of chondrosarcoma involving the right petrous apex in a 62-year-old man who presented with dizziness, diplopia, and dysphagia. Contrast-enhanced T1 MRI (**a**) axial and (**b**) coronal. Noncontrast CT (**c**) axial and (**d**) coronal

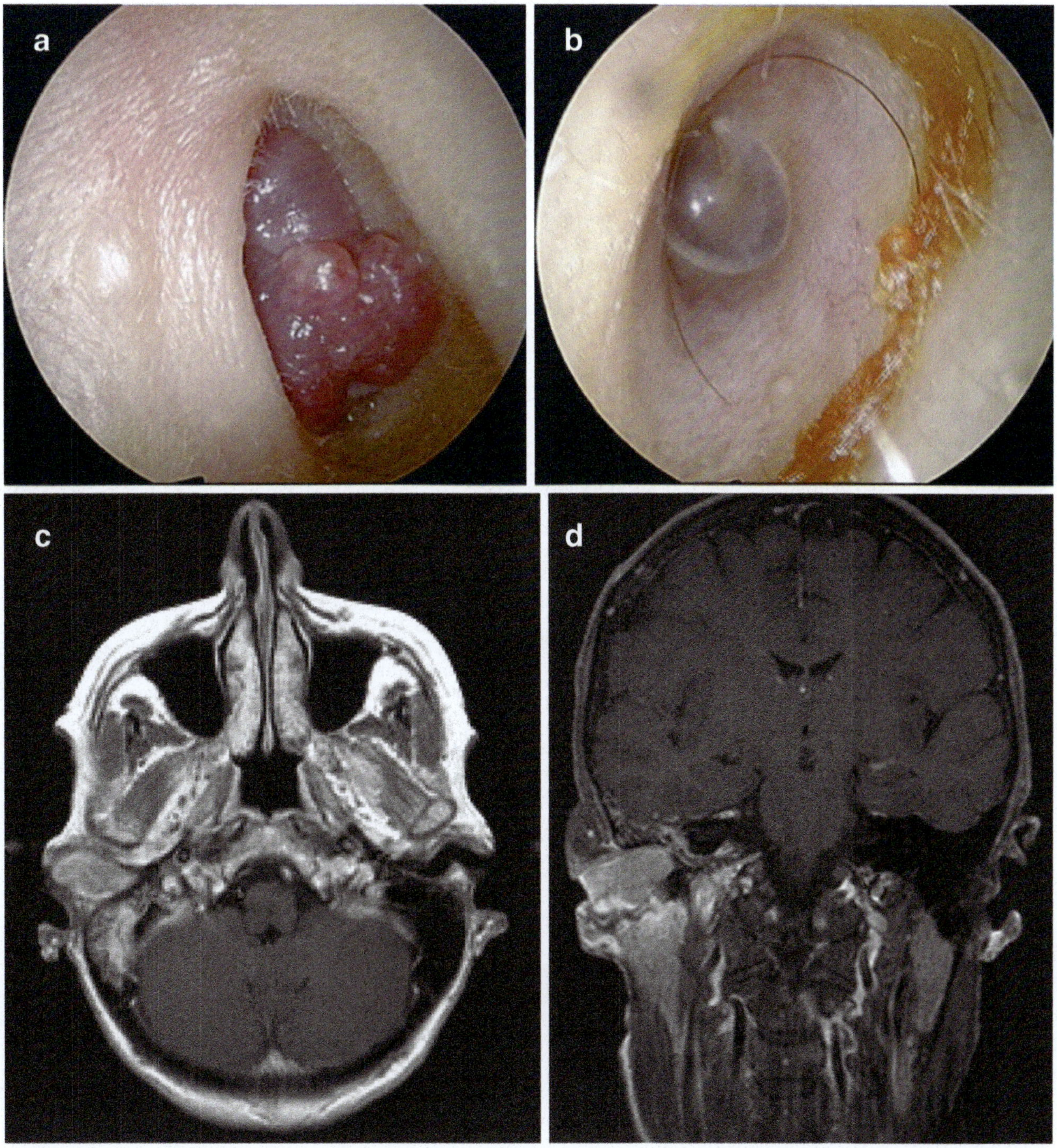

Fig. 13.9 Leiomyosarcoma of the right temporal bone. Otoendoscopic view of (**a**) right and (**b**) left ear canal. Contrast-enhanced MRI (**c**) axial and (**d**) coronal

References

1. Siegel RL, Miller KD, Jemal A. Cancer statistics, 2016. CA Cancer J Clin. 2016;66(1):7–30.
2. Potter BO, Sturgis EM. Sarcomas of the head and neck. Surg Oncol Clin N Am. 2003;12(2):379–417.
3. Jo VY, Doyle LA. Refinements in sarcoma classification in the current 2013 World Health Organization classification of tumours of soft tissue and bone. Surg Oncol Clin N Am. 2016;25(4):621–43.
4. Hui JY. Epidemiology and Etiology of sarcomas. Surg Clin North Am. 2016;96(5):901–14.
5. Shellenberger TD, Sturgis EM. Sarcomas of the head and neck region. Curr Oncol Rep. 2009;11(2):135–42.
6. Huh WW, Fitzgerald N, Mahajan A, Sturgis EM, Beverly Raney R, Anderson PM. Pediatric sarcomas and related tumors of the head and neck. Cancer Treat Rev. 2011;37(6):431–9.
7. Peng KA, Grogan T, Wang MB. Head and neck sarcomas: analysis of the SEER database. Otolaryngol Head Neck Surg. 2014;151(4):627–33.
8. Monroe MM, Guadagnolo BA, Ravi V, Wang W, Sturgis EM. Sarcomas and soft tissue tumors of the head and neck. In: Myers JN, Hanna EYN, Myers EN, editors. Cancer of the head and neck. 5th ed. Philadelphia: Wolters Kluwer; 2017.
9. Leonetti JP, Marzo SJ. Malignancy of the temporal bone. Otolaryngol Clin North Am. 2002;35(2):405–10.
10. Morris LG, Mehra S, Shah JP, Bilsky MH, Selesnick SH, Kraus DH. Predictors of survival and recurrence after temporal bone resection for cancer. Head Neck. 2012;34(9):1231–9.
11. Gidley PW, DeMonte F. Temporal bone malignancies. Neurosurg Clin N Am. 2013;24(1):97–110.
12. Hahn SS, Kim JA, Goodchild N, Constable WC. Carcinoma of the middle ear and external auditory canal. Int J Radiat Oncol Biol. 1983;9(7):1003–7.
13. Gloria-Cruz TI, Schachern PA, Paparella MM, Adams GL, Fulton SE. Metastases to temporal bones from primary nonsystemic malignant neoplasms. Arch Otolaryngol Head Neck Surg. 2000;126(2):209–14.
14. Gidley PW, Thompson CR, Roberts DB, DeMonte F, Hanna EY. The oncology of otology. Laryngoscope. 2012;122(2):393–400.
15. Hizli O, Salduz A, Kaya S, Paparella MM, Cureoglu S. A rare location for sarcoma metastasis: the temporal bone. Am J Otolaryngol. 2015;36(6):772–7.
16. Scholsem M, Raket D, Flandroy P, Sciot R, Deprez M. Primary temporal bone angiosarcoma: a case report. J Neurooncol. 2005;75(2):121–5.
17. Al-Daraji W, Lasota J, Foss R, Miettinen M. Synovial sarcoma involving the head: analysis of 36 cases with predilection to the parotid and temporal regions. Am J Surg Pathol. 2009;33(10):1494–503.
18. Cross JP Jr, Ladaga LA. Peripheral synovial sarcoma metastatic to the temporal bone. Am J Otol. 1986;7(3):169–71.
19. Hsieh ST, Guo YC, Tsai TL, Li WY, Lin CZ. Parosteal osteosarcoma of the mastoid bone following radiotherapy for nasopharyngeal carcinoma. J Chin Med Assoc. 2004;67(6):314–6.
20. Sharma SC, Handa KK, Panda N, Banerjee AK, Mann SB. Osteogenic sarcoma of the temporal bone. Am J Otolaryngol. 1997;18(3):220–3.
21. Seo T, Nagareda T, Shimano K, Saka N, Kashiba K, Mori T, et al. Liposarcoma of temporal bone: a case report. Auris Nasus Larynx. 2007;34(4):511–3.
22. Agarwal PN, Mishra SD, Pratap VK. Primary liposarcoma of the mastoid. J Laryngol Otol. 1975;89(10):1079–82.
23. Coatesworth AP, Martin-Hirsch DP, MacDonald A. Post-irradiation liposarcoma of the temporal bone. J Laryngol Otol. 1996;110(8):779–81.
24. Charlton CA, Leiomyosarcoma of the external auditory canal. Br J Surg. 1964;51:24–5.
25. Rasp G, Holtmann S, Wiebecke B. Leiomyosarcoma of the external ear canal. Laryngorhinootologie. 1991;70(3):164–6.
26. Lambert EM, Gunn GB, Gidley PW. Effects of radiation on the temporal bone in patients with head and neck cancer. Head Neck. 2016;38(9):1428–35.
27. Goh YH, Chong VF, Low WK. Temporal bone tumours in patients irradiated for nasopharyngeal neoplasm. J Laryngol Otol. 1999;113(3):222–8.
28. Lambert EM, Garden AS, DeMonte F, Roberts DB, Gidley PW. Radiation-associated malignancies of the ear canal and temporal bone. Laryngoscope. 2015;125(5):1198–204.
29. Patel SR. Radiation-induced sarcoma. Curr Treat Options Oncol. 2000;1(3):258–61.
30. Lustig LR, Jackler RK, Lanser MJ. Radiation-induced tumors of the temporal bone. Am J Otol. 1997;18(2):230–5.
31. Nakanishi H, Tomita Y, Myoui A, Yoshikawa H, Sakai K, Kato Y, et al. Mutation of the p53 gene in postradiation sarcoma. Lab Invest. 1998;78(6):727–33.
32. Pisters PW, Weiss M, Maki RG, Raut CP. Soft-tissue sarcomas. In: Edge SB, Byrd DR, Compton CC, Fritz AG, Greene FL, Trotti A, editors. AJCC cancer staging manual. 7th ed. New York: Springer; 2010. p. 291–6.
33. Shuman AG, Brennan MF, Palmer FL, Kuk D, Moraco N, Singer S, et al. Soft tissue sarcoma of the head & neck: nomogram validation and analysis of staging systems. J Surg Oncol. 2015;111(6):690–5.
34. O'Sullivan B, Maki RG, Agulnik M, Patel SG, Lazar AJ, Jones RL, et al. Soft tissue sarcoma of the head and neck. In: Amin MB, Edge SB, Greene FL, Byrd DR, Brookland RK, Washington MK, et al., editors. AJCC cancer staging manual. 8th ed. Switzerland: Springer; 2017. p. 499–505.
35. Coffin CM, Davis JL, Borinstein SC. Syndrome-associated soft tissue tumours. Histopathology. 2014;64(1):68–87.
36. Turner JH, Richmon JD. Head and neck rhabdomyosarcoma: a critical analysis of population-based incidence and survival data. Otolaryngol Head Neck Surg. 2011;145(6):967–73.
37. Reilly BK, Kim A, Pena MT, Dong TA, Rossi C, Murnick JG, et al. Rhabdomyosarcoma of the head and neck in children: review and update. Int J Pediatr Otorhinolaryngol. 2015;79(9):1477–83.
38. Durve DV, Kanegaonkar RG, Albert D, Levitt G. Paediatric rhabdomyosarcoma of the ear and temporal bone. Clin Otolaryngol Allied Sci. 2004;29(1):32–7.
39. Sbeity S, Abella A, Arcand P, Quintal MC, Saliba I. Temporal bone rhabdomyosarcoma in children. Int J Pediatr Otorhinolaryngol. 2007;71(5):807–14.
40. Malempati S, Hawkins DS. Rhabdomyosarcoma: review of the Children's oncology group (COG) soft-tissue sarcoma committee experience and rationale for current COG studies. Pediatr Blood Cancer. 2012;59(1):5–10.
41. Gluth MB. Rhabdomyosarcoma and other pediatric temporal bone malignancies. Otolaryngol Clin North Am. 2015;48(2):375–90.
42. Jaffe BF, Fox JE, Batsakis JG. Rhabdomyosarcoma of the middle ear and mastoid. Cancer. 1971;27(1):29–37.
43. Raney RB Jr, Lawrence W Jr, Maurer HM, Lindberg RD, Newton WA Jr, Ragab AH, et al. Rhabdomyosarcoma of the ear in childhood. A report from the Intergroup Rhabdomyosarcoma Study—I. Cancer. 1983;51(12):2356–61.
44. Le Deley MC, Delattre O, Schaefer KL, Burchill SA, Koehler G, Hogendoorn PC, et al. Impact of EWS-ETS fusion type on disease progression in Ewing's sarcoma/peripheral primitive neuroectodermal tumor: prospective results from the cooperative Euro-E.W.I.N.G. 99 trial. J Clin Oncol Off J Am Soc Clin Oncol. 2010;28(12):1982–8.
45. Hoglund M, Gisselsson D, Mandahl N, Mitelman F. Ewing tumours and synovial sarcomas have critical features of karyotype evolution in common with epithelial tumours. Int J Cancer. 2005;116(3):401–6.

46. Ludwig JA. Ewing sarcoma: historical perspectives, current state-of-the-art, and opportunities for targeted therapy in the future. Curr Opin Oncol. 2008;20(4):412–8.
47. Allam A, El-Husseiny G, Khafaga Y, Kandil A, Gray A, Ezzat A, et al. Ewing's sarcoma of the head and neck: a retrospective analysis of 24 cases. Sarcoma. 1999;3(1):11–5.
48. Siegal GP, Oliver WR, Reinus WR, Gilula LA, Foulkes MA, Kissane JM, et al. Primary Ewing's sarcoma involving the bones of the head and neck. Cancer. 1987;60(11):2829–40.
49. Kadar AA, Hearst MJ, Collins MH, Mangano FT, Samy RN. Ewing's sarcoma of the petrous temporal bone: case report and literature review. Skull Base. 2010;20(3):213–7.
50. Hara N, Kaneko H, Inoue K, Watanabe M. Primary Ewing's sarcoma of the temporal bone—case report (author's transl). No Shinkei Geka Neurol Surg. 1980;8(6):557–62.
51. Davidson MJ. Ewing's sarcoma of the temporal bone. A case report. Oral Surg Oral Med Oral Pathol. 1991;72(5):534–6.
52. Watanabe H, Tsubokawa T, Katayama Y, Koyama S, Nakamura S. Primary Ewing's sarcoma of the temporal bone. Surg Neurol. 1992;37(1):54–8.
53. Kuzeyli K, Akturk F, Reis A, Cakir E, Baykal S, Pekince A, et al. Primary Ewing's sarcoma of the temporal bone with intracranial, extracranial and intraorbital extension. Case report. Neurosurg Rev. 1997;20(2):132–4.
54. Desai K, Goel A, Nadkarni TD. Primary petrous bone Ewing's sarcoma. Br J Neurosurg. 2000;14(2):143–5.
55. Souviron Encabo R, Arenas Britez O, Gil R, Perez-Luengo E, Scola Yurrita B. Primitive neuroectodermal tumor/extraosseus Ewing sarcoma of the temporal bone. Acta Otorrinolaringol Esp. 2005;56(1):38–40.
56. Nandi M, Bhattacharya J, Goswami S, Goswami C. Primary Ewing's sarcoma of the squamous part of temporal bone in a young girl treated with adjuvant volumetric arc therapy. J Cancer Res Ther. 2015;11(4):1015–7.
57. Whaley JT, Indelicato DJ, Morris CG, Hinerman RW, Amdur RJ, Mendenhall WM, et al. Ewing tumors of the head and neck. Am J Clin Oncol. 2010;33(4):321–6.
58. Carroll R, Miketic LM. Ewing sarcoma of the temporal bone: CT appearance. J Comput Assist Tomogr. 1987;11(2):362–3.
59. Raney RB, Asmar L, Newton WA Jr, Bagwell C, Breneman JC, Crist W, et al. Ewing's sarcoma of soft tissues in childhood: a report from the Intergroup Rhabdomyosarcoma Study, 1972 to 1991. J Clin Oncol Off J Am Soc Clin Oncol. 1997;15(2):574–82.
60. Grevener K, Haveman LM, Ranft A, van den Berg H, Jung S, Ladenstein R, et al. Management and outcome of Ewing sarcoma of the head and neck. Pediatr Blood Cancer. 2016;63(4):604–10.
61. Moore DD, Luu HH. Osteosarcoma. Cancer Treat Res. 2014;162:65–92.
62. Mirabello L, Troisi RJ, Savage SA. Osteosarcoma incidence and survival rates from 1973 to 2004: data from the surveillance, epidemiology, and end results program. Cancer. 2009;115(7):1531–43.
63. Hansen MF, Koufos A, Gallie BL, Phillips RA, Fodstad O, Brogger A, et al. Osteosarcoma and retinoblastoma: a shared chromosomal mechanism revealing recessive predisposition. Proc Natl Acad Sci U S A. 1985;82(18):6216–20.
64. Kansara M, Thomas DM. Molecular pathogenesis of osteosarcoma. DNA Cell Biol. 2007;26(1):1–18.
65. Laurin N, Brown JP, Morissette J, Raymond V. Recurrent mutation of the gene encoding sequestosome 1 (SQSTM1/p62) in Paget disease of bone. Am J Hum Genet. 2002;70(6):1582–8.
66. Smith RB, Apostolakis LW, Karnell LH, Koch BB, Robinson RA, Zhen W, et al. National Cancer Data Base report on osteosarcoma of the head and neck. Cancer. 2003;98(8):1670–80.
67. Kassir RR, Rassekh CH, Kinsella JB, Segas J, Carrau RL, Hokanson JA. Osteosarcoma of the head and neck: meta-analysis of nonrandomized studies. Laryngoscope. 1997;107(1):56–61.
68. Laskar S, Basu A, Muckaden MA, D'Cruz A, Pai S, Jambhekar N, et al. Osteosarcoma of the head and neck region: lessons learned from a single-institution experience of 50 patients. Head Neck. 2008;30(8):1020–6.
69. Ha PK, Eisele DW, Frassica FJ, Zahurak ML, McCarthy EF. Osteosarcoma of the head and neck: a review of the Johns Hopkins experience. Laryngoscope. 1999;109(6):964–9.
70. Mark RJ, Sercarz JA, Tran L, Dodd LG, Selch M, Calcaterra TC. Osteogenic sarcoma of the head and neck. The UCLA experience. Arch Otolaryngol Head Neck Surg. 1991;117(7):761–6.
71. Guadagnolo BA, Zagars GK, Raymond AK, Benjamin RS, Sturgis EM. Osteosarcoma of the jaw/craniofacial region: outcomes after multimodality treatment. Cancer. 2009;115(14):3262–70.
72. Patel SG, Meyers P, Huvos AG, Wolden S, Singh B, Shaha AR, et al. Improved outcomes in patients with osteogenic sarcoma of the head and neck. Cancer. 2002;95(7):1495–503.
73. Rand CW. Osteosarcoma of left temporal bone followed by development of an astrocytoma of underlying temporal lobe. Thirty year review of an unusual case. Bull Los Angel Neuro Soc. 1961;26:23–31.
74. Gertner R, Podoshin L, Fradis M. Osteogenic sarcoma of the temporal bone. J Laryngol Otol. 1983;97(7):627–31.
75. Sataloff RT, Myers DL, Spiegel JR, Roberts BR, Telian S. Total temporal bone resection for osteogenic sarcoma. Ear Nose Throat J. 1988;67(9):626–7, 30–2, 34 passim.
76. Kellie SJ, Hutchison RE, Robertson JT, Pratt CB. Successful treatment of a radiation-associated extradural osteosarcoma with chemotherapy in an adolescent girl. Med Pediatr Oncol. 1989;17(6):514–9.
77. Iemoto Y, Ushigome S, Ikegami M, Koide K. Case report 648: Parosteal osteosarcoma arising from the right temporal bone. Skelet Radiol. 1991;20(1):59–61.
78. Smeele LE, Kostense PJ, van der Waal I, Snow GB. Effect of chemotherapy on survival of craniofacial osteosarcoma: a systematic review of 201 patients. J Clin Oncol Off J Am Soc Clin Oncol. 1997;15(1):363–7.
79. Daw NC, Mahmoud HH, Meyer WH, Jenkins JJ, Kaste SC, Poquette CA, et al. Bone sarcomas of the head and neck in children: the St Jude Children's research hospital experience. Cancer. 2000;88(9):2172–80.
80. Leddy LR, Holmes RE. Chondrosarcoma of bone. Cancer Treat Res. 2014;162:117–30.
81. Barnes R, Catto M. Chondrosarcoma of bone. J Bone Joint Surg. 1966;48(4):729–64.
82. Verdegaal SH, Bovee JV, Pansuriya TC, Grimer RJ, Ozger H, Jutte PC, et al. Incidence, predictive factors, and prognosis of chondrosarcoma in patients with Ollier disease and Maffucci syndrome: an international multicenter study of 161 patients. Oncologist. 2011;16(12):1771–9.
83. Burningham Z, Hashibe M, Spector L, Schiffman JD. The epidemiology of sarcoma. Clin Sarcoma Res. 2012;2(1):14.
84. Ruark DS, Schlehaider UK, Shah JP. Chondrosarcomas of the head and neck. World J Surg. 1992;16(5):1010–5. discussion 5-6.
85. Burkey BB, Hoffman HT, Baker SR, Thornton AF, McClatchey KD. Chondrosarcoma of the head and neck. Laryngoscope. 1990;100(12):1301–5.
86. Ellis MA, Gerry DR, Byrd JK. Head and neck chondrosarcomas: analysis of the Surveillance, Epidemiology, and End Results database. Head Neck. 2016;38(9):1359–66.
87. Koch BB, Karnell LH, Hoffman HT, Apostolakis LW, Robinson RA, Zhen W, et al. National cancer database report on chondrosarcoma of the head and neck. Head Neck. 2000;22(4):408–25.
88. Lustig LR, Sciubba J, Holliday MJ. Chondrosarcomas of the skull base and temporal bone. J Laryngol Otol. 2007;121(8):725–35.
89. Yagisawa M, Ishitoya J, Tsukuda M, Sakagami M. Chondrosarcoma of the temporal bone. Auris Nasus Larynx. 2007;34(4):527–31.
90. Raghu M, Moumoulidis I, De R, Moffat D. Chondrosarcomas of the temporal bone: presentation and management. J Laryngol Otol. 2004;118(7):551–5.

91. Tao D, Hoffman MR, Chen B. Temporal bone chondrosarcoma: presentation of 4 cases and review of the literature. Ear Nose Throat J. 2014;93(12):494–500.
92. Coltrera MD, Googe PB, Harrist TJ, Hyams VJ, Schiller AL, Goodman ML. Chondrosarcoma of the temporal bone. Diagnosis and treatment of 13 cases and review of the literature. Cancer. 1986;58(12):2689–96.
93. Aneiros-Fernandez J, Antonio Retamero J, Husein-Elahmed H, Ovalle F, Aneiros-Cachaza J. Primary cutaneous and subcutaneous leiomyosarcomas: evolution and prognostic factors. Eur J Dermatol. 2016;26(1):9–12.
94. Wanebo HJ, Koness RJ, MacFarlane JK, Eilber FR, Byers RM, Elias EG, et al. Head and neck sarcoma: report of the Head and Neck Sarcoma Registry. Society of Head and Neck Surgeons Committee on Research. Head Neck. 1992;14(1):1–7.
95. Farhood AI, Hajdu SI, Shiu MH, Strong EW. Soft tissue sarcomas of the head and neck in adults. Am J Surg. 1990;160(4):365–9.
96. Freedman AM, Reiman HM, Woods JE. Soft-tissue sarcomas of the head and neck. Am J Surg. 1989;158(4):367–72.
97. Eloy JA, Mortensen M, Gupta S, Lewis MS, Brett EM, Genden EM. Metastasis of uterine leiomyosarcoma to the thyroid gland: case report and review of the literature. Thyroid. 2007;17(12):1295–7.
98. Cassoni A, Terenzi V, Bartoli D, Zadeh OR, Battisti A, Pagnoni M, et al. Metastatic uterine leiomyosarcoma in the upper buccal gingiva misdiagnosed as an epulis. Case Rep Oncol Med. 2014;2014:402342.
99. Tomasini D, Niccoli A, Crivelli F, Scandroglio I. Cutaneous scalp metastasis as the first indication of a clinically silent retroperitoneal leiomyosarcoma and of its further relapse as metastatic widespread disease. Eur J Dermatol. 2014;24(2):264–5.
100. Nusrath MA, Kendall CH, Avery CM. Metastatic uterine leiomyosarcoma masquerading as a primary lesion of the masseter muscle. Int J Oral Maxillofac Surg. 2006;35(5):466–8.
101. Vora NM, Levin RJ. Metastatic leiomyosarcoma to the tongue. Otolaryngol Head Neck Surg. 2003;128(4):601–2.
102. Annest NM, Grekin SJ, Stone MS, Messingham MJ. Cutaneous leiomyosarcoma: a tumor of the head and neck. Dermatol Surg. 2007;33(5):628–33.
103. Yadav J, Bakshi J, Chouhan M, Modi R. Head and neck leiomyosarcoma. Ind J Otolaryngol Head Neck Surg. 2013;65(Suppl 1): 1–5.
104. Eppsteiner RW, DeYoung BR, Milhem MM, Pagedar NA. Leiomyosarcoma of the head and neck: a population-based analysis. Arch Otolaryngol Head Neck Surg. 2011;137(9):921–4.
105. Zbaren P, Ruchti C. Leiomyosarcoma of the middle ear and temporal bone. Ann Otol Rhinol Laryngol. 1994;103(7):537–41.
106. Ursick JA, Linthicum FH. Leiomyosarcoma of the temporal bone. Otol Neurotol. 2011;32(4):e30–1.
107. Kim BG, Kim J, Lee WS. Leiomyosarcoma of the middle ear and temporal bone. Clin Exp Otorhinolaryngol. 2013;6(4):254–8.
108. Nilles R, Plinkert PK, Ruck P. Leiomyosarcoma of the temporal bone. Laryngorhinootologie. 1995;74(1):54–6.
109. Izumi K, Maeda T, Cheng J, Saku T. Primary leiomyosarcoma of the maxilla with regional lymph node metastasis. Report of a case and review of the literature. Oral Surg Oral Med Oral Pathol Oral Radiol Endod. 1995;80(3):310–9.
110. Farshid G, Pradhan M, Goldblum J, Weiss SW. Leiomyosarcoma of somatic soft tissues: a tumor of vascular origin with multivariate analysis of outcome in 42 cases. Am J Surg Pathol. 2002;26(1):14–24.

Temporal Bone Malignancies in Children

14

Elton Lambert

Introduction

Malignancies of the temporal bone are rare in children. Presenting signs and symptoms may be vague, and there may be great difficulty differentiating signs and symptoms of these tumors from the common ear issues that children have. The most common pediatric malignancies of the temporal bone include rhabdomyosarcoma and Langerhans cell histiocytosis (LCH). Management of temporal bone malignancies should occur within the context of a multidisciplinary team as the pathology involved may require consideration of chemotherapy, radiotherapy, and/or surgery. Rehabilitation efforts must take into account age appropriate developmental considerations.

Assessment

Signs and Symptoms

The assessment of a child with a potential temporal bone tumor can be very challenging. Ear complaints such as acute otitis media and chronic otitis media are especially common before age 5. These can occur above age 5, but older children especially those who regularly swim can develop acute otitis externa. The recognition of ear pain in children is not always obvious. Small children cannot vocalize their symptoms, so other signs – including ear tugging, hitting of the head, placing the finger in the ear, or head tilting – must be used.

Ear drainage is another common complaint in acute/chronic otitis media, when associated with tympanic membrane perforation or otitis media with effusion. A range of temporal bone pathology including cholesteatoma and LCH are associated with ear drainage. The color and odor of the drainage are non-specific characteristics. Bloody drainage may be concerning, but may be associated with acute otitis media (AOM). Clear ear drainage, especially when pulsatile in nature, should raise suspicions for a cerebrospinal fluid (CSF) leak.

Temporal bone tumors can also be associated with hearing loss. Speech delay may be the only presenting sign of hearing loss, although this may not be present in unilateral hearing loss. It is not until children are of school age that they may be able to complain of hearing loss. Parents may notice that a child may favor one ear for hearing. Any concerns for hearing loss or speech delay should be investigated through audiometry.

Ear pain and ear drainage are common symptoms, but context and timing may be helpful clues to differentiate common etiologies from more worrisome ones. Ear pain or ear drainage that is refractory to standard treatment must alert the physician to an underlying condition. Sbeity et al. in their series of temporal bone rhabdomyosarcoma noted that 66% of patients presented with chronic otitis media refractory to treatment [1].

Common ear symptoms can be associated with pediatric temporal bone tumors, but there are more worrisome symptoms that must be recognized. A postauricular mass can be an indication of a temporal bone process, but the characterization of these masses is very important. A solid mobile mass, not fixed to the temporal bone proper, could be a benign process, such as a dermoid cyst or benign postauricular lymphadenopathy. Masses that are fixed to the temporal bone with less discrete borders are more troubling.

Malignant lesions often distort the integrity of the temporal bone. Any lesion that causes signs and symptoms of temporal bone erosion should be considered a potential malignancy until proven otherwise. LCH commonly presents with lytic skulls lesion, which leaves the affected areas devoid of the bone. Signs and symptoms showing interruption of the organs and structures within the temporal bone are especially worrisome. Temporal bone malignancies may present with unilateral facial nerve paresis or paralysis due to disruption of

E. Lambert, M.D.
Pediatric Otolaryngology, Texas Children's Hospital/Baylor College of Medicine, Houston, TX, USA
e-mail: emashela@texaschildrens.org

P. W. Gidley, F. DeMonte (eds.), *Temporal Bone Cancer*, https://doi.org/10.1007/978-3-319-74539-8_14

the facial nerve along its course through the temporal bone. Facial nerve paresis or paralysis may be hard to elucidate in very young children. It is difficult to prompt infants to make volitional facial movements. Signs of facial nerve paralysis in children include the inability to close the eye, especially when crying, loss of the nasolabial fold, oral incompetence as evidenced by drooling, oral spilling of food, or difficulty maintaining good suck-swallow coordination.

The temporal bone houses the hearing and balance organs. Once again, in young children hearing and balance complaints may be difficult to ascertain. Children with hearing loss may have speech delay, but this may not occur in unilateral processes. Injury to the labyrinth may produce nystagmus. Subtle balance issues may be present and may be revealed by frequent falling, delay, or regression in walking.

Diagnostic Studies

Cross-sectional imaging is necessary both to characterize a lesion and to determine its extent. Temporal bone lesions can spread locally and intracranially, to deep neck spaces, subcutaneous tissue, or the temporomandibular joint. Depending on the location, an assessment of regional lymphadenopathy and distant metastasis is prudent for treatment and prognosis. Plain X-rays may show signs of temporal bone lesions, e.g., punched out skull lesions in LCH but are not as important for treatment planning. One should not underestimate the importance of plain films and ultrasound in the diagnosis of lesions and neck metastasis, but they will not be discussed in this chapter.

Computer tomography (CT) and magnetic resonance imaging (MRI) are often complementary in the diagnosis and management of temporal bone lesions. The complementary role is highlighted by the relative strengths and weaknesses of each modality.

Temporal bone lesions often destroy the integrity of the temporal bone. CT scanning has the advantage of delineating the bony structures within the temporal bone. With a CT scan, the ossicles, skull base, bony labyrinth, vestibule, internal auditory canal, mastoid air cells, fallopian/facial nerve canal, Eustachian tube, and petrous apex can be evaluated. There is often a clear difference between a lesion, such as a dermoid cyst which has a pushing border, versus destructive lesions, such as LCH or rhabdomyosarcoma. CT helps to narrow the differential diagnosis, but one can only deduce so much from the interaction of the lesion with the surrounding bony structures. When the lesion spreads outside the limits of the temporal bone, it can be difficult to delineate the true limit of the lesion as it enters the soft tissue or the brain. Intracranial spread or perineural invasion may not be readily recognized. Even with these limitations, CT is a valuable tool in assessing cervical lymphadenopathy. In children, temporal bone CT exposes the child to radiation; the long-term risks, of which, are not completely understood.

Magnetic resonance imaging (MRI) has the disadvantage that it does not display bony destruction/replacement as well as CT scan. However, the resolution of CT cannot be compared to the resolution on MRI for lesions that are infiltrating the brain, parotid space, masticator space, parapharyngeal space, infratemporal fossa, and subcutaneous tissue. The multiple imaging sequences of MRI refine the differential diagnosis, including T1-, T2-, and diffusion-weighted (DWI) and echo planar, just to name a few. Gadolinium contrast can help to differentiate the wide array of pathologies that can affect the temporal bone. Young children usually need to be sedated for an MRI, and the effect of sedation and anesthesia on the neurocognitive development of children is an area of concern that demands further research. MRI does come with an increased cost. Table 14.1 shows CT and MRI characteristics of common pediatric temporal bone malignancies.

Table 14.1 Differential diagnosis of temporal bone masses and imaging characteristics on CT and MRI

Pathology	CT	MRI
Chloroma	Expansile, homogenous	T1 hypointense, enhancement with Gd, T2 isointense
Chondrosarcoma	Infiltrative bony destruction with bony spicules, matrix calcifications	T1 hypointense/isointense, variable enhancement with Gd, T2 hyperintense
Chordoma	Lobulated, bony destruction	T1 hypointense/isointense, variable enhancement with Gd, T2 hyperintense
Ewing sarcoma	Well circumscribed with hyperostosis	T1 hypointense, no enhancement with Gd, T2 with mixed intensities
Fibrosarcoma	Expansile with calcification	T1 hypointense, strong enhancement with Gd, T2 hyperintense
Lymphoma	Irregular with smooth margins	T1 hypointense, variable enhancement with Gd, T2 isointense
Metastasis	Bony erosion	T1 variable intensity, enhances with gadolinium, T2 variable intensity
Osteosarcoma	Radiolucent	T1 irregular hypointense/isointense, irregular enhancement with Gd, T2 mixed enhancement
Rhabdomyosarcoma	Destructive and infiltrative	T1 hypointense/isointense, enhances with Gd, T2 Hyperintense
Squamous cell carcinoma	Destructive, invasive	T1 isointense, enhancement with Gd, T2 hyperintense

Adapted from Gluth et al., 2015 [2]

Suspected or confirmed malignancies may require further imaging. This is especially true of tumor pathologies that have a high likelihood of metastasis. Cervical and distant metastasis can be accessed via positron emission tomography (PET), where the uptake of the radioactive dye fluorodeoxyglucose may show areas of spread. PET/CT is particularly helpful in identifying a primary site when the temporal bone mass is a site of distant metastasis. PET/CT is very useful for proper staging in lymphoma. In any confirmed or suspected malignancy, consultation with a pediatric hematologist/oncologist is appropriate to guide further staging studies such as bone marrow aspiration.

Pathology and Management

Rhabdomyosarcoma

Rhabdomyosarcoma is the most common soft tissue malignancy in children. It originates from skeletal muscle and accounts for approximately 3.5% of cancer cases in children below the age of 14 [3, 4]. Thirty to seventy percent of rhabdomyosarcoma occurs within the head and neck with 8–10% of these occurring with the middle ear and mastoid [5] (Fig. 14.1).

The origin of middle ear and mastoid rhabdomyosarcoma is controversial. They may originate from embryonal mesenchymal cells, immature myoblastic tissue, or muscles of the middle ear [1]. Pathologically, rhabdomyosarcoma displays small, anaplastic, round- and spindle-shaped cells with hyperchromic nuclei and granular eosinophilic nuclei [6]. The four histologic subtypes of rhabdomyosarcoma are embryonal, alveolar, botryoid, and pleomorphic. The embryonal subtype is the most common in the head and neck, including the middle ear and temporal bone subsites. There is some phenotypic variation in the embryonal subtype with cytoplasmic variability representing different stages of skeletal muscle differentiation. Immunohistochemistry and genetic studies are becoming increasingly important in the diagnosis of rhabdomyosarcoma. Desmin- and muscle-specific actin are special stains used to identify rhabdomyosarcoma. Molecular studies have shown loss of heterozygosity within the short arm of chromosome 11 to be characteristic of the embryonal subtype, while mutations in FOX and PAX7 are associated with the alveolar subtype. Molecular subtyping is becoming increasing important in determining prognosis [7].

Rhabdomyosarcoma is locally invasive, which is important to note within the temporal bone where many important structures are confined to a small anatomic space. Destruction of the fallopian canal and facial paralysis can occur with involvement of the middle ear. Intracranial involvement can occur via skull base destruction or through perineural spread. Local invasion can extend to the soft tissue of the neck, labyrinth, cochlea, jugular bulb, carotid artery, Eustachian tube, and nasopharynx. Both hematogenous spread and lymphatic spread can occur with rhabdomyosarcoma; however, hematogenous spread is more common than lymphatic spread in temporal bone rhabdomyosarcoma.

Staging of rhabdomyosarcoma has implications for treatment, prognosis, and investigative research. The TNM staging for the ear and temporal bone has been described elsewhere. The Intergroup Rhabdomyosarcoma Studies (IRS) Group and Soft Tissue Sarcoma Committee of the Children's Oncology Group have developed staging systems for rhabdomyosarcoma shown in Table 14.2.

An important point evidenced by the IRS modified system is that para-meningeal involvement results in more advanced staging. The middle ear and temporal bone are considered para-meningeal sites. Since temporal bone and middle ear rhabdomyosarcoma are rare, consensus treatment protocols are difficult to develop. Para-meningeal sites such as the temporal bone and middle ear are similar to the nasopharynx and sinuses in the fact that complete surgical resection is difficult to achieve. The IRS studies have shown considerable survival advantage for tumors where complete resection can be achieved, but this must be balanced against the expected surgical morbidity especially with respect to temporal bone resections.

Multimodality therapy with chemotherapy with or without radiation is considered foremost in temporal bone and middle ear tumors when complete surgical resection cannot be achieved. Classically rhabdomyosarcoma has been treated with a combination vincristine, Adriamycin, and cyclophosphamide (VAC) with radiation dosages of 50–60 Gy. When considering para-meningeal sites such as the temporal bone and middle ear, one advantage of the IRS standards for stratification is the allowance for relative intensification or de-intensification of chemotherapy and radiation. This has led to the addition of etoposide or ifosfamide in advanced cases or elimination of cyclophosphamide or Adriamycin in low-risk cases. The initial IRS-1 study reported in 1983 included 24 cases of temporal bone rhabdomyosarcoma with a 4-year survival rate of 41% [9]. IRS- II, IRS-III, and IRS-IV representing progressive studies of chemotherapy and radiotherapy protocols using risk stratification showed 3-year overall survival of 70%, 65%, and 88%, respectively [10]. Ongoing research continues to focus on intensification and de-intensification protocols of chemotherapy and radiotherapy with respect to site, histology, and molecular studies. Efficacy and side effects of proton radiotherapy are of special interest in the treatment of para-meningeal rhabdomyosarcomas such as those in the temporal bone and middle ear [11].

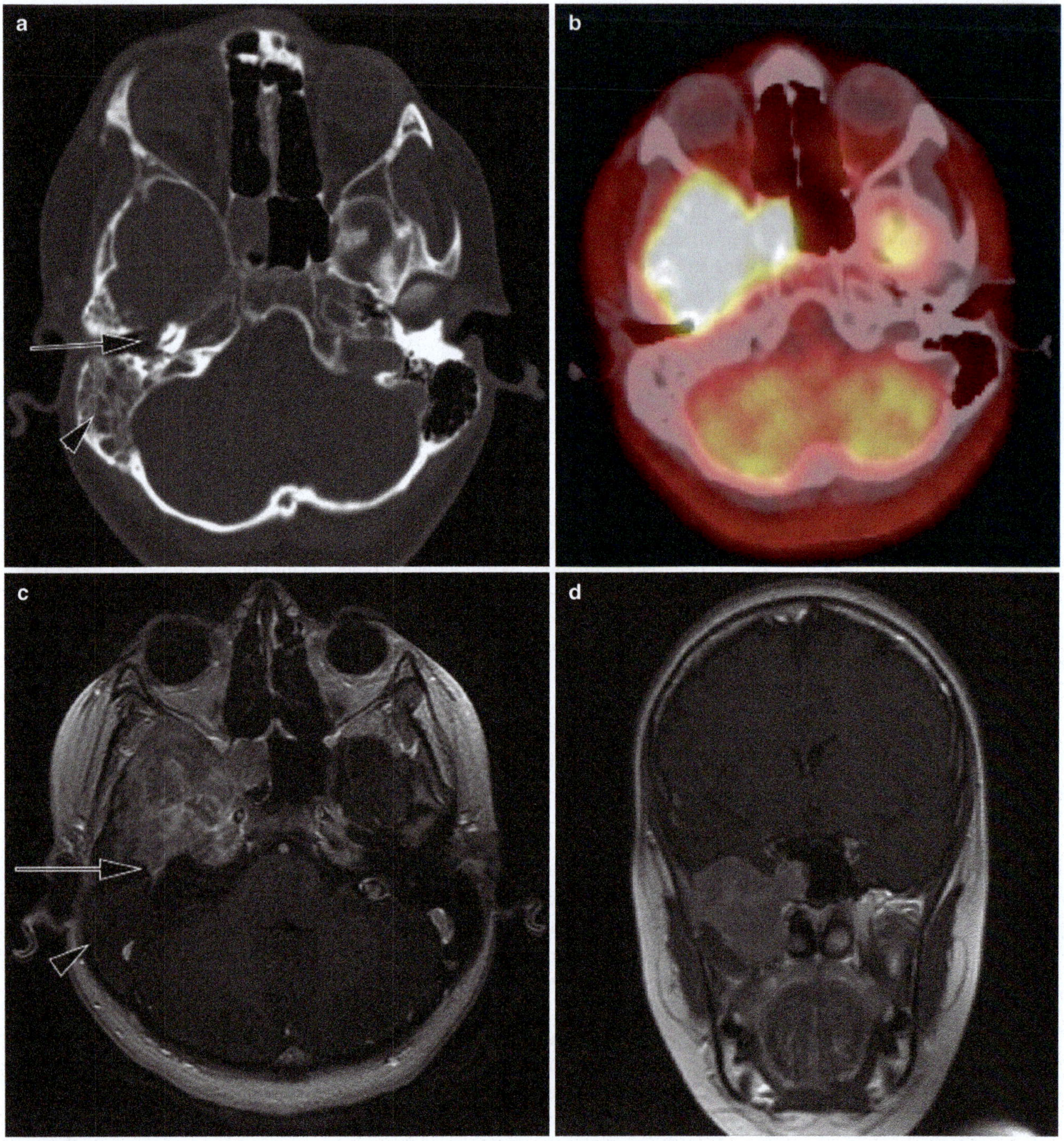

Fig. 14.1 *Rhabdomyosarcoma of the right infratemporal fossa with secondary involvement of* the middle ear. Facial paralysis was the presenting symptom in this 13-year-old girl. (**a**) Axial CT at the level of the basal turn of the cochlea. Arrow shows tumor within the middle ear; arrowhead shows mastoid opacification from obstructive serous otitis media. (**b**) PET/CT showing hypermetabolic tumor, approximately same level as in A. (**c**) Axial T1 contrast MRI at approximate same level as in A. White arrow shows tumor within the middle ear; white triangle shows mastoid opacification from obstructive serous otitis media. (**d**) Coronal T1 contrast MRI, showing disease in the middle cranial fossa, sphenoid, and infratemporal fossa (Photos courtesy of Paul Gidley, MD)

Table 14.2 Staging of rhabdomyosarcoma using the Intergroup Rhabdomyosarcoma Study and Soft Tissue Sarcoma Committee of the Children's Oncology Group (COG) Systems

IRS clinical group
Group I: Describes a tumor that can be completely removed by surgery
Group II: Describes a tumor that has been removed with surgery, but cancer cells remain at the edge of the tissue that surrounded the tumor (called a margin), and/or cancer cells are in the regional lymph nodes (lymph nodes near the site of the tumor)
Group III: Describes a local tumor. A local tumor is a tumor that has not spread outside of the area where it started and cannot be removed by surgery
Group IV: Describes distant metastases. A distant metastasis is cancer that has spread through the lymph system or blood to other parts of the body
IRS-modified TNM stage
Stage 1: Describes a local tumor in the orbit (the area near the eye); head and neck area, except for para-meningeal sites; or a genitourinary tract tumor, except for a tumor in the bladder or prostate
Stage 2: Describes a small local tumor in any part of the body not in Stage 1. The tumor is smaller than 5 centimeters (cm), and there is no spread to regional lymph nodes
Stage 3: Describes a local tumor in any part of the body not included in Stage 1 that is larger than 5 cm in diameter and/or has spread to regional lymph nodes
Stage 4: Distant metastases are present at diagnosis. The primary tumor can be of any size or location
Recurrent: Recurrent cancer is cancer that has come back after treatment. If there is a recurrence, the cancer may need to be staged again (called restaging) using the system above

Langerhans Cell Histiocytosis

LCH is a rare but important tumor that can affect the temporal bone of the pediatric patient. It is caused by clonal proliferation of Langerhans cells or histiocytes, although the true origin of these cells is not completely understood. It can occur in many sites, but temporal bone presentation is well described. There are three distinct manifestations of the disease: eosinophilic granuloma (EG), Hand-Schuller-Christian disease, and Letterer-Siwe disease. EG is a unifocal lesion, osteolytic in nature without associated systemic symptoms. Hand-Schuller-Christian disease occurs in children under the age of 5 with multifocal lytic lesions, typically within the skull with limited organ involvement. A chronic draining ear, multifocal lytic lesions, exophthalmos, and diabetes insipidus are common features of Hand-Schuller-Christian. Temporal bone involvement and multiple punched out lesions are usually present (Fig. 14.2). Letterer-Siwe disease carries the worst prognosis with multi-organ system involvement [12]. Surgery is usually reserved for unifocal disease when that the lesion can be adequately resected without risk of significant morbidity. Chemotherapy as single-modality therapy is more common in multifocal disease, but neoadjuvant therapy may be employed in unifocal disease. Steroids and vinblastine are considered first-line therapy. Radiation is not considered to be first-line therapy due to limited efficacy with risk of undue side effects [13]. Patients with systemic disease are less likely to respond to therapy and more likely to relapse.

Osteosarcoma, Ewing's Sarcoma, and Chondrosarcoma

Osteosarcoma is an aggressive malignancy of primary mesenchymal origin arising from bone. Osteosarcoma usually occurs in long bones, but can occur within the cranial vault (Fig. 14.3). The mean age of diagnosis of cranial osteosarcoma is about 12 years. Osteosarcoma is characterized by spindle cells morphology and excessive production of immature bone or osteoid. Skull base osteosarcoma is associated with lower rates of metastasis when compared to those arising from long bones.

Principles of therapy are based on degree of resectability. Resectability is more difficult with cranial vault and skull base locations like the temporal bone when compared to axial and facial sites including maxilla and mandible. Dural or cerebral involvement can make total resection more difficult in cases of temporal bone involvement. Neoadjuvant chemotherapy is regularly employed in patients where gross total resection is not possible. High-grade osteosarcomas are treated with high-dose, multi-agent chemotherapy including doxorubicin, cisplatin, methotrexate, and ifosfamide. Radiation therapy is typically reserved for unresectable cases [14].

Ewing's sarcoma is the second most common primary bone cancer in children. It is also of mesenchymal origin and is thought to originate from the medullary cavity. Like osteosarcoma, Ewing's sarcoma is more common in long bones, but cranial and temporal bone involvement has been described. Early lung metastasis is a hallmark of Ewing's sarcoma; but like other sarcomas involving the skull, there may be a lower propensity for metastasis for temporal bone Ewing's sarcoma. The pathology of Ewing's sarcoma displays lobulated small round blue cells with varying degrees of neuroectodermal differentiation. Just as in the case of osteosarcoma, neoadjuvant chemotherapy followed by surgical resection is preferred treatment. Vincristine and cyclophosphamide are mainstays of therapy, and the addition of ifosfamide, doxorubi-

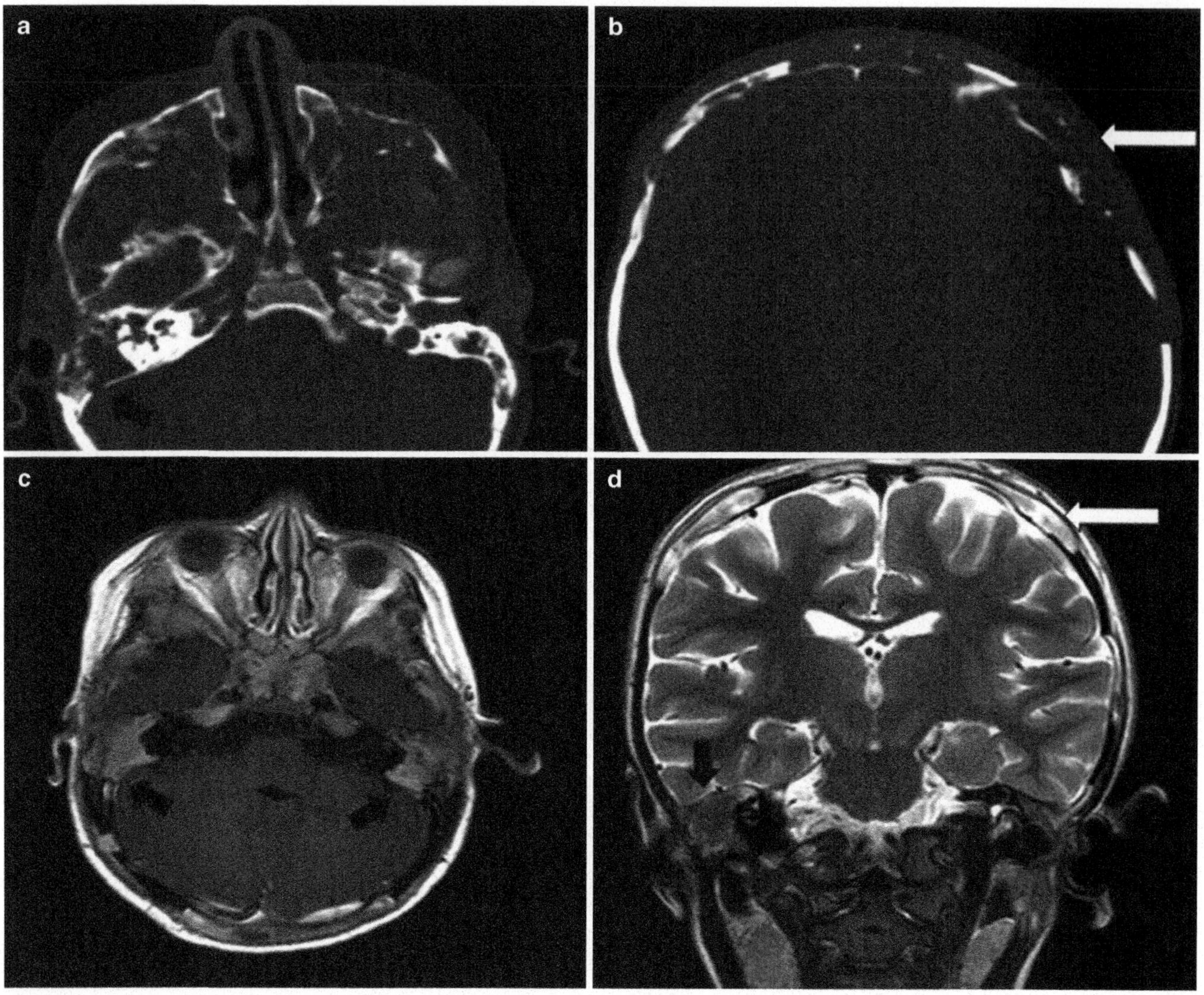

Fig. 14.2 Computer tomography (**a**, **b**) and magnetic resonance (**c**, **d**) images of a 3-year-old female with Langerhans cell histiocytosis (LCH). Temporal bone involvement is indicated by the black arrows, while white arrows show characteristic "punched out" skull lesions characteristic of the disease

cin, and/or etoposide may be helpful. Radiotherapy, once again, is used in unresectable cases but is not preferred due to potential late side effects [15].

Chondrosarcoma is a malignant tumor of cartilage-forming tissues. They may arise from structures formed by endochondral ossification like the temporal bone. They do not typically metastasize. The middle cranial fossa is the most common region of the skull base affected due to tumors arising from the petroclival, petro-occipital, spheno-occipital, and sphenopetrosal synchondroses. Chondrosarcomas can be classified using a grading scale from 1 to 4. Grade 1 chondrosarcomas are on a continuum with the benign entity chondroma with progressively higher grades displaying a greater proportion of undifferentiated cells. Chondrosarcomas pathologically are composed of malignant cartilage-forming cells. Surgical therapy is the mainstay of treatment [16].

The temporal bone can also be affected by even rarer pathologies including fibrosarcomas (originating from fibroblasts) and pleomorphic sarcoma. Surgical treatment is usually advocated when possible.

Lymphoma and Leukemic Tumors

There have been reports of both Hodgkin's and Non-Hodgkin's lymphoma occurring within the ear and temporal bone of children. Lymphoma occurs when there is malignant proliferation of the lymphoreticular system. These normally occur in lymph node basins. The temporal bone is an extranodal site which is more common with non-Hodgkin's lymphoma especially in diffuse large-cell malignant lymphoma. NHLs are further subdivided into T-cell, B-cell, low-grade, and high-grade lymphomas [17].

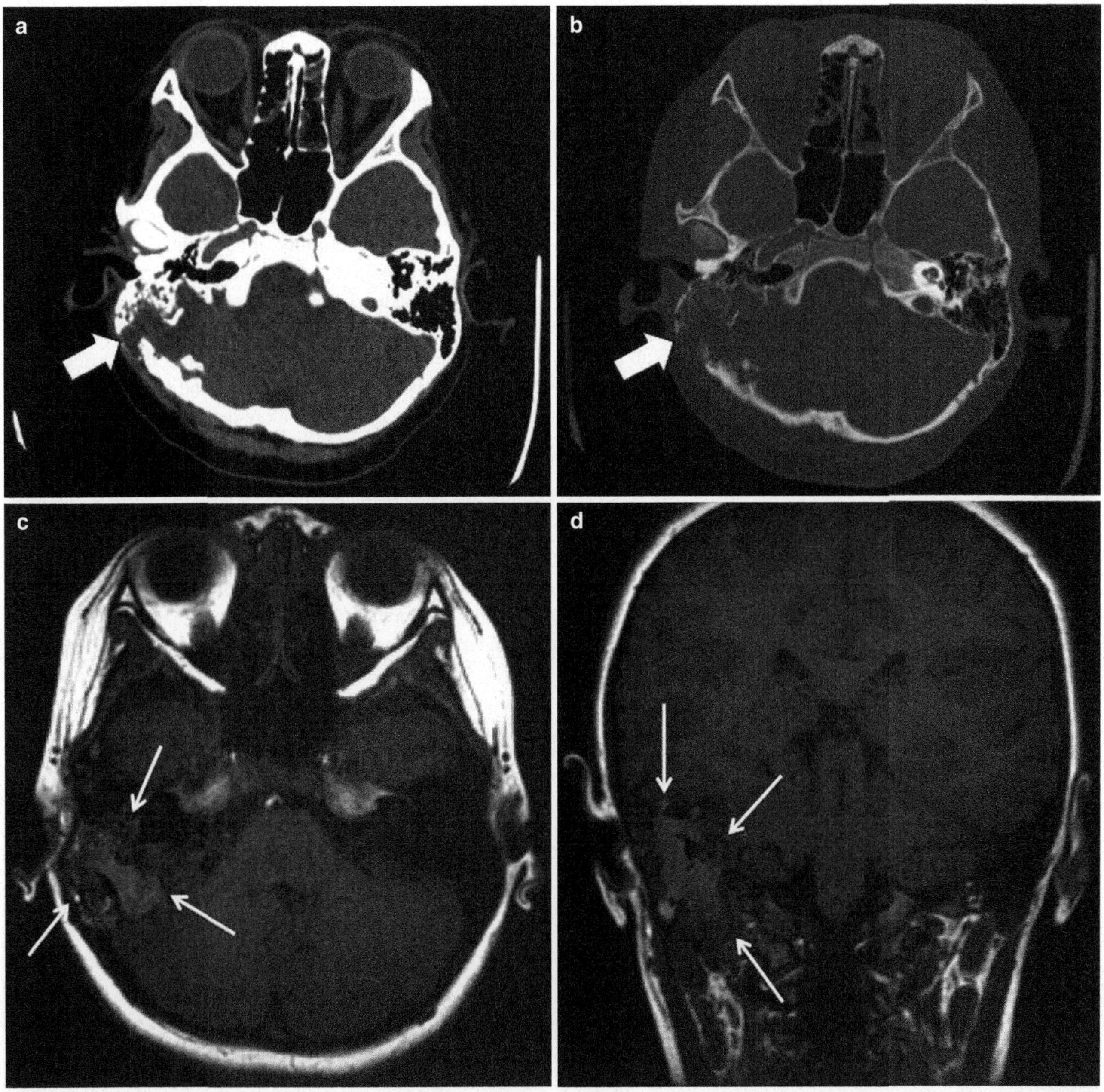

Fig. 14.3 Osteosarcoma of the mastoid in a 9-year-old girl that presented with facial paralysis. (**a**) Axial CT soft tissue and (**b**) axial CT bone windows. Mastoid destruction noted by white arrows. Contrast-enhanced T1 MRI (**c**) axial and (**d**) coronal. White arrows highlighting tumor extent (Photos courtesy of Paul Gidley, MD.)

Leukemia is one of the most common malignancies in children and is also within the continuum of cancers of the lymphoreticular system. Acute lymphocytic leukemia (ALL) is the most common form in children. Up to 40% of patients with ALL may have otologic manifestations that include pain, drainage, aural polyps, and even facial nerve paralysis [18]. These are thought to occur due to leukemic infiltrates within the middle ear and temporal bone and can be a sign of initial presentation or relapse. In addition to leukemic infiltrates, solitary masses can occur. Chloromas or myeloid sarcomas are composed of myeloblasts or immature white blood cells. Plasmacytomas are discrete solitary masses of plasma cells associated with multiple myeloma. These can affect calvarial bone including the temporal bone. Biopsy is typically the only role of surgery in these malignancies of the lymphoreticular system, with diagnosis made via immunohistochemistry and flow cytometry.

Late Effects of Treatment of Temporal Bone Cancers in Children

The effects of temporal bone cancer in children are not limited to surgical treatment of these tumors. Wound complications, hearing loss (both conductive and sensorineural), tinnitus, cerebrospinal fluid leak, cranial neuropathies, and recurrences are some of the negative effects that can occur with chemotherapy and radiotherapy. Depending on the age, cranial neuropathies and hearing loss can have a detrimental effect on speech development. Aural rehabilitation should be offered as early as possible to limit the impact on speech and language development. Nutritional support is also an important consideration to ensure adequate growth. Children, who may lack an understanding of the issues surrounding the management of their tumors, may have severe nutritional impairment if their age appropriate psychosocial issues are not addressed.

Chemotherapy and radiotherapy can also have lasting side effects for children. The myriad of chemotherapy agents can have their own unique side effects. Some chemotherapeutic agents can lead to sensorineural hearing loss, issues with fertility, and growth. With these long-term issues in mind, many de-intensification protocols are being investigated in order to balance adequate treatment with prevention of these side effects.

The efficacy of radiotherapy is questionable in many sarcomas and lymphoreticular malignancies. This coupled with the numerous late-term side effects should lead the multidisciplinary team charged with the care of a child with a temporal bone malignancy to take great caution in recommending radiotherapy. Effects of temporal bone radiation in children include radiation-associated sensorineural hearing loss due to cochleotoxic effects; middle ear and mastoid effusions due to mucosal and Eustachian tube injury; chronic otitis externa, otorrhea; xerostomia due to salivary gland radiation; cranial neuropathies; endocrinopathies due to pituitary gland involvement; and disturbance of craniofacial growth. Proton therapy protocols are being developed to minimize these effects.

Temporal bone osteoradionecrosis and radiation-associated malignancies are potentially more dangerous sequelae to temporal bone irradiation (Fig. 14.4). Temporal bone osteoradionecrosis can range from very limited bony exposure necessitating only conservative management to large sequestrate requiring aggressive surgery. Sarcomas are common secondary malignancies (Fig. 14.4). These effects are especially important to note for children as there can be significant latency associated with the development of these entities. The development of secondary malignancies of the temporal bone can develop on average about 13 years after radiation. The greater years of life expectancy in younger children can put them at an increased risk developing secondary malignancies [19].

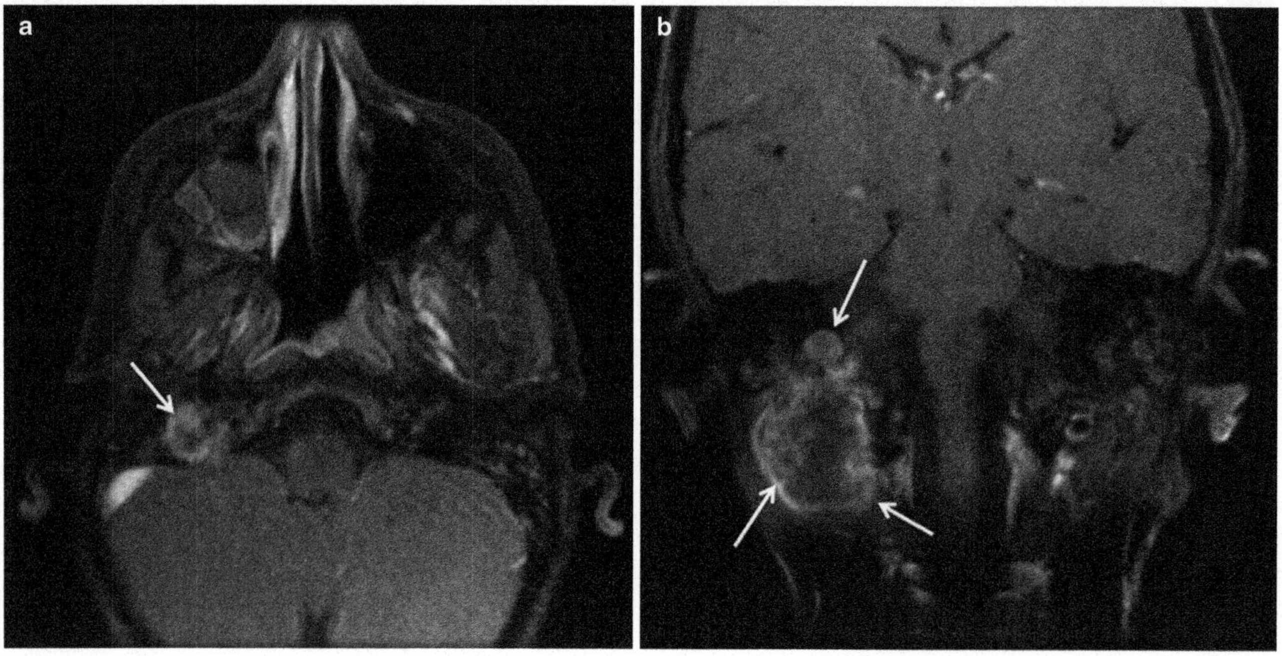

Fig. 14.4. Axial (**a**) and coronal (**b**) MRI of 9-year-old boy who developed radiation-associated osteosarcoma (white arrows) of the right neck and temporal bone 6 years following chemotherapy and radiotherapy for rhabdomyosarcoma of the right buccal mucosa (Images courtesy of Paul Gidley, MD)

Conclusion

Although temporal bone malignancies are rare in children, vigilance is needed by the clinician as presenting symptoms can be very similar to common ear complaints in the pediatric population. It is true that temporal bone malignancies can begin with ear pain, ear drainage, and hearing loss; but symptoms including a postauricular mass, bony erosion, and facial nerve weakness are especially concerning. CT and MRI are complimentary in evaluating temporal bone tumors with respect to integrity of the bony structures and the soft tissue, respectively. Special attention must be paid to radiation exposure for CT and anesthetic risk of MRI in children. Rhabdomyosarcoma and Langerhans cell histiocytosis are the most common temporal bone malignancies. Lymphoma and leukemia may directly involve the temporal bone or secondary to infiltration by malignant cells. Children may succumb to many side effects of treatment for temporal bone malignancies, and these effects must be balanced when deciding upon an optimal treatment plan.

References

1. Sbeity S, Abella A, Arcand P, Quintal MC, Saliba I. Temporal bone rhabdomyosarcoma in children. Int J Pediatr Otorhinolaryngol. 2007;71(5):807–14. https://doi.org/10.1016/j.ijporl.2007.02.002.
2. Gluth MB. Rhabdomyosarcoma and other Pediatric temporal bone malignancies. Otolaryngol Clin North Am. 2015;48(2):375–90. https://doi.org/10.1016/j.otc.2014.12.010.
3. Gurney JG, Severson RK, Davis S, Robison LL. Incidence of cancer in children in the United States. Sex-, race-, and 1-year age-specific rates by histologic type. Cancer. 1995;75(8):2186–95. https://doi.org/10.1002/1097-0142(19950415)75:8<2186::AID-CNCR2820750825>3.0.CO;2-F.
4. Maurer HM, Gehan EA, Beltangady M, et al. The intergroup rhabdomyosarcoma study-II. Cancer. 1993;71(5):1904–22. https://doi.org/10.1002/1097-0142(19930301)71:5<1904::AID-CNCR2820710530>3.0.CO;2-X.
5. Durve DV, Kanegaonkar RG, Albert D, Levitt G. Paediatric rhabdomyosarcoma of the ear and temporal bone. Clin Otolaryngol Allied Sci. 2004;29(1):32–7. https://doi.org/10.1111/j.1365-2273.2004.00764.x.
6. Parham DM. Pathologic classification of rhabdomyosarcomas and correlations with molecular studies. Mod Pathol. 2001;14(5):506–14. https://doi.org/10.1038/modpathol.3880339.
7. De Giovanni C, Landuzzi L, Nicoletti G, Lollini P-L, Nanni P. Molecular and cellular biology of rhabdomyosarcoma. Future Oncol. 2009;5(9):1449–75. https://doi.org/10.2217/fon.09.97.
8. Manning SC, Bloom DC, Perkins JA, Gruss JS, Inglis A. Diagnostic and surgical challenges in the Pediatric Skull Base. Otolaryngol Clin North Am. 2005;38(4):773–94. https://doi.org/10.1016/j.otc.2005.03.001.
9. Raney RBJ, Lawrence WJ, Maurer HM, et al. Rhabdomyosarcoma of the ear in childhood. A report from the intergroup Rhabdomyosarcoma Study-I. Cancer. 1983;51(12):2356–61.
10. Hawkins DS, Anderson JR, Paidas CN, et al. Improved outcome for patients with middle ear rhabdomyosarcoma: a children's oncology group study. J Clin Oncol. 19(12):3073–9. http://ovidsp.ovid.com/ovidweb.cgi?T=JS&CSC=Y&NEWS=N&PAGE=fulltext&D=med4&AN=11408504.
11. Childs SK, Kozak KR, Friedmann AM, et al. Proton radiotherapy for parameningeal rhabdomyosarcoma: clinical outcomes and late effects. Int J Radiat Oncol Biol Phys. 2012;82(2):635–42. https://doi.org/10.1016/j.ijrobp.2010.11.048.
12. Saliba I, Sidani K, El Fata F, Arcand P, Quintal MC, Abela A. Langerhans' cell histiocytosis of the temporal bone in children. Int J Pediatr Otorhinolaryngol. 2008;72(6):775–86. https://doi.org/10.1016/j.ijporl.2008.02.001.
13. Haupt R, Minkov M, Astigarraga I, et al. Langerhans cell histiocytosis (LCH): guidelines for diagnosis, clinical work-up, and treatment for patients till the age of 18 years. Pediatr Blood Cancer. 2013;60(2):175–84. https://doi.org/10.1002/pbc.24367.
14. Hadley C, Gressot LV, Patel AJ, et al. Osteosarcoma of the cranial vault and skull base in pediatric patients. J Neurosurg Pediatr. 2014;13(4):380–7. https://doi.org/10.3171/2013.12.PEDS13359.
15. Goudarzipour K, Shamsian S, Alavi S, Nourbakhsh K, Aghakhani R, Eydian Z, Arzanian MT. Primary Ewing's sarcoma of the temporal bone in an infant. Int J Hematol Stem Cell Res. 2015;9(2):104.
16. Mosier SM, Patel T, Strenge K, Mosier AD. Chondrosarcoma in childhood: the radiologic and clinical conundrum. J Radiol Case Rep. 2012;6(12):32–42. https://doi.org/10.3941/jrcr.v6i12.1241.
17. Lang EE, Walsh RM, Leader M. Primary middle-ear lymphoma in a child. J Laryngol Otol. 2003;117(3):205–7. https://doi.org/10.1258/002221503321192520.
18. Terao K, Cureoglu S, Schachern PA, et al. Pathologic correlations of otologic symptoms in acute lymphocytic leukemia. Am J Otolaryngol Head Neck Med Surg. 2011;32(1):13–8. https://doi.org/10.1016/j.amjoto.2009.08.006.
19. Lambert EM, Garden AS, Demonte F, Roberts DB, Gidley PW. Radiation-associated malignancies of the ear canal and temporal bone. Laryngoscope. 2015;125:1198–204. https://doi.org/10.1002/lary.25071.

Metastatic Lesions to the Temporal Bone

15

Paul W. Gidley and Marc-Elie Nader

Introduction

The prevalence of temporal bone metastasis is more than 20% in large autopsy series of cancer patients. Breast, lung, kidney, stomach, and prostate cancers are the most common malignancies to metastasize to the temporal bone [1–4]. More recent autopsy studies include melanoma and cervical cancer into this list [5].

While metastases to the temporal bone are considered rare in clinical practice, they are more common than reported for several reasons: (1) temporal bone metastases are a sign of late-stage disease, (2) the symptoms are not disabling and are often overshadowed by more urgent needs, (3) otologic examination is not performed routinely on patients with widely metastatic disease, and (4) histologic examination of the temporal bone is not a routine part of postmortem examination [6, 7]. Gloria-Cruz et al. estimated a 22% prevalence of temporal bone metastasis in a large series of autopsies performed at an academic center [5].

Patterns of Involvement

According to Berlinger et al. [8], there are five patterns of temporal bone involvement from malignant tumors: (1) isolated metastases from a distant primary tumor by hematogenous spread, (2) direct extension from a regional tumor, (3) direct meningeal extension from an intracranial primary tumor, (4) leptomeningeal extension, and (5) leukemic or lymphomatous infiltration. However, only three patterns of temporal bone involvement truly apply for metastatic disease to the temporal bone: (1) seeding of marrow spaces by hematogenous spread, (2) perineural spread, and (3) CSF dissemination leading to leptomeningeal spread [9].

P. W. Gidley, M.D., F.A.C.S. (✉) · M.-E. Nader, M.D., M.Sc.
Department of Head and Neck Surgery, The University of Texas M.D. Anderson Cancer Center, Houston, TX, USA
e-mail: pwgidley@mdanderson.org; mnader@mdanderson.org

The temporal bone has a rich blood supply but a sluggish blood flow that makes it a likely site for hematogenous seeding of tumor cells [8, 10–13]. The marrow spaces of the petrous apex supposedly filter out tumor cells in circulation, and the sluggish flow in the sinusoidal capillaries favors tumor cell deposition [7]. Clinically, these petrous apex metastases remain asymptomatic until tumor growth produces symptoms similar to mastoiditis [14, 15].

Perineural spread is a common finding in head and neck tumors, especially squamous cell carcinoma and adenoid cystic carcinoma (Fig. 15.1). Perineural extension via the facial nerve can involve the temporal bone from a parotid or cutaneous primary. Clinically, this spread of disease is signaled by facial weakness and paralysis. Isolated facial nerve branch deficit should immediately raise the suspicion for perineural disease. Bell's palsy that does not resolve with standard therapy should also raise the suspicion for perineural disease, especially in patients with a history of skin cancer.

Subarachnoid (leptomeningeal) spread is characterized by diffuse metastatic involvement of the pia and arachnoid [15]. This can lead to bilateral internal auditory canal involvement (Fig. 15.2).

Autopsy and Histopathologic Studies

The literature on temporal bone metastasis consists primarily of case reports or small case series [16]. Several studies have demonstrated temporal bone metastasis on autopsy studies [3, 5, 17–22]. Many of these patients had no symptoms related to the ear or hearing [23].

While these reports help to clarify the clinical presentation, larger postmortem studies have illuminated the pathophysiology of temporal bone metastasis. The incidence of temporal bone metastases is probably much higher than reported in the literature due to the lack of temporal bone histopathologic study on routine autopsy [6, 24].

Schuknect et al. (1968) reported the histopathologic results in ten patients and a literature review of an additional

P. W. Gidley, F. DeMonte (eds.), *Temporal Bone Cancer*, https://doi.org/10.1007/978-3-319-74539-8_15

63 cases of secondary malignancies of the temporal bone [7]. They reported that the breast, kidney, lung, stomach, and larynx were the most common sites for primary tumors. They observed that the otic capsule is relatively resistant to metastatic growth. They found that metastatic lesions are similar to the primary tumor but often less well differentiated [7].

Adams et al. (1971) reported on 15 patients with metastatic tumors in the temporal bone including the histopathologic features in six patients [25]. The petrous apex and osseous labyrinth were the most commonly involved areas. Although the otic capsule was involved in four cases, in no case did metastatic disease extend through the endosteum.

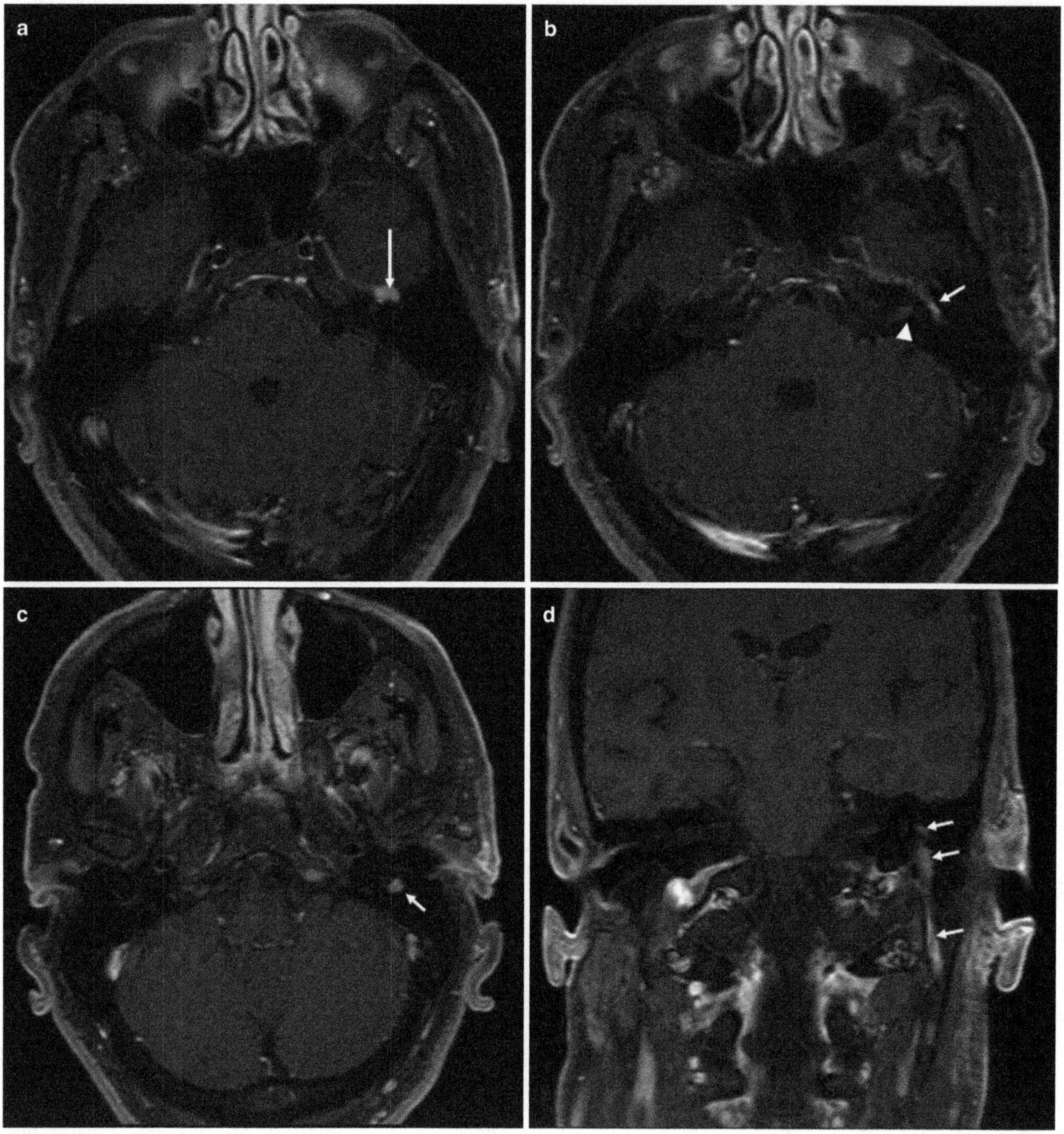

Fig. 15.1 Perineural spread along facial nerve. This 44-year-old man had a 5-year history of left "Bell's palsy" before a left parotid tumor was found. At parotidectomy, he was found to have an adenoid cystic carcinoma with tubular and cribriform patterns. (**a–c**) Contrast-enhanced axial T1 MRI. (**d**) Contrast-enhanced coronal T1 MRI. White arrows mark the course of the facial nerve. Triangle marks perineural disease along the facial nerve into the internal auditory canal

Hoshino et al. (1972) reported the pattern of inner ear involvement from a case of metastatic lung cancer [16]. This patient developed left facial nerve paralysis and right true vocal fold paralysis and bilateral hearing loss. She died 5 months after presentation, and at autopsy, leptomeningeal disease with bilateral internal auditory canal involvement was identified. Tumor cells infiltrated CNs VII and VIII. Metastatic cells were identified in the cochlea, while the vestibular organs were relatively spared except the singular nerve [16].

Jahn et al. (1979) examined 19 temporal bones from 11 patients with metastatic disease from a distant primary [26]. They observed that most of these metastases were occult (seven out of ten documented cases), that melanoma was a significant source of metastatic disease (three out of ten cases), and that clinical features correlated poorly with pathologic features. They attributed all metastases to just two distinct modes of spread: (1) hematogenous spread to the petrous apex, mastoid, middle ear, or external canal and (2) perineural spread to nerves in the IAC. They did not identify any case of leptomeningeal spread.

Saito et al. (1988) examined 47 temporal bones in patients who died of malignant tumors; 38% of these temporal bones had either metastasis or invasion [27]. Facial canal destruction was found in six patients; however, only half of these

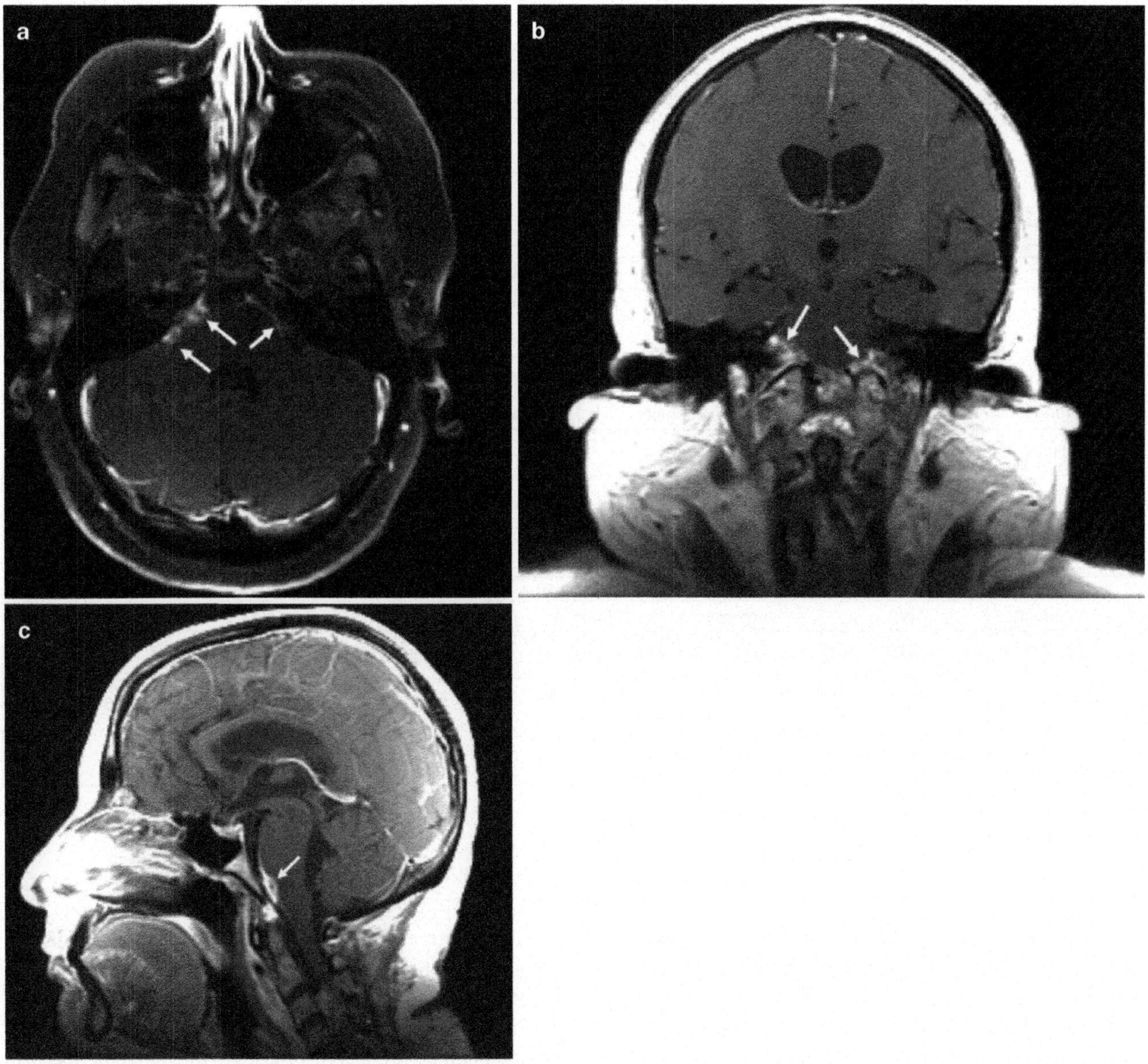

Fig. 15.2 Leptomeningeal spread. This 40-year-old woman presented with tinnitus and vertigo. She had a history of anaplastic ependymoma treated by surgical resection and craniospinal radiation 5 years earlier. Contrast-enhanced T1 MRI shows disease along the skull base. (**a**) Axial view at level of the IACs. (**b**) Coronal view through the IAC. (**c**) Midline sagittal view. (**d**) Audiogram

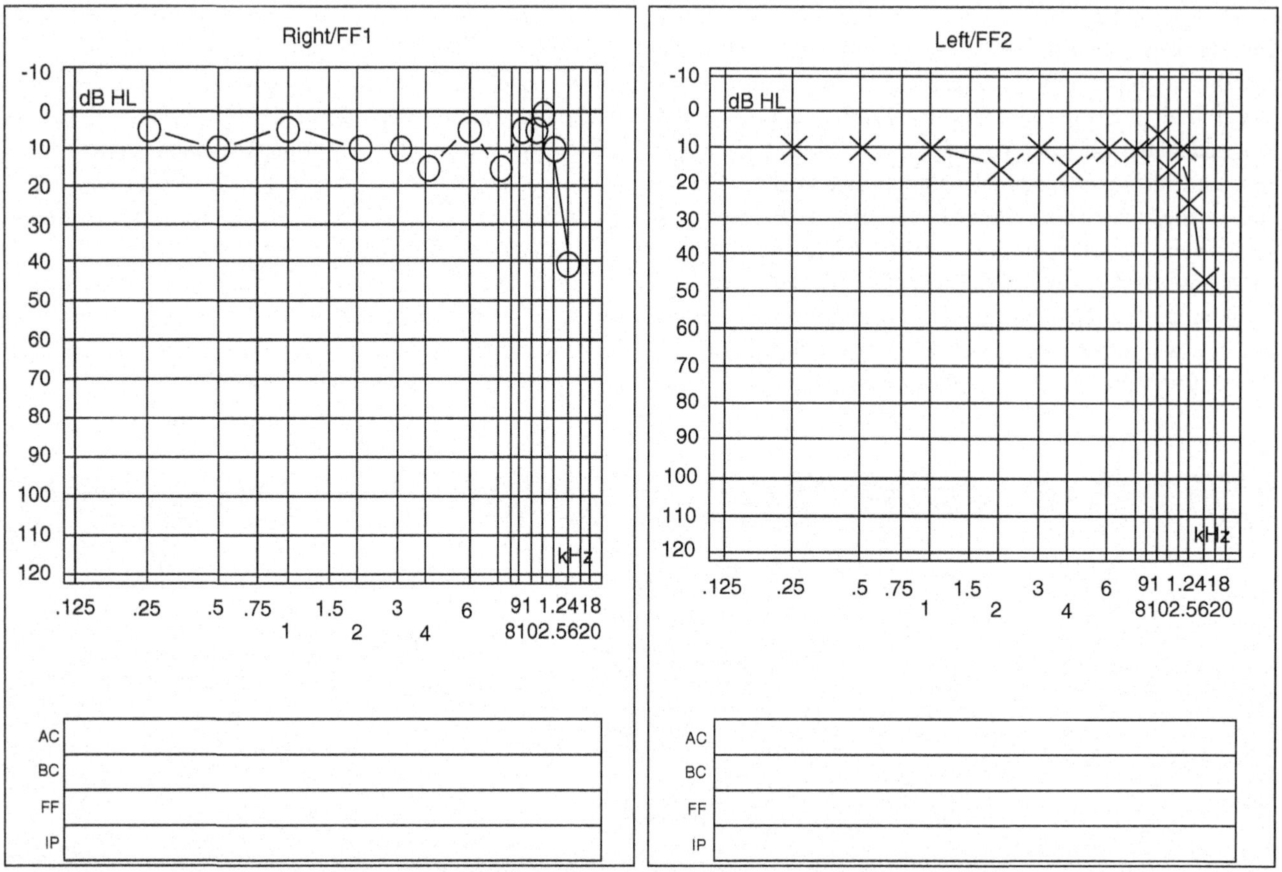

SRT PTA Right: - PTA Left: -					
Transducer	Test type	Intensity	Masking	Aided	ISF440 list
Right	HL	0			Spondee A
Left	HL	5			Spondee B

WR PTA Right: - PTA Left: -						
Transducer	WR	Intensity	Masking	Score	Aided	ISF440 List
Left	WR1	45		100		NU-6 LIST 1A
Right	WR1	45		100		NU-6 LIST 2A

Fig. 15.2 (continued)

patients had clinical facial paralysis. Facial paralysis occurred when the tumor cells invaded the nerve beyond the epineural sheath.

Nelson and Hinojosa (1991) evaluated 60 temporal bones in 33 patients with temporal bone metastases [11]. Bilateral metastases were found in 27 cases (82%). The breast was the most common primary tumor location (8/33). Only 10 out of 33 (30.3%) patients had otologic symptoms.

Gloria-Cruz et al. (2000) reported the largest study of temporal bone histopathologic findings on 212 patients with primary solid malignant neoplasm (i.e., lymphoma, leukemia, and multiple myeloma excluded) [5]. Forty-seven patients (76 temporal bones) had metastases to the temporal bone. All patients with temporal bone metastasis had metastasis in other body locations, indicating the systemic nature of the disease. These patients had 20 different primary tumors. In their series, breast, lung, prostate, melanoma, and cervical cancers were the most common sites of primary tumors. (There was only one case of renal cell carcinoma in their series of 212 patients, and this patient did not have a temporal bone metastasis.) Adenocarcinoma was the most common histopathological tumor type. Interestingly, squamous cell carcinoma of head and neck origin accounted for 8.5% of these patients. Bilateral temporal bone involvement was identified in 62% (29 patients). Of the 47 patients, 19 had hearing loss, 7 had vertigo or dizziness, 7 had facial asymmetry, and 17 patients (36%) had no otologic symptoms.

Yildirim-Baylan et al. (2011) reported a case of metastatic bladder cancer to both temporal bones. The patient had no otologic symptoms. Both temporal bones showed tumor infiltration of the petrous apex and the elastic layer of the internal carotid artery. One temporal bone also showed infiltration of the Eustachian tube, internal auditory canal, and tensor tympani muscle [23].

Histologic Tumor Types

Temporal bone metastases are most likely to come from tumors that have a predilection for bony metastasis. In a landmark study, Hill and Kohut reviewed the world literature in 1976 and compiled 102 cases of metastases to the temporal bone. They reported the breast, lung, kidney, stomach, and larynx as the most common primary sites for metastases to the temporal bone [24]. Breast cancer has a 56% rate for bone metastasis, renal cell carcinoma has a 33% rate, and lung cancer has a 20% rate [28]. Breast cancer makes up about 30% of the temporal bone metastasis, followed by lung cancer (11%) [29]. Nelson and Hinojosa compiled a list of metastatic temporal bone lesions from a comprehensive review of the literature: breast (31/148), lung (15/148), kidney (11/148), prostate (10/148), stomach (8/148), pharynx, and nasopharynx (6/148) [11]. According to Streitmann and Sistmanis, the six primary tumor sites account for more than 70% of temporal bone metastases: the breast (24.8%), lung (11.3%), kidney (9.2%), stomach (6.4%), bronchus (5.7%), and prostate (5.7%) [3, 13]. Gloria-Cruz et al. reported that breast, lung, prostate, melanoma, and cervical cancers were the most common sites of primary tumors [5].

Twenty-three cases of metastatic prostate cancer to the temporal bone have been reported [13, 30–33]. These metastases typically occur in the petrous apex.

Since laryngeal cancer is the most common head and neck tumor site, this tumor location accounts for the most temporal bone metastasis from a head and neck primary [34]. Two cases of hypopharyngeal squamous cell carcinoma have been reported with temporal bone metastases [35].

Rare tumors to have metastasis to the temporal bone include osteosarcoma of the tibia [36] and seminoma [30].

Clinical Presentation

The mechanism for otologic symptoms includes bony invasion producing Eustachian tube obstruction, compression of the nerves within the internal auditory canal, or direct invasion of the inner ear [37]. Hearing loss, otorrhea, otalgia, and facial paralysis are the most common symptoms for temporal bone metastasis [13, 38]; however, these signs are much more commonly associated with primary otologic disease, such as chronic otitis media. A high degree of suspicion must be maintained when examining a patient with a past history of malignant disease and these symptoms.

The metastatic lesion to the temporal bone can also be the presenting sign of underlying, undiagnosed cancer. Maddox reported four cases of metastatic temporal bone involvement initially diagnosed as mastoiditis, and in each case, the temporal bone metastasis was the presenting sign of a distant primary tumor [6]. Multiple cases have been reported where the temporal bone metastasis or otologic symptom was the presenting symptom or sign of a metastatic cancer [1, 32, 33, 37–39]. In cases where otologic symptoms were the presenting symptoms of metastatic disease, patient demise often quickly followed [15, 22, 40–42].

Overall, hearing loss is the most common sign of metastatic lesion (Fig. 15.3) [3, 37]. Rapidly progressive and sudden hearing losses have been reported with metastatic involvement of the internal auditory canal. Return of hearing has been reported in one case following radiotherapy to the IAC [3].

Facial paralysis that does not respond to medical therapy requires further evaluation with either CT or MRI (Fig. 15.4). Facial paralysis and ear pain are an especially worrisome combination for malignant disease, and this symptom cluster has been described as the presenting sign of widely metastatic lung cancer, breast cancer, and hepatocellular carcinoma [4, 39, 43, 44].

The incidence of facial paralysis with metastatic lesions to the temporal bone has been reported in 15–50% of patients [4–7]. Metastatic tumors have been described as involving the facial canal throughout its mastoid portion [45]. Other research has reported that the facial nerve is equally involved in the mastoid and intralabyrinthine segments [5]. Roughly only half of those patients who were found at autopsy to have facial nerve involvement had clinical facial paralysis [27]. In order to manifest facial paralysis clinically, the tumor invasion must be beyond the epineural sheath [5, 27, 45].

Weiss et al. reported two cases of facial nerve involvement in patients with metastatic adenocarcinoma (Fig. 15.5) [46]. Facial paralysis from temporal bone metastasis has been reported 1 year after treatment for uroendothelial bladder cancer [47].

Generally, cranial nerve involvement is a sign of poor prognosis, with average survival of only about 6 months

[12, 48]. Cranial nerves V, VI, and XII are the most common nerves involved [41, 49]. Isolated cases of temporal bone metastasis have been reported causing multiple cranial nerve deficits (Fig. 15.6) [1, 39]. When patients present with deficits of the facial nerve or lower cranial nerves, metastatic lesions have been mistaken for paraganglioma and schwannoma [50, 51].

While many clinical signs can point to temporal bone metastasis, perhaps as many as 40% of patients with metastasis to the temporal bone are asymptomatic [5, 8, 23, 52, 53].

Metastatic lesions to the temporal bone have been reported many years after the original primary tumor was diagnosed and treated. Metastatic prostate cancer has been reported more than 10 years after diagnosis in three cases [13]. Breast metastasis to the skull base producing vertigo has been reported as late as 33 years after original diagnosis [54].

Sites of Involvement

The most common sites for metastasis to the temporal bone are the petrous portion (83%), internal auditory canal (28%), and mastoid process (28%), followed by the middle ear (21%) and facial nerve (20%) [5, 53, 55]. Multiple sites of invasion occur in roughly a quarter of cases [3]. Metastatic involvement of pneumatized spaces of the temporal bone is unusual from hematogenous spread but can be involved from direct extension [24].

In patients with widely metastatic cancer, the symptoms of temporal bone metastases can be overshadowed by much more disabling problems [24]. This might account for the much higher incidence of temporal bone metastasis in autopsy series than has been reported in purely clinical studies.

External Ear

External ear canal metastasis is very rare; perhaps only a dozen or so cases have been reported (Fig. 15.7) [40, 55, 56]. When the external ear canal is involved, symptoms such as hearing loss, pressure, and bleeding provoke patients to seek medical attention quickly. The most common primary site has been reported as the kidney followed by the esophagus. An external auditory canal tumor was reported as the presenting sign of metastatic bronchogenic carcinoma in one case [55]. Metastatic small cell lung cancer has been reported to cause external auditory canal metastasis [57]. Two cases of metastatic hepatocellular carcinoma to the ear canal and TM have been reported [40, 58]. Yasumatsu et al. described

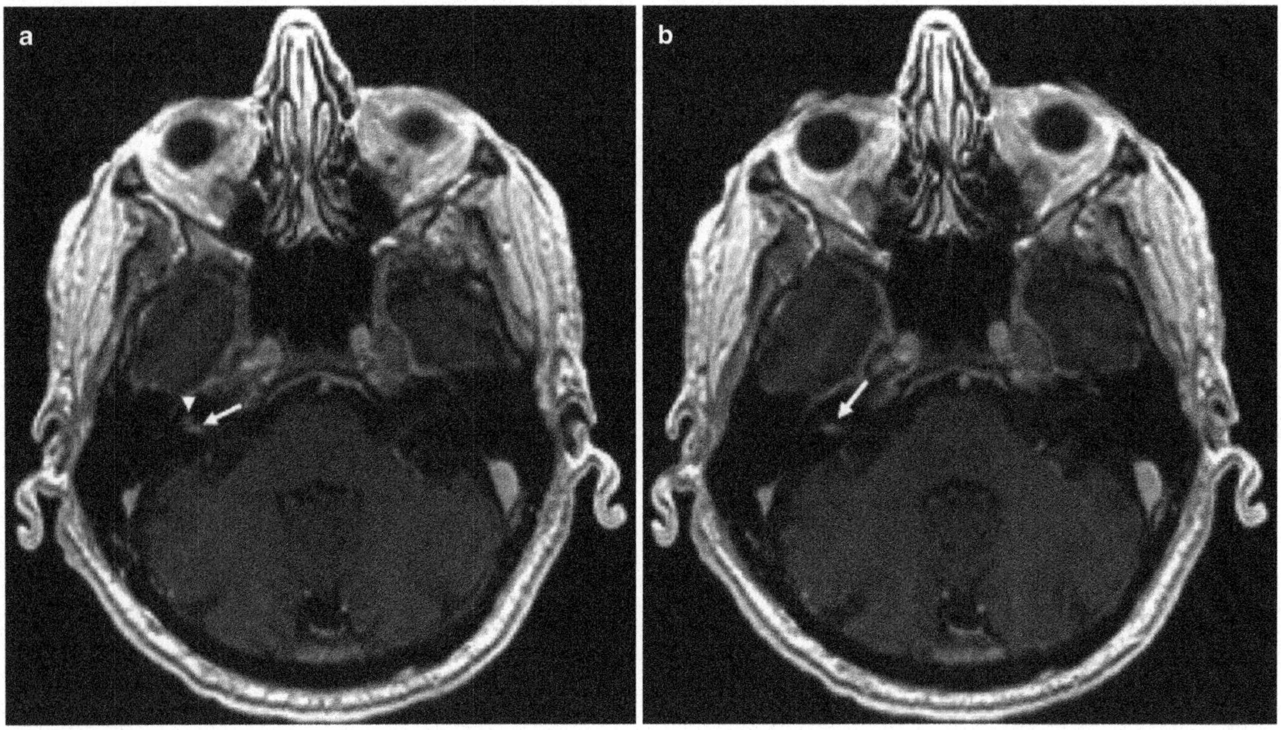

Fig. 15.3 Metastatic adenocarcinoma of the lung to the right IAC and cochlea. This 65-year-old man presented with a 4-month history of progressive right-sided hearing loss and tinnitus. He was diagnosed with metastatic adenocarcinoma of the lung 6 months earlier. (**a, b**) Contrast-enhanced high-resolution axial T1 MRI. Triangle shows disease in the cochlea, and arrow shows disease in the IAC. (**c**) Audiogram showing profound hearing loss in the right ear. This patient had multiple cranial nerve deficits (left CN-V and right CN-X) along with hearing loss. He died 9 months later

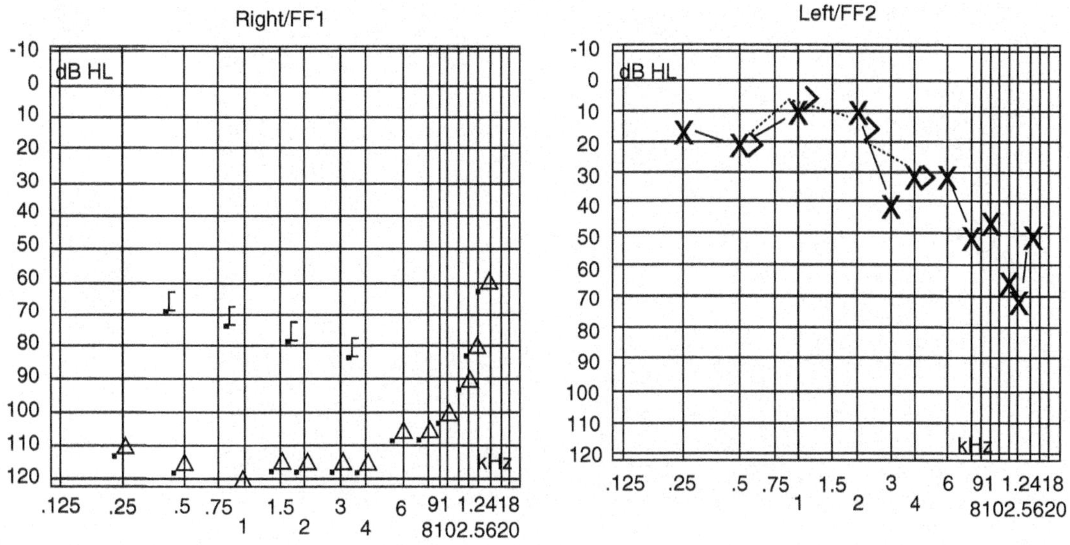

	Right
AC	40 70 70 60 60 60 60 60 60 40 40
BC	85 65 70 65
FF	
IP	

	Left
AC	
BC	
FF	
IP	

SRT PTA Right: - PTA Left:-					
Transducer	Test type	Intensity	Masking	Aided	ISF440 list
Left	HL	15			Spondee A
Right	HL	NR			Spondee B

WR PTA Right: - PTA Left: -						
Transducer	WR	Intensity	Masking	Score	Aided	ISF440 List
Left	WR1	55		100		NU-6 LIST 1A

Fig. 15.3 (continued)

a case of hepatocellular carcinoma to the external auditory canal (EAC) that presented with a protuberant, bleeding tumor and was treated with surgical debulking followed by postoperative intracavitary irradiation [40]. Metastatic melanoma has also been described to produce external auditory canal metastasis (Fig. 15.8) [59].

Middle Ear

Middle ear involvement by metastatic lesion can produce signs and symptoms confused with chronic otitis media and mastoiditis [60, 61]. Lan et al. reported a case of metastatic breast cancer that presented with right-sided otalgia, otorrhea, and facial paralysis. CT scan showed soft tissue density within the mastoid [4].

Mastoid

Given its relatively poor supply, the mastoid is rarely involved by hematogenous spread of malignancy. When involved, however, the air cell system gives little resistance to the rapid spread of tumor. Mastoid involvement usually leads to symptoms of hearing loss, aural fullness, and pain, and these symptoms prompt medical evaluation.

Petrous Apex

The petrous apex is the most common site of metastatic spread in the temporal bone (Fig. 15.9). In their series, Gloria-Cruz et al. reported that the petrous apex was the only site of metastasis in 31% [5]. The petrous apex has

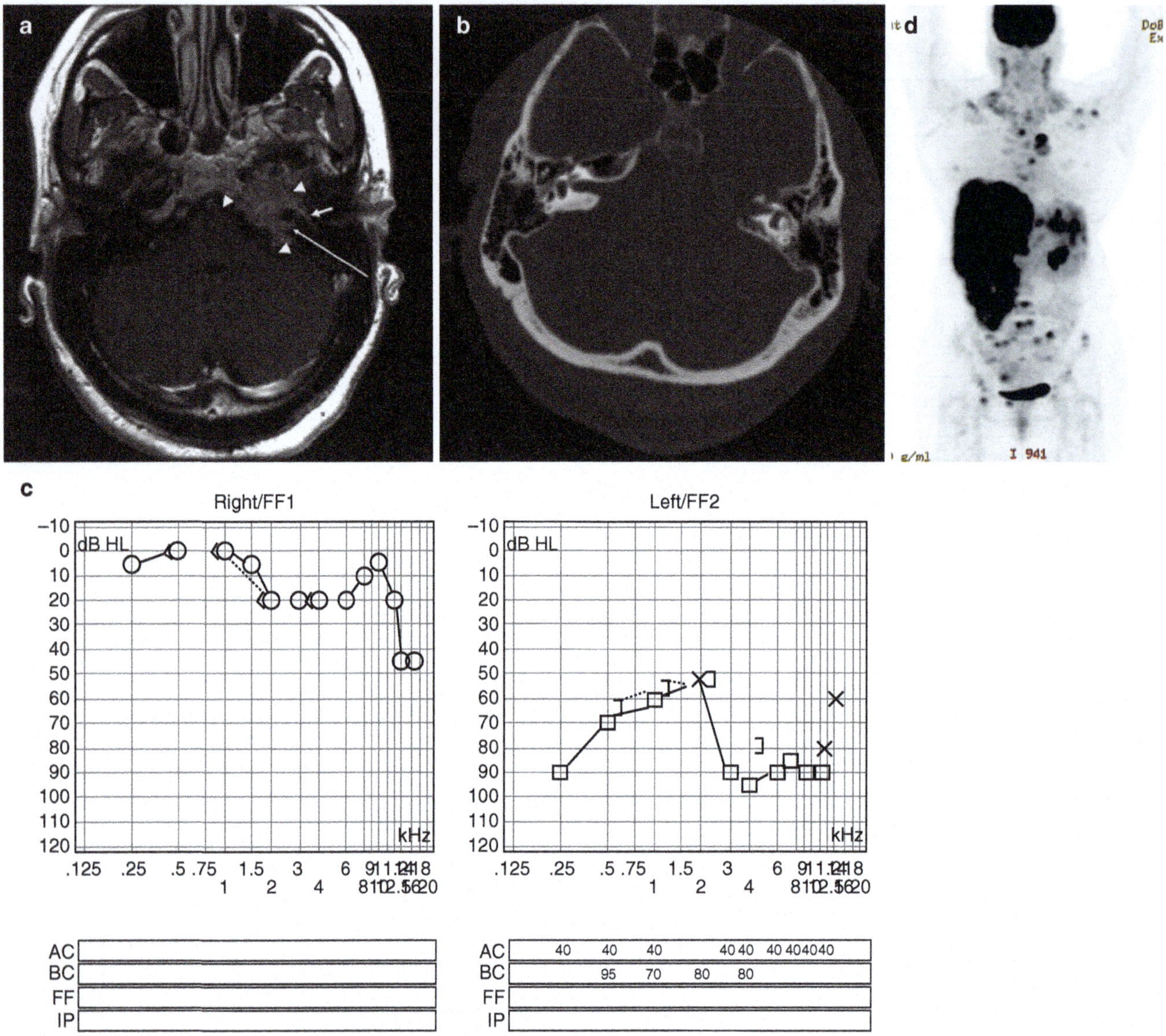

SRT PTA Right:- PTA Left:-

Transducer	Test type	Intensity	Masking	Aided	ISF440 List
Right	HL	0			N/A
Left	HL	65	35		N/A

WR PTA Right:- PTA Left:-

Transducer	WR	Intensity	Masking	Score	Aided	ISF440 List
Right	WR1	40		96		N/A
Left	WR1	90	60	92		N/A

Fig. 15.4 Facial paralysis as presenting complaint for widespread metastatic breast cancer. This 50-year-old woman presented with left facial paralysis and dizziness. She had ignored a left breast mass for 2 years. (**a**) Contrast-enhanced MRI showing extensive left petrous apex involvement (surrounded by triangles). Long white arrow shows disease in the IAC, short fat arrow shows disease in the tympanic segment of the facial nerve. (**b**) CT scan at roughly the same level as MRI showing osteolytic changes in the petrous apex from tumor. (**c**) Audiogram showing moderate to profound hearing loss in the left ear, yet word recognition scores are preserved. (**d**) PET image showing widespread metastases

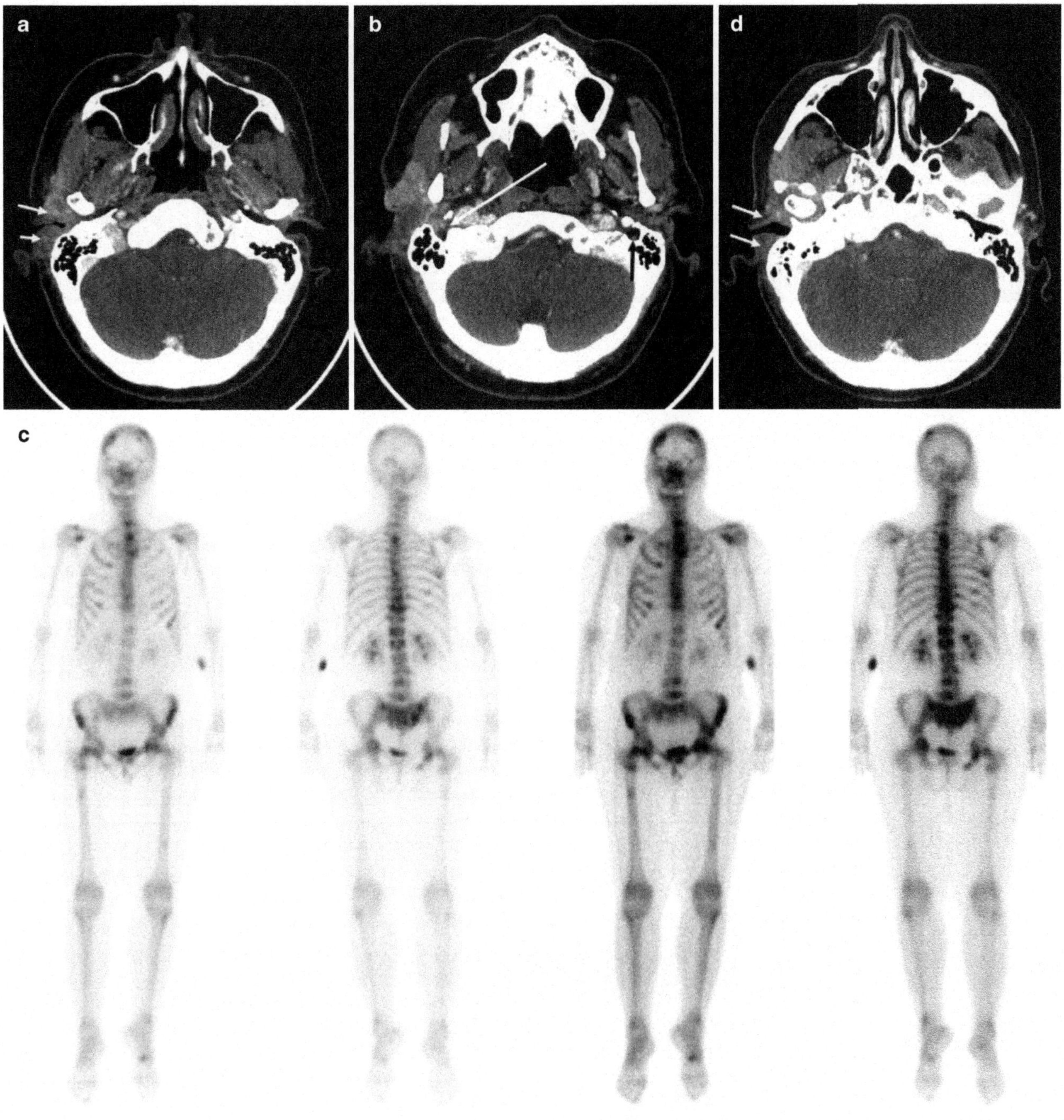

Fig. 15.5 This 63-year-old woman was referred for right facial paralysis and a right ear canal tumor, which was initially interpreted as adenocarcinoma (**a**). (**b**) CT shows tumor at the stylomastoid foramen. Further history revealed a right breast cancer, and biopsy of the breast revealed a high-grade invasive ductal carcinoma, high nuclear grade, and Nottingham histologic grade 3. (**c**) Whole-body bone scan showed diffuse bone metastases. (**d**) CT scan 7 months after starting letrozole, showing resolution of disease around the right ear canal. She lived for another 5 years

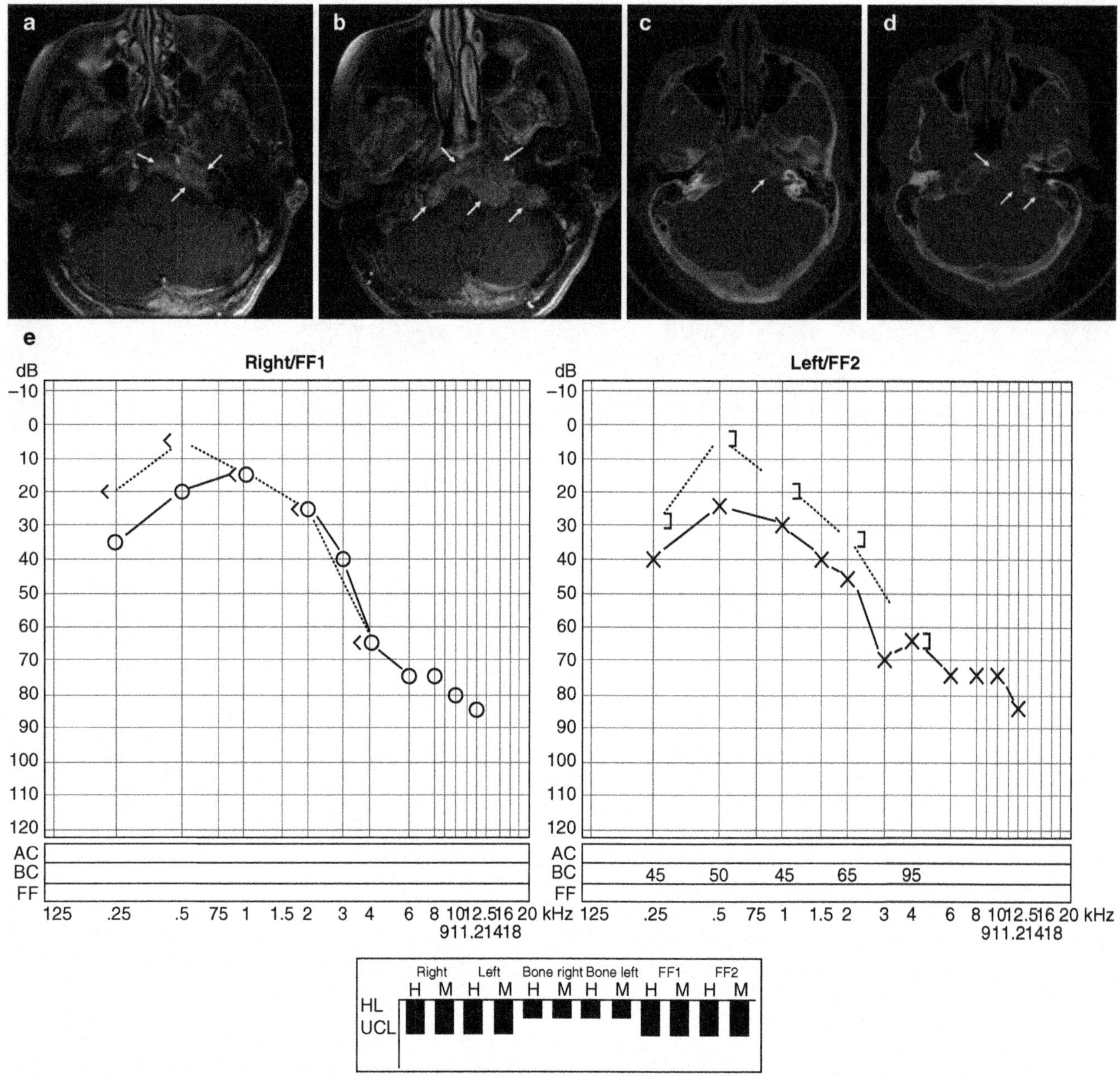

SRT Right/Masking/UCL						SRT Left/Masking/UCL						SRT FF1	SRT FF2
AC			BC			AC			BC			FF	FF
25dB						35dB							

SDS % / Right / Masking						SDS % / Left / Masking						SDS % / FF1		SDS % / FF2	
AC			BC			AC			BC			FF		FF	
96%	60dB					96%	75dB								

Fig. 15.6 Metastatic lung cancer presenting with lower cranial nerve deficits. This 72-year-old woman with a distant history of cervical cancer, presented with a 3-month history of hoarseness and tinnitus. On examination, she was found to have a left CN IX, X, and XII deficit. CT-guided lung biopsy found small cell carcinoma. (**a**, **b**) Contrast-enhanced T1 MRI, arrows outline metastatic lesion in the skull base. (**c**, **d**) CT scan of the same level as MRI. (**e**) Audiogram showing left-sided mild sloping to severe mixed hearing loss. (**f**) Whole-body bone scan showing extensive bony metastatic disease. She refused any treatment and died 12 months later

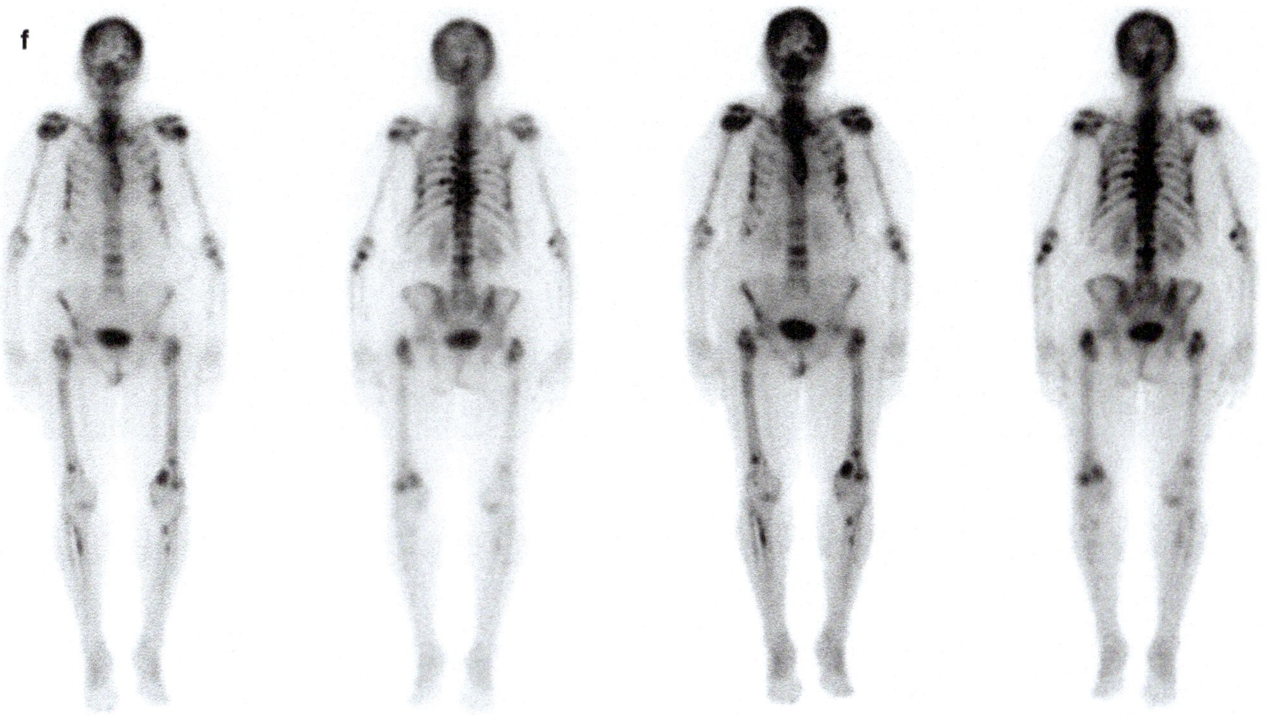

Fig. 15.6 (continued)

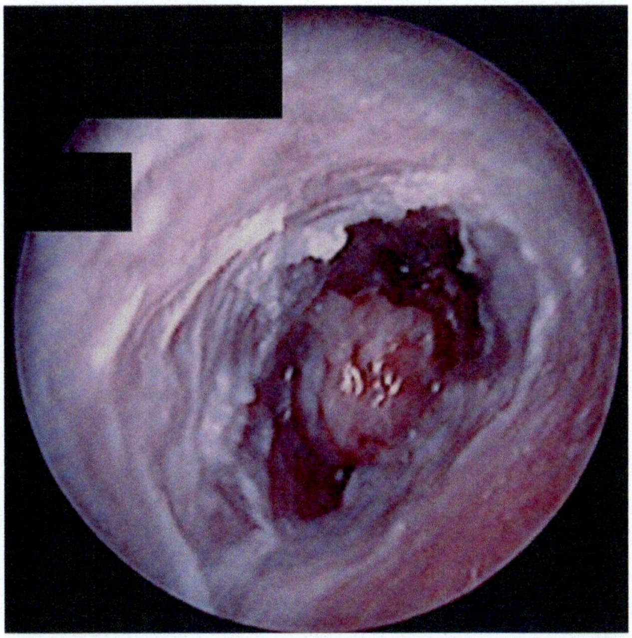

Fig. 15.7 Metastatic squamous cell carcinoma to the right external auditory canal and middle ear 8 months after treatment from an oral cavity primary

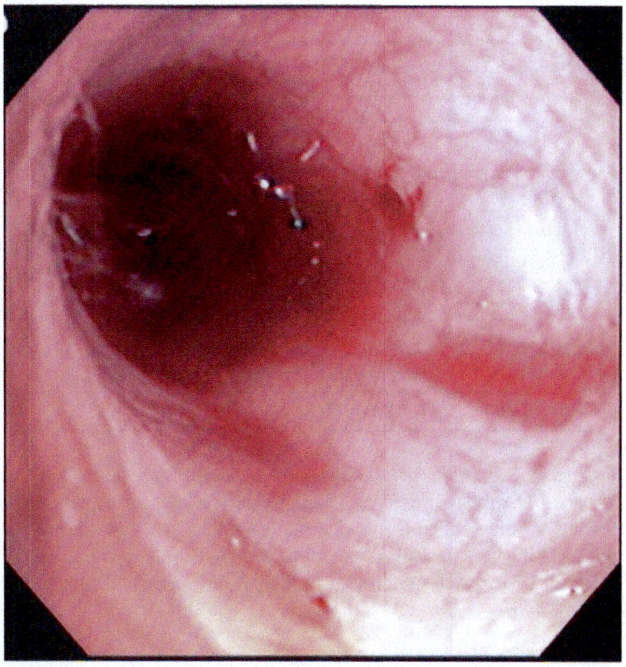

Fig. 15.8 Otoendoscopic photograph of metastatic melanoma to the external auditory canal

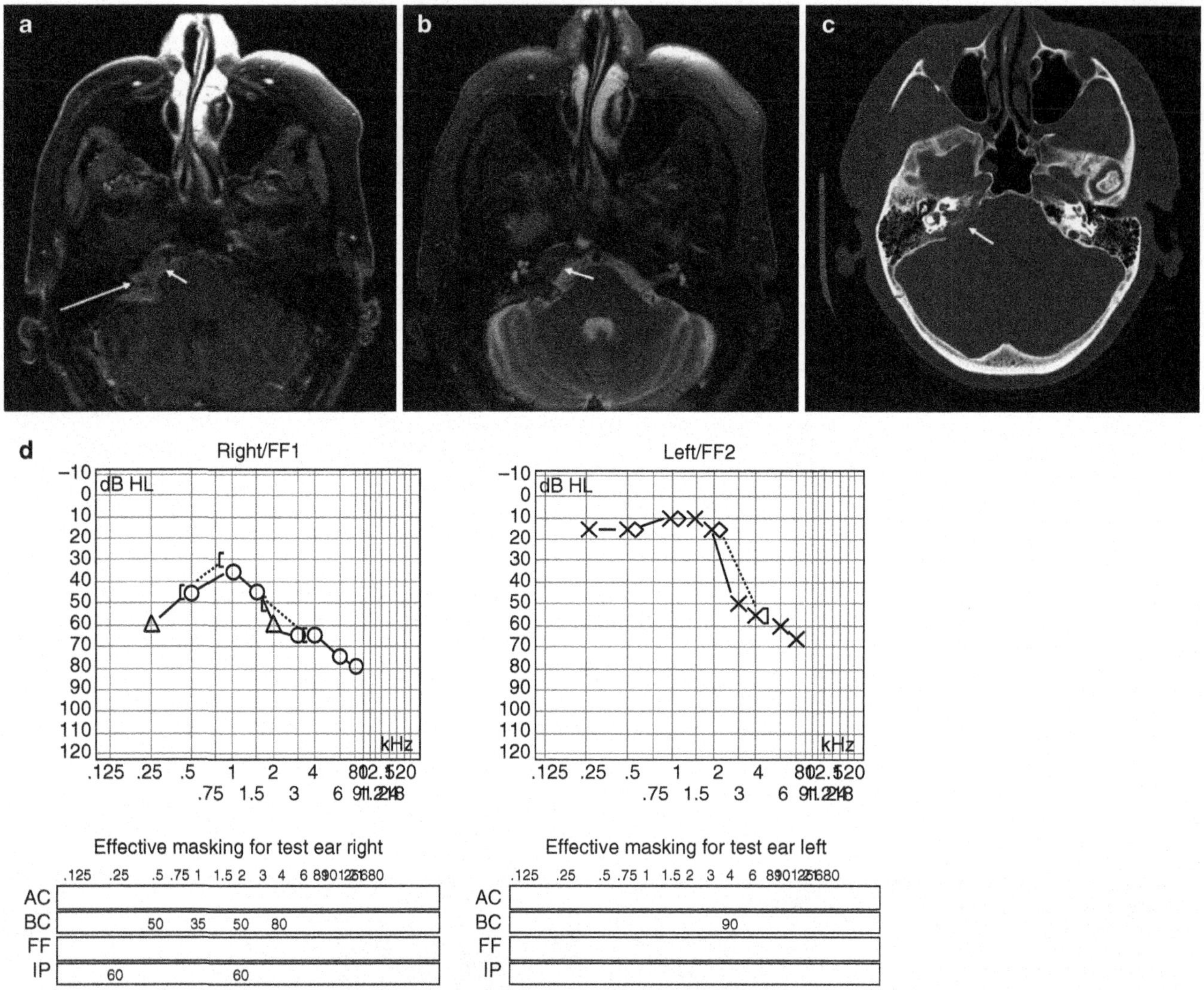

SRT PTA Right: 46.7 PTA Left: 13.3

Transducer	Test type	Intensity	Masking	Aided	Binaural	ISF440 List
Insert Right	HL	45	25			Spondee B
Insert Left	HL	15	--			Spondee A

WR PTA Right: 46.7 PTA Left: 13.3

Transducer	WR	Intensity	Masking	Score	Aided	Binaural	ISF440 List
Insert Right	WR1	85	45	60			NU-6 LIST 2A
Insert Left	WR1	55		100			NU-6 LIST 1A

Fig. 15.9 Metastatic breast cancer to the right temporal bone. This 78-year-old woman presented with a 1-year history of dizziness and a feeling of being pulled to one side while walking. She later developed tinnitus and hearing loss in the right ear. (**a**) Contrast-enhanced T1 MRI; short arrow shows disease in the petrous apex, and long arrow shows disease in the IAC. (**b**) T2 MRI; arrow shows interface between tumor and CSF. (**c**) Non-contrast axial CT of the temporal bone shows destruction of the petrous apex (arrow). (**d**) Audiogram showing asymmetric sensorineural hearing loss. This lesion was biopsied through a retrolabyrinthine approach, and her remaining hearing was preserved

bone marrow that is fed by a slow-flow capillary network, and for this reason, it is more commonly involved than the mastoid or internal auditory canals [13, 38, 62, 63]. Furthermore, petrous apex lesions remain asymptomatic until they reach the mastoid. For this reason, temporal bone metastases are relatively silent and clinically very rare. The bony labyrinth appears to be resistant to metastatic involvement, indicating that sensorineural hearing loss in the setting of metastasis is usually from direct nerve involvement.

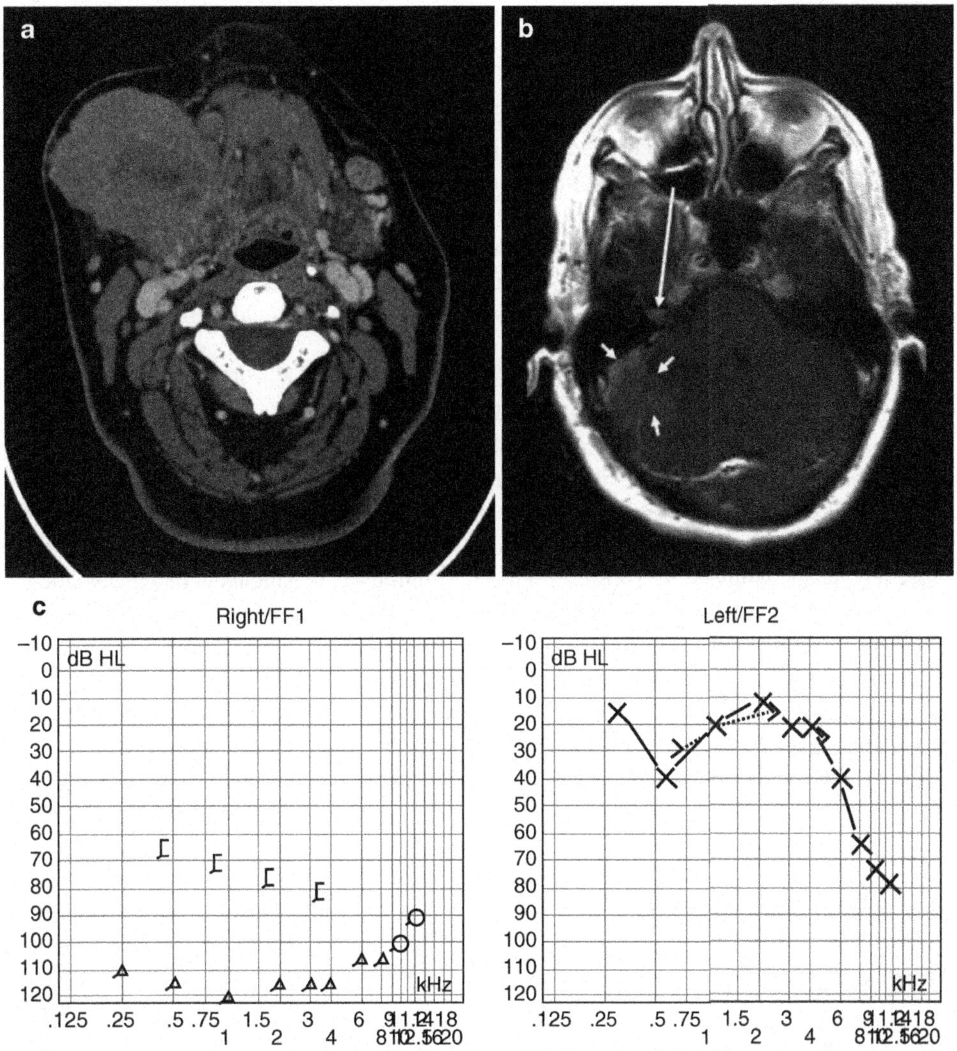

	Right		Left
AC	45 65 60 60 6060 6060	AC	
BC	85 65 65 65	BC	
FF		FF	
IP		IP	

SRT PTA Right:- PTA Left:-

Transducer	Test type	Intensity	Masking	Aided	ISF440 List
Left	HL	10			
Right	HL	90	60	No Response	

WR PTA Right:- PTA Left:-

Transducer	WR	Intensity	Masking	Score	Aided	ISF440 List
Left	WR1	50		100		

Fig. 15.10 Metastatic neuroendocrine carcinoma to the cerebellopontine angle. This 59-year-old woman presented with a right neck mass. (**a**) Contrast-enhanced CT of the neck showing right submandibular tumor at presentation. This mass was biopsied and found to be neuroendocrine carcinoma. She was treated with induction chemotherapy of cisplatin and etoposide followed by concurrent cisplatin and etoposide and radiation therapy. She had complete remission from this disease, until 1 year later when she presented with dizziness, gait disturbance, nausea, and vomiting. (**b**) Contrast-enhanced T1 MRI showing cerebellar (small arrows) and IAC metastasis (long arrow). (**c**) Audiogram showing profound hearing loss in the right ear. A suboccipital craniotomy was performed to resect the cerebellar tumor. She was then treated with whole-brain radiation (30 Gy). She died 3 months later

Cerebellopontine Angle

Brackmann and Bartels defined the presenting signs and symptoms that should make a clinician suspect metastatic lesion to the cerebellopontine angle (CPA). These signs include rapid hearing loss, headache, and lower cranial nerve findings in a patient with a previous diagnosis of malignancy [64]. Lung cancer is the most common source of CPA metastasis, followed by breast, gastrointestinal, and melanoma (Fig. 15.10) [65].

Internal Auditory Canal

Internal auditory canal involvement has been reported in 18–28% of cases of metastatic disease to the temporal bone, with bilateral IAC involvement occurring in about half of patients [3]. In older publications, carcinomatous involvement of the internal auditory canal has been called *otitis interna carcinomatosa* [42]. These metastases can appear as solitary metastasis, bilateral IAC metastasis, or associated with leptomeningeal disease. Facial paralysis and sudden hearing loss are common findings [41, 66]. IAC metastases were associated with brain metastases in 25% and meningeal carcinomatosis in 36% of cases [3]. Fewer than 1% of hepatocellular carcinoma (HCC) metastases involve the skull, but HCC characteristically involves the temporal bone as IAC metastases [40, 41].

The symptoms of bilateral internal auditory canal metastases are facial paralysis in 100%, progressive tinnitus in more than 50%, and sudden hearing loss in about 20% of cases [3]. Hearing loss is asymmetric and progressive. Bilateral internal auditory canal masses have been reported in colon cancer [67], pancreatic adenocarcinoma [15, 22, 68], and melanoma [69, 70]. Bilateral temporal bone metastases have been described in one case of uterine cervical cancer [20].

Diagnostic Investigation

Laboratory Studies

Calcium, alkaline phosphatase, lactate dehydrogenase (LDH), and liver function tests can be useful in identifying patients with widely metastatic disease; however, for the patient with an isolated temporal bone lesion, these tests are likely to be unrevealing [13, 47]. Prostate-specific antigen (PSA) should be tested in patients with a prior history of prostate cancer, and increasing PSA levels usually correlate to larger tumor volumes.

CSF Studies

CSF cytology studies are important in the evaluation of leptomeningeal disease. The hallmark of leptomeningeal disease is multiple cranial nerve deficits, usually anatomically disparate nerves.

Open Biopsy and Surgery

Imaging studies can indicate the diagnosis of a metastatic lesion, especially in cases where other metastatic disease has been identified, but in cases with only one metastasis, the diagnosis depends on histologic confirmation.

In the setting of multiple metastases, open biopsy does not have a role, since the diagnosis is usually obvious or other metastasis than the temporal bone lesion might be more accessible. However, if imaging does not disclose other metastasis or if there is not a prior diagnosis of cancer or an obvious primary tumor, then open biopsy via a transcanal, transtympanic, transmastoid, or transtemporal approach is indicated. Biopsy should be performed through the least morbid approach.

The goal of surgery for a metastatic lesion is different than when a primary temporal bone tumor is encountered. Generally, the most direct approach that will provide an adequate tissue is taken to avoid additional morbidity (see case description in Fig. 15.9). Frozen section is performed on biopsies to try to provide a diagnosis and to assure that adequate tissue has been obtained for special studies. Given that patients with a metastatic lesion have systemic disease, gross total tumor resection is generally not the goal.

Audiometric and Vestibular Evaluation

Audiometry is indicated in any patient with hearing loss, tinnitus, vertigo, or facial paralysis. Sensorineural, conductive, and mixed hearing loss patterns can be seen with metastatic disease. Asymmetric hearing loss, especially with impaired word recognition, can be seen with metastasis [13]. When available, previous audiograms should be sought out and compared to the present testing to determine if the hearing loss is progressing rapidly.

Radiographic Evaluation

Since most of the temporal bone is not amenable to direct inspection, cross-sectional imaging is essential for the diagnosis and management of lesions occurring therein. An osteolytic lesion in the temporal bone should raise the suspicion of malignancy, and a metastatic lesion should be included in the differential diagnosis. CT scan is useful in evaluating patients that present with symptoms similar to Eustachian tube dysfunction or mastoiditis. CT can demonstrate the extent of bony destruction due to a metastatic lesion. Asymmetric hearing loss is often evaluated by contrast-enhanced MRI, and it can be very useful in diagnosing metastatic lesion or leptomeningeal disease.

Temporal bone tumors are rare, and a broad differential diagnosis should be entertained. Primary temporal bone cancer, paraganglioma, chondrosarcoma, chordoma, plasmacytoma or multiple myeloma, endolymphatic sac tumor, and metastatic tumor should be considered in the differential. Metastatic lesions (from thyroid, breast, renal cell, and hepatocellular carcinomas) have been confused for paraganglioma and schwannoma on clinical examination (pulsating, retrotympanic mass), MRI, and CT scan [21, 50, 51, 71]. An accurate history or identifying a second tumor helps to rule out these benign pathologies [51].

The development of whole-body PET/CT has been useful to identify metastatic disease. This study has permitted a rapid means of identifying systemic disease, and it has made the identification of possible primary tumors where previously a biopsy of the temporal bone lesion might be required for diagnosis.

Technetium-99m scintigraphy bone scan can be helpful when only skeletal metastasis is suspected, i.e., prostate cancer or breast cancer. As shown in many of the case histories attached, whole-body bone scanning can be very useful and less costly than PET/CT to diagnose systemic disease.

Treatment

For the patient with temporal bone metastasis, the treatment is palliative. Surgery, chemotherapy, or radiotherapy might be indicated depending on the clinical scenario. Most lesions are beyond surgical excision, and radiotherapy is given for local control [47, 54]. With newer chemotherapy regimens, some patients are able to enjoy significant life spans after diagnosis (see case depicted in Fig. 15.5).

Conclusion

Metastatic lesions to the temporal bone are relatively rare in clinical practice, but the temporal bone is often found to be involved by metastatic disease in autopsy studies. Breast, lung, prostate, melanoma, kidney, and stomach cancers are the most likely primary tumors to produce temporal bone metastases. Hearing loss, otorrhea, vertigo, and facial paralysis are the most common symptoms of temporal bone metastasis; however, a large proportion of metastatic lesions to the temporal bone are asymptomatic. The most common site for metastatic involvement is the petrous portion of the temporal bone, which is clinically silent until neurologic deficit or mastoid invasion occurs. In the patient with a history of malignant disease, the differential diagnosis should include metastasis when patients present with otologic complaints. Diagnostic imaging with CT and MRI gives an excellent appreciation of disease within the temporal bone. PET/CT or whole-body bone scan help identify systemic disease. Open biopsy is required in only a paucity of cases. Surgical resection of metastatic disease in the temporal bone is not warranted because temporal bone metastases are usually a sign of widespread metastatic disease.

References

1. Bakhos D, Chenebaux M, Lescanne E, Lauvin M-A, Cormier B, Robier A. Two cases of temporal bone metastases as presenting sign of lung cancer. Eur Ann Otorhinolaryngol Head Neck Dis. 2012;129(1):54–7.
2. Yoda S, Cureoglu S, Paparella MM. Pulmonary carcinoma metastasis to the internal auditory canal. Otol Neurotol. 2011;32(6):e48.
3. Streitmann MJ, Sismanis A. Metastatic carcinoma of the temporal bone. Am J Otol. 1996;17(5):780–3.
4. Lan M-Y, Shiao A-S, Li W-Y. Facial paralysis caused by metastasis of breast carcinoma to the temporal bone. J Chin Med Assoc. 2004;67(11):587–90.
5. Gloria-Cruz TI, Schachern PA, Paparella MM, Adams GL, Fulton SE. Metastases to temporal bones from primary nonsystemic malignant neoplasms. Arch Otolaryngol Head Neck Surg. 2000;126(2):209–14.
6. Maddox HE 3rd. Metastatic tumors of the temporal bone. Ann Otol Rhinol Laryngol. 1967;76(1):149–65.
7. Schuknecht HF, Allam AF, Murakami Y. Pathology of secondary malignant tumors of the temporal bone. Ann Otol Rhinol Laryngol. 1968;77(1):5–22.
8. Berlinger NT, Koutroupas S, Adams G, Maisel R. Patterns of involvement of the temporal bone in metastatic and systemic malignancy. Laryngoscope. 1980;90:619–27.
9. Deroee AF, Joglekar S, Paparella MM. Malignant melanoma metastasis to temporal bone. Otol Neurotol. 2009;30(2):248–9.
10. Proctor B, Lindsay JR. Tumors involving the petrous pyramid of the temporal bone. Arch Otolaryngol. 1947;46:180–94.
11. Nelson EG, Hinojosa R. Histopathology of metastatic temporal bone tumors. Arch Otolaryngol Head Neck Surg. 1991;117(2):189–93.
12. Laigle-Donadey F, Taillibert S, Martin-Duverneuil N, Hildebrand J, Delattre J-Y. Skull-base metastases. J Neurooncol. 2005;75(1):63–9.
13. Faucett EA, Richins H, Khan R, Jacob A. Metastatic prostate cancer to the left temporal bone: a case report and review of the literature. Case Rep Otolaryngol. 2015;2015:250312.
14. Kedjanyi WK, Bath AP, Ball RY, Hosni AA, Wickstead M. Metastatic adenocarcinoma of the temporal bone. J Laryngol Otol. 1994;108(8):710–2.
15. Wu C, Kaga K, Ohira Y, Suzuki J. Histopathology of multiple temporal bone metastasis from pancreatic adenocarcinoma: a case showing bilateral hearing loss and Bechterew's phenomenon. Otolaryngol Head Neck Surg. 2000;122(4):613–5.
16. Hoshino T, Hiraide F, Nomura Y. Metastatic tumour of the inner ear: a histopathological report. J Laryngol Otol. 1972;86(7):697–707.
17. Kumagami H. Cases of malignant lymphosarcoma metastasizing into the temporal bone. Jibiinkoka. 1971;43(8):579–82.
18. Janczewski G, Fujita S. Metastasis of prostatic adenocarcinoma to the temporal bone. Otolaryngol Pol. 1972;26(1):81–5.
19. Sienkiewicz H, Berezowski S. Neoplastic metastases to the temporal bone. Otolaryngol Pol. 1974;28(5):585–90.
20. Katsarkas A, Seemayer TA. Bilateral temporal bone metastases of a uterine cervix carcinoma. J Otolaryngol. 1976;5(4):315–8.
21. Sasaki J, Katoh N, Ishida M, Yoshida H, Mori S, Satoh M, et al. A case of thyroid carcinoma with temporal bone metastasis. Gan No Rinsho. 1984;30(2):162–6.
22. Ohira Y, Kaga K, Kodama A. A case of bilateral sudden hearing loss and vertigo caused by bilateral temporal bone metastasis from pancreatic carcinoma—comparison of clinical findings and temporal bone pathological findings. Nippon Jibiinkoka Gakkai Kaiho. 1991;94(1):9–15.
23. Yildirim-Baylan M, Erdogmus N, Cureoglu S, Paparella MM. Bladder cancer metastases to the temporal bone. Otol Neurotol. 2011;32(5):e40–e1.
24. Hill BA, Kohut RI. Metastatic adenocarcinoma of the temporal bone. Arch Otolaryngol. 1976;102(9):568–71.

25. Adams GL, Paparella MM, el-Fiky FM. Primary and metastatic tumors of the temporal bone. Laryngoscope. 1971;81(8):1273–85.
26. Jahn AF, Farkashidy J, Berman JM. Metastatic tumors in the temporal bone—a pathophysiologic study. J Otolaryngol. 1979;8(1):85–95.
27. Saito H, Chinzei K, Furuta M. Pathological features of peripheral facial paralysis caused by malignant tumour. Acta Otolaryngol Suppl. 1988;446:165–71.
28. Robbins SL, editor. Pathology. 4th ed. Philadelphia: WB Saunders; 1972.
29. Cumberworth V, Friedmann I, Glover G. Late metastasis of breast carcinoma to the external auditory canal. J Laryngol Otol. 1994;108(09):808–10.
30. Kobayashi K, Igarashi M, Ohashi K, McBride RA. Metastatic seminoma of the temporal bone. Arch Otolaryngol Head Neck Surg. 1986;112(1):102–5.
31. Grubbe Gregersen K, Hansen S. Metastasis to the temporal bone may cause acute peripheral vestibular syndrome and impaired hearing. Ugeskr Laeger. 2013;175(22):1576–7.
32. Sahin AA, Ro JY, Ordonez NG, Luna MA, Weber RS, Ayala AG. Temporal bone involvement by prostatic adenocarcinoma: report of two cases and review of the literature. Head Neck. 1991;13(4):349–54.
33. Dogan E, Erdag TK, Sarioglu S, Guneri EA. Metastatic adenocarcinomas of the temporal bone: a report of three cases. Kulak Burun Bogaz Ihtis Derg. 2011;21(5):285–9.
34. Vize G. Laryngeal metastasis to the temporal bone causing facial paralysis. J Laryngol Otol. 1974;88(2):175–7.
35. Nakamura M, Kaga K, Ohira Y. Metastatic hypopharyngeal carcinoma to the temporal bone. Eur Arch Otorhinolaryngol. 1996;253(3):185–8.
36. Pfleiderer AG, Molyneux AJ, Tee MK. Metastatic spread of osteosarcoma to the temporal bone in a patient with Paget's disease: a case report. J Otolaryngol. 1992;21(2):112–4.
37. Thirunavukarasu V, Carter T, Dezso A, Holland C. Post-aural ache: an unusual presentation of a metastatic temporal bone lesion from a primary adenocarcinoma of the lung. J Laryngol Otol. 2013;127(10):1017–9.
38. Djeric D, Boricic I, Tomanovic N, Cvorovic L, Blazic S, Folic M, et al. The facial palsy as first symptom of the temporal bone lung cancer metastasis. Braz J Otorhinolaryngol. 2017;83(6):720–2.
39. Yang JI, Kang JM, Byun HJ, Chung GE, Yim JY, Park MJ, et al. Metastatic hepatocellular carcinoma presenting as facial nerve palsy and facial pain. Korean J Hepatol. 2011;17(4):319–22.
40. Yasumatsu R, Okura K, Sakiyama Y, Nakamuta M, Matsumura T, Uehara S, et al. Metastatic hepatocellular carcinoma of the external auditory canal. World J Gastroenterol. 2007;13(47):6436–8.
41. Nagai M, Yamada H, Kitamoto M, Ikeda J, Mori Y, Monzen Y, et al. Facial nerve palsy due to temporal bone metastasis from hepatocellular carcinoma. J Gastroenterol Hepatol. 2005;20(7):1131–2.
42. Bergstrom LV, Baker BB, Sando I. Sudden deafness and facial palsy from metastatic bronchogenic carcinoma. J Laryngol Otol. 1977;91(9):787–93.
43. Choi SH, Park IS, Kim YB, Hong SM. Unusual presentation of a metastatic tumor to the temporal bone: severe otalgia and facial paralysis. Korean J Audiol. 2014;18(1):34–7.
44. Teschner M, Durisin M, Mangold A, Lenarz T, Stover T. Peripheral facial palsy as the first symptom of a metastatic bronchogenic carcinoma. Laryngorhinootologie. 2006;85(7):512–6.
45. Kitajiri M, Sando I, Takahara T, Klau M. Metastatic squamous cell carcinoma in the neck invading the facial canal—a case report. Auris Nasus Larynx. 1984;11(3):171–6.
46. Weiss MD, Kattah JC, Jones R, Manz HJ. Isolated facial nerve palsy from metastasis to the temporal bone: report of two cases and a review of the literature. Am J Clin Oncol. 1997;20(1):19–23.
47. Garcia-Garcia P, Laguna-del-Estal P, Gonzalez-Lois C, Brea-Alvarez B. Facial paralysis secondary to single metastasis to the temporal bone from bladder cancer. Acta Otorrinolaringol Esp. 2015;66(2):122–3.
48. Mitsuya K, Nakasu Y, Horiguchi S, Harada H, Nishimura T, Yuen S, et al. Metastatic skull tumors: MRI features and a new conventional classification. J Neurooncol. 2011;104(1):239–45.
49. O'Sullivan JM, Norman AR, McNair H, Dearnaley DP. Cranial nerve palsies in metastatic prostate cancer—results of base of skull radiotherapy. Radiother Oncol. 2004;70(1):87–90.
50. Hugh SC, Enepekides D, Wong J, Yeung R, Lin VY. Metastasis of follicular variant of papillary thyroid carcinoma masquerading as primary temporal bone tumour. J Laryngol Otol. 2011;125(5):528–32.
51. Suryanarayanan R, Dezso A, Ramsden RT, Gillespie JE. Metastatic carcinoma mimicking a facial nerve schwannoma: the role of computerized tomography in diagnosis. J Laryngol Otol. 2005;119(12):1010–2.
52. Cureoglu S, Tulunay O, Ferlito A, Schachern PA, Paparella MM, Rinaldo A. Otologic manifestations of metastatic tumors to the temporal bone. Acta Otolaryngol. 2004;124(10):1117–23.
53. Razek AA, Huang BY. Lesions of the petrous apex: classification and findings at CT and MR imaging. Radiographics. 2012;32(1):151–73.
54. Tsunoda A, Tanaka Y, Sato T, Kirimura S, Kitamura K. Vertigo by breast cancer metastasis 33 years after treatment. Intern Med. 2016;55(3):311–3.
55. Vasileiadis I, Kapetanakis S, Vasileiadis D, Petousis A, Karatzas T. External auditory canal mass as the first manifestation of a bronchogenic carcinoma: report of a rare case. Ann Otol Rhinol Laryngol. 2013;122(6):378–81.
56. Saldanha CB, Bennett JD, Evans JN, Pambakian H. Metastasis to the temporal bone, secondary to carcinoma of the bladder. J Laryngol Otol. 1989;103(6):599–601.
57. Hain M, Feldberg E, Halperin D. Case report: metastatic small-cell lung carcinoma of the external auditory canal. Ear Nose Throat J. 2012;91(11):476–8.
58. Wu ZS, Li SC, Ho HC, Tseng JE, Lin YH, Su YC. Metastatic hepatocellular carcinoma in the tympanic membrane. Jpn J Clin Oncol. 2011;41(2):272–4.
59. Khan I, Mohamad S, Shakeel M, Jaramillo MJ. Aural metastasis from a nasal malignant melanoma: case report with literature review. J Laryngol Otol. 2011;125(12):1290–3.
60. Merrick Y. Metastatic colon adenocarcinoma of the middle ear. Arch Otorhinolaryngol. 1983;238(2):103–5.
61. Feinmesser R, Libson Y, Uziely B, Gay I. Metastatic carcinoma to the temporal bone. Am J Otol. 1986;7(2):119–20.
62. Barnes L. Metastases to the head and neck: an overview. Head Neck Pathol. 2009;3(3):217–24.
63. Chapman PR, Shah R, Curé JK, Bag AK. Petrous apex lesions: pictorial review. Am J Roentgenol. 2011;196(3_Suppl):WS26–37.
64. Brackmann DE, Bartels LJ. Rare tumors of the cerebellopontine angle. Otolaryngol Head Neck Surg. 1980;88(5):555–9.
65. Hariharan S, Zhu J, Nadkarni MA, Donahue JE. Metastatic lung cancer in the cerebellopontine angles mimicking bilateral acoustic neuroma. J Clin Neurosci. 2005;12(2):184–6.
66. Della Puppa A, Rossetto M, Berti F, Zustovich F, Manara R, Gardiman MP, et al. Internal auditory canal metastasis. J Neurosurg Sci. 2010;54(4):159–62.
67. Nazim K, Mehmet Y, Tuna ED, Marlen MA. Bilateral internal acoustic canal mass. J Craniofac Surg. 2013;24(5):1863.
68. Ziegler EA, Bohl J, Maurer J. Bilateral progressive hearing loss as the first manifestation of metastatic carcinoma of the head of the pancreas. Case report. Laryngorhinootologie. 2001;80(8):436–8.
69. Yang AS, Bird P. Intracranial metastatic melanoma presenting with bilateral hearing loss. Otol Neurotol. 2009;30(2):243–4.
70. Gerganov VM, Hore N, Herold C, Wrede K, Stan AC, Samii A, et al. Bilateral malignant melanoma metastases to the internal auditory canal/cerebellopontine angle: surgical management and preservation of function. J Neurosurg. 2008;108(4):803–7.
71. De Vos C, Gerard JM, Decat M, Gersdorff M. Metastatic renal cell carcinoma to the temporal bone: case report. B-ENT. 2005;1(1):43–6.

Mastoidectomy and Facial Nerve Decompression

16

Paul W. Gidley

Mastoidectomy and Facial Nerve Decompression

Temporal bone surgery is an important adjunct for the treatment of advanced or recurrent parotid gland tumors [1]. Primary parotid tumors are rare, and they make up about 3–6% of all head and neck cancers [2]. Of these, perhaps only about 5% of patients have disease so advanced that a temporal bone procedure is required. Primary parotid malignancy and metastatic tumors to the parotid gland can involve the facial nerve either through direct extension or through perineural invasion [1].

In a large series of cancers affecting the temporal bone, the rate of facial nerve weakness at presentation approaches 40% [3]. Mastoidectomy and facial nerve decompression provide an excellent avenue to approach parotid tumors that involve the facial nerve or that extend into the stylomastoid foramen.

In patients where parotid malignancy has already produced facial paralysis, mastoidectomy allows access to the nerve proximal to the site of involvement and in an area where the nerve is not involved by the extratemporal tumor. In the subset of parotid malignancies that involve the mastoid or temporal bone, the rate of facial nerve sacrifice approaches 70% [1]. By identifying the facial nerve away from the primary tumor, the facial nerve can be sampled and a negative margin achieved. The addition of temporal bone surgery to the treatment of advanced parotid tumors increases the negative margin rate from 37% up to 80% [1, 4].

Additionally, in cases where the facial nerve will be sacrificed, a proximal stump in the mastoid allows for nerve grafting to distal branches of the nerve.

Mastoidectomy is an essential part of temporal bone surgery. The key to successful temporal bone surgery is identification of landmarks within the mastoid. From these key landmarks, all of the transtemporal approaches can be accomplished.

This chapter will discuss the basics of mastoidectomy and facial nerve decompression in the setting of parotid malignancy. The goals of this surgery are to identify the facial nerve in an area where it is uninvolved by tumor or unscarred from previous surgery, to achieve a negative margin on the facial nerve, and to prepare a facial nerve stump for grafting. For this chapter, parotid malignancy encompasses both primary parotid tumors and metastatic disease (usually squamous cell carcinoma or melanoma from the ipsilateral temple or cheek) [1, 2]. While preoperative facial paralysis is a known poor prognostic sign, the absence of facial weakness does not connote an absence of perineural invasion.

Indications

A key step in parotidectomy is facial nerve identification. While there are many landmarks for the extratemporal portion of the facial nerve, these landmarks are either absent or obscured by advanced parotid malignancies and thus not available for finding the facial nerve.

There are five primary indications for mastoidectomy and facial nerve decompression in the setting of parotid malignancy: (1) revision parotidectomy, (2) large bulky parotid tumor, (3) parotid tumor with facial paralysis, (4) parotid tumor with extension into the stylomastoid foramen or positive facial nerve margin at the stylomastoid foramen, and (5) deep lobe parotid tumors.

Revision parotidectomy in the setting of recurrent or persistent disease is the most common reason to perform mastoidectomy for facial nerve identification (Table 16.1). Usually these patients have normal or near-normal facial function, and the surgical team strives for facial nerve preservation whenever oncologically feasible. Previous surgery, and especially previous radiation, creates scarring around the nerve making its identification and preservation difficult.

P. W. Gidley, M.D., F.A.C.S.
Department of Head and Neck Surgery, The University of Texas M.D. Anderson Cancer Center, Houston, TX, USA
e-mail: pwgidley@mdanderson.org

P. W. Gidley, F. DeMonte (eds.), *Temporal Bone Cancer*, https://doi.org/10.1007/978-3-319-74539-8_16

Mastoidectomy and facial nerve decompression are performed in order to identify the facial nerve in an unoperated area so that it can be traced through the previously dissected tissue and scar and help to preserve its function.

Large parotid tumors can invade the external auditory canal. In this circumstance, lateral temporal bone resection, and not mastoidectomy alone, should be performed.

Adenoid cystic carcinoma and squamous cell carcinoma may be associated with perineural spread. Perineural spread along the facial nerve can produce one or several branch deficits or whole face paresis or paralysis. In this circumstance, facial nerve decompression permits identification of the facial nerve proximal to the site of involvement, and thus a negative margin on the facial nerve can be achieved. Facial nerve grafting can then be performed if viable distal branches of the facial nerve are present.

Table 16.1 MD Anderson experience of mastoidectomy and facial nerve decompression

Location primary tumor		
Site	*N*	%
Parotid gland	88	71.5
Periauricular skin	33	26.8
Skull base	2	1.6
Disease status at presentation		
Untreated	57	46.3
Recurrent disease	50	40.7
Persistent disease	16	13.0
Tumor size		
Average	3.4 cm (0.1–8.0 cm)	
Tumor type		
Malignant	101	82.1
Benign	22	17.9
Pathology		
Squamous cell carcinoma	27	22.0
Acinic cell carcinoma	13	10.6
Adenoid cystic carcinoma	12	9.8
Salivary duct carcinoma	9	7.3
Basaloid carcinoma	8	6.5
Mucoepidermoid carcinoma	8	6.5
Carcinoma ex PMA	4	3.2
Myoepithelial carcinoma	4	3.2
Adenocarcinoma	3	2.4
Melanoma	3	2.4
Basal cell carcinoma	2	1.6
Undifferentiated carcinoma	2	1.6
Neuroendocrine carcinoma	2	1.6
No tumor	2	1.6
Atypical lipomatous tumor	1	0.8
Oncocytic carcinoma	1	0.8
Pleomorphic adenoma (PMA)	17	13.8
Warthin's tumor	3	2.4
Lymphoepithelioma	1	0.8
Canalicular adenoma	1	0.8

Some parotid tumors grow toward the stylomastoid foramen without infiltrating the facial nerve or causing facial paralysis. Mastoidectomy and facial nerve decompression removes the mastoid tip and allows microdissection of the tumor off of the facial nerve in such cases. Sampling the tissue at the stylomastoid foramen can help in making the decision for facial nerve sacrifice. When the nerve is infiltrated at the stylomastoid foramen, facial nerve sacrifice with nerve grafting is performed [5].

Lastly, mastoidectomy and facial nerve decompression can help in the setting of deep lobe parotid tumors. Many of these tumors can be approached transcervically by dividing the digastric and gaining access to the deep lobe. In other patients, the mastoid tip can make this dissection difficult, and removal of the mastoid tip with identification of the facial nerve at the outset can improve access and help with facial nerve preservation.

Preoperative Assessment

Following a head and neck examination, these patients are examined closely for their facial nerve function. Each branch of the facial nerve is carefully assessed. In cases where facial paralysis exists, placing a thumb on the midline can help to eliminate distortion from the intact side. While many different scales have been developed for assessing facial function, the House-Brackmann scale still remains the easiest one to use [6]. Rates of facial nerve dysfunction (HBII–VI) vary in this clinical situation from 65 to 75% of patients [1, 5]. While preoperative facial paralysis is a known poor prognostic sign, the absence of facial weakness does not connote an absence of perineural invasion (Table 16.2) [1, 5].

The ear canals are examined under the otomicroscope to ensure that disease does not involve the ear canal.

Basic audiometry including pure-tone testing, speech audiometry, and immittance testing is performed. This testing is important to establish a baseline and to counsel the patient about hearing loss. Acoustic reflex testing measures facial nerve function proximal to the stapedius muscle; how-

Table 16.2 Preoperative facial nerve function in the MD Anderson series of mastoidectomies

House-Brackmann score	*N*, pts	%
I	59	48.0
II	31	25.2
III	10	8.1
IV	3	2.4
V	3	2.4
VI	17	13.8

ever, this testing is not a reliable marker for facial nerve involvement by occult disease [5].

CT and MRI are performed to evaluate the extent of disease [1, 5]. CT scan is particularly useful in disclosing the bony anatomy of the temporal bone. Anomalies, such as high-riding jugular bulb (Fig. 16.1), are important to identify preoperatively. MRI can show enhancement of the facial nerve in cases where facial paralysis exists [1] (Fig. 16.2).

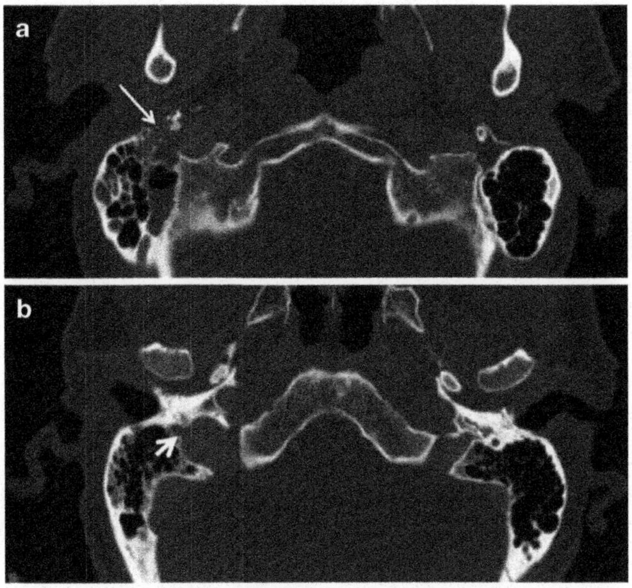

Fig. 16.1 CT scan of parotid cancer affecting the right facial nerve. (**a**) Bony erosion at the stylomastoid foramen (white arrow). (**b**) A higher level section shows the facial nerve (short arrow) in intimate contact with the jugular bulb

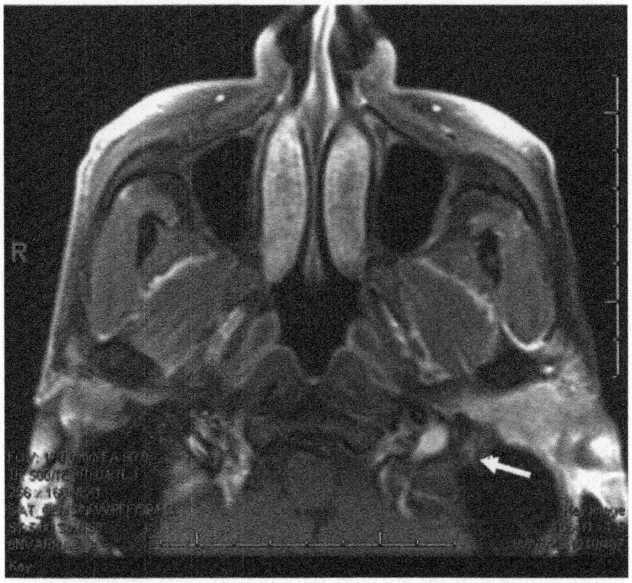

Fig. 16.2 MRI showing enhancement of the facial nerve in the left stylomastoid foramen

Either imaging modality can demonstrate if the tumor is in the superficial or deep lobe or both, if it involves the stylomastoid foramen or mastoid tip, or if it involves the tympanic or labyrinthine segments of the nerve [1].

Surgical Setup

These procedures are all performed under general anesthesia. The patient's physical health needs to be acceptable to undergo such surgery. Appropriate IV access and monitoring needs to be set up for a potentially long duration procedure. Arterial lines are useful for monitoring during such long procedures.

Once general endotracheal anesthesia and appropriate monitoring have been achieved, the patient is padded and strapped to the operating room table, and the table is turned 180° so that the head is away from the anesthesia station (Fig. 16.3). This maneuver allows the surgical team full access to the head and neck; but conversely, the anesthesia team does not have ready access to the airway, and care must be taken to secure the endotracheal tube properly. Excessive rotation of the head from side to side should be avoided.

During an otologic procedure, this table orientation allows the scrub nurse to be across from the surgeon while working under the microscope. The scrub nurse can readily hand instruments to the surgeon and can monitor the face for any facial movements during the facial nerve dissection.

Intraoperative facial nerve monitoring is employed during these procedures, even in cases where there is some preoperative facial nerve weakness. While facial nerve monitoring does not necessarily help in finding the facial nerve, the feedback provided by the monitor helps to minimize trauma to the nerve. The electrodes are placed in the lateral brow and upper lip and oriented so that the wires do not cross the affected side of the face (Fig. 16.4). The monitor is placed near the surgeon so that the screen is visible and the warning tones are audible.

These procedures often involve multiple teams: neurotology, head and neck surgery, and plastic surgery. The patient is positioned and prepared so that each of these teams can perform the necessary procedure without cross-contamination and without the need to re-prep or redrape.

Prophylactic antibiotics are administered prior to the initial incision and are re-dosed every 4 h during the procedure. Sequential compression devices and thromboembolic hosiery are used to avoid the complications of deep vein thrombosis and thromboembolic events.

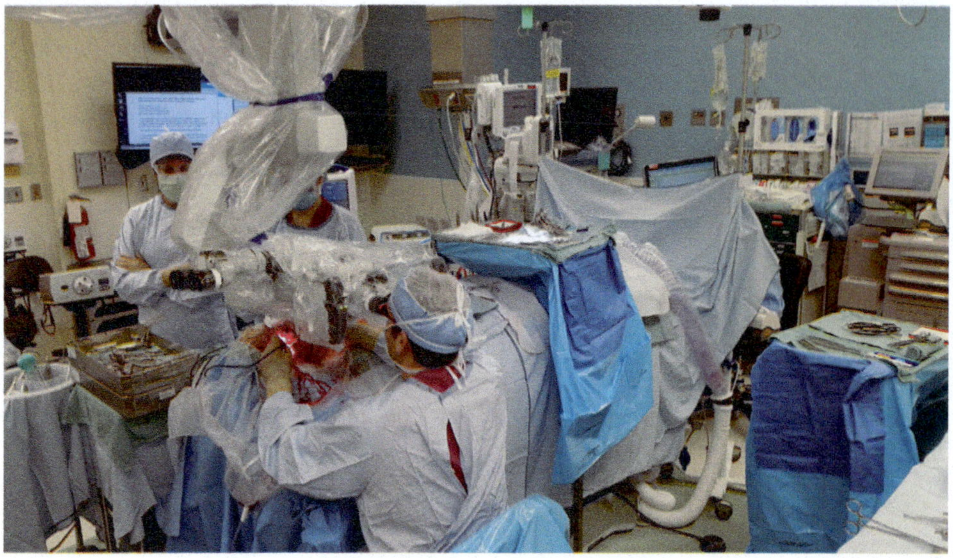

Fig. 16.3 Operating room arrangement for temporal bone surgery

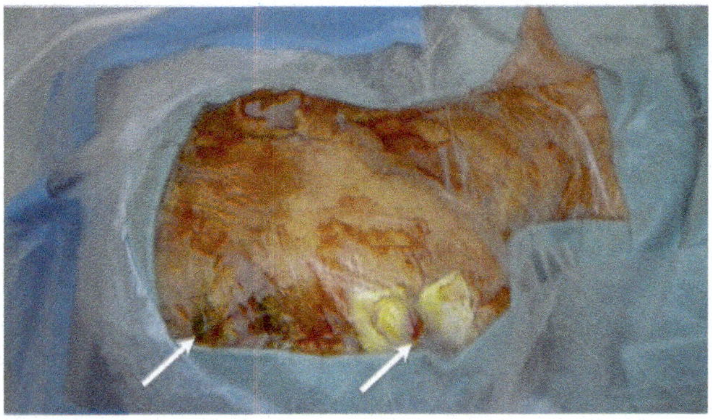

Fig. 16.4 Facial nerve electrodes (arrows) are placed at the eyebrow and corner of the mouth. Ground electrodes are placed below the clavicles on the opposite chest

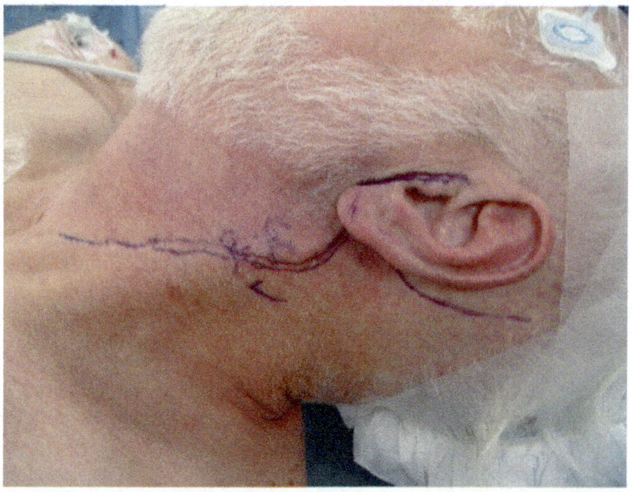

Fig. 16.5 Incisions for mastoidectomy with parotidectomy with mastoidectomy. This patient is undergoing revision parotidectomy, and the scar is marked for excision

Procedure

Incision

Incision planning is usually straightforward, since a modified Blair incision is used for parotidectomy. This incision extends from the sideburn area along the preauricular sulcus and lobule and then curves upward under the lobule for a centimeter or so before gently curving down toward the neck following a skinfold crease. The neck incision is generally planned to be about 2–3 fingerbreadths below the angle of the mandible, but the exact location depends on which levels of the neck need to be dissected.

A postauricular incision extends off the parotidectomy incision, being placed 1 fingerbreadth behind the ear, and continues until the temporal line. This incision is made rather straight and not curved in order to maintain the blood supply to the auricle. (Fig. 16.5). Having an incision in front and behind the auricle does present some hazard to the blood supply to the auricle. Thankfully the structures of the head and neck have a rich anastomotic blood supply. The blood supply to the outer ear has contributions from the superficial temporal artery, the occipital artery, and the internal maxillary artery via the ear canal.

In patients that have received prior radiation, however, the blood supply is already compromised, and these incisions might compromise the blood supply further leading to ischemia and necrosis. Necrosis of the lobule, inferior half, or entire pinna can occur, and patients need to be forewarned about this possibility.

Once the postauricular skin incision has been made, soft tissue work continues as for routine mastoidectomy. A large Palva flap is outlined and elevated (Fig. 16.6). The temporalis

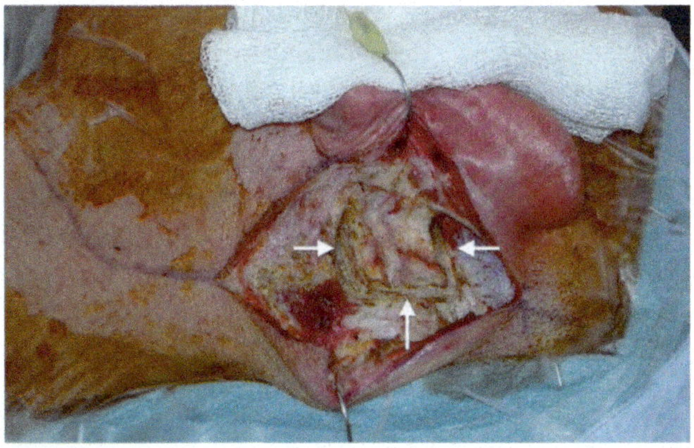

Fig. 16.6 Palva flap (outlined by arrows) is elevated prior to left mastoidectomy

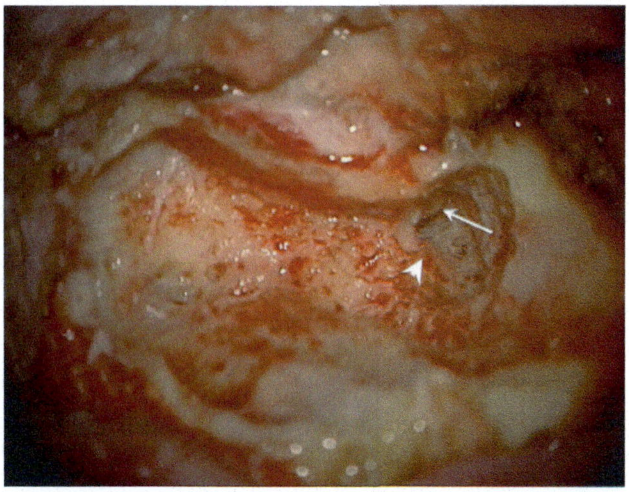

Fig. 16.7 Simple left mastoidectomy completed, antrum opened, exposing horizontal semicircular canal (arrowhead) and incus (arrow)

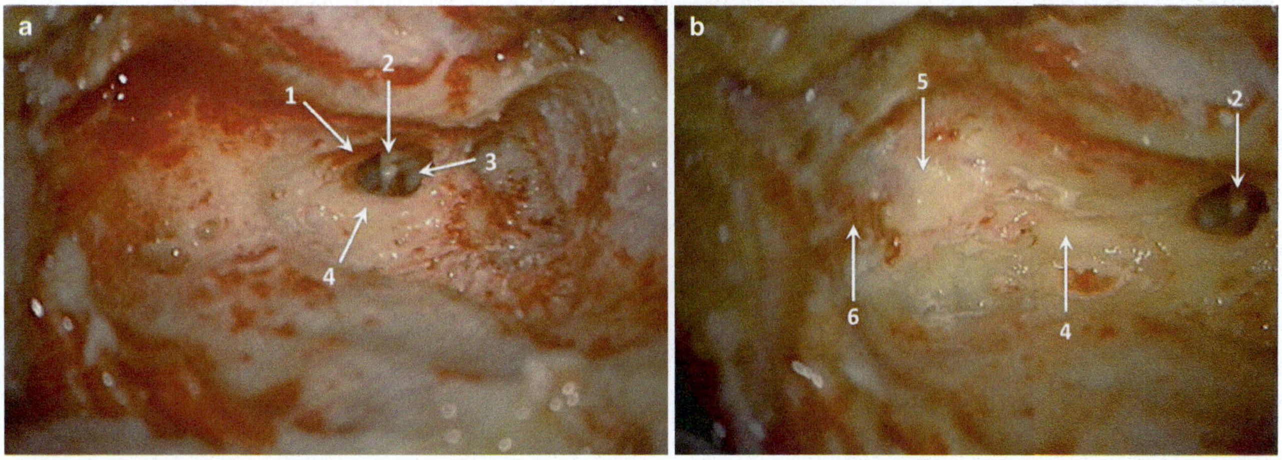

Fig. 16.8 Left facial recess and facial nerve. (**a**) Facial recess opened showing tympanic portion of facial nerve. (**b**) Facial nerve course is outlined to the stylomastoid foramen. Key: (*1*) chorda tympani nerve, (*2*) lenticular process of incus, (*3*) tympanic portion of facial nerve, (*4*) mastoid portion of facial nerve, (*5*) stylomastoid foramen, (*6*) digastric muscle

muscle is elevated and retracted away. Mastoid periosteum posteriorly and around the mastoid tip is elevated and retracted. The posterior attachment of the digastric muscle is identified.

Mastoidectomy

Mastoidectomy is performed with large cutting bur and suction-irrigation. The mastoid tegmen, sigmoid sinus, and digastric ridge are identified. The antrum is opened and the horizontal semicircular canal is identified. The operating microscope is brought into place and used for the remainder of the procedure. The antrum is widened further until the incus is identified (Fig. 16.7).

The incus is used as a landmark for the facial recess, since the body of the incus acts like an arrow pointing to the facial recess. The posterior ear canal wall is thinned down. Using continuous suction-irrigation and progressively smaller diamond burs, with strokes paralleling the course of the facial nerve, the facial recess is opened. Care is taken to avoid being too lateral to the facial nerve, since this might lead to the ear canal and not the middle ear and may damage the tympanic membrane.

The facial recess is widened until the chorda tympani nerve is seen. The incus buttress is thinned down to permit a view of the tympanic portion of the facial nerve (Fig. 16.8a). The tympanic portion of the facial nerve is used as a landmark for the second genu and mastoid portion of the facial nerve. The facial nerve can then be followed along its mastoid course to the stylomastoid foramen (Fig. 16.8b). The digastric ridge is thinned down until the underlying muscle becomes visible. This always points to the stylomastoid foramen and it can be used as a landmark for the facial nerve. The drill is used to widen the stylomastoid foramen.

A bony cut is made lateral to the stylomastoid foramen and inferior to the ear canal. This action frees up the mastoid tip. It can then be safely removed by elevating the tip away from the mastoid and facial nerve and dividing the soft tissue attachments on the mastoid tip with electrocautery (Fig. 16.9). The facial nerve is bound down to the mastoid by periosteum at the stylomastoid foramen, preventing it from being elevated with the tip. This step is important to unify the mastoid and neck, allowing the facial nerve to be followed from the mastoid into the neck.

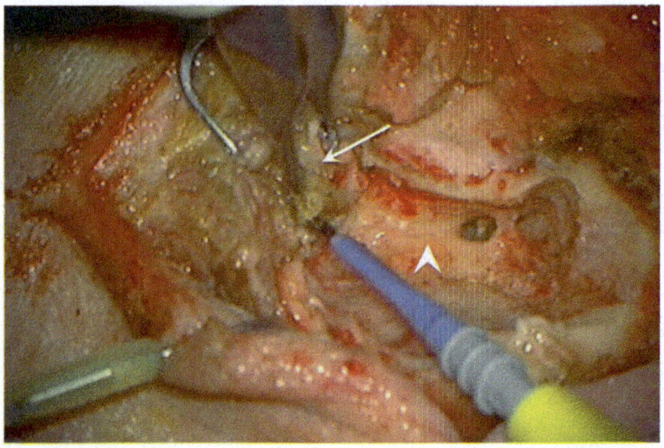

Fig. 16.9 Left mastoid tip removal. Mastoid tip (arrow) is grasped and pulled away from facial nerve (arrowhead)

Facial nerve decompression is then performed by extending the facial recess. The chorda tympani nerve is divided. Drill strokes parallel to the nerve are used to remove bone around the circumference of the nerve. If nerve identification alone is needed, then only about 180° of the circumference of the nerve needs to be exposed. If facial nerve sacrifice and grafting are required, then most of the bone (270° or more) around the nerve must be removed. Fisch instruments are useful in removing the last thin shell of bone on the facial nerve (Fig. 16.10a).

Once the nerve is exposed, it needs to be traced into the neck. Fisch instruments are useful to open the periosteal ring at the stylomastoid foramen. The thin adipose tissue around the nerve can be bluntly dissected to expose the nerve plainly. A fine Jacobsen's hemostat is placed parallel to the nerve and opened. The soft tissue lateral to the nerve is divided with bipolar electrocautery and a #12 blade (Fig. 16.10b). Once the nerve has been identified extratemporally, parotidectomy and neck dissection can be performed.

The decision to sacrifice the facial nerve is always difficult, especially if the patient has normal or near-normal function preoperatively. This decision is usually based on several conditions: (1) preoperative function, (2) tumor histology, (3) tumor location, and (4) appearance of the nerve.

Patients who present with facial paralysis will have facial nerve sacrifice in order to try to achieve a negative margin on the facial nerve. It is reasonable to take sequential proximal segments of the nerve to achieve a negative margin; however, with each subsequent segment, the proximal stump becomes shorter and facial nerve grafting becomes more difficult. A negative margin can be achieved in the majority of patients by the level of the mastoid segment of the facial nerve; fewer

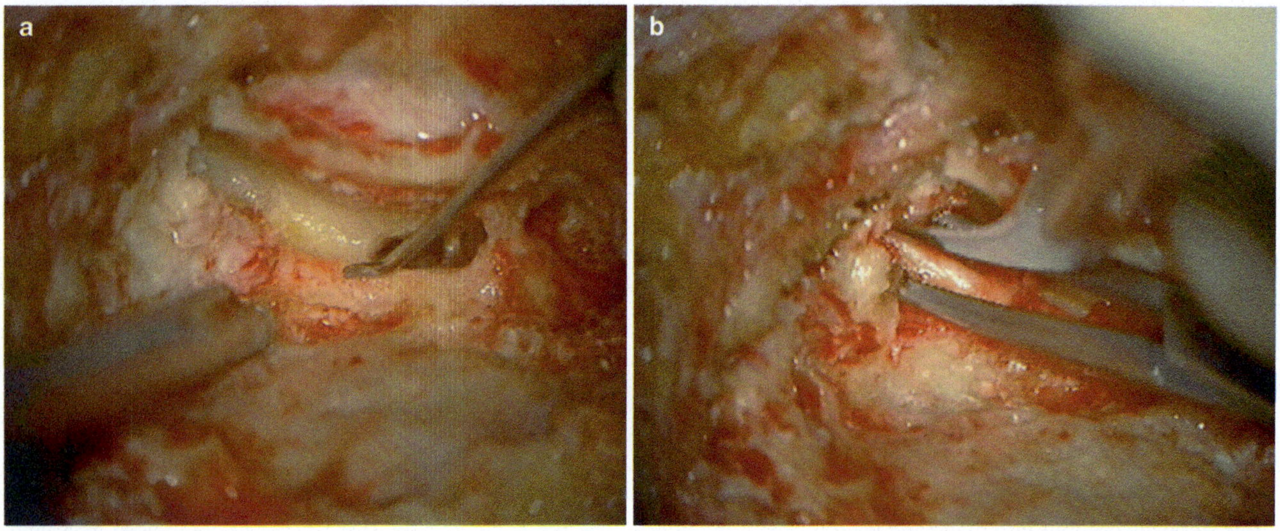

Fig. 16.10 Left facial nerve decompression. (**a**) Bone covering the facial nerve is removed with Fisch instruments. (**b**) Soft tissue over the facial nerve is opened with a fine hemostat and #12 blade

than 25% have disease involving either the tympanic segment or more proximal facial nerve [5].

In the MD Anderson series of mastoidectomies, facial nerve sacrifice was performed in 66 patients (53.7%). In six of these patients, only a division (either upper or lower) or an isolated branch or two was sacrificed. Facial nerve grafting was performed in 50 patients (75.6%).

A positive margin on the nerve does not preclude grafting the nerve [7]. In their series, Wax and Kaylie (2007) describe 19 patients who underwent facial nerve sacrifice, of which 8 patients had a positive neural margin. No significant difference in facial nerve outcome was seen between these two groups [7].

While achieving a negative margin on the facial nerve is a laudable goal, this goal does not justify labyrinthectomy to chase microscopic perineural disease in the facial nerve [5]. The added morbidity of profound hearing loss and vestibular loss is not outweighed by the perceived benefit of a potential negative margin. Postoperative radiotherapy with or without chemotherapy will be used in such patients with perineural disease, regardless of the final margin status for the facial nerve [1]. Tumors that exhibit this aggressive behavior, such as intratemporal facial nerve perineural invasion, usually have positive margins at other locations and patients usually die from local, regional, or distant disease (skin, parotid, or neck) [1].

Risks and Complications

The risks for mastoidectomy are well known: hearing loss, tinnitus, dizziness or vertigo, facial weakness or paralysis, and distorted or loss of taste on the ipsilateral tongue. Additional possible risks are tympanic membrane perforation, caused by drilling the facial recess too far laterally, and loss of some or all of the pinna, as described above.

The rate of hearing loss, tinnitus, and dizziness are very low. Sensorineural hearing loss can be caused by trauma to the inner ear, and conductive hearing loss can be caused by trauma to the ossicular chain. Severe to profound hearing loss can occur when performing facial nerve decompression and sacrifice of the tympanic segment of the facial nerve. Separating the incudostapedial joint can help to prevent transmitted movements of the chain into the inner ear.

Dizziness and vertigo occur rarely (<2%) after mastoidectomy in this clinical setting, since the labyrinth can be preserved [1] (Table 16.3).

Loss of taste will occur since the chorda tympani nerve is sacrificed in facial nerve decompression. However, most patients do not notice or report a change in taste following this surgery.

Given the nature of the surgery and the tumor characteristics, postoperative facial function tends to be worse than preoperative facial function. Gidley et al. reported that almost 60% of patients had poor facial function (HBIV–VI) at last follow-up [3]. Many of these patients will require ancillary procedures, such as gold weights or static slings, to address facial paralysis (Table 16.4).

Table 16.3 Complications encountered in MD Anderson series of mastoidectomy

Complications in 123 mastoidectomies	*N*, pts	%
Neck hematoma	4	3.3
Mental status change	4	3.3
Donor site hematoma	2	1.6
Respiratory insufficiency	1	0.8
Compartment syndrome, leg	1	0.8
Tympanic membrane perforation	1	0.8
Atrial fibrillation	1	0.8

Table 16.4 House-Brackmann facial nerve function at last follow-up

House-Brackmann Score	*N*, pts	%
I	28	22.8
II	14	11.4
III	17	13.8
IV	5	4.1
V	2	1.6
VI	44	35.8
Unknown	13	10.6
Total	123	100

Table 16.5 Adjuvant therapy in MD Anderson mastoidectomy series

Indicators for adjuvant therapy	Patients (%)
Perineural invasion	52 (42.3%)
Lymphovascular invasion	12 (9.8%)
Extracapsular spread	18 (14.6)
Soft tissue invasion	62 (50.4)
Radiotherapy	
Preop XRT	3 (2.4%)
Post-op XRT	87 (70.7%)
Dose	Avg = 60.4Gy (30–70 Gy)
Chemotherapy	
Preop chemo	5 (4.1%)
Post-op chemo	22 (17.9%)
Pre- and Post-op chemo	3 (2.4%)

Preop XRT, preoperative radiotherapy; *post-op XRT*, postoperative radiotherapy; *preop hemo*, preoperative chemotherapy; *post-op chemo*, postoperative chemotherapy

Adjuvant Therapy

Indications for postoperative radiotherapy include perineural invasion, lymphovascular invasion, extracapsular spread, more than one positive lymph node, recurrent tumor, or positive surgical margin (Table 16.5).

Conclusions

Mastoidectomy and facial nerve decompression is an important step for patients with advance parotid malignancy, with preoperative facial nerve dysfunction, or with recurrent disease. The goals of this surgery are to identify the facial nerve in an area where it is uninvolved by tumor or unscarred from previous surgery, to achieve a negative margin on the facial nerve, and to prepare a facial nerve stump for grafting. There are five primary indications for mastoidectomy and facial nerve decompression in the setting of parotid malignancy: (1) revision parotidectomy, (2) large bulky parotid tumor, (3) parotid tumor with facial paralysis, (4) parotid tumor with extension into the stylomastoid foramen or positive facial nerve margin at the stylomastoid foramen, and (5) deep lobe parotid tumors.

References

1. Gidley PW, Thompson CR, Roberts DB, Weber RS. The results of temporal bone surgery for advanced or recurrent tumors of the parotid gland. Laryngoscope. 2011;121(8):1702–7.
2. Bron LP, Traynor SJ, McNeil EB, O'Brien CJ. Primary and metastatic cancer of the parotid: comparison of clinical behavior in 232 cases. Laryngoscope. 2003;113(6):1070–5.
3. Gidley PW, Thompson CR, Roberts DB, DeMonte F, Hanna EY. The oncology of otology. Laryngoscope. 2012;122(2):393–400.
4. Garden AS, el-Naggar AK, Morrison WH, Callender DL, Ang KK, Peters LJ. Postoperative radiotherapy for malignant tumors of the parotid gland. Int J Radiat Oncol Biol Phys. 1997;37(1):79–85.
5. Carlson ML, Patel NS, Modest MC, Moore EJ, Janus JR, Olsen KD. Occult temporal bone facial nerve involvement by parotid malignancies with perineural spread. Otolaryngol Head Neck Surg. 2015;153(3):385–91.
6. House JW, Brackmann DE. Facial nerve grading system. Otolaryngol Head Neck Surg. 1985;93(2):146.
7. Wax MK, Kaylie DM. Does a positive neural margin affect outcome in facial nerve grafting? Head Neck. 2007;29(6):546–9.

Lateral Temporal Bone Resection

17

Paul W. Gidley

Lateral Temporal Bone Resection

The lateral temporal bone resection (LTBR) is the workhorse procedure for dealing with tumors of the ear canal and temporal bone. Parotid, periauricular, and skull base tumors can involve the temporal bone in such a way that removal of the ear canal might be required, either to enhance an approach or to create a negative margin.

The observations in this chapter are based on personal experience of more than 200 LTBR performed by the author.

Indications

The primary indication for LTBR is cancer within the ear canal. LTBR removes the ear canal as a single, intact specimen. This resection removes the ear canal, eardrum, malleus, and incus, while the facial nerve, stapes, and inner ear are preserved. This resection allows en bloc removal of tumor within the ear canal without tumor spillage. LTBR alone is curative for patients with Pittsburgh stage T1 temporal bone tumor [1].

Using a canal wall-down mastoidectomy approach, Moore et al. described a non-en bloc temporal bone resection. They had residual disease in 46% [2]. Thirty-four percent developed local recurrence. Using an en bloc approach helps to minimize the chance for local recurrence.

In the MD Anderson series, primary ear canal cancers constituted only about 25% of the total number of LTBR. LTBR alone might be sufficient for low-grade malignancies within the ear canal. However, LTBR is usually combined with parotidectomy and neck dissection for primary ear canal cancers that have a potential for direct extension to the parotid or metastatic spread to regional lymph nodes.

The most common indication for LTBR in the MD Anderson series was for advanced stage parotid, external ear, or periauricular skin cancers that invaded the ear canal or temporal bone secondarily. Parotidectomy and neck dissection are usually combined with LTBR, especially for parotid and periauricular skin cancers. More extensive cancers might require the addition of mandibular condylectomy, infratemporal fossa dissection, and craniotomy.

Lastly, LTBR might be the first stage in a larger operation to remove a more medially situated tumor. Advanced temporal bone cancers that involve the ear canal, middle ear, and labyrinth often required LTBR to gain access to more medially placed structures.

Definitions

The lateral temporal bone resection (LTBR) is defined as the en bloc removal of the ear canal, eardrum, malleus, and incus; and the facial nerve, stapes, and labyrinth are left undisturbed. Several other terms have been used in association with lateral temporal bone resection, and these terms add confusion to the literature.

Local canal resection (LCR) is used to denote a procedure to remove a lesion within the ear canal. Oftentimes this term is used synonymously with "sleeve resection" which connotes removal of the ear canal skin. Sleeve resection can include removal of the tympanic membrane. The defect is reconstructed with a split-thickness skin graft. The skin of the ear canal is very thin, on average 0.2 mm thick. By its very nature, removal of the ear canal skin is not a cancer operation since there is no way to remove a tumor with an adequate deep margin. Local canal resection has been linked to high recurrence rate for invasive squamous cell carcinoma of the ear canal [3].

P. W. Gidley, M.D., F.A.C.S.
Department of Head and Neck Surgery, The University of Texas M.D. Anderson Cancer Center, Houston, TX, USA
e-mail: pwgidley@mdanderson.org

P. W. Gidley, F. DeMonte (eds.), *Temporal Bone Cancer*, https://doi.org/10.1007/978-3-319-74539-8_17

Moody et al. describe a “modified” LTBR, which leaves an uninvolved tympanic membrane intact [1]. In their series of 32 patients, 3 underwent a modified LTBR. All three patients had T1 lesions, and all three were NED at last follow-up (84–116 months).

Medina et al. described four types of LTBR [4]. Type I consists of removal of the ear canal and tympanic bone lateral to the tympanic membrane. This procedure matches the “modified LTBR” above. Type II resection is removal of the ear canal en bloc lateral to the facial nerve, and it matches the classic LTBR description. Type III resection includes the classic LTBR and further includes resection of the facial nerve, fallopian canal, mastoid tip, styloid process, and stylomastoid foramen. Type IV resection entails removal of only the mastoid tip and inferior portion of the tympanic bone. This procedure is a complete mastoidectomy with facial nerve dissection, as described in Chap. 16. Since it does not resect the ear canal, type IV should not be considered a temporal bone resection. While this paper does describe these procedures in detail, the classification scheme is confusing and misleading.

Gacek and Goodman (1977) published a series of 31 patients from the Massachusetts Eye and Ear Infirmary and used the term “partial temporal bone resection,” which they use to describe either a classic LTBR or a modified LTBR [5]. Arriaga et al. also used the term “partial temporal bone resection” without defining the limits of the resection [6].

Moffat et al. describe an “extended temporal bone resection” [7]. This resection removes a wider area of the skin and soft tissue than LTBR, and it requires a middle and posterior fossa craniotomy. By its nature, this resection is closer in description to a subtotal temporal bone resection, since the labyrinth is removed. Leong et al. used the term “extended temporal bone resection” to describe a procedure that includes a LTBR with additional resection of the ascending ramus, head, and coronoid of the mandible [8].

“Composite LTBR” might be a better descriptor for the procedure in which the ear canal, external ear, parotid gland, condyle of the mandible, and neck dissection are removed en bloc (Fig. 17.1). Given the variability in including one or more of these extratemporal structures, the best practice is still to list these procedures as individual components rather than trying to lump them all under one moniker.

Preoperative Assessment

LTBR takes several hours to perform under general anesthesia, and patients need to be in good physical health to undergo this procedure. While this procedure does not involve major fluid shifts or endocrinologic derangements, the population requiring LTBR has an average age of 67 years (range 3–91 years) and often has multiple underlying medical comorbidities. Simple lateral temporal bone resection and temporalis flap reconstruction take about 4 h. When combined with parotidectomy, neck dissection, and microvascular free flap, the procedure can take 10–12 h; and it is imperative that patients be in good physical shape to tolerate such a long procedure.

The physical examination should include close examination of the external ear and ear canal to determine the lateral extension of the tumor. Tumors that involve the outer ear will require partial or total auriculectomy for complete excision. Careful cranial nerve examination is required. Facial weakness or paralysis must be noted, since these signs often indicate direct or perineural invasion of the facial nerve. Facial numbness from trigeminal involvement can be seen in periauricular skin cancers that involve the auriculotemporal nerve. Tumors that involve this nerve can extend along V3 through the foramen ovale and continue onto the trigeminal ganglion (Fig. 17.2). Patients with such significant perineural

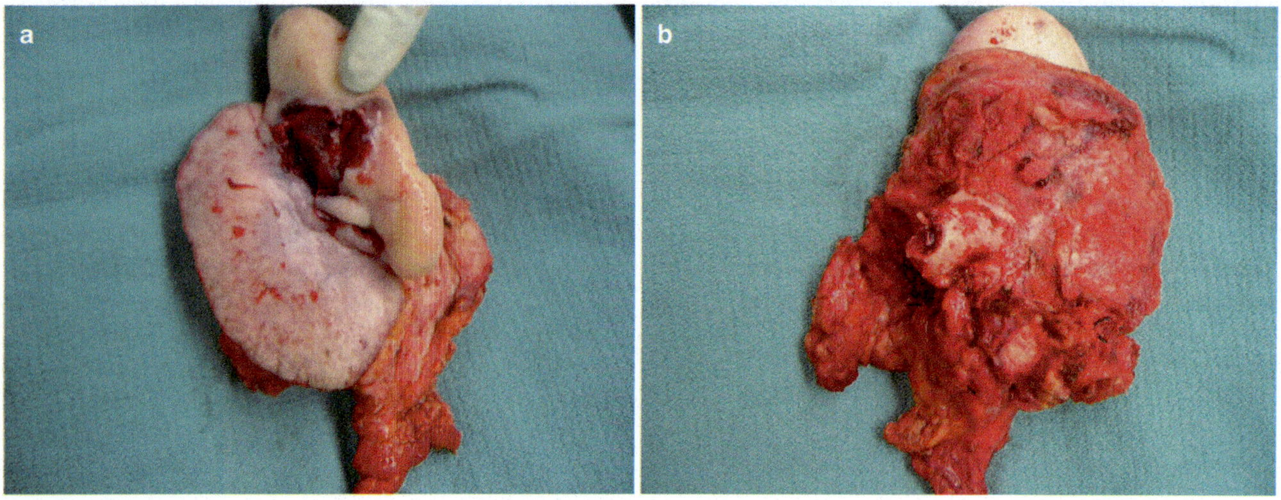

Fig. 17.1 Composite resection of the temporal bone, including the outer ear, ear canal, parotid, and neck dissection. (**a**) Lateral surface. (**b**) Medial surface. Note the intact tympanic membrane and malleus

spread are not good candidates for lateral temporal bone resection. Additionally, patients with deficits in the lower cranial nerves (IX, X, XI, XII) are not good surgical candidates. These patients are best treated with combination chemotherapy and radiotherapy.

Audiometric assessment is essential for any patient prior to an ear operation. Since a maximum conductive hearing loss is the expected outcome of LTBR, it is important to know the bone thresholds in order to counsel the patient and to make plans for auditory rehabilitation. Likewise, an

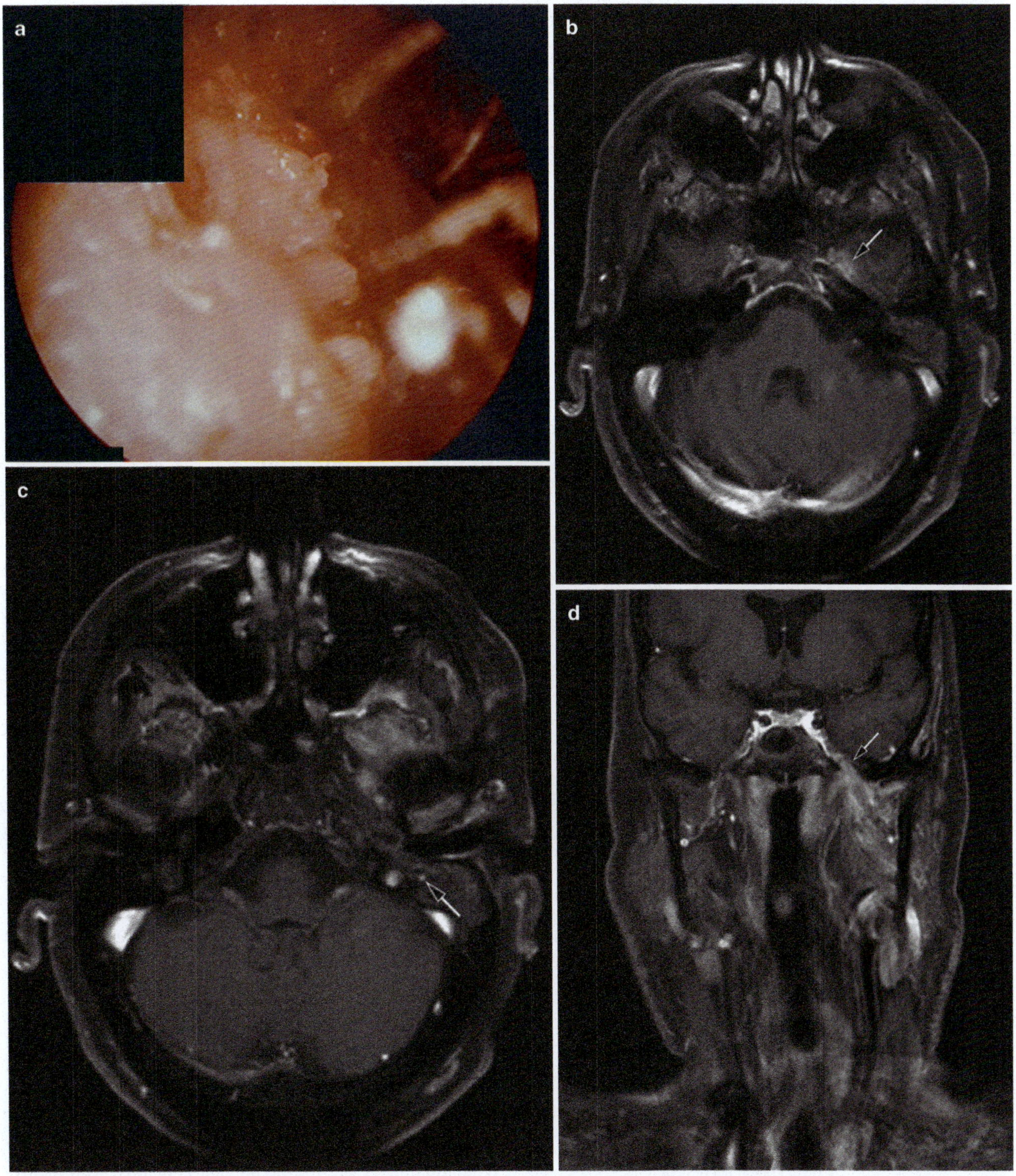

Fig. 17.2 Perineural spread in cranial nerves V and VII from squamous cell carcinoma of the left ear canal. (**a**) Oto-endoscopic photo of lesion in the left ear canal. Contrast-enhanced axial T1 MRI showing disease in Meckel's cave (**b**) and intratemporal facial nerve (**c**). (**d**) Coronal MRI showing disease in trigeminal nerve

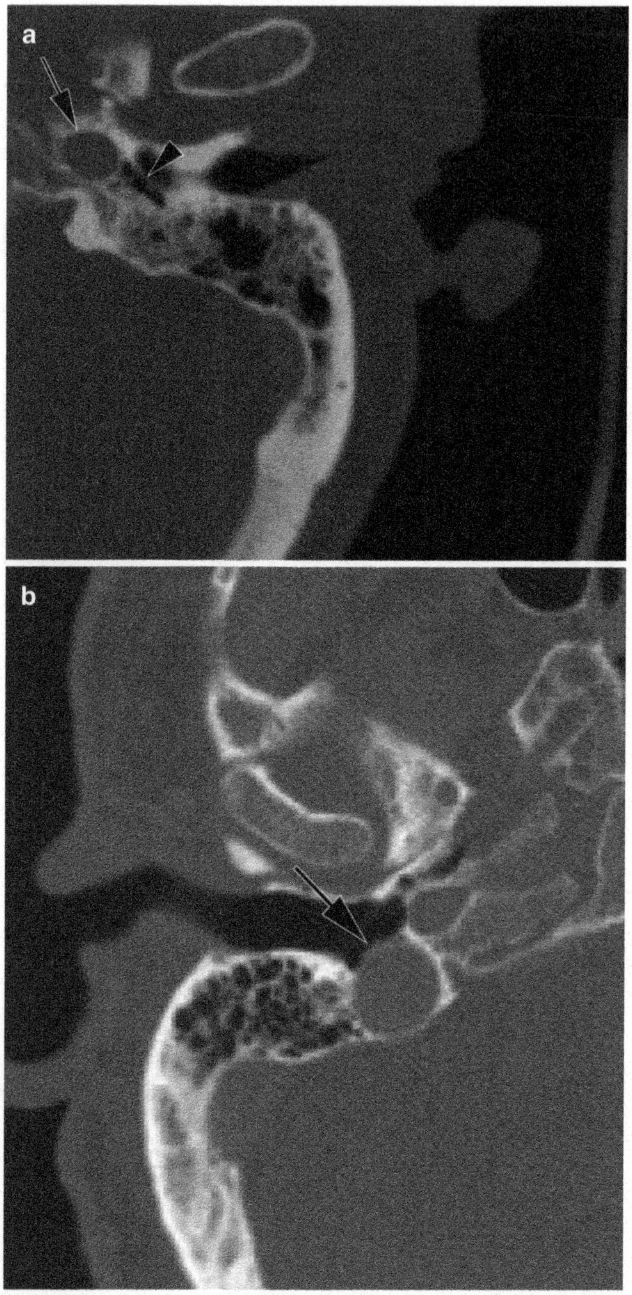

Fig. 17.3 (**a**) CT scan showing the inferior tympanic ring abutting the carotid canal in a patient with recurrent, metastatic squamous cell carcinoma in the left parotid gland. Arrowhead = inferior annulus. Arrow = carotid canal. (**b**) High-riding jugular bulb (arrow) in a patient with metastatic squamous cell carcinoma to the parotid and ear canal

Table 17.1 Contraindications for surgery

Systemic disease	Advanced local disease
Poor overall health	Carotid artery encasement or invasion
Distant metastasis	Brain invasion
	Lower cranial nerve deficit
	Perineural spread along CN V or CN VII intracranially

assessment of the opposite, uninvolved ear is important, since the affected ear might be the better (or only) hearing ear. Surgery in an only hearing ear is not an absolute contraindication to LTBR, since the surgery can be performed while preserving cochlear hearing and the hearing can be rehabilitated with an osseointegrated implant for cochlear stimulation. The alternative to surgery (radiotherapy with or without chemotherapy) can destroy hearing and does not offer better tumor control.

Preoperative assessment must include diagnostic imaging. Contrast-enhanced CT is the preferred initial test since it gives exquisite detail of the structures of the ear canal, eardrum, ossicles, facial nerve, inner ear, and the vascular structures of the temporal bone. The surgeon should examine the CT looking for a high-riding jugular bulb or aberrant carotid artery, since these anomalies have a major impact when performing a LTBR (Fig. 17.3). CT should also include the parotid gland and cervical lymph nodes. MRI has the distinct advantage over CT for assessment of dural involvement around the temporal bone. See Table 17.1 for contraindications for surgery.

Operative Preparation

The patient is taken to the operating room and placed on the operating table in supine position. After sufficient level of anesthetic, the patient is orally endotracheally intubated. In patients with restricted mouth opening due to trismus, a fiber-optic intubation might be required. The patient is then padded with the arms tucked at the sides. At least three straps are placed across the patient to secure the patient to the operating table to allow the table to be tilted during the procedure. The operating table is then turned 180°.

Turning the table 180° places the patient's feet at the anesthesia station. The head of the table is fully accessible by members of the surgical team. This allows the scrub nurse to be directly across the table from the surgeon. While under the microscope, instruments can be easily passed from nurse to surgeon. This table positioning also allows the plastic surgery team sufficient access to raise an anterior lateral thigh (ALT) flap (Fig. 17.4).

Facial nerve monitoring is used for all temporal bone procedures. Electrodes for the facial nerve monitor are placed in the orbicularis oculi and orbicularis oris muscles. Patients must not be given long-acting paralytics for induction, and this fact must be communicated to the anesthesia team.

Since a maximum conductive hearing loss is a result of the surgery, an osseointegrated implant is used for auditory rehabilitation. A site for the implant is marked with methylene blue 5.5 cm behind the external auditory canal at the temporal line (Fig. 17.5).

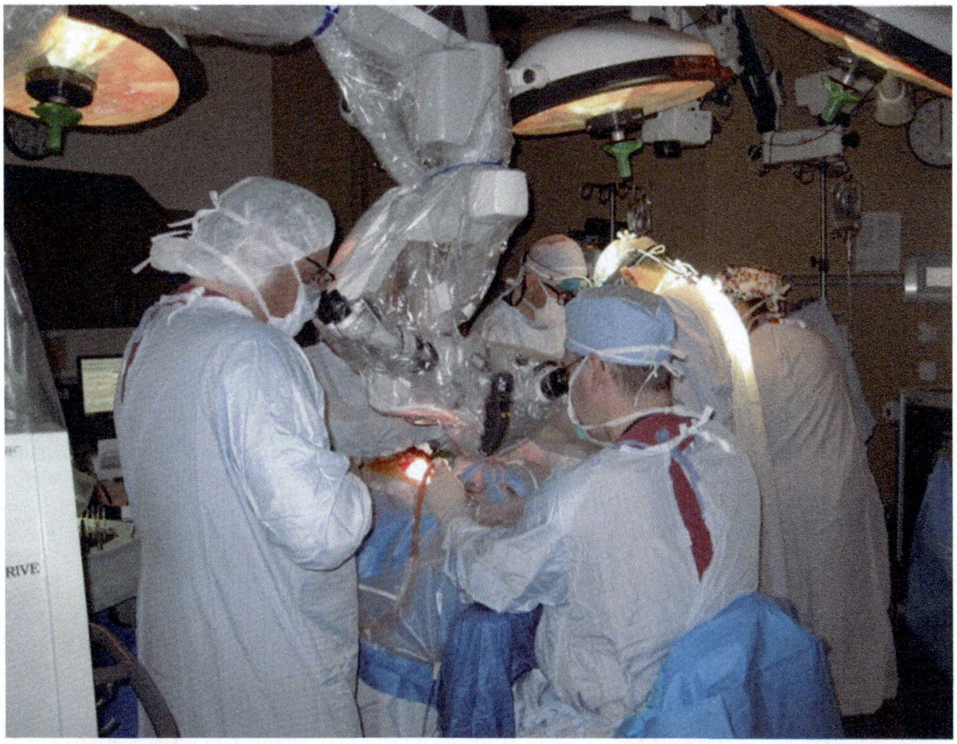

Fig. 17.4 Plastic surgery team elevating anterolateral thigh flap during lateral temporal bone resection

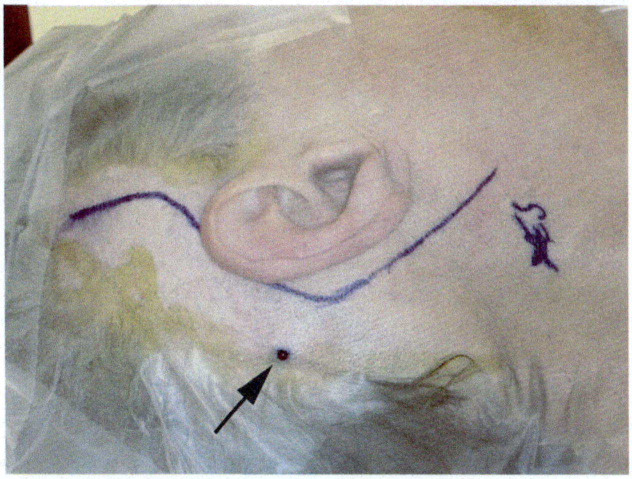

Fig. 17.5 Site (arrow) for osseointegrated implant is marked 5.5 cm behind the external auditory meatus at the temporal line

Incisions

Incision planning is crucial for temporal bone procedures. The incision must allow sufficient access to the temporal bone, parotid gland, neck, and perhaps the mandible, middle cranial fossa or infratemporal fossa.

The choice of incision is influenced by at least three factors: (1) location and extent of tumor, (2) location of previous incisions, and (3) history of previous radiation. When planning to save the auricle, incisions must be placed to avoid compromising blood flow to the auricle. When the ear has been radiated previously, its blood supply is compromised, and its elevation may be poorly tolerated. In this situation, preserving as much blood supply to the auricle as possible is necessary to maintain a healthy pinna. In spite of every good intention and planning, some auricles do not survive the procedure. Either these ears are resected at the time of closure or they necrose and require excision and wound revision in a second-stage operation. In preparation for such an outcome, every patient undergoing temporal bone resection must be made aware that loss of the pinna is a possibility and recognized risk of the procedure (Fig. 17.6).

Three main incision types are used for temporal bone surgery: (1) postauricular C-shaped incision; (2) an anterior, pretragal incision; or (3) a circumferential incision around the entire auricle. All three incisions can be extended into the neck and/or temporal hairline as needed for either neck dissection or temporalis muscle flap.

When tumors are located only within the ear canal, an incision at the external auditory meatus lateral to the tumor is combined with a postauricular incision. The postauricular incision is usually placed at the hairline or about two fingerbreadths behind the postauricular sulcus (Fig. 17.7). The postauricular skin flap is raised in the loose fascial plane superficial to the temporalis muscle, over the mastoid periosteum, and superficial to the sternocleidomastoid muscle and parotid gland. The canal incision is encountered, the tragal cartilage is divided, and flap elevation continues in a plane superficial to the parotid gland.

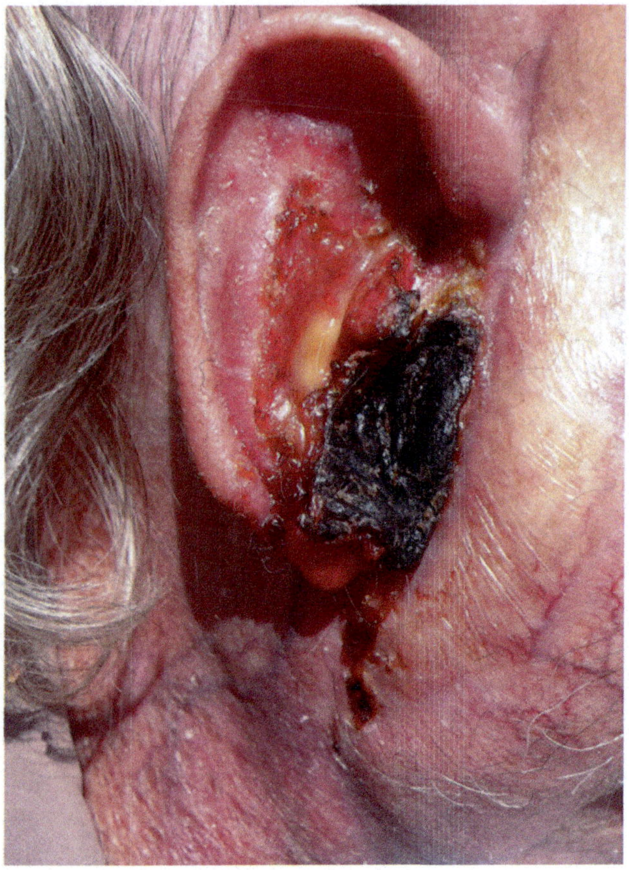

Fig. 17.6 Partial necrosis of the pinna in an ear irradiated prior to lateral temporal bone resection

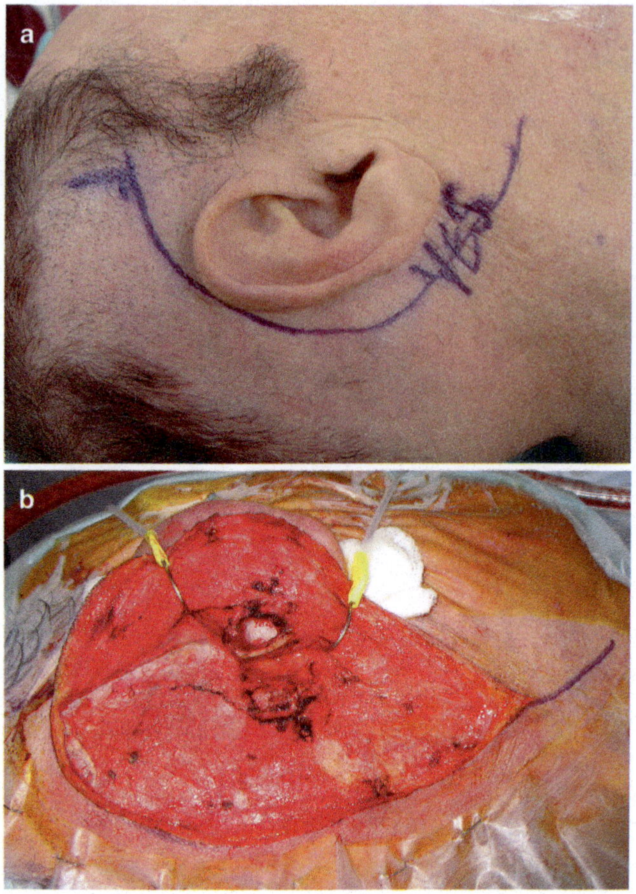

Fig. 17.7 Postauricular incision for lateral temporal bone resection. (**a**) Planned incision. (**b**) Flap raised, and external canal is divided lateral to the tumor

When the tumor extends anteriorly into the parotid gland or when prior parotidectomy has been performed, an anterior pretragal incision can be used. The incision encompasses the external auditory meatus, and it extends superiorly into the temporal scalp and inferiorly into the neck following a skinfold crease (Fig.17.8a). This approach works very well and gives good access for parotidectomy, upper neck dissection, and temporalis muscle flap. The difficulty with this approach is that the external ear is elevated from an anterior to posterior direction, and this mode of elevation is very foreign to most otologists. However, a plane of dissection is easily established over the head of the sternocleidomastoid muscle and the temporalis fascia, which is continuous with the mastoid periosteum. If the tumor does not involve the membranous canal, then the membranous canal can be preserved and closed onto itself (Fig. 17.8b).

When tumors involve the entire pinna and extend into the ear canal, total auriculectomy is usually required. An incision that completely encircles the outer ear is required, and it can be extended into the neck for neck dissection and parotidectomy and into temporal hairline, as needed (Fig. 17.9). Before the flaps are raised, margins from the ear canal or surrounding skin are sent for frozen section analysis.

Flaps are developed over the temporalis fascia superiorly, mastoid periosteum posteriorly, parotid gland anteriorly, and sternocleidomastoid muscle inferiorly. The posterior flap is raised until the methylene blue marking for osseointegrated implant is identified. The flaps are held in place with self-retaining or fish hook retractors.

The mastoid bone is exposed by raising a mastoid periosteal (Palva) flap and exposing the mastoid cortex and root of the zygoma (Fig. 17.10). The Palva flap is sewn over the ear canal defect to prevent tumor spillage. The temporalis muscle is elevated and retracted to identify the zygomatic root. The soft tissue of the temporomandibular joint is identified just below the root of the zygoma. The sternocleidomastoid muscle is elevated off the mastoid tip. The attachment of the digastric muscle in the posterior digastric ridge is identified.

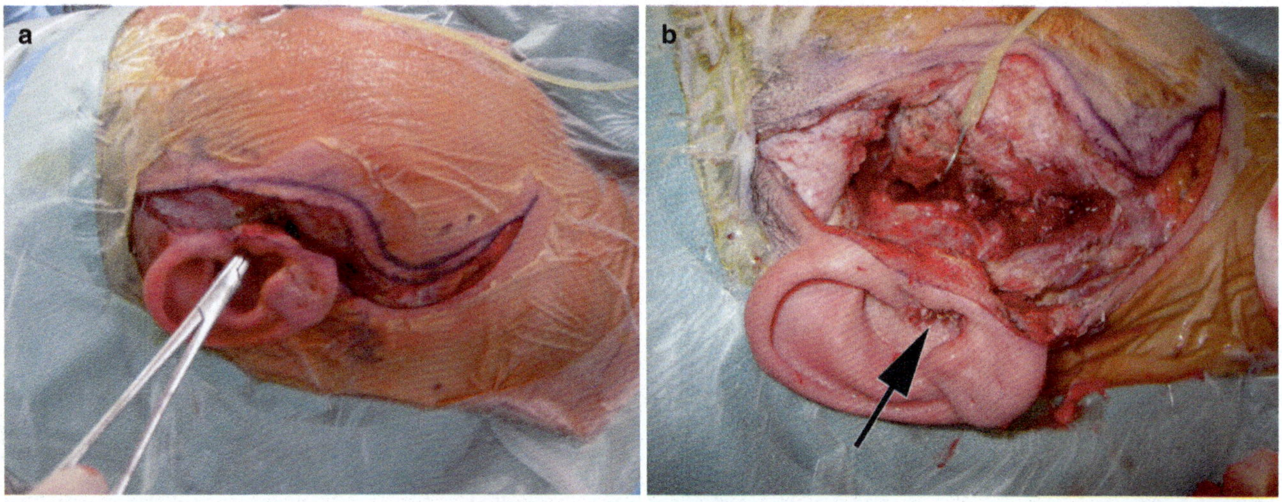

Fig. 17.8 (**a**) Anterior pretragal incision for LTBR in a patient with pleomorphic adenoma metastatic to the ear canal. (**b**) Membranous canal has been closed onto itself (arrow)

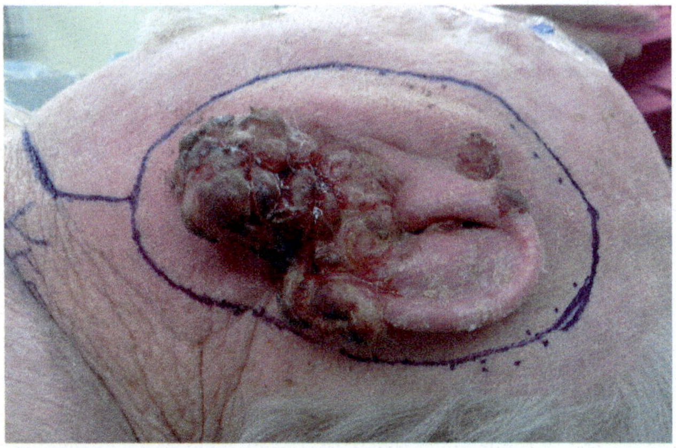

Fig. 17.9 Incision including total auriculectomy

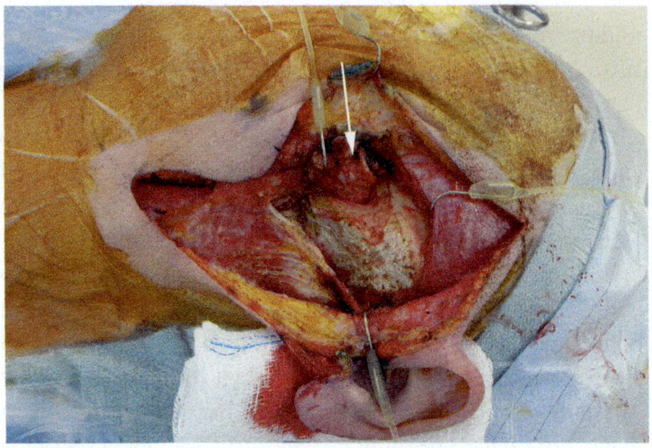

Fig. 17.10 Temporal bone exposure. The Palva flap is sewn over the cut edge of the ear canal (arrow) to avoid tumor spillage

Mastoidectomy

Complete mastoidectomy, including facial recess approach and facial nerve identification, is performed as described in Chap. 16.

Superior Canal Cut

Drilling continues anteriorly through zygomatic air cells removing the bone between the ear canal and middle fossa dura until the temporomandibular joint capsule is reached. Drilling is performed lateral to the ossicular chain. The incus can be disarticulated to avoid transmitting drill vibratory trauma to the inner ear. Care is taken to avoid injury to the dura. Occasionally, the dura is very close to the ear canal bone. In this case, additional ear canal bone is drilled away to avoid tearing the dura and causing a CSF leak. The temporomandibular joint capsule marks the anterosuperior extent of the dissection (Fig. 17.11).

Facial Recess and Facial Nerve Identification

Under high-power magnification and using continuous suction irrigation, the facial recess is drilled out. The middle ear is inspected. If the middle ear is free of disease, then lateral temporal bone resection will be sufficient. If tumor has breached the eardrum, then a subtotal temporal bone resection needs to be performed (Chap. 18). The facial nerve is then identified at the tympanic segment and in the floor of the

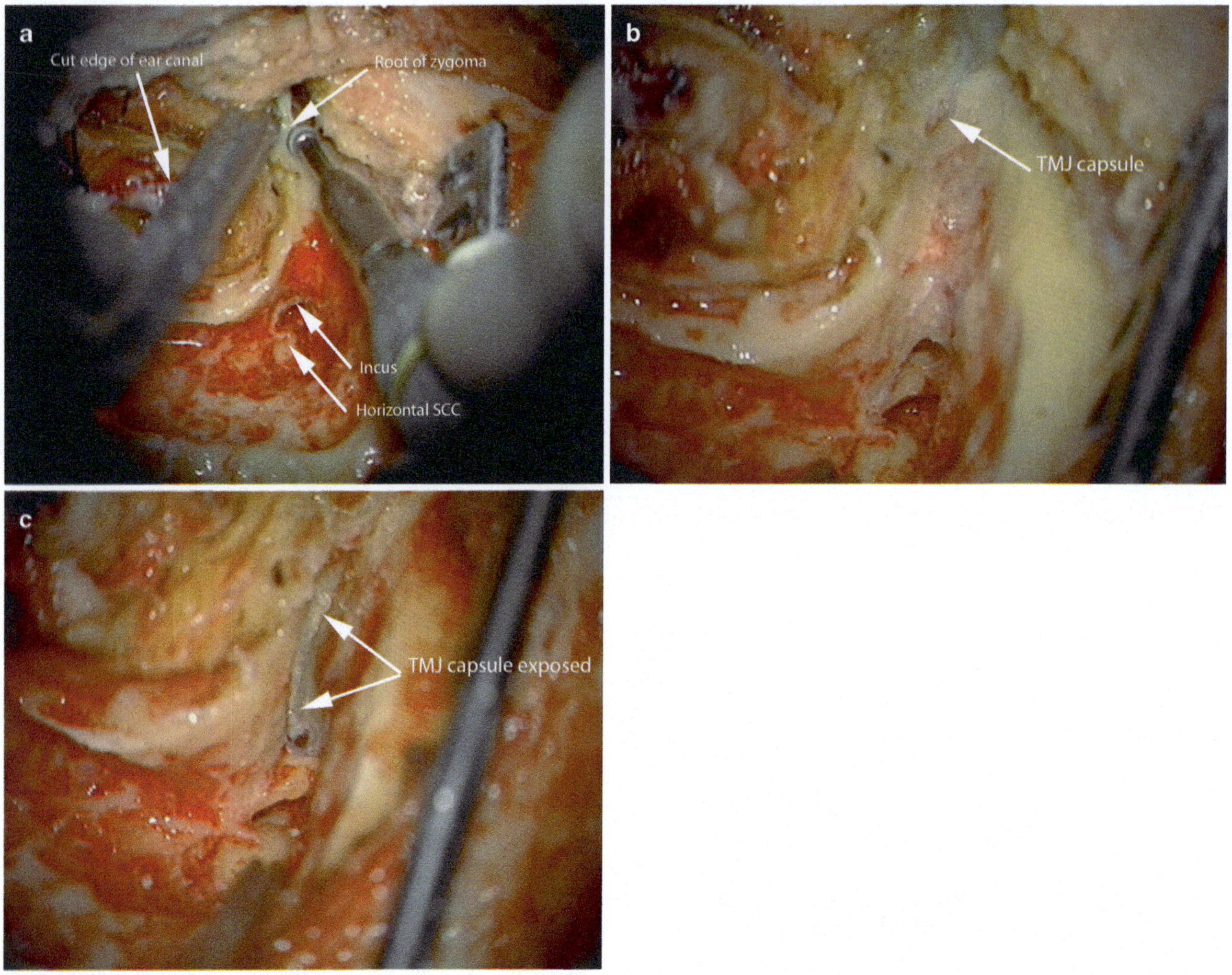

Fig. 17.11 Anterior-superior canal cut. (**a**) Root of the zygoma is drilled down (SCC = semicircular canal). (**b**) Lateral temporomandibular joint (TMJ) capsule is identified. (**c**) The bone is removed along the TMJ capsule

facial recess and followed past the second genu into its mastoid portion. The facial nerve is followed along its mastoid portion to the stylomastoid foramen (Fig. 17.12). The stylomastoid foramen is widened, and the bone of the digastric ridge is removed. A trough is drilled lateral and anterior to the facial nerve, extending the facial recess. This allows identification of the chorda tympani nerve, which is later sacrificed.

Mastoid Tip Removal

Mastoid tip removal is performed in all cases to allow unobstructed dissection of the facial nerve from its mastoid segment to its extratemporal branches (Fig. 17.13). Furthermore, removal of the mastoid tip permits dissection at the skull base, medial to the facial nerve. Lastly, removal of the mastoid tip makes closure with a temporalis flap easier, since the surrounding soft tissues can be mobilized and sutured to the flap.

The bone along the digastric ridge is drilled away to expose the underlying muscle. Widening the stylomastoid foramen naturally exposes the digastric muscle near the facial nerve. Drilling is performed through the bone inferior to the ear canal and anterior and lateral to the facial nerve until soft tissue of the TMJ is reached. Doing so frees the last bony attachment of the mastoid tip, having already divided the bone posteriorly along and through the digastric ridge. The mastoid tip is then elevated, and the soft tissue attachments are divided beginning posteriorly. The facial nerve is held in the stylomastoid foramen by its periosteal attachments and does not elevate with the mastoid tip. No attempt is made to identify the extratemporal portion of the facial nerve prior to removal of the mastoid tip.

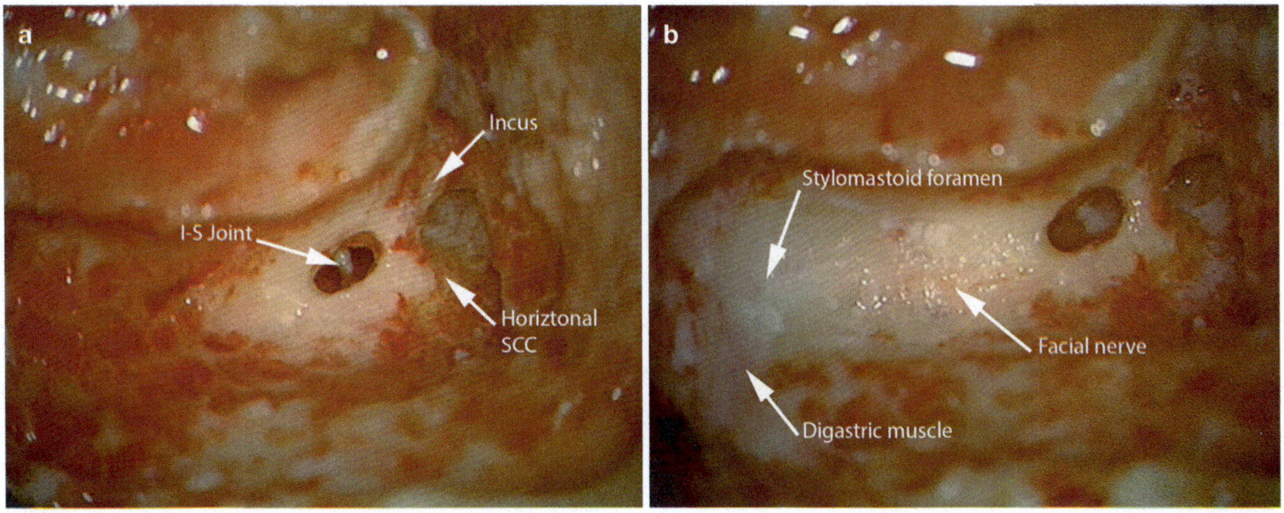

Fig. 17.12 Facial nerve dissection. (**a**) Facial recess opened. I-S joint = incudostapedial joint. (**b**) Digastric muscle and stylomastoid foramen identified

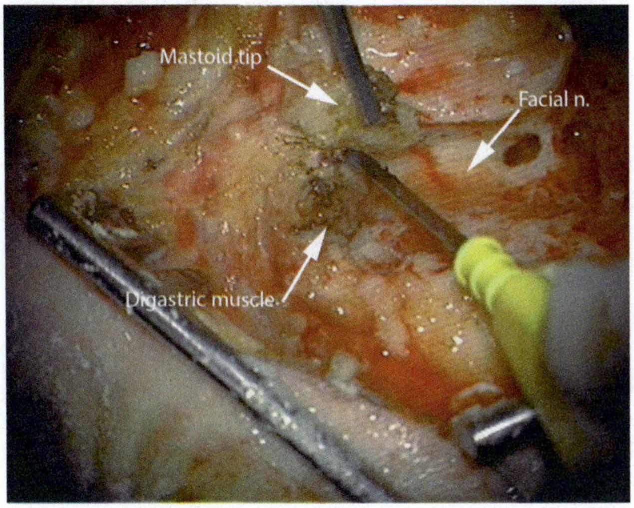

Fig. 17.13 Mastoid tip is removed

Inferior Canal Cut

Once the mastoid tip is removed, then the inferior tympanic ring can be drilled away. The facial recess is extended, and bone is removed between the facial nerve and the annulus (Fig. 17.14). The annulus is then followed inferiorly, and drilling is performed through the hypotympanic air cells. At this point, care must be taken to avoid having the shaft of the drill rest on the facial canal.

The author has found that some patients have either a deep annulus or a superficial facial nerve, meaning that the facial nerve lies in a plane lateral to the level of the annulus. In this circumstance, drilling between the facial nerve and the annulus must be done with great care to avoid having the shaft of the drill rest on the facial nerve. If the shaft does rest on the facial nerve, the facial nerve can be burned by the drill's shaft. The facial nerve monitor will not fire in this event, and there will be no warning to the surgeon. Only constant vigilance and care can prevent this type of injury.

The surgeon must also be cognizant of a high-riding jugular bulb and/or a high or dehiscent carotid artery. Preoperative CT imaging will alert the surgeon of these anatomical variants. The high-riding jugular bulb should be suspected when the sigmoid sinus is more anterior and lateral than normal. Occasionally, the jugular bulb lies dehiscent just below the facial nerve. The dehiscent carotid artery is encountered and first noticed when drilling out hypotympanic air cells. A bulge in the anterior hypotympanic air cells is a telltale sign (Fig. 17.15). Care must be taken when drilling medial to the annulus since the artery can lie just below it. The classic description of LTBR (by Gacek and Goodman(5)) involves using an osteotome to make the anterior canal cut. Placing an osteotome medial to the annulus in the setting of an aberrant carotid artery could be disastrous.

Mobilizing the External Bony Canal

At this point, the ear canal is held principally by only a thin shell of the bone anteriorly. The incus is disarticulated, and the incus bar is removed. The tensor tympani muscle is divided. Thumb pressure on the external auditory canal allows it to fracture off anteriorly (Fig. 17.16).

Using a Freer elevator, the surgeon can assure that the canal is completely freed. Care must be exercised not to use the facial canal or tegmen as a fulcrum for the elevator. Occasionally, the anterior bony annulus does not fracture off in continuity with the canal, and it can be removed with the drill or rongeurs. Failure to remove the anterior tympanic ring risks leaving tumor or squamous epithelium behind.

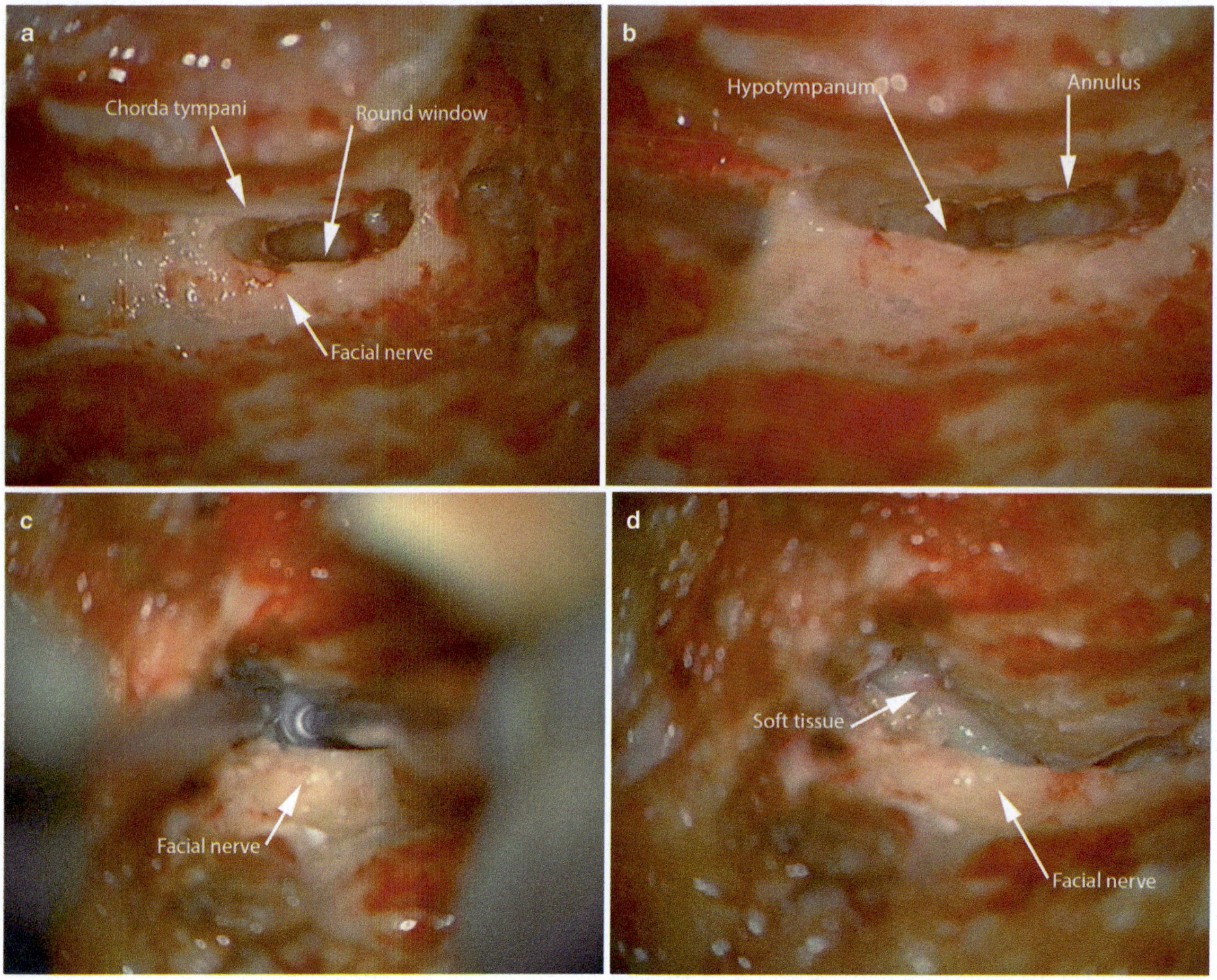

Fig. 17.14 Inferior canal cut. (**a**) Facial recess is extended. (**b**) Hypotympanic air cells are opened. (**c**) Drill shaft must not touch facial nerve. (**d**) Canal cut is complete when soft tissue is reached

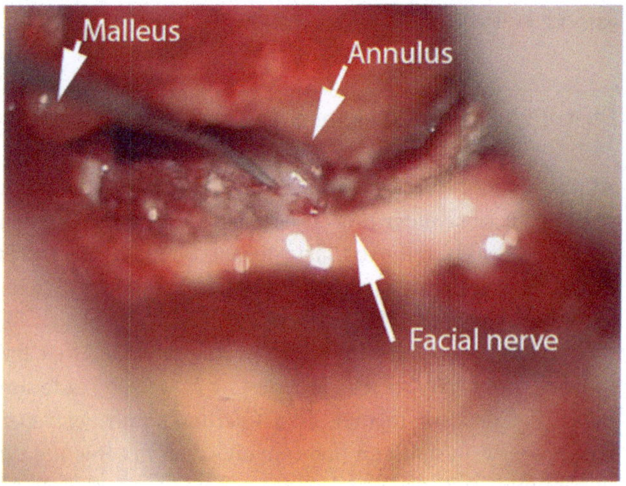

Fig. 17.15 Tympanic ring at level of carotid canal. Rosen needle points to carotid canal. See temporal bone CT in Fig. 17.3a

Both tissue types have the potential to grow and cause problems (cancer or cholesteatoma, respectively).

If tumor is confined only to the ear canal and parotidectomy or neck dissection is not planned, then the ear canal can be removed by developing a plane of dissection between the parotid gland and the ear canal (Fig. 17.17), producing a "simple" lateral temporal bone specimen. Bridging blood vessels to the ear canal are cauterized with bipolar electrocautery. Blunt and sharp dissection staying close to the bony ear canal will allow the specimen to be removed, and facial nerve injury can be avoided.

For larger tumors, especially tumors of the external ear, auriculectomy, parotidectomy, and neck dissection are performed. A large "composite" specimen is produced by including the external ear, ear canal, parotid, and neck nodes (Fig. 17.18).

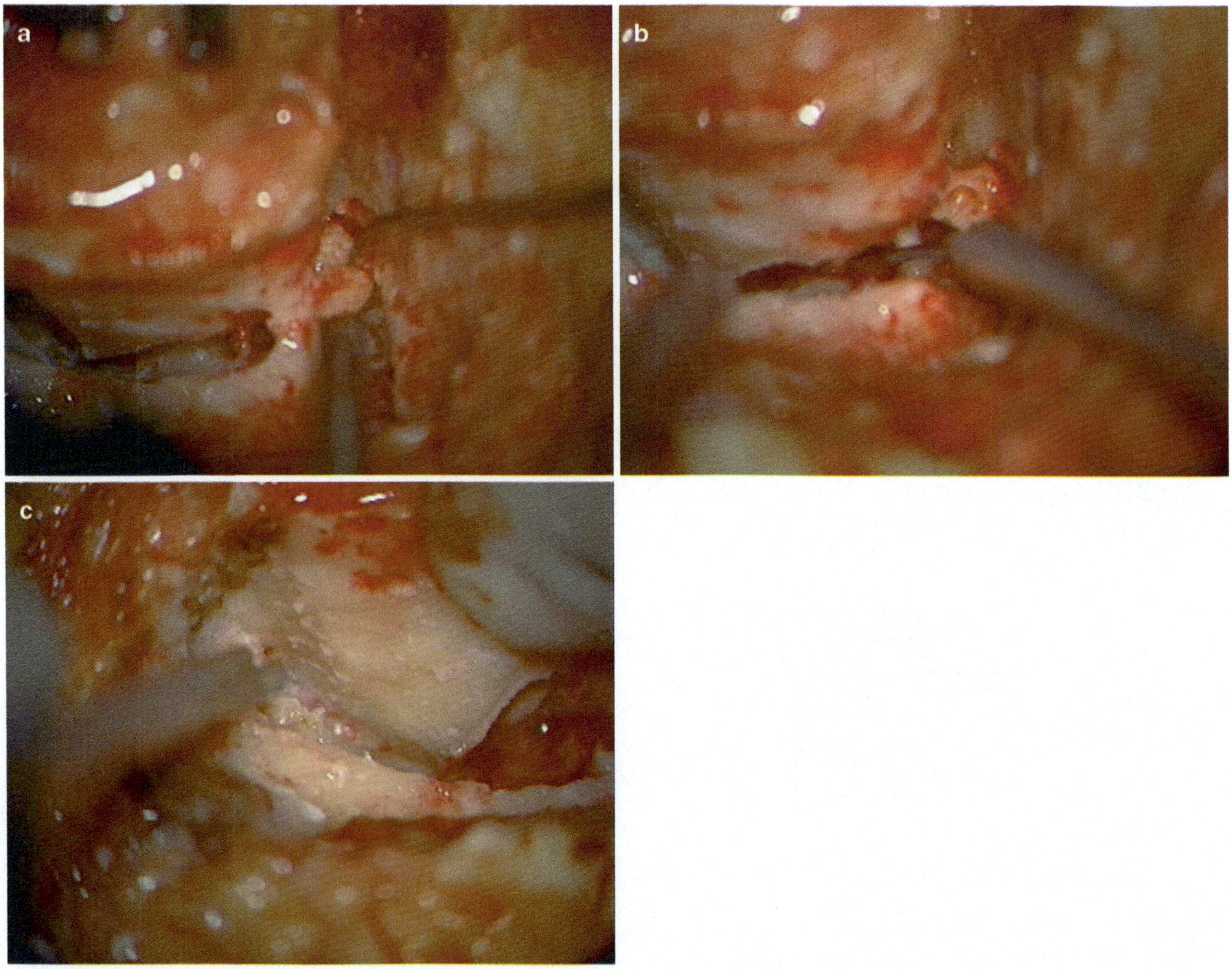

Fig. 17.16 Ear canal mobilization. (**a**) Incus is disarticulated. (**b**) Tensor tendon is cut with Bellucci scissors. (**c**) Thumb pressure fractures the canal anteriorly

Facial Nerve Management

Many times the lateral temporal bone resection is combined with parotidectomy for advanced parotid cancers. In this circumstance, the facial nerve can be decompressed in preparation for parotidectomy or mobilized if nerve sacrifice and grafting are required.

Facial nerve decompression is required in at least three circumstances: (1) when facial weakness is identified preoperatively, since this connotes facial nerve involvement by tumor, (2) when tumor is located at the stylomastoid foramen and the nerve will need to be mobilized or sacrificed, or (3) when scarring from previous parotidectomy is suspected.

Facial nerve decompression has at least three purposes: (1) to identify the facial nerve at an uninvolved segment, (2) to obtain a negative margin on an infiltrated nerve, and (3) to permit facial nerve grafting if facial nerve sacrifice is required.

After the ear canal is mobilized, the ear canal can be left attached to the soft tissue of the parotid and TMJ. The bone of the facial canal is removed with fine diamond burrs and continuous suction irrigation. The bone is removed for 270 degrees around the nerve until only a thin layer remains. Fisch instruments or other suitable raspatories are used to remove this last layer of the bone. At the stylomastoid foramen, the periosteal cuff is opened, and the facial nerve is identified extratemporally (Fig. 17.19). Blunt dissection along the length of the nerve with a Jacobson hemostat and sharp dissection with bipolar electrocautery and a #12 blade exposes the extratemporal portion of the facial nerve. The nerve is traced out until the pes anserinus is identified or until tumor is encountered. Parotidectomy can then proceed.

The decision for facial nerve sacrifice is always difficult, and it can be made based on inspection of the nerve. Frozen section pathology is required for this decision-making. Facial nerve sacrifice is performed in at least three circumstances: (1) there is obvious disease involving the nerve (Fig. 17.20),

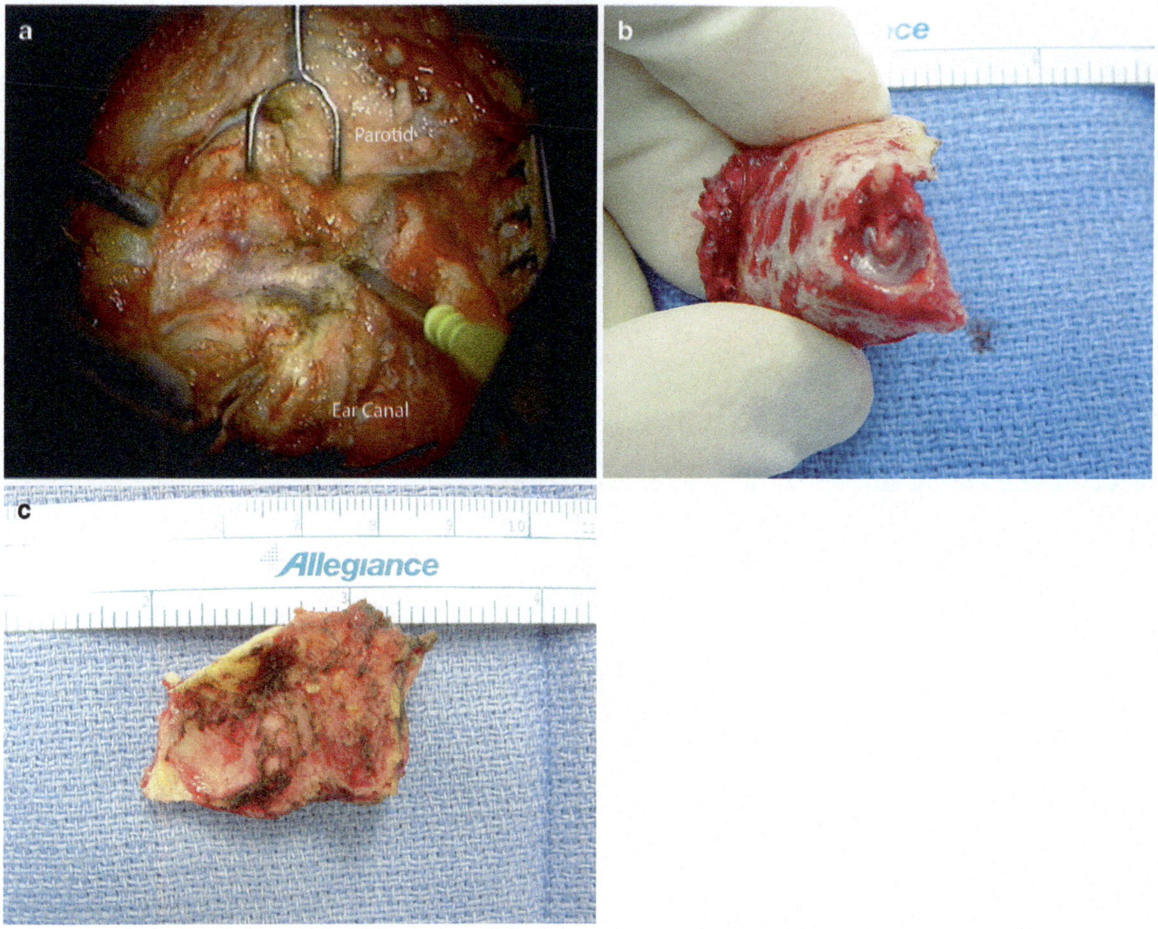

Fig. 17.17 Canal removal. (**a**) Dissection in the soft tissue plane anterior to the ear canal. "Simple" lateral temporal bone specimen. (**b**) Medial surface. (**c**) Anterior surface

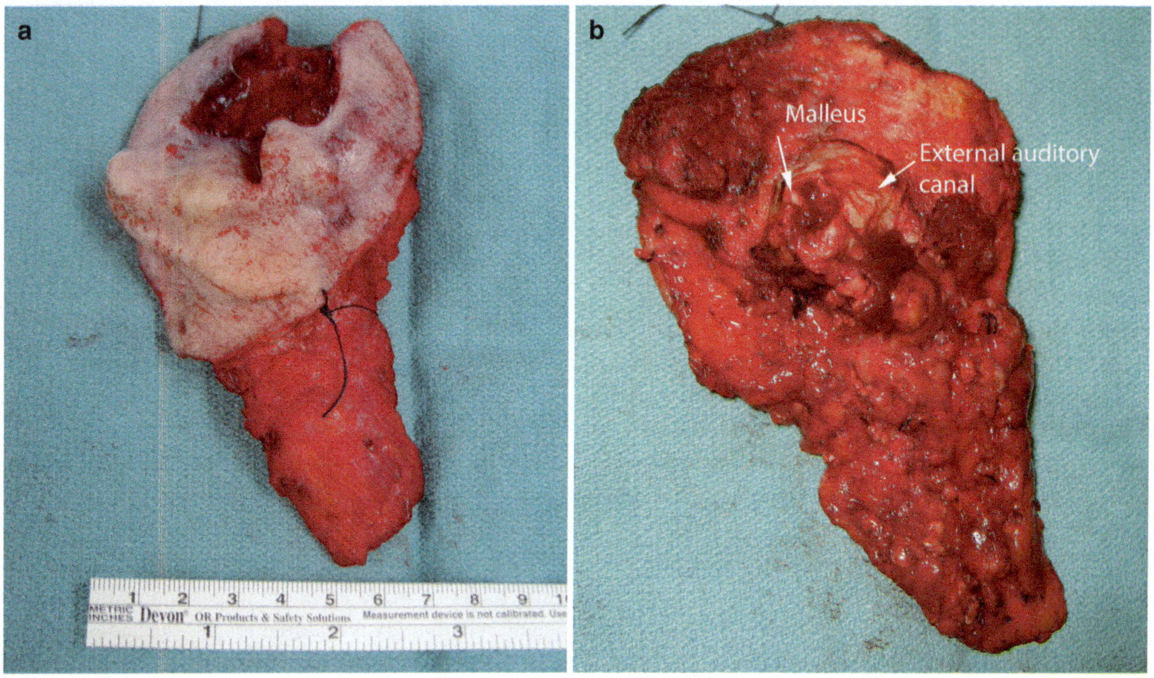

Fig. 17.18 Composite resection of ear canal, parotid, and neck nodes. (**a**) Lateral surface. (**b**) Medial surface

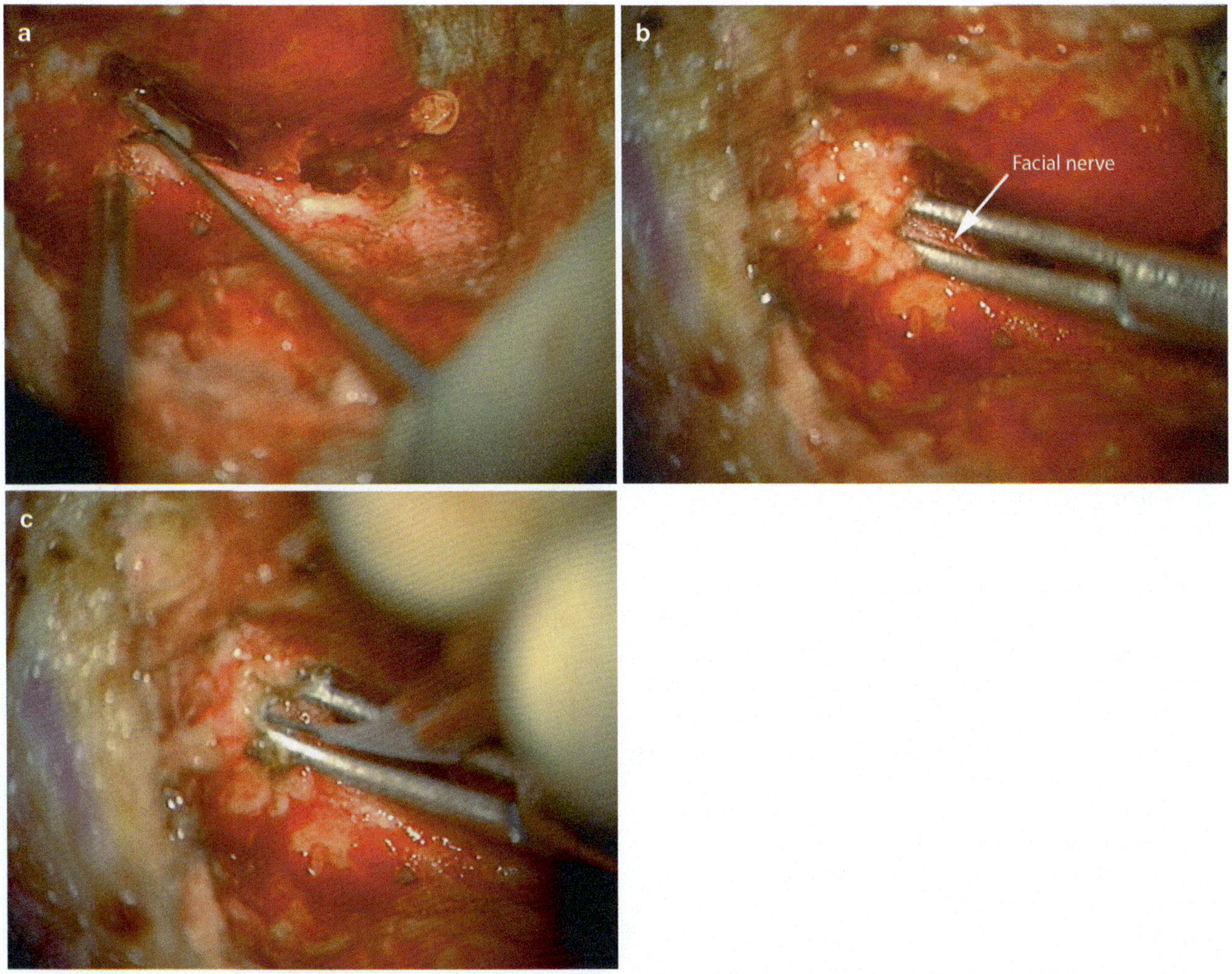

Fig. 17.19 Facial nerve dissection. (**a**) Fisch instrument opens periosteal cuff at the stylomastoid foramen. (**b**) A fine Jacobson's hemostat bluntly dissects along the facial nerve. (**c**) A no. 12 blade divides the soft tissue lateral to the nerve

(2) there is disease involving the tissue surrounding the nerve, or (3) there is preoperative facial nerve paralysis, which indicates perineural spread along the nerve. Branch defects of the nerve might require only one extratemporal branch to be sacrificed. In the MD Anderson series, facial nerve sacrifice was required in 93 (40.7%) of the cases, of which 14 were sacrifice of only a branch or division of the nerve.

When facial nerve sacrifice is performed, an initial cut in the nerve is performed just above the stylomastoid foramen and a second cut more proximally in an area that appears normal. The nerve is marked with ink proximally to orient the pathologist; and frozen section is performed to determine the margin. Multiple segments of the nerve can be sent until the margin is negative. In practice, if the margin is still positive with microscopic disease at the geniculate ganglion, no further surgery is performed. In such a circumstance, labyrinthectomy has been recommended to obtain a negative margin [9]. However, this procedure creates the undue morbidity of profound hearing loss and vertigo. Instead, these patients will be treated with postoperative radiotherapy, and this treatment should be sufficient to control the microscopically positive margin on the nerve. Facial nerve grafting is not impeded by a positive facial nerve margin [10]. Facial nerve grafting can be considered depending on the amount of remaining intratemporal and any extratemporal branches.

Osseointegrated Implant for Auditory Rehabilitation

Since all of these patients develop a maximum conductive hearing loss, an osseointegrated implant for cochlear stimulation is very effective for auditory rehabilitation. Many different brands have been developed, but the basic principles of implantation remain the same. In this setting, a two-stage process is used for these implants. An implant is placed in the bone followed by the conical cover screw. Transcutaneous abutments are placed in a second-stage procedure.

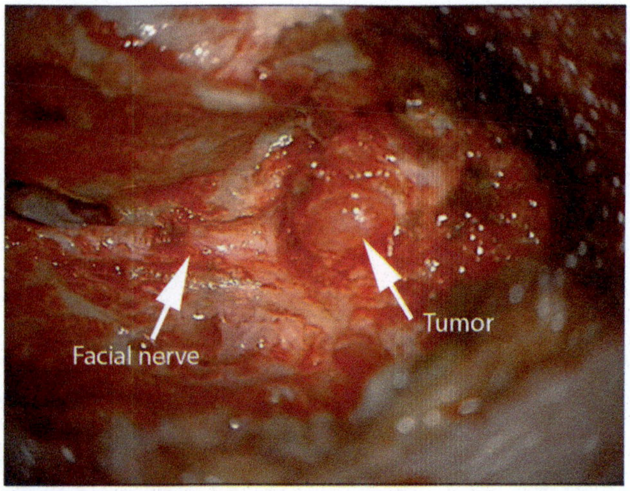

Fig. 17.20 Cancer in the facial nerve at stylomastoid foramen

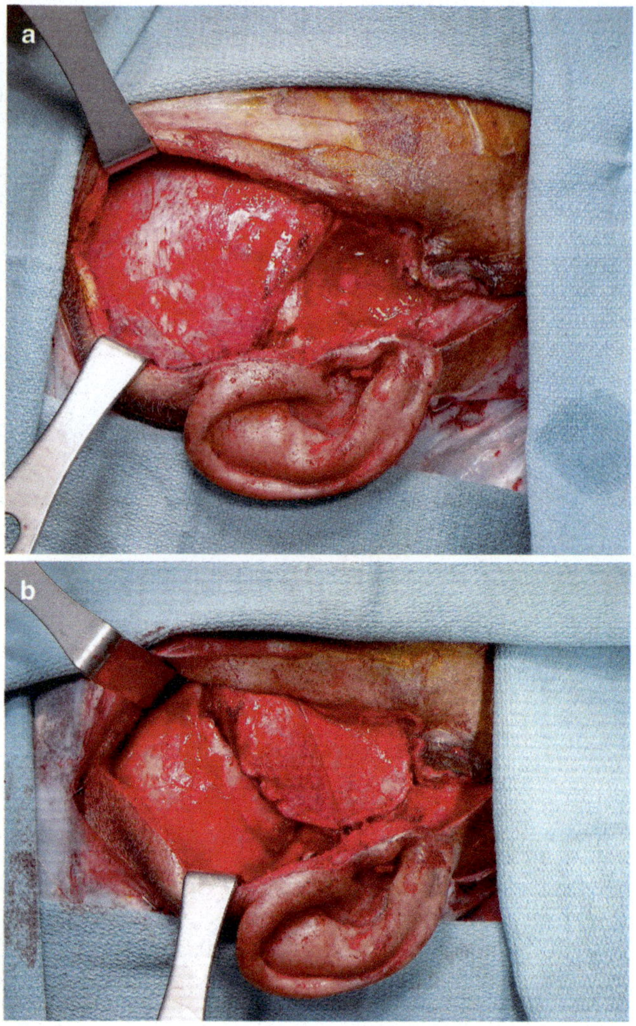

Fig. 17.21 Temporalis muscle flap. (**a**) Temporalis muscle is exposed. (**b**) Flap rotated into place

Implants are placed at the time of the initial extirpative surgery for two reasons: (1) to start the process of osseointegration and (2) to improve the outcome and osseointegration process since implants placed prior to radiotherapy do better than those implants placed after radiotherapy [11]. The second stage is performed at 3 or 6 months depending on the use of postoperative radiotherapy.

The decision to give postoperative radiation is predicated on the results found on the final pathology report. The bone or cartilage invasion, perineural invasion, recurrent cancer, and positive lymph nodes are all indicators for postoperative radiotherapy. Radiation has a major role to play in treating ear canal cancers, and more than 60% of patient will receive radiation. Radiation has a major impact on these implants. Radiation affects the length of time given for osseointegration, and irradiated bone is given 6 months to osseointegrate with the implant. Without radiotherapy, the abutment can be placed at 3 months. This second-stage procedure usually takes about 15 min to perform and can be done under local anesthesia. Details of the implantation process are given in Chap. 27.

Wound Closure

The temporal bone defect can be closed in a variety of ways: skin graft, temporalis flap, or microvascular free flap. Some authors have written about creating an open cavity covered by a split-thickness skin graft [12]. Skin graft is laid over the exposed bone, and the cavity is packed with antibiotic impregnated gauze, as is done for chronic ear disease. Morita et al. have described reconstructing the ear canal with rolled split-thickness skin graft [13]. This author has not used either one of these techniques; and these techniques should be reserved only for those cases in which radiotherapy is not planned, since radiotherapy can result in a chronic draining ear [14].

The temporalis flap is a commonly used to close the defect when the ear canal alone is removed and the external ear and surrounding skin is preserved. Temporalis muscle flap was performed in about 25% of the cases in the MD Anderson series. Its bulk allows protection of the temporal bone for radiation. The flap is measured, cut, elevated, and rotated into the defect. Removal of the posterior attachment of the zygomatic arch can help to free up the muscle and makes rotation easier; however, this maneuver is rarely needed. The flap is sewn to the mastoid periosteum, the sternocleidomastoid muscle, and the parotid fascia (Fig. 17.21). The author also places sutures from the undersurface of the pinna to the temporalis muscle to suspend the outer ear and to avoid the inevitable sag that happens without an ear canal. A closed suction wound drain is necessary to prevent a hematoma.

Larger defects, as in the case of total auriculectomy, might require free flap coverage. Microvascular free flaps, primarily the anterior lateral thigh flap, were performed in 75% of the cases in the MD Anderson series. Please see Chap. 25 for details on this reconstruction.

The Eustachian tube is not obliterated or packed as described by some authors, unless there is a dural opening and risk of CSF leak. Most of these patients have normal Eustachian tube function preoperatively, and postoperatively they develop an aerated middle ear. This air space helps to define and delineate recurrent tumors if they occur in the middle ear [8, 15].

Postoperative Care

Given that the average patient is elderly, consider admitting patients to an intensive care unit for the first night if there are pre-existing medical problems or if a microvascular free flap has been performed. Younger patients will not need this level of attention or support.

Eye care is important for patients with facial weakness or paralysis. Liberal use of eye moisturizers is necessary to prevent corneal drying and ulceration. Early consultation with an oculoplastic surgeon is helpful in managing the eye after facial nerve sacrifice.

Conductive hearing loss is an expected outcome of the surgery. In a few patients, the operated ear was the only hearing ear. For these individuals, the speech processor for the bone-anchored hearing aid is placed with a soft headband on the first postoperative day. This device gives these patients an immediate connection with the speaking world.

Dizziness and vertigo have not been encountered as a postoperative complication in this patient population. Tinnitus can occur in some patients after LTBR. Closure of the ear canal and creation of a maximal conductive loss can block out masking noises and uncover tinnitus. Patients with this type of tinnitus fare very well with an osseointegrated hearing aid.

Hospitalization continues until the patient meets criteria for dismissal. Patients are usually discharged after 2 days when uncomplicated surgery without free flap is performed. Microvascular free flap patients generally stay 5–7 days after surgery.

Due to removal of the ear canal and/or rotation of the temporalis muscle, some patients will develop difficulty with mouth opening. These patients should be instructed to start mouth opening stretching exercises about 10 days to 2 weeks following surgery.

Conclusion

The lateral temporal bone resection is the most common procedure for cancers of the ear canal and temporal bone. The indications for this procedure are enumerated. The goal is complete en bloc resection of the ear canal along with the disease within it. The steps for this procedure are illustrated and discussed. The facial nerve is dissected and decompressed. The rationale for facial nerve sacrifice is given. Reconstructive techniques are outlined. The inner ear is spared, and patients are good candidates for hearing rehabilitation using an osseointegrated implant. Complications and postoperative management are highlighted.

References

1. Moody SA, Hirsch BE, Myers EN. Squamous cell carcinoma of the external auditory canal: an evaluation of a staging system. Am J Otol. 2000;21(4):582–8.
2. Moore MG, Deschler DG, McKenna MJ, Varvares MA, Lin DT. Management outcomes following lateral temporal bone resection for ear and temporal bone malignancies. Otolaryngol Head Neck Surg. 2007;137(6):893–8.
3. Zhang T, Li W, Dai C, Chi F, Wang S, Wang Z. Evidence-based surgical management of T1 or T2 temporal bone malignancies. Laryngoscope. 2013;123(1):244–8.
4. Medina JE, Park AO, Neely JG, Britton BH. Lateral temporal bone resections. Am J Surg. 1990;160(4):427–33.
5. Gacek RR, Goodman M. Management of malignancy of the temporal bone. Laryngoscope. 1977;87(10 Pt 1):1622–34.
6. Arriaga M, Curtin H, Takahashi H, Hirsch BE, Kamerer DB. Staging proposal for external auditory meatus carcinoma based on preoperative clinical examination and computed tomography findings. Ann Otol Rhinol Laryngol. 1990;99(9 Pt 1):714–21.
7. Moffat DA, Wagstaff SA, Hardy DG. The outcome of radical surgery and postoperative radiotherapy for squamous carcinoma of the temporal bone. Laryngoscope. 2005;115(2):341–7.
8. Leong SC, Youssef A, Lesser TH. Squamous cell carcinoma of the temporal bone: outcomes of radical surgery and postoperative radiotherapy. Laryngoscope. 2013;123(10):2442–8.
9. Leonetti JP, Benscoter BJ, Marzo SJ, Borrowdale RW, Pontikis GC. Preauricular infratemporal fossa approach for advanced malignant parotid tumors. Laryngoscope. 2012;122(9):1949–53.
10. Wax MK, Kaylie DM. Does a positive neural margin affect outcome in facial nerve grafting? Head Neck. 2007;29(6):546–9.
11. Nader ME, Beadle BM, Roberts DB, Gidley PW. Outcomes and complications of osseointegrated hearing aids in irradiated temporal bones. Laryngoscope. 2016;126(5):1187–92.
12. Renton JP, Wetmore SJ. Split-thickness skin grafting in postmastoidectomy revision and in lateral temporal bone resection. Otolaryngol Head Neck Surg. 2006;135(3):387–91.
13. Morita S, Nakamaru Y, Homma A, Sakashita T, Masuya M, Fukuda S. Hearing preservation after lateral temporal bone resection for early-stage external auditory canal carcinoma. Audiol Neurootol. 2014;19(6):351–7.
14. Nadol JB Jr, Schuknecht HF. Obliteration of the mastoid in the treatment of tumors of the temporal bone. Ann Otol Rhinol Laryngol. 1984;93(1 Pt 1):6–12.
15. Masterson L, Rouhani M, Donnelly NP, Tysome JR, Patel P, Jefferies SJ, et al. Squamous cell carcinoma of the temporal bone: clinical outcomes from radical surgery and postoperative radiotherapy. Otol Neurotol. 2014;35(3):501–8.

Subtotal and Total Temporal Bone Resection

18

Paul W. Gidley and Franco DeMonte

Indications

Subtotal temporal bone resection (STBR) is required for tumors that involve the mastoid, middle ear, inner ear, or lateral skull base (i.e., jugular foramen) [1]. A STBR is performed when there is evidence of invasion medial to the tympanic membrane or into the mastoid [2]. Subtotal temporal bone resection removes the otic capsule. The total temporal bone resection proceeds after the STBR to include removal of the petrous apex [2]. STBR has also been called "extended temporal bone resection" [3–5]. Moffat et al. describe an "extended temporal bone resection" [4]. This resection removes a wider area of skin and soft tissue than LTBR, and it requires a middle and posterior fossa craniotomy. By its nature, this resection is closer in description to a subtotal temporal bone resection, since the labyrinth is removed. Subtotal temporal bone resection has been described as either a piecemeal resection [2, 5, 6] or en bloc resection [4, 7–14].

The direction and extent of dissection depends on the location of the tumor. These tumors are often extensive, and a team approach is necessary. Typically, our team consists of a neurotologist, neurosurgeon, head and neck surgeon, and plastic reconstructive surgeon. When sacrifice of cranial nerves IX through XI is contemplated, a preoperative speech and swallowing evaluation should be performed.

Prasad and Janecka showed that when SCCa is in the middle ear, a 5-year survival is better for patients who had subtotal temporal bone resection (41.7%) over lateral temporal bone resection (28.7%) [15]. Conversely, Zanoletti et al. reported results of 17 patients who developed recurrence after primary tumor resection with negative margins. Postoperative radiotherapy was administered to only eight of these patients. They observed that lateral temporal bone resection (LTBR) had a longer disease-free survival (DFS) and disease-specific survival (DSS) than patients who underwent subtotal temporal bone resection (STBR); however, this comparison and associated outcomes may be more indicative of the difficulty in assessing margins in temporal bone surgery and the impact of disease burden rather than the results of the two procedures themselves [16].

In a meta-analysis, Takenaka et al. analyzed 752 cases of SCC of the temporal bone and found that STBR and TTBR obtained 5-year survival rate of 45.7% [17]. Okada et al. reported a 78% 5-year survival rate in their patients who underwent en bloc subtotal temporal bone resection [12]. More recent developments in the management of large T3 and T4 tumors involve the use of preoperative chemotherapy and radiotherapy, as initially proposed by Nakagawa et al. in 2006 [11]. A larger trial involving 66 patients with advanced SCC of the temporal bone has been published showing improved outcomes when preoperative chemotherapy and radiotherapy are given [18].

In general, there seems to be four classes of tumors that require STBR: (1) tumors that involve the middle ear and have limited mastoid disease, (2) tumors that extend into the labyrinth, (3) tumors that extend below the otic capsule into the jugular foramen, and (4) tumors that have replaced the otic capsule and entered the cochlea. These tumors are the most dangerous due to the involvement of the carotid artery. These tumors usually have replaced the mastoid completely prior to involving the labyrinth.

Adequate preoperative evaluation must be performed to determine the extent of carotid involvement. Surgery is not offered to patients with high-grade malignancy who have tumors that encase the carotid artery.

En bloc subtotal temporal bone resection has been described [4, 7–14]. We consider this procedure as engendering excessive morbidity and typically do not support its use.

P. W. Gidley, M.D., F.A.C.S. (✉)
Department of Head and Neck Surgery, The University of Texas M.D. Anderson Cancer Center, Houston, TX, USA
e-mail: pwgidley@mdanderson.org

F. DeMonte, M.D.
Department of Neurosurgery, The University of Texas M.D. Anderson Cancer Center, Houston, TX, USA
e-mail: fdemonte@mdanderson.org

P. W. Gidley, F. DeMonte (eds.), *Temporal Bone Cancer*, https://doi.org/10.1007/978-3-319-74539-8_18

It is our opinion that a margin-negative piecemeal resection offers the same patient outcomes at a significantly reduced risk. Similarly, some authors have described total temporal bone resection as an en bloc procedure. To date, en bloc resection has not been shown to produce any lengthening of disease-free survival and thus has little to recommend it given the significant morbidity associated with this procedure.

Management decisions for advanced temporal bone cancer are complicated. The most difficult decision is related to the resectability of the tumor. Criteria that typically contraindicate surgical therapy include (1) extensive brain involvement including involvement of the vein of Labbé, (2) carotid encasement, (3) treatment failure following LTBR and radiotherapy, (4) distant metastatic disease, and (5) moribund patient.

Intratemporal carotid artery involvement is a challenge. Tumors that are within 1.8 mm of the carotid artery or that encompass more than 180° of the artery have much poorer survival than those situated farther away [19]. While carotid artery resection and bypass grafting has been described [20], these procedures are fraught with significant morbidity and mortality and have resulted in little appreciable improvements in patient outcome [21, 22]. It is our practice not to perform carotid artery sacrifice when the internal carotid artery (ICA) is involved by high-grade malignancy since this, in our patient population, has not resulted in improved oncologic outcomes and carries significant risks of morbidity. In this circumstance, quality of life outweighs any potential extension of life. For these patients, chemotherapy and radiotherapy provide an alternative approach.

Subtotal temporal bone resection differs from lateral temporal bone resection in at least one of five ways: (1) the posterior fossa plate is removed, exposing the sigmoid sinus and posterior fossa dura; (2) the labyrinth is removed, either partially or totally; (3) the retrofacial air cell tract and jugular bulb bone are exenterated, as a prelude to possible jugular bulb resection; (4) the cochlea is removed; and (5) the carotid artery is skeletonized.

These procedures usually produce a large defect in the skull base, and careful reconstructive planning is necessary. The temporal bone defect communicates with the neck. Although an abdominal fat graft might be sufficient with smaller defects and uncomplicated cases without a prior history of radiotherapy, free microvascular flap reconstruction is usually required for closure of larger, complicated skull base defects.

Preoperative Assessment

All patients undergo rigorous history and physical examination to identify the extent of the disease, to document cranial nerve deficits, and to ensure good overall health (Fig. 18.1). CT scan of the head and neck is the usual first step for radiographic demonstration of the extent of disease. MRI scan is useful with larger tumors to identify dural involvement. Preoperative angiography is needed to understanding the extent or lack of arterial and venous collateral and to assess the venous outflow pattern since many patients will require ligation of the sigmoid sinus. A freely communicating torcular herophili lessens the risk associated with ligation of the sigmoid sinus [23].

Patient Preparation and Positioning

These procedures are performed with the patient placed supine on the operating table. The table is turned so that the anesthesia stand is at the foot of the bed. The head is fixed in a Mayfield head holder and positioned to allow access to the temporal bone and neck. Rigid fixation of the head is necessary for intraoperative stereotactic guidance systems. Intraoperative stereotactic guidance systems can be helpful in determining extent of surgical exposure required. The arms are tucked at the patient's side, and the patient is strapped to the table with three straps. A site for abdominal fat graft harvest is exposed, if required. Otherwise, a donor site for microvascular flap is prepared.

Facial nerve and laryngeal monitoring should be considered when these nerves have normal preoperative function, and an attempt will be made to preserve their function. This fact needs to be communicated to the anesthesia team so that long-acting paralytics are not given. Many of these patients already have facial paralysis, and facial nerve monitoring is not required.

Operative Procedure

Incisions

A large C-shaped incision that extends into the neck is made (Fig. 18.2). This incision gives the needed exposure for craniotomy, neck dissection, and parotidectomy. The skin flap is raised superficial to the temporalis muscle, mastoid periosteum, and sternocleidomastoid muscle.

Canal incisions are dictated by the lateral extent of the tumor. Biopsies are taken from the ear lateral canal to be certain that the margin is clear. In general, tumors that require STBR and TTBR tend to have limited ear canal involvement, and an incision is made at the bony-cartilaginous junction, and the membranous canal skin is everted and closed primarily (Fig. 18.3). Often for these more medially placed temporal bone tumors, the ear canal skin is normal and can be elevated and an incision made medial to the bony-cartilaginous junction.

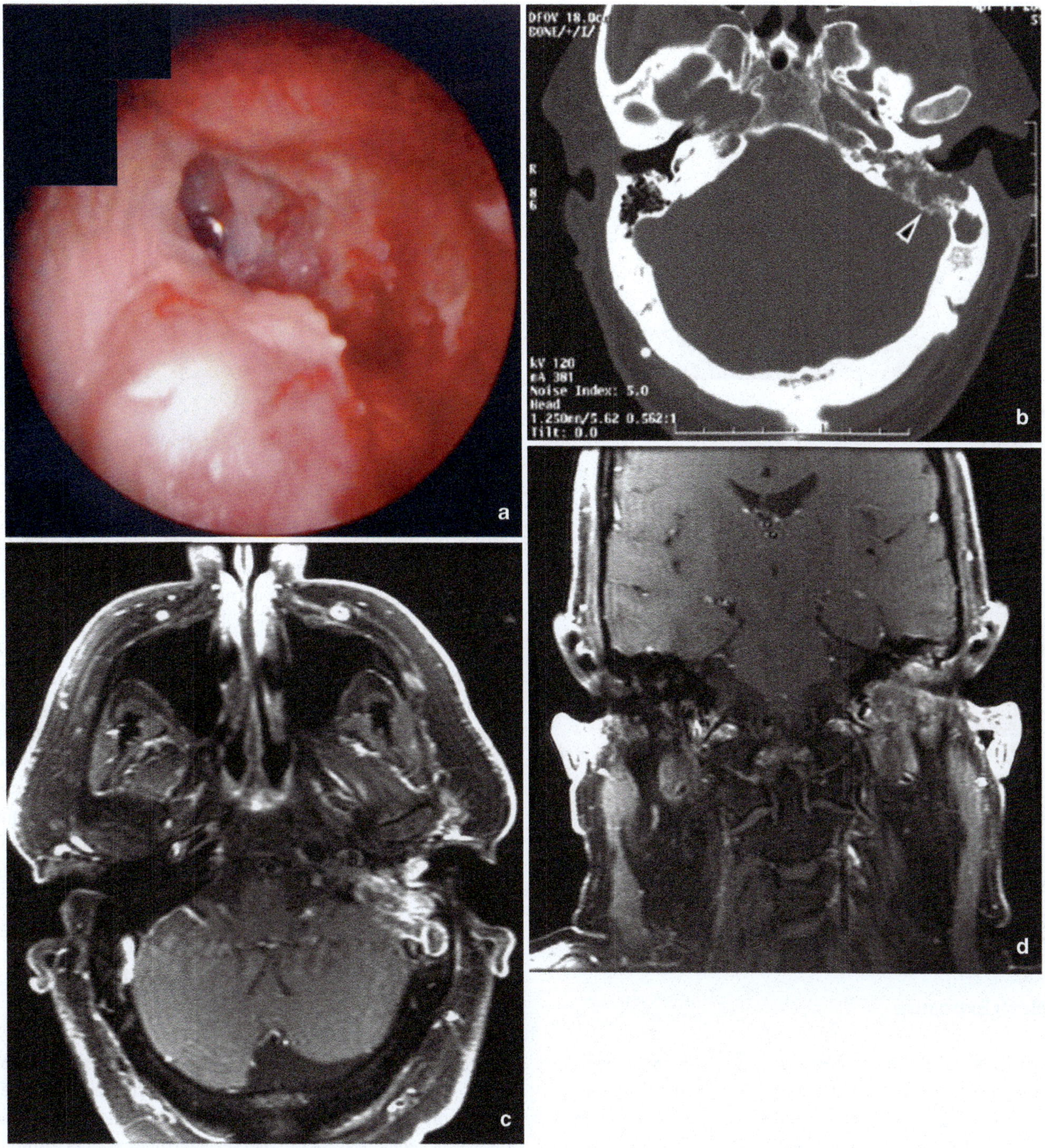

Fig. 18.1 T4 squamous cell carcinoma of the left temporal bone. This man presented with left facial paralysis and otorrhea. A tympanostomy tube was placed by his referring physician. He had a history of childhood brain radiation therapy. He received one dose of Paclitaxel prior to surgery. (**a**) Oto-endoscopic view of the left ear canal. (**b**) Axial CT showing destruction of the left temporal bone. (**c**) Axial and (**d**) coronal contrast-enhanced MRI. He remains free of disease 10 years following subtotal temporal bone resection and postoperative radiotherapy

The tragal cartilage is elevated off the anterior tympanic ring, and the flap is raised superficial to the parotid gland. The skin of the external auditory meatus is undermined and everted and oversewn in a water-tight fashion. The Palva flap can be sewn to the tragal cartilage to create a second layer of closure on the ear canal. Alternatively, the Palva flap is raised and is sewn to the anterior ear canal cartilage and used to cover the bony canal to prevent tumor spillage. The skin flap is held forward with self-retaining or fish hook retractors.

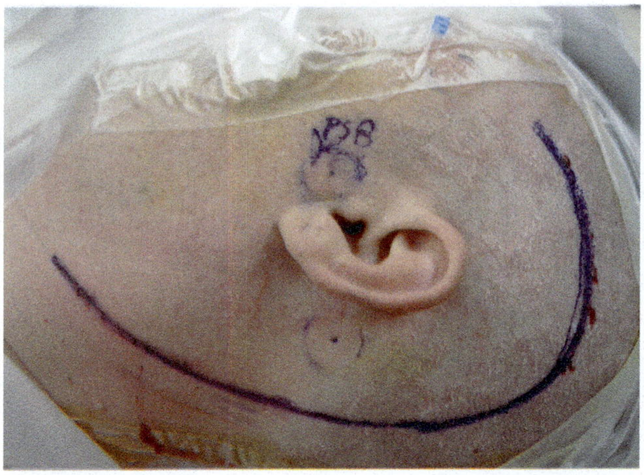

Fig. 18.2 Large postauricular C-shaped incision is planned for subtotal temporal bone resection. Note electrode for facial nerve monitoring

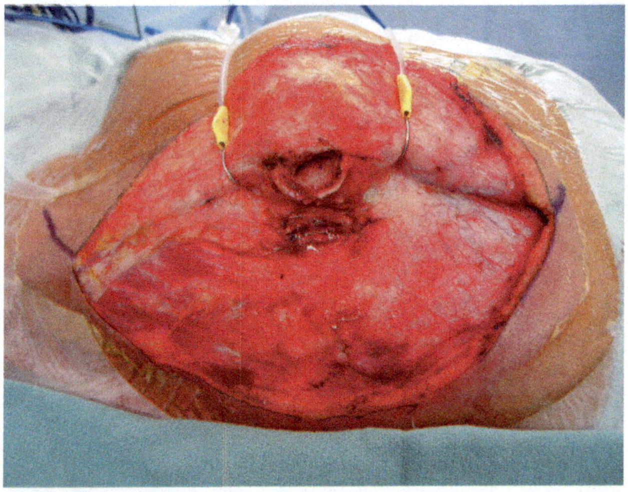

Fig. 18.3 The canal is incised lateral to the visible margin of the tumor. Margins on the ear canal are sent for frozen section

Neck Exposure

For subtotal temporal bone resection, the neck exposure should precede the temporal bone dissection. Once the lymphoareolar tissues of level II and III are removed, the jugular vein, carotid artery, and cranial nerves IX, X, XI, and XII are identified. The great vessels are then isolated with vessel loops (Fig. 18.4). This maneuver is performed in case of inadvertent injury to the carotid or if the jugular bulb needs to be resected.

Temporal Bone Dissection

Mastoidectomy is performed to identify the tegmen and posterior fossa dura. The middle fossa and posterior fossa dura are important landmarks to identify since they represent the limits of resection. The external bony ear canal can be removed as described for lateral temporal bone resection. Removal of the canal gives an unobscured view of the disease in the middle ear.

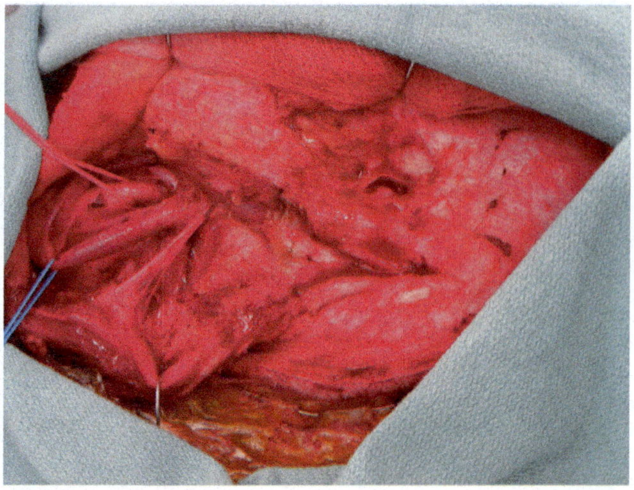

Fig. 18.4 Neck dissection is performed and the vessels are isolated and looped. The lower cranial nerves are identified

Many times, due to the extent of tumor in the mastoid, landmarks can be difficult to find. The dura can be identified in an uninvolved area and followed to identify the sigmoid sinus. The Eustachian tube is an important landmark for the carotid artery. Mohri et al. emphasize the point that the Eustachian tube needs to be completely resected for these tumors [10]. The cochleariform process, the horizontal semicircular canal, the digastric ridge, and the chorda tympani nerve are important landmarks for the facial nerve. Tumor is debulked as needed for exposure.

Identifying and Managing the Facial Nerve

Palpation of the ear canal, bony labyrinth, and/or cochlea should be performed to identify these structures. From these structures, one can try to find the facial nerve. Oftentimes, these tumors have already produced facial paralysis, and so facial nerve sacrifice is performed. Proximal and distal margins of the facial nerve are sent for frozen section (Fig. 18.5). Frequently, given the pre-existing facial paralysis, these patients are not candidates for facial nerve grafting.

When the facial nerve is intact preoperatively and not involved by tumor, an attempt can be made to preserve its function. This is especially true for low-grade tumors, such as endolymphatic sac tumors.

When the jugular bulb region is involved, the facial nerve can be left in its bony canal by drilling medial and anterior to it. This creates a bridge with the facial nerve protected within

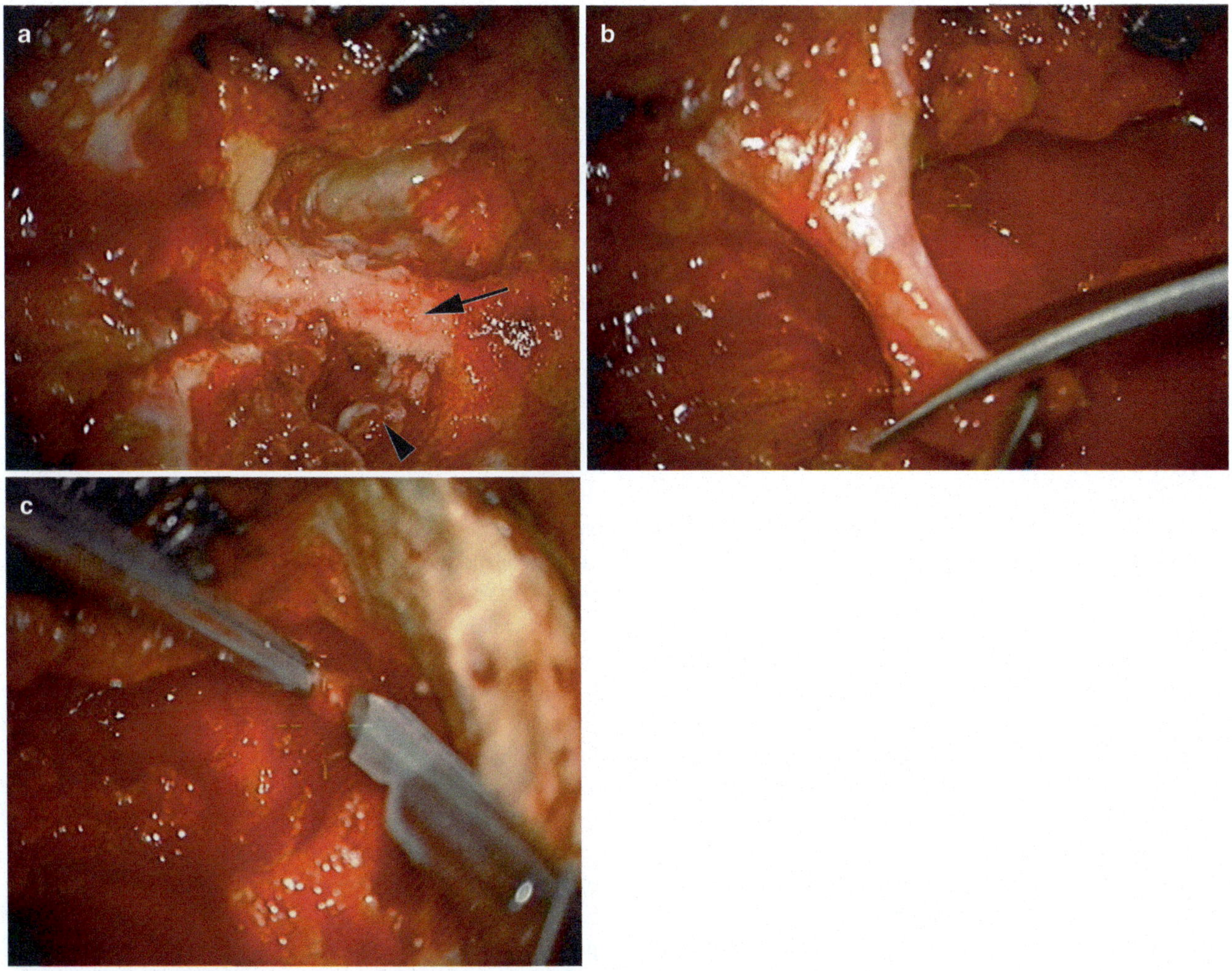

Fig. 18.5 Facial nerve. (**a**) Infiltrated facial nerve (arrow) and tumor filling the retrofacial air cells (arrowhead). (**b**) Distal facial nerve is cut and margin is sent. (**c**) Proximal facial nerve margin is sent

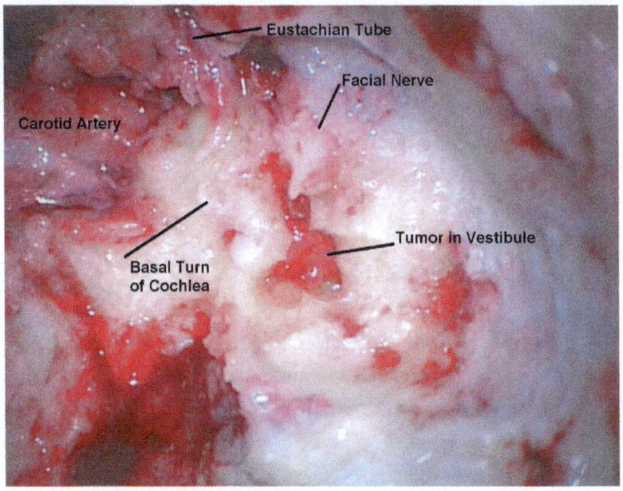

Fig. 18.6 Cancer in the labyrinth

the bone of its canal. Alternatively, the facial nerve can be transposed by removing the bone surrounding the nerve, dissecting the extratemporal portion of the nerve, and elevating the nerve out of its canal. The nerve is sewn to parotid fascia with a silk suture placed in the periosteal cuff from the stylomastoid foramen.

Labyrinthectomy

Disease that involves the labyrinth, oval or round windows, or cochlea will require labyrinthectomy and/or cochlectomy (Fig. 18.6). The bone of the labyrinth is removed and the internal auditory canal (IAC) is identified. If the facial nerve is being preserved, care must be taken not to disturb the nerve in the internal auditory canal. If the IAC is involved, then facial nerve sacrifice is undertaken.

Carotid Artery

Once the labyrinth is removed, dissection around the carotid artery is undertaken. The carotid artery is readily identified in the temporal bone by drilling in the floor of the Eustachian tube (identifying the lateral wall of the carotid artery). Alternatively, the carotid artery can be identified anteriorly through the temporomandibular joint (method of Lempert [24]). En bloc subtotal temporal bone resection makes use of this technique to avoid tumor spillage and to preserve the carotid artery during osteotomy.

Once the cochlea is removed, drilling can be performed posterior and medial to the carotid artery. Disease around the carotid artery is removed in a piecemeal fashion. In our practice, no attempt is made to resect the carotid artery.

Managing the Jugular Bulb

Unlike the carotid artery, jugular bulb resection is performed to eradicate disease. The morbidity associated with jugular bulb resection includes possible injury to cranial nerves IX–XI and the potential for increased intracranial pressure from venous outflow clamping. The patient must be made aware of these significant potential morbidities. Preoperative MRI and MRV are helpful to demonstrate contralateral sigmoid sinus flow.

Prior to sigmoid ligation, a retrosigmoid dural incision is made to evaluate for any intradural disease. The sigmoid sinus is doubly ligated, and the lateral wall of the sinus is removed. Dividing the sigmoid as a planned procedure has not been associated with neurologic deficit [23]. The digastric muscle is divided and the upper jugular vein is then ligated. Disease involving the jugular bulb can then be removed.

Tumor debulking in the region of the jugular bulb is often very bloody. Extra-luminal compression of the sigmoid (or ligation of the sigmoid) and delayed ligation of the jugular can help to minimize blood loss in this area. Bleeding continues through the superior and inferior petrosal sinuses until these are secured. These sinuses are gently packed with surgical or occluded with a fibrin sealant.

Care is taken to identify and preserve the cranial nerves IX–XI when possible. Malignancies at this location rarely make this possible, however.

En Bloc Subtotal Temporal Bone Resection

Several authors have described en bloc subtotal temporal bone resection [7, 11, 12, 14, 25]. While several surgical variations exist, the principle technique remains the same. A large postauricular C-shaped incision is made that extends into the neck. The ear canal is transected and sutured close.

Neck dissection is performed to remove the cervical lymph nodes and to identify the internal carotid artery, jugular vein, and lower cranial nerves. The distal branches of the facial nerve are cut outside of the parotid gland. The zygomatic arch is divided. The condyle or ascending ramus of the mandible is cut to allow access to the temporomandibular joint so that the carotid artery can be followed superiorly without violating the tumor in the middle ear.

Temporal and occipital craniotomies are performed to elevate the middle and posterior fossa dura. If dural and brain invasion has occurred, then the involved dura and brain is separated from the main temporal bone resection and addressed separately in a piecemeal fashion. In the middle fossa, the arcuate eminence, greater superficial petrosal nerve (GSPN), foramen spinosum and middle meningeal artery, and posterior petrous ridge are identified. The middle meningeal artery is coagulated and divided. The greater superficial petrosal nerve is identified and used as a landmark for the horizontal petrous carotid artery. The bony carotid canal is drilled away so that the artery can be transposed laterally and anteriorly.

On the occipital side, the sigmoid sinus and petrous dura are separated from the posterior aspect of the temporal bone. The jugular bulb is exposed in a posterior transcondylar approach.

Four basic osteotomies are required: (1) a subtemporal osteotomy from the carotid canal to the posterior edge of the temporal bone through the proximal third of the internal auditory canal, (2) an occipital osteotomy from the petrous bone to the jugular foramen sparing its medial wall, (3) from the jugular foramen to the carotid canal, and (4) from the carotid canal to the glenoid fossa. Most surgeons describe using a high-speed drill for these osteotomies. A diamond threadwire saw, which has the benefit of making fine cuts, has been described as helpful to make the osteotomy cuts [14].

This bony block can be kept in continuity with the parotid gland and neck dissection, so that the tumor is not breeched. The carotid artery and jugular vein are preserved if oncologically sound; however, the sigmoid sinus and jugular vein can be ligated and resected if the bulb is infiltrated. Significant bleeding has been described when the specimen is removed en bloc. This bleeding is usually from tearing the jugular bulb and is readily controlled with packing [25].

Total Temporal Bone Resection

Total temporal bone resection (TTBR) connotes complete removal of the temporal bone and extends the dissection of a subtotal temporal bone resection to the petrous apex. This dissection can be accomplished as either a piecemeal dissection or en bloc resection.

As detailed above, patients with malignant tumors all have extensive disease that typically produces facial paralysis and hearing loss. Since the facial nerve is already paralyzed and since the petrous apex will be removed in the resection, no proximal stump is available for facial nerve grafting. Occasionally, low-grade tumors, such as endolymphatic sac tumor, produce extensive disease with preserved facial function. A TTBR can be accomplished preserving the facial nerve in its bony canal, but tumor dissection is limited or inaccessible in the anterior-medial temporal bone (Kawase's triangle). The alternative is to reroute the facial nerve out of the internal auditory canal by severing the GSPN. This technique is accompanied by dense temporary facial paralysis that improves to no greater than HBIII function with time.

In our series, TTBR was accomplished following the same steps as outlined above for STBR. The petrous apex is drilled away, and the carotid artery is followed along its horizontal and vertical portions with tumor being removed piecemeal until uninvolved bone is encountered. If extensive dural removal is required, repair is necessary. Dural grafts, fat grafts, and microvascular free flaps have all been used to close off this dural defect.

The classic description of en bloc TTBR is from Graham et al. [26] Originally described in 1984 and modified in 1987 [27], the en bloc TTBR resection involves carotid artery sacrifice, division of cranial nerves VI through XII, and adjacent structures. Since carotid artery sacrifice is planned, balloon occlusion test (BOT) is performed preoperatively. Despite the results of BOT, the chance of significant stroke remains at about 20%, and carotid artery sacrifice is associated with high mortality and morbidity [27].

Given that these patients historically have a bad overall prognosis with a short survival despite extensive surgery, our team avoids sacrificing the carotid artery so as to avoid the potential for stroke. Additionally, the added morbidity of lower cranial nerve deficit following en bloc TTBR significantly impairs quality of life for these patients.

Since our team does not perform the en bloc resection, the interested reader is referred to several articles written about this technique and its modifications [26–29].

Complications associated with TTBR are similar to those enumerated for STBR and include the possibility of carotid artery injury, abducens nerve palsy, and substantially greater incidence of CSF leakage [25].

As early as 1977, the advantage of TTBR over the resection over STBR was questioned [25]. As discussed above, for these patients with poor overall prognosis and short survival following treatment, consideration must be given to overall quality of life. The newer treatment paradigm of preoperative chemotherapy (Taxane, Platinum, and 5-FU, so-called TPF) with or without radiotherapy offers new hope to these patients with T3 and T4 disease.

Reconstruction

The principal goal of reconstruction is to achieve a watertight dural closure. Small dural defects in the middle fossa can be closed with allografts (Fig. 18.7). Temporalis fascia and abdominal fat graft are good choices for a limited posterior fossa and jugular foramen dural defect. The temporalis muscle flap can be rotated to cover the abdominal fat graft and create another layer of closure. Soft tissue coverage is usually not required since many of these patients will have normal skin. Larger defects, especially in the postradiation setting, will require microvascular tissue transfer.

Postoperative care

These patients are always admitted to an intensive care unit for at least one night of close observation. Eye care is important for patients with facial weakness or paralysis. Liberal use of eye moisturizers is necessary to prevent corneal drying and ulceration.

Voice and swallowing problems will need to be diagnosed and addressed. Close cooperation with a speech and

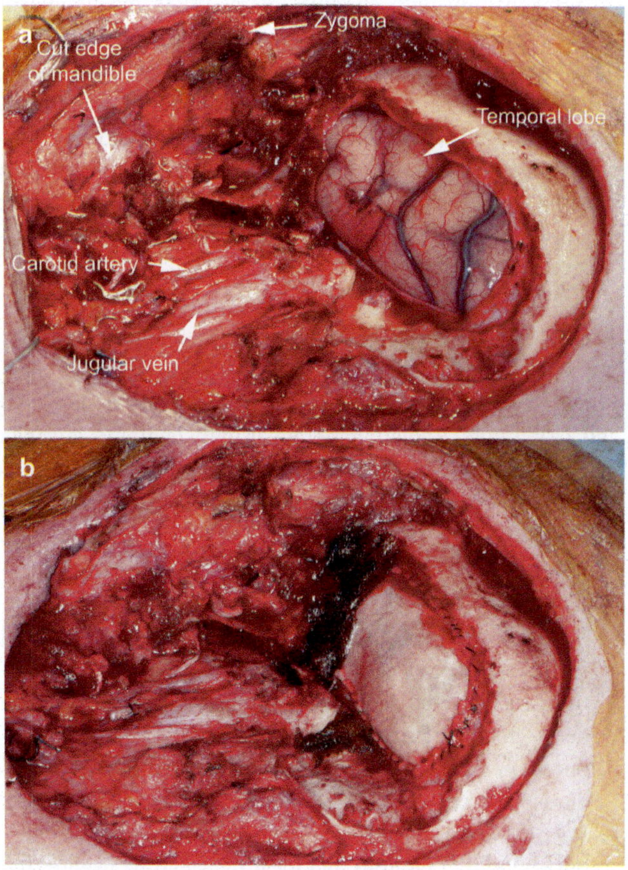

Fig. 18.7 Dural closure. (**a**) Total temporal bone defect. (**b**) Dural repair

swallowing therapist is essential. Modified barium swallow (MBS) can be performed when the patient's condition permits. Patients who fail MBS need to have a gastrostomy tube placed. Vocal fold augmentation or medialization might be required to help with phonation and protection from aspiration.

Hospitalization continues until the patient meets criteria for dismissal. Patients are usually discharged after 7–10 days.

Complications

Facial paralysis, profound hearing loss, and vestibular loss are expected outcomes of subtotal and total temporal bone resections. Postoperative complications include CSF leak, meningitis, lower cranial nerve deficit, trigeminal nerve deficit, flap necrosis, and wound infection [3, 12, 25, 30, 31]. Rates of postoperative complications can be high (28%), especially if an en bloc technique is used [12]. As a result of lower cranial nerve deficits, thyroplasty, tracheostomy, and gastrostomy tubes are occasionally required [4]. Operative mortality rates have been reported from 0 to 18% [3, 12, 15, 25].

Subtotal and total temporal bone resection should be undertaken only with curative intent. When the neoplasm extends to the ICA or intradurally, especially with involvement of the vein of Labbe, an alternative surgical approach, along with a complete plan of multimodal management, should be used. Given the extent of resection and the typically universal need for adjuvant therapies, reconstruction must be a planned integral part of the procedure and is most appropriately addressed with free microvascular transfer.

Adjuvant Therapy

Postoperative radiotherapy is given to all advanced-stage (T3 and T4) tumors. Radiation therapy usually begins 3–4 weeks postoperatively. Concomitant chemotherapy should be considered in patients with multiple adverse pathologic findings.

Conclusion

Subtotal and total temporal bone resection are required for late-stage cancers. The indications and contraindications for these procedures are discussed. Patients need to be in good physical condition to undergo these procedures. A multidisciplinary team is used for these procedures. The critical steps of tumor resection are outlined. Reconstruction usually involves a microvascular free flap, but abdominal fat graft and local flaps can be used in the appropriate circumstance. Postoperative radiotherapy is given to all patients.

References

1. Gidley PW, DeMonte F. Temporal bone malignancies. Neurosurg Clin N Am. 2013;24(1):97–110.
2. Moody SA, Hirsch BE, Myers EN. Squamous cell carcinoma of the external auditory canal: an evaluation of a staging system. Am J Otol. 2000;21(4):582–8.
3. Moffat DA, Grey P, Ballagh RH, Hardy DG. Extended temporal bone resection for squamous cell carcinoma. Otolaryngol Head Neck Surg. 1997;116(6 Pt 1):617–23.
4. Moffat DA, Wagstaff SA, Hardy DG. The outcome of radical surgery and postoperative radiotherapy for squamous carcinoma of the temporal bone. Laryngoscope. 2005;115(2):341–7.
5. Masterson L, Rouhani M, Donnelly NP, Tysome JR, Patel P, Jefferies SJ, et al. Squamous cell carcinoma of the temporal bone: clinical outcomes from radical surgery and postoperative radiotherapy. Otol Neurotol. 2014;35(3):501–8.
6. Bacciu A, Clemente IA, Piccirillo E, Ferrari S, Sanna M. Guidelines for treating temporal bone carcinoma based on long-term outcomes. Otol Neurotol. 2013;34(5):898–907.
7. Mazzoni A, Danesi G, Zanoletti E. Primary squamous cell carcinoma of the external auditory canal: surgical treatment and long-term outcomes. Acta Otorhinolaryngol Ital. 2014;34(2):129–37.
8. Yamada S, Schuh FD, Harvin JS, Perot PL Jr. En bloc subtotal temporal bone resection for cancer of the external ear. J Neurosurg. 1973;39(3):370–9.
9. Somekawa Y, Asano K, Hata M. En bloc resection of the temporal bone for middle ear carcinoma extending to the cranial base. Nippon Jibiinkoka Gakkai Kaiho. 1997;100(7):782–9.
10. Mohri M, Nagashima T, Tahara S, Amatsu M. Significance of tubal resection in surgical treatment of middle ear carcinoma. Eur Arch Otorhinolaryngol. 1997;254(4):208–11.
11. Nakagawa T, Kumamoto Y, Natori Y, Shiratsuchi H, Toh S, Kakazu Y, et al. Squamous cell carcinoma of the external auditory canal and middle ear: an operation combined with preoperative chemoradiotherapy and a free surgical margin. Otol Neurotol. 2006;27(2):242–8. discussion 9.
12. Okada T, Saito K, Takahashi M, Hasegawa Y, Fujimoto Y, Terada A, et al. En bloc petrosectomy for malignant tumors involving the external auditory canal and middle ear: surgical methods and long-term outcome. J Neurosurg. 2008;108(1):97–104.
13. Chi FL, Gu FM, Dai CF, Chen B, Li HW. Survival outcomes in surgical treatment of 72 cases of squamous cell carcinoma of the temporal bone. Otol Neurotol. 2011;32(4):665–9.
14. Jimbo H, Kamata S, Miura K, Masubuchi T, Ichikawa M, Ikeda Y, et al. En bloc temporal bone resection using a diamond threadwire saw for malignant tumors. J Neurosurg. 2011;114(5):1386–9.
15. Prasad S, Janecka IP. Efficacy of surgical treatments for squamous cell carcinoma of the temporal bone: a literature review. Otolaryngol Head Neck Surg. 1994;110(3):270–80.
16. Zanoletti E, Marioni G, Franchella S, Lovato A, Giacomelli L, Martini A, et al. Recurrent squamous cell carcinoma of the temporal bone: critical analysis of cases with a poor prognosis. Am J Otolaryngol. 2015;36(3):352–5.
17. Takenaka Y, Cho H, Nakahara S, Yamamoto Y, Yasui T, Inohara H. Chemoradiation therapy for squamous cell carcinoma of the external auditory canal: a meta-analysis. Head Neck. 2015;37(7):1073–80.
18. Morita S, Homma A, Nakamaru Y, Sakashita T, Hatakeyama H, Kano S, et al. The outcomes of surgery and chemoradiotherapy for temporal bone cancer. Otol Neurotol. 2016;37(8):1174–82.
19. Yoo GH, Hocwald E, Korkmaz H, Du W, Logani S, Kelly JK, et al. Assessment of carotid artery invasion in patients with head and neck cancer. Laryngoscope. 2000;110(3 Pt 1):386–90.
20. Urken ML, Biller HF, Haimov M. Intratemporal carotid artery bypass in resection of a base of skull tumor. Laryngoscope. 1985;95(12):1472–7.

21. Snyderman CH, D'Amico F. Outcome of carotid artery resection for neoplastic disease: a meta-analysis. Am J Otolaryngol. 1992;13(6):373–80.
22. Kalani MY, Kalb S, Martirosyan NL, Lettieri SC, Spetzler RF, Porter RW, et al. Cerebral revascularization and carotid artery resection at the skull base for treatment of advanced head and neck malignancies. J Neurosurg. 2013;118(3):637–42.
23. Zanoletti E, Cazzador D, Faccioli C, Martini A, Mazzoni A. Closure of the sigmoid sinus in lateral skull base surgery. Acta Otorhinolaryngol Ital. 2014;34(3):184–8.
24. Lempert J. Complete apicectomy (mastoidotympano-apicectomy). Arch Otolaryngol Head Neck Surg. 1937;25(2):144–77.
25. Gacek RR, Goodman M. Management of malignancy of the temporal bone. Laryngoscope. 1977;87(10 Pt 1):1622–34.
26. Graham MD, Sataloff RT, Kemink JL, Wolf GT, McGillicuddy JE. Total en bloc resection of the temporal bone and carotid artery for malignant tumors of the ear and temporal bone. Laryngoscope. 1984;94(4):528–33.
27. Sataloff RT, Myers DL, Lowry LD, Spiegel JR. Total temporal bone resection for squamous cell carcinoma. Otolaryngol Head Neck Surg. 1987;96(1):4–14.
28. Sataloff RT, Myers DL, Spiegel JR, Roberts BR, Telian S. Total temporal bone resection for osteogenic sarcoma. Ear Nose Throat J. 1988;67(9):626–7. 30–2, 34 passim.
29. Komune N, Komune S, Morishita T, Rhoton AL Jr. Microsurgical anatomy of subtotal temporal bone resection en bloc with the parotid gland and temporomandibular joint. Neurosurgery. 2014;10(2):334–56.
30. Lewis JS. Temporal bone resection. Review of 100 cases. Arch Otolaryngol. 1975;101(1):23–5.
31. Zhang B, Tu G, Xu G, Tang P, Hu Y. Squamous cell carcinoma of temporal bone: reported on 33 patients. Head Neck. 1999;21(5):461–6.

Jugular Foramen Approach

19

Paul W. Gidley and Franco DeMonte

Introduction

Cancers of the jugular foramen are relatively rare. While squamous cell carcinoma of the middle ear and temporal bone often involve the jugular foramen, primary tumors in this location are unusual. While this chapter is dedicated to the management of malignant neoplasms at the jugular foramen, the techniques used for management of paragangliomas and other more common skull base tumors are similar.

In the MD Anderson series, 35 patients had malignancy involving the jugular foramen. The average patient age was 53 years (range 9–79 years). There were 22 men and 13 women. The right side was involved in 18 patients; the left side in 17 patients. Seventeen patients presented with untreated disease; 5 patients had persistent disease, and 13 patients had recurrent disease. Seven patients (20%) had radiation-associated tumors. The most common symptoms were hearing loss in 22 (62.8%), facial nerve dysfunction in 18 (51.4%), and otalgia in 11 (31.4%). The most common tumor type was sarcoma in 15/35 patients (Table 19.1).

These tumors grow superiorly into the middle ear, anteriorly into the parotid or along the carotid artery, inferiorly along the jugular and lower cranial nerves, posteriorly into the sigmoid sinus, medially into the dura and intracranial space, or laterally into the facial nerve, middle ear, and ear canal (Fig. 19.1).

Neck dissection is an important step in jugular foramen surgery for control of the vessels in the neck and identification of the lower cranial nerves. While all lymph node dissections are sent for pathologic examination, positive lymph nodes were only found in cases of squamous cell carcinoma and high-grade salivary duct carcinoma.

P. W. Gidley, M.D., F.A.C.S. (✉)
Department of Head and Neck Surgery, The University of Texas M.D. Anderson Cancer Center, Houston, TX, USA
e-mail: pwgidley@mdanderson.org

F. DeMonte, M.D.
Department of Neurosurgery, The University of Texas M.D. Anderson Cancer Center, Houston, TX, USA
e-mail: fdemonte@mdanderson.org

Patient Evaluation

These tumors are usually confined to the middle ear and temporal bone and usually do not involve the ear canal to a great extent. Noting the ear canal portion is important when considering skin incisions. Although hearing preservation approaches to the jugular foramen have been described for benign tumors, the presence of malignancy requires the removal of the ear canal in order to have adequate access to the intratemporal carotid artery and jugular vein [1–3]. Since the patient will subsequently have a maximal conductive hearing loss, an osseointegrated hearing aid should be considered in such cases and can be placed at the time of the original surgery.

Cranial nerve examination is critical in these patients since nerves VII thru XII are potentially at risk. Various neuropathies affecting the lower cranial nerves have been described and are listed in Table 19.2.

Table 19.1 Tumor types seen in jugular foramen

Histology		N (%)
Sarcoma 42.7%	Chondrosarcoma	5 (14.3)
	Osteosarcoma	4 (11.4)
	Ewing sarcoma/PNET	3 (8.6)
	Pleomorphic sarcoma	2 (5.7)
	Sarcoma NOS	1 (2.9)
Epithelial tumors 22.9%	Squamous cell carcinoma	5 (14.3)
	Basal cell carcinoma	2 (5.7)
	Basosquamous carcinoma	1 (2.9)
Salivary gland 20.1%	Adenocarcinoma	3 (8.6)
	Salivary duct carcinoma	2 (5.7)
	Adenoid cystic carcinoma	1 (2.9)
	Mucoepidermoid carcinoma	1 (2.9)
Chordoma		2 (5.7)
Neuroendocrine carcinoma		1 (2.9)
Other		2 (5.7)
Total		35

P. W. Gidley, F. DeMonte (eds.), *Temporal Bone Cancer*, https://doi.org/10.1007/978-3-319-74539-8_19

A reasonable effort should be made to preserve intact cranial nerve function; however, intraoperative findings may dictate sacrifice of one or more of these cranial nerves. Patients need to be counseled about the potential problems that arise from sacrifice of each of these nerves.

These patients may develop temporary or permanent vocal cord paralysis. A preoperative evaluation by a speech pathologist is important, and these patients will require their services postoperatively.

These procedures are typically long (i.e., 8–12 h, if a free flap is performed), and patients need to be in good overall health to undergo such a procedure.

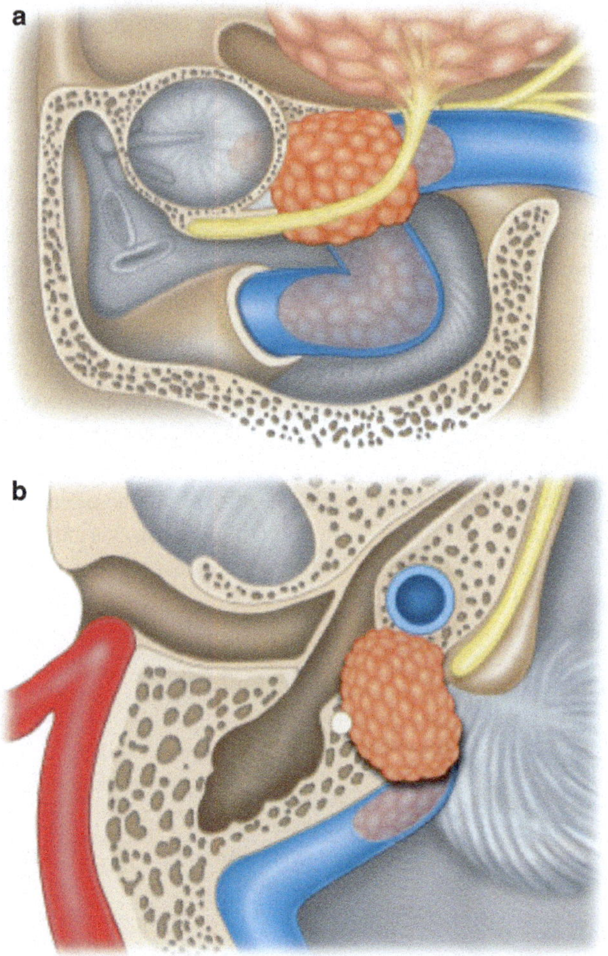

Fig. 19.1 Growth patterns for jugular foramen tumors. (**a**) Showing superior, anterior, inferior, and posterior growth, (**b**) showing medial and lateral growth

Table 19.2 Jugular foramen neurological syndromes

Observed neuropathies	Syndromic nomenclature
CN IX, X, XI	Vernet's syndrome
CN IX, X, XI, XII	Collet-Sicard syndrome
CN IX, X, XI, XII and sympathetics (Horner's syndrome)	Villaret's syndrome

Diagnostic Imaging

The most common lesions in the jugular foramen are benign tumors, such as paragangliomas, schwannomas, and meningiomas. Diagnostic imaging has an important role in discerning these benign tumors from malignant tumors [4]. Furthermore, imaging can help in differentiating primary from metastatic lesions to the jugular foramen [5–9]. The interested reader is referred to the excellent treatise by Lowenheim et al. [10]

Contrast-enhanced CT and MRI are essential to understand the tumor's relationship to the regional anatomy and for surgical planning. CT scanning provides excellent bony detail, while MRI provides excellent soft tissue detail. Axial CT imaging is important to map out the course of the facial nerve and to observe the relation of the tumor to the jugular foramen and the carotid canal. Coronal imaging shows the relationship of the mass to the hypotympanum and labyrinth [5] (Fig. 19.2).

Angiography is useful to help differentiate these malignant lesions from paraganglioma and schwannoma [11]. Embolization is helpful for highly vascular tumors [12]. When carotid sacrifice is contemplated, balloon occlusion

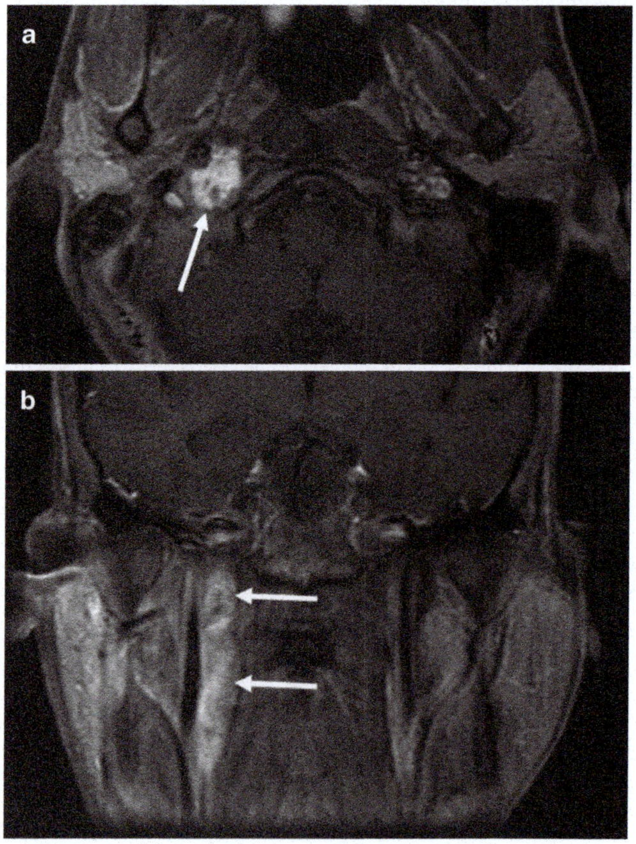

Fig. 19.2 Axial (**a**) and coronal (**b**) contrast-enhanced MRI of jugular foramen and carotid space sarcoma (white arrows) arising from the vagus nerve

test has been advocated [13]. MR venography is performed prior to ligation of the jugular vein to determine the extent of venous collateral and connectivity of the transverse sinuses.

Surgical Procedure

The patient is placed supine on the operating table. General anesthesia is induced, and a nerve-monitoring endotracheal tube is placed. Since nerve monitoring will be performed, the anesthesia team needs to avoid using long-term paralytics. Arterial line are IV lines are placed. Continuous monitoring of end-tidal CO_2, oxygen saturation, and intra-arterial blood pressures are carried out throughout the procedure. A Foley catheter is placed, and compression stockings and sequential compression devices are placed on both calves to minimize the chance of thromboembolic event.

The anesthesiologist is instructed to hyperventilate the patient down to an arterial pCO_2 of 28. Dexamethasone (10 mg) is given IV and repeated every 8 h during the procedure. A broad spectrum antibiotic (e.g., ampicillin/sulbactam) is given prior to incision and repeated every 4 h during the procedure.

The patient is padded and strapped to the operating room table, and the table is turned 180° from the anesthesia stand. A shoulder roll can be placed to help extend the neck. The head is placed in a Mayfield head holder and rotated 30–45° to the opposite side and the vertex is slightly tipped toward the floor. Electrotrodes for facial nerve monitoring are placed. Electrodes can also be placed in the sternocleidomastoid/trapezius muscles and tongue in order to monitor the accessory (CN XI) and hypoglossal nerves (CNXII), respectively.

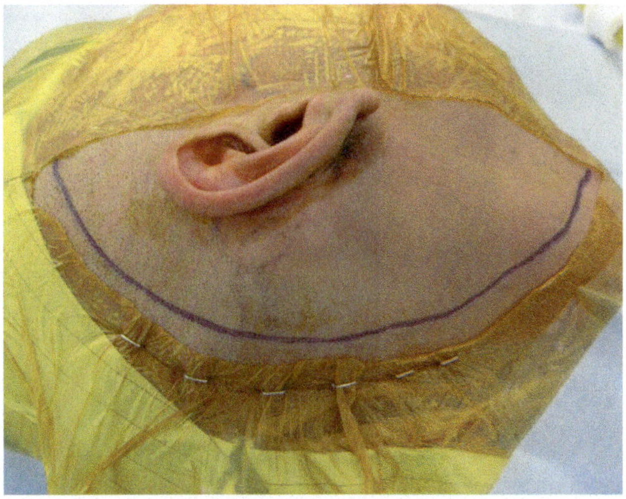

Fig. 19.3 Postauricular C-shaped incision for jugular foramen approach

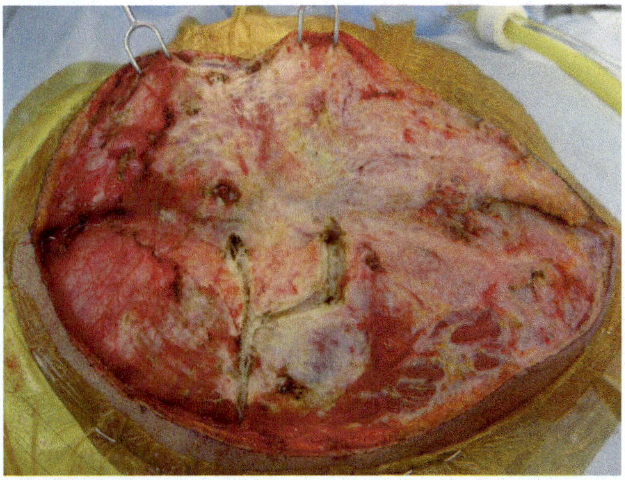

Fig. 19.4 Skin flap is elevated over the temporalis fascia, mastoid periosteum, and sternocleidomastoid muscle. A Palva periosteal flap is outlined

Skin Incisions and Soft Tissue Exposure

Skin incision is planned to accommodate neck dissection, parotidectomy, temporal bone resection, and craniotomy. A large C-shaped incision is usually used, since this gives access to the areas listed above and since the overlying skin, outer ear, and ear canal are otherwise normal (Fig. 19.3). This C-shaped incision is placed 2–3 fingerbreadths above and behind the ear, and then the incision curves gently into the neck following a skinfold crease at about the level of the larynx. The patient is sterilely prepped and draped for head and neck exposure and for free flap harvesting, if required.

The skin incisions are made with Bovie electrocautery. Raney clips are not used since they may contribute to skin necrosis with such a long procedure. The skin flap is raised in a subplatysmal plane in the neck and superficial to the temporalis fascia and mastoid periosteum in the head. In the neck, the greater auricular nerve and external jugular vein are identified and preserved. The greater auricular nerve can be mobilized, divided distal to the bifurcation, and preserved in case a nerve graft is required (Fig. 19.4).

A large Palva flap is elevated from the mastoid periosteum. The skin of the bony ear canal is divided medial to the bony-cartilaginous junction. If the tumor involves the ear canal, the canal incision is made lateral to the tumor. The cartilage of the ear canal is elevated away from the bone (Fig. 19.5). The skin flap is raised anteriorly by following, and remaining superficial to, the parotid fascia. The skin of the membranous ear canal is undermined, everted, trimmed, and closed on itself. The medial edge of the ear canal skin is sent as a margin, especially if tumor is identified in the bony ear canal. The skin flap is held forward with fishhook retractors.

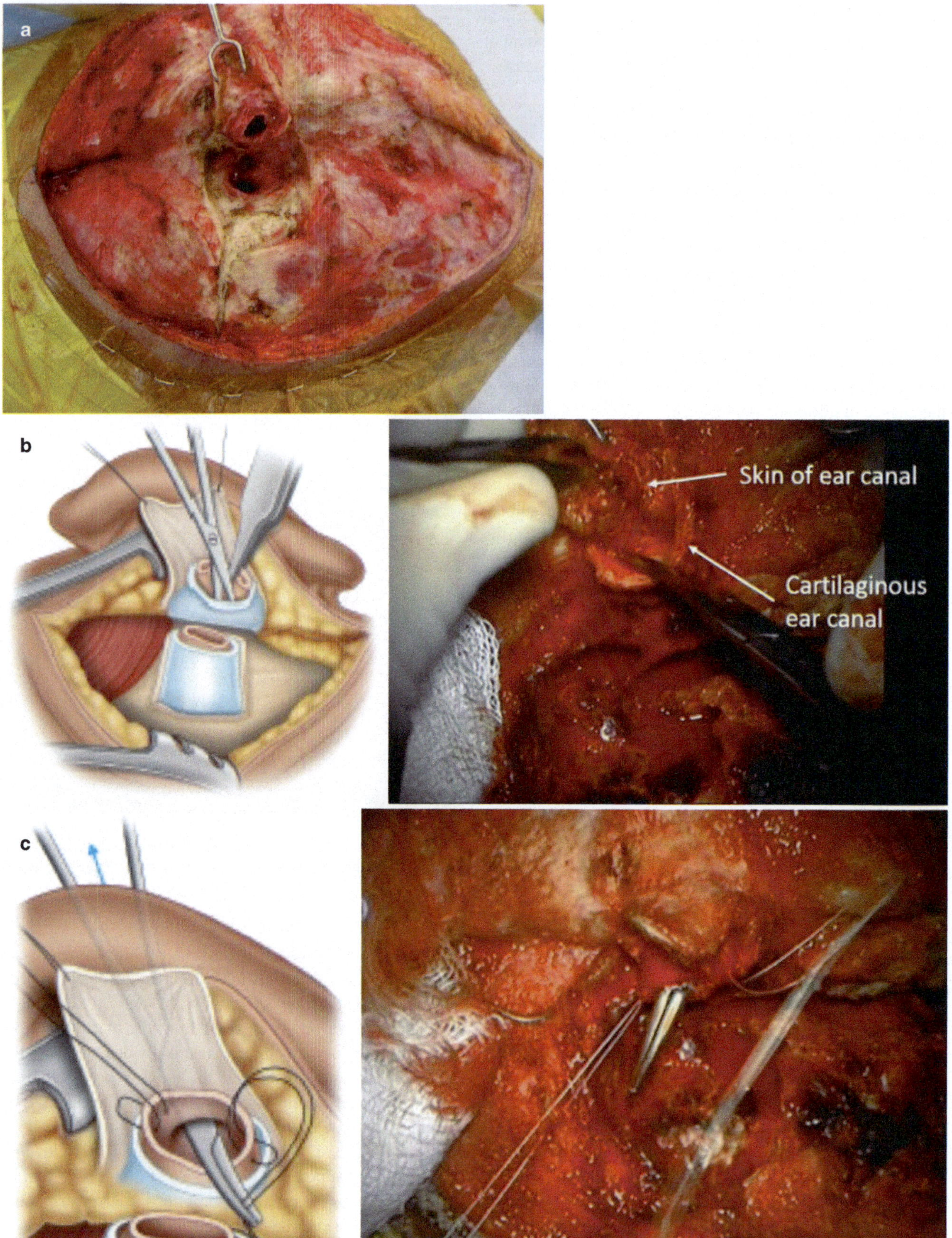

Fig. 19.5 Dividing and closing the ear canal. (**a**) The ear canal is transected medial to the bony-cartilaginous junction. (**b**) The ear canal skin is then undermined, (**c**) everted, and (**d**) closed. (**e**) The Palva flap (held by double skin hook) is used as a second layer of closure

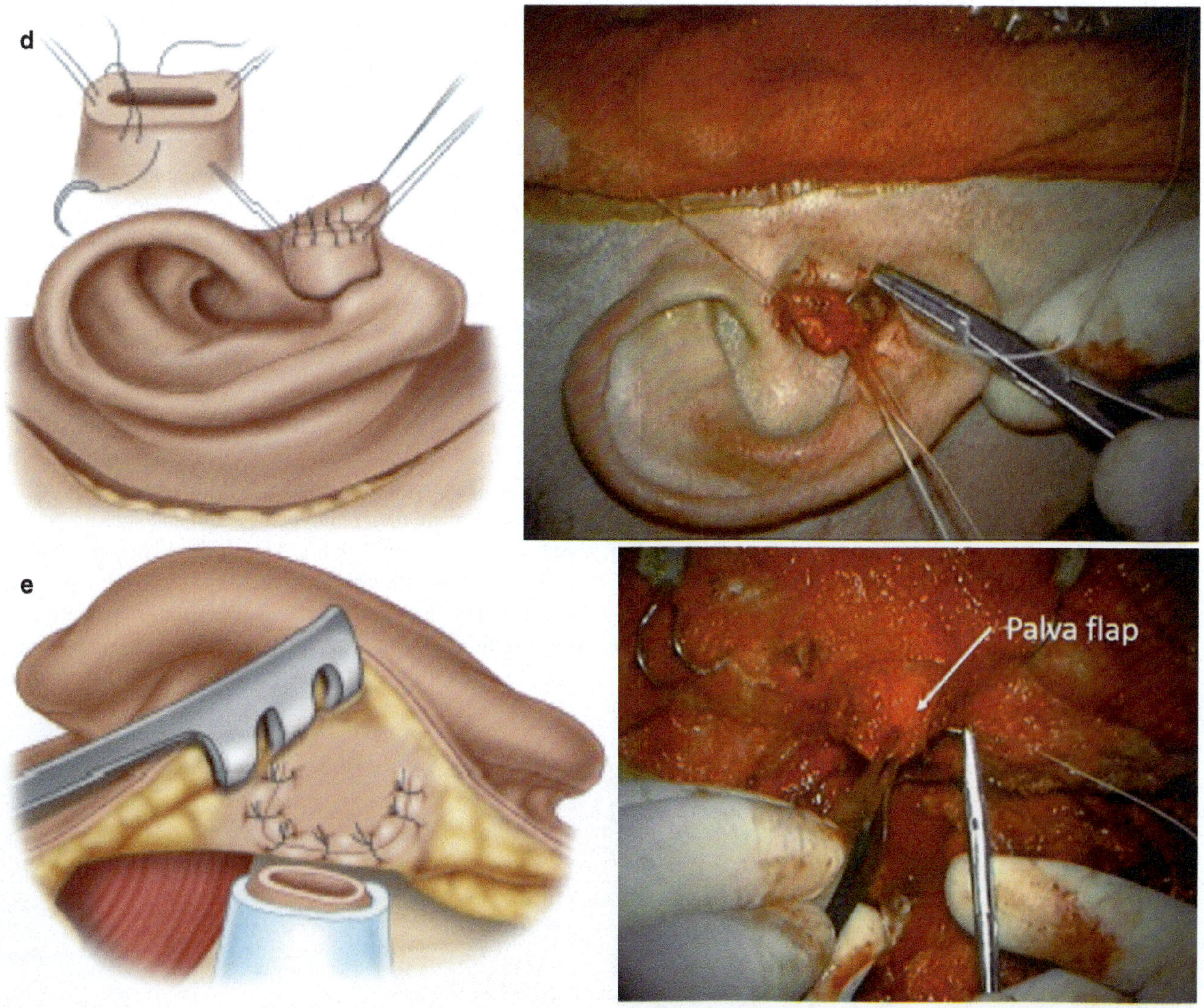

Fig. 19.5 (continued)

Neck Exposure

A subplatysmal flap is raised superiorly in the right neck. An incision is made along the anterior border of the sternocleidomastoid muscle. The spinal accessory nerve (CN XI) is identified running posteriorly lateral to the internal jugular vein (IJV) to supply the sternocleidomastoid muscle (SCM) and preserved. The lymph node contents of level IIB are resected off the floor of the neck. The hypoglossal nerve (CN XII) is typically identified as it turns anteriorly at the level of the carotid bifurcation and transposed superiorly out of the operating field. The IJV is identified and traced superiorly.

The anterior belly of the digastric and stylohyoid muscles are delineated and then cut for better exposure of the parapharyngeal space. The carotid bifurcation is identified. The vagus (CN X) is identified running vertically between the IJV and internal carotid artery (ICA). The IJV and ICA are traced superiorly into the parapharyngeal space. Vessel loops are placed around the internal jugular vein and internal carotid artery (Fig. 19.6).

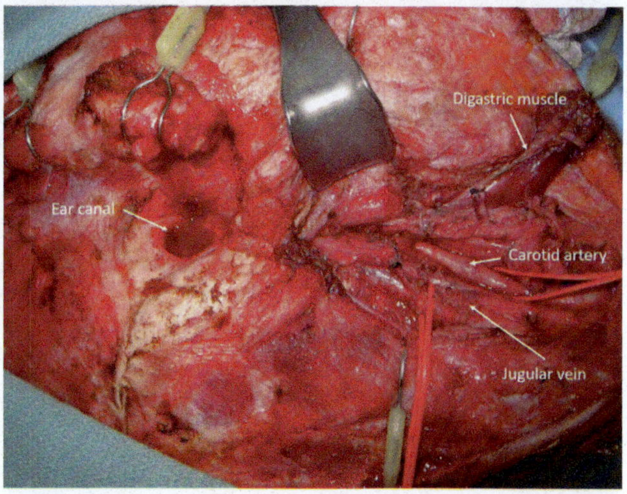

Fig. 19.6 Neck dissection has been completed. The digastric muscle is divided and retracted. The carotid artery and jugular vein have been isolated and tagged with vessel loops

Temporal Bone Exposure

The temporalis muscle is elevated and retracted superiorly with fish-hook retractors. The mastoid periosteum is reflected off of the bone and held with fish-hook retractors. The mastoid cortex is then widely exposed. A complete mastoidectomy is performed. The tegmen and sigmoid sinus are identified and skeletonized. The bone behind the sigmoid sinus is removed to expose 1 cm of retrosigmoid dura. The antrum is opened and widened, and the horizontal semicircular canal and body of the incus are identified and preserved throughout the procedure.

The operating microscope is used for the remaining portions of the procedure. Under high-power magnification, using continuous suction-irrigation and fine diamond burs, the facial recess is opened (Fig. 19.7a). The facial nerve is then followed from its tympanic portion to the second genu and then through the mastoid to the stylomastoid foramen (Fig. 19.7b). The stylomastoid foramen is widened with the drill. The digastric ridge is drilled away to expose the underlying posterior belly of the digastric muscle. If the middle ear and mastoid are engulfed in tumor, then the digastric muscle is a reliable landmark to identify the facial nerve at the stylomastoid foramen.

A bony cut is made inferior to the ear canal and lateral to the facial nerve; this liberates the mastoid tip. Removing the mastoid tip helps to unify the temporal bone field with the neck dissection, and it helps to permit complete visualization of the jugular and carotid as they exit and enter the temporal bone. The remaining soft tissue attachments to the mastoid tip are divided with Bovie electrocautery, and the mastoid tip is sent to pathology (Fig. 19.7c). The retrofacial air cells are drilled away (Fig. 19.7d); this maneuver will make it easier to decompress and transpose the facial nerve and to follow the sigmoid to the jugular bulb.

The skin of the ear canal and tympanic membrane are then elevated and removed. The incus is disarticulated. The tensor tympani tendon is divided and the entire eardrum and ear canal skin are then removed as a unit and sent for permanent pathology (Fig. 19.8a). The drill or rongeurs can be used to remove the posterior ear canal wall. Having done this, the bone of the anterior mesotympanum is then drilled down until the vertical petrous carotid artery is identified. Drilling is performed in the posterior mesotympanum to

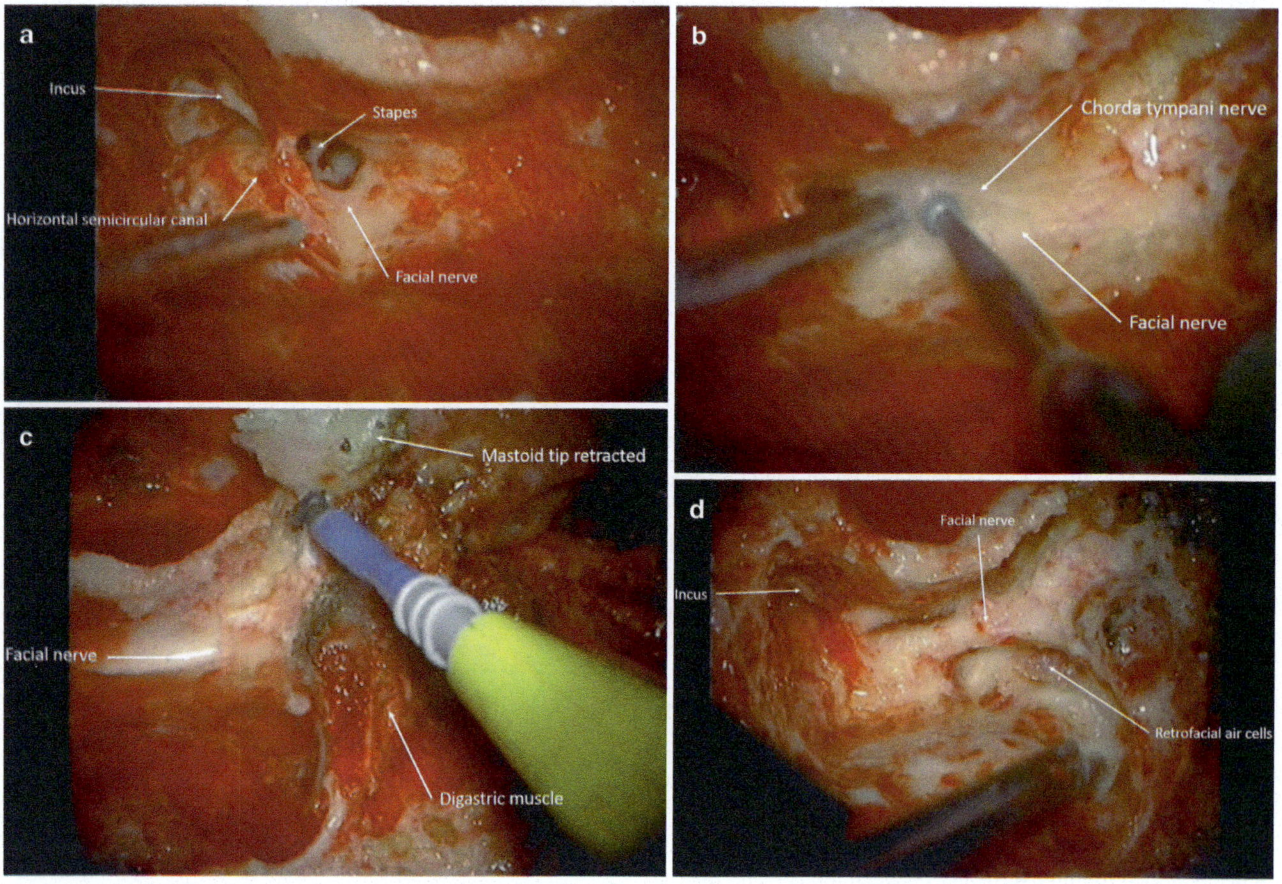

Fig. 19.7 A complete mastoidectomy is performed. The facial recess is opened (**a**). The facial nerve is traced and skeletonized to the stylomastoid foramen (**b**). The mastoid tip is removed (**c**). Retrofacial air cells are opened (**d**)

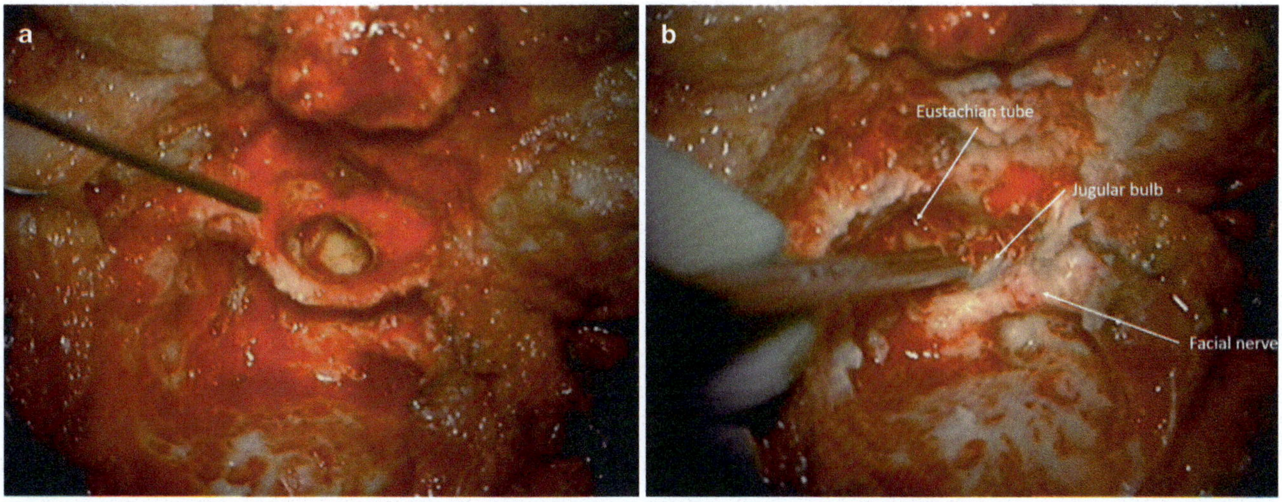

Fig. 19.8 The skin of the ear canal is removed in preparation to take down the posterior ear canal wall (**a**). Once the ear canal is removed, the jugular bulb can be seen anterior to the facial nerve (**b**)

identify the jugular bulb (Fig. 19.8b). The sigmoid sinus is followed to the jugular bulb.

Assessment can be made about the status of the labyrinth. If the patient has no signs of labyrinthine invasion (i.e., good hearing, no vestibular symptoms, and no evidence of bony erosion into the labyrinth), then the labyrinth should be preserved. However, if the patient has signs and symptoms of labyrinthine dysfunction, then labyrinthectomy is performed. Each of the three semicircular canals is identified and exenterated. The bone covering the posterior fossa dura is removed down to the jugular bulb. This dissection can be carried to the internal auditory canal as dictated by the extent of the disease.

If the cochlea is eroded and involved with tumor, then cochlectomy can be performed at this point. This is easier to perform at this stage rather than after the facial nerve has been elevated out of its canal. Identification of the carotid artery is important here to avoid inadvertent injury to the artery. The carotid artery can easily be found in the floor (i.e., lateral wall) of the Eustachian tube. Small curettes are helpful in the task of removing the bone along the carotid artery.

Assessment is made about the status of the facial nerve. If it is intact preoperatively, then every effort should be made to preserve its function. However, if it is nonfunctional (i.e., preoperative facial function is House-Brackmann VI/VI), then facial nerve sacrifice is performed. The distal and proximal margins on the nerve are sent for frozen section.

When the nerve is to be preserved, facial nerve decompression is performed in order to mobilize the nerve out of its canal. The bone along the mastoid portion of the facial nerve is thinned down and removed with Fisch instruments (Fig. 19.9a). At the stylomastoid foramen, Fisch instruments are used to open the soft tissue envelope around the facial nerve. Dissection with a fine Jacobson hemostat, bipolar and a #12 blade are used to follow the facial nerve extratemporally until the pes anserinus is encountered (Fig. 19.9b). Blunt dissection around the facial nerve separates it from the surrounding soft tissues. The digastric muscle and a cuff of periosteum are then sharply divided to use as a handle to allow elevation of the facial nerve out of its canal (Fig. 19.9c). This cuff of tissue and the facial nerve are then sewn to the parotid tail with a 2-O silk (Fig. 19.9d). This maneuver gives clear exposure to the jugular bulb (Fig. 19.10).

Carotid Canal and Jugular Foramen Access

The goal of the next steps is to continue to unify the temporal bone with the neck dissection and to remove any and all bone of the skull base so that the tumor can be seen and dissected. With the facial nerve transposed anteriorly, better access is gained to the lateral aspect of the jugular foramen. The soft tissue attachments of the styloid process are sharply divided, and the process removed with rongeurs. The ICA, located medial to the styloid process, is followed superiorly to its entry into the carotid canal. Care is needed to identify the glossopharyngeal nerve as it courses anteriorly just lateral to the ICA near its entry into the skull base. The bone lateral to the jugular bulb and carotid canal can be removed with a diamond drill. It is important to note that a dense fibrous ring is present around the ICA as it enters the carotid canal. This band is tightly attached to the periosteum of the canal and the introduction of instruments into the canal risks injury to the ICA.

The bone overlying the sigmoid sinus is removed with rongeurs down to the level of the jugular bulb. A shelf of the bone is left over the sigmoid sinus superiorly, so that extraluminal packing could be placed, if needed.

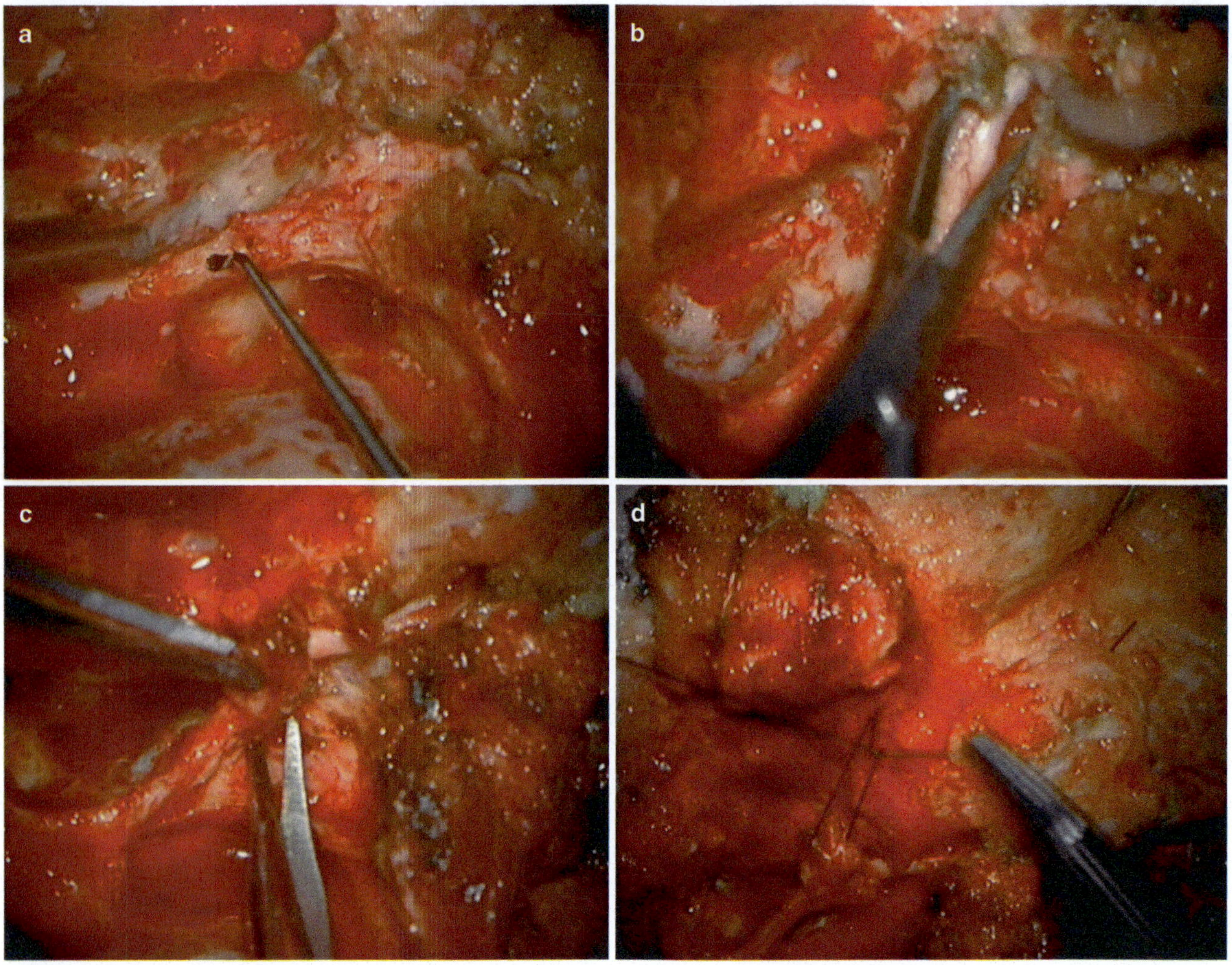

Fig. 19.9 Facial nerve transposition. (**a**) Fisch instrument is used to remove the bone of the facial canal to the second genu. (**b**) Jacobson hemostat and #12 blade scalpel are used to divide the soft tissue over the facial nerve. (**c**) The digastric muscle is divided and used to elevate the facial nerve, while tenotomy scissors are used to divide the soft tissue attachments medial to the facial nerve. (**d**) A 2-0 silk stitch is used to sew the facial nerve to the parotid gland

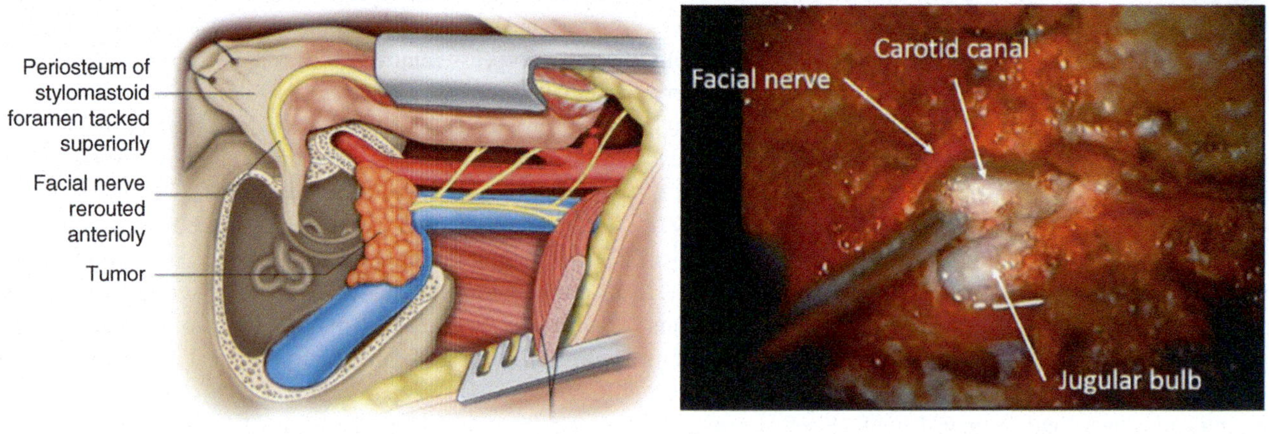

Fig. 19.10 View of jugular bulb after transposition of the facial nerve

With the unification of the surgical fields of the temporal bone and neck, full access to the extradural component of the tumor is acquired. The primary goal in the resection of malignancies of this region is preservation of the ICA. Cranial nerve preservation is not possible with infiltrative tumors, if a complete tumor resection is to be achieved. If the plan is for a subtotal resection, then a bulky tumor is removed piecemeal; but the cranial nerves are left anatomically intact to preserve any remaining function. Sarcomatous tumors, especially malignant peripheral nerve sheath tumors (MPNST), can be relatively well demarcated, and every attempt should be made to preserve the surrounding cranial nerves that are not encompassed within the tumor. The tumor is sharply dissected from the ICA and IJV.

The next steps give access to any intradural component of the tumor and allow resection of the sigmoid sinus-jugular bulb-IJV and dural complex.

Sigmoid Sinus and Dural Resection

The sigmoid sinus is ligated proximally by making dural incisions anterior and posterior to the sinus. The sinus is doubly ligated with 2-O silk sutures. In the neck, the jugular vein is doubly ligated distal to the tumor (Fig. 19.11a). Closure of the sigmoid sinus is generally well tolerated and without significant complication [14].

The dura is opened and the sigmoid sinus is divided and reflected anteriorly and inferiorly. The intradural component of the tumor is assessed (Fig. 19.11b). If the tumor is involving the cranial nerves, then these nerves are sacrificed in order to resect the tumor completely. The dural resection continues inferiorly to the jugular bulb. The jugular bulb is resected leaving its medial wall intact if lower cranial nerve function still remains. The jugular bulb and the attached tumor are sharply dissected from the surrounding tissues and

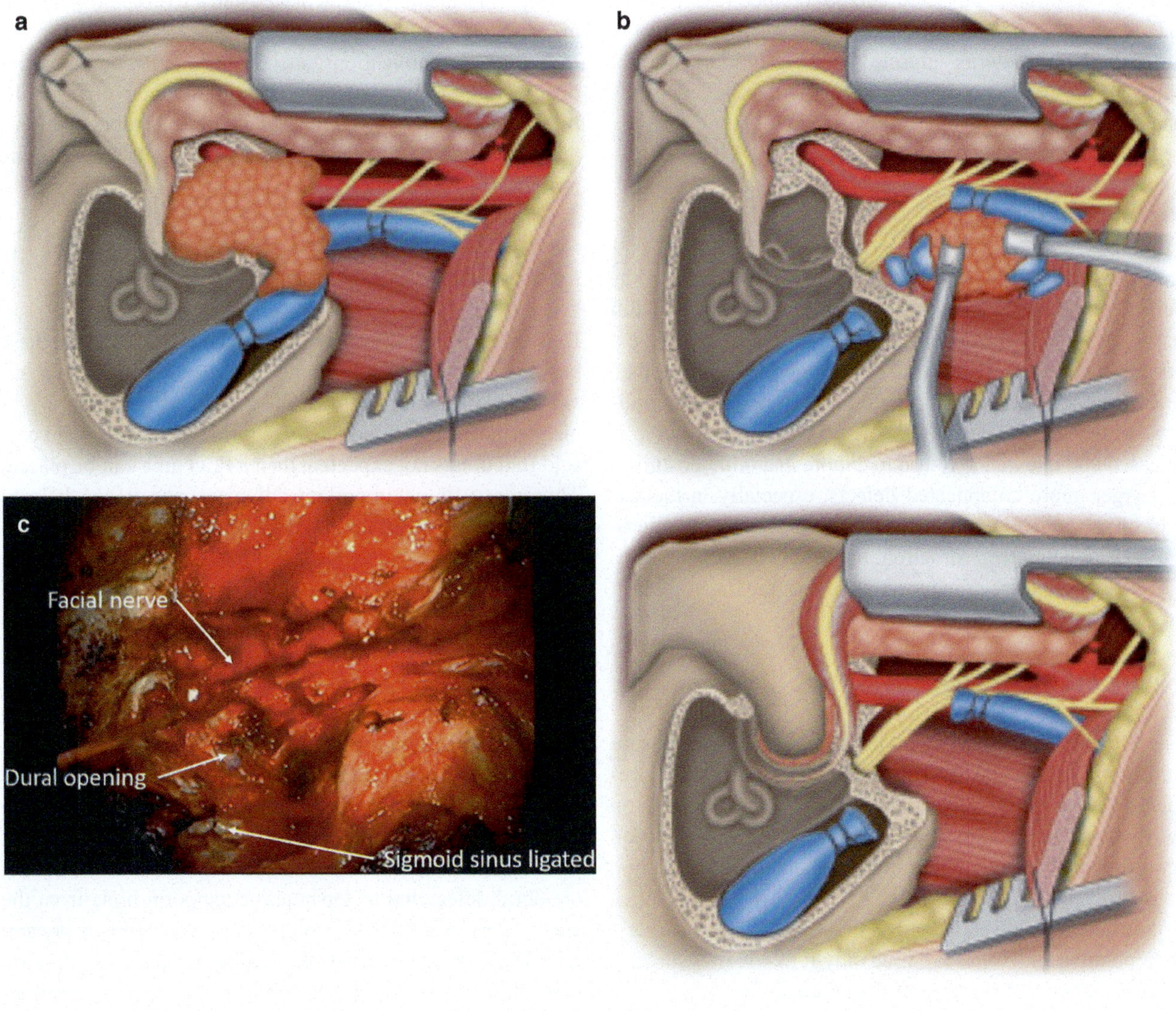

Fig. 19.11 Tumor removal. (**a**) The sigmoid sinus and jugular vein are doubly ligated. (**b**) The tumor is removed. (**c** and **d**) Appearance of defect following tumor removal

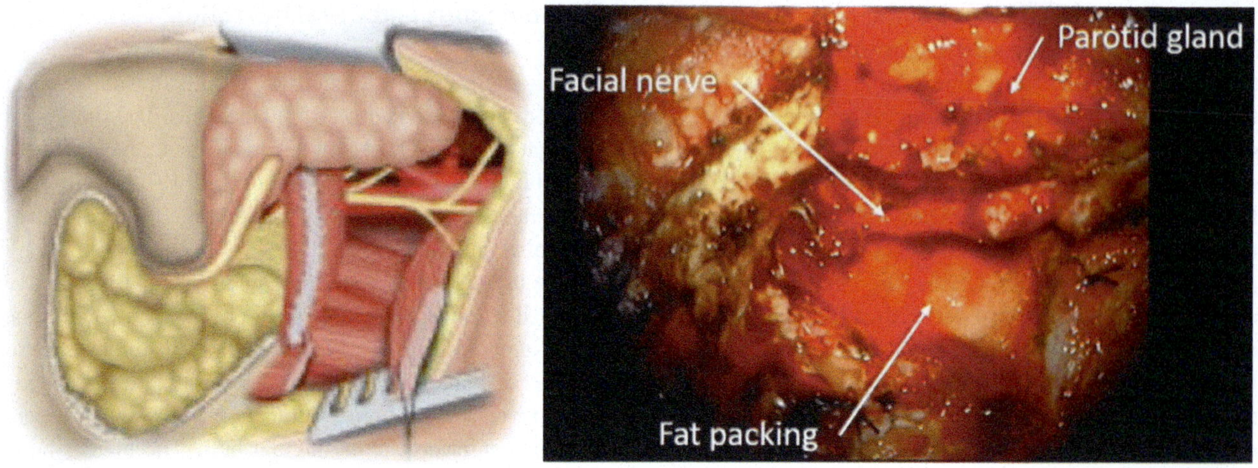

Fig. 19.12. Fat graft is used to seal the dural defect

removed. Caution needs to be exercised when resecting the IJV as the vertebral artery lies just posterior to it, posterior to the rectus capitis lateralis muscle. Bleeding from the inferior petrosal sinuses can be significant and is controlled by gentle packing with Surgicel.

Reconstruction

Reconstruction depends on the size and complexity of the defect. The Eustachian tube is sealed off with layers of soft tissue and Surgicel to avoid CSF rhinorrhea. If the patient has not had prior radiation and there is no dural defect, then reconstruction with an abdominal fat graft and a temporalis muscle flap is reasonable (Fig. 19.12). The facial nerve is released and allowed to return to a more anatomic position.

Larger, more complicated defects, especially in the setting of previous radiation treatment, usually require microvascular free flap reconstruction. In the MD Anderson series, 21 (60%) patients required microvascular free flaps.

Postoperative Management

These patients are observed overnight in the intensive care unit. Vital signs and neurologic status are checked frequently. Postoperative imaging is performed routinely on the following day. Any signs of neurologic deterioration require urgent CT imaging to rule out hematoma, ischemia, or hydrocephalus.

Steroids are given for the first 24 h after surgery. Perioperative antibiotics are used only for 24 h after surgery. Nausea and vomiting are controlled with antiemetics.

Most patients will have difficulty swallowing, and some may have trouble protecting their airway. For these patients, a temporary feeding tube is placed and a gastrostomy may be necessary. Tracheostomy is rarely needed.

To avoid complications, such as deep vein thrombosis or pneumonia, patients are mobilized out of bed to chair on the first postoperative day. Physical therapy and occupational therapy consults are beneficial in improving strength and mobility.

Complications

Deficits of cranial nerves IX–XI can be expected when these nerves are involved with tumor. As mentioned above, preventing aspiration pneumonia is mandatory; and the use of an alternate route of feeding is required. If recovery of vocal fold function is not expected, then a PEG tube can be placed. Thyroplasty is an important adjunct, since it can help to improve voice quality and strengthen cough to help protect the airway.

Facial nerve weakness and paralysis are managed with attention to eye care to avoid exposure keratopathy. Artificial tears during the day and ointment at night help to keep the cornea protected. Adjunctive procedures, such as gold weight and tarsorrhaphy, are helpful. These patients are referred to an oculoplastic surgeon for management of the eye.

CSF leak is a distinctive possibility for these patients. The rate of CSF leak is higher for jugular foramen surgery than for translabyrinthine surgery given that the surgical defect includes the temporal bone and neck. It is difficult to seal off the dural defect and to separate the temporal bone from the neck. Using vascularized, bulky flaps can help to prevent CSF leak. However, when these leaks do occur, temporary CSF drainage with a lumbar drain is helpful. A few refractory cases might require permanent CSF diversion with a VP shunt.

Adjuvant Therapy

Most of these patients will receive postoperative radiotherapy. In the MD Anderson series, postoperative radiotherapy was given 71% of patients, mostly to patients with tumors from epithelial and salivary gland origin. This number includes three patients who received re-irradiation to the site following microvascular free flap reconstruction.

Postoperative radiotherapy was not given to sarcoma patients who had radiation-associated tumors, completely excised tumors, or low-grade chondrosarcoma.

Conclusion

This chapter discussed the jugular foramen approach for malignant tumors. The preoperative evaluation and indications for this procedure are discussed. The procedure is illustrated and described in detail. Postoperative management, complications, and adjuvant therapy are highlighted.

References

1. Kim CJ, Yoo SJ, Nam SY, Kim SY. A hearing preservation technique for the resection of extensive jugular foramen tumors. The Laryngoscope. 2001;111(11 Pt 1):2071–6.
2. Gold SR, Kamerer DB Jr. Preservation of conductive hearing in approaches to tumors of the jugular foramen. Otol Neurotol. 2006;27(8):1126–30.
3. Sanna M, Bacciu A, Falcioni M, Taibah A. Surgical management of jugular foramen schwannomas with hearing and facial nerve function preservation: a series of 23 cases and review of the literature. The Laryngoscope. 2006;116(12):2191–204.
4. Megerian CA, McKenna MJ, Nadol JB Jr. Non-paraganglioma jugular foramen lesions masquerading as glomus jugulare tumors. Am J Otol. 1995;16(1):94–8.
5. Lo WW, Solti-Bohman LG, Lambert PR. High-resolution CT in the evaluation of glomus tumors of the temporal bone. Radiology. 1984;150(3):737–42.
6. Greenberg HS, Deck MD, Vikram B, Chu FC, Posner JB. Metastasis to the base of the skull: clinical findings in 43 patients. Neurology. 1981;31(5):530–7.
7. Chao CK, Sheen TS, Lien HC, Hsu MM. Metastatic carcinoma to the jugular foramen. Otolaryngol Head Neck Surg. 2000;122(6):922–3.
8. Shine NP, O'Sullivan P. Collet-Sicard syndrome: a rare presentation of metastatic prostate adenocarcinoma. Auris Nasus Larynx. 2005;32(3):315–8.
9. Chacon G, Alexandraki I, Palacio C. Collet-sicard syndrome: an uncommon manifestation of metastatic prostate cancer. South Med J. 2006;99(8):898–9.
10. Lowenheim H, Koerbel A, Ebner FH, Kumagami H, Ernemann U, Tatagiba M. Differentiating imaging findings in primary and secondary tumors of the jugular foramen. Neurosurg Rev. 2006;29(1): 1–11. discussion 2–3.
11. Weber A, McKenna M. Radiologic evaluation of the jugular foramen. Anatomy, vascular variants, anomalies, and tumors. Neuroimaging Clin N Am. 1994;4(3):579–98.
12. Rosenbloom JS, Storper IS, Aviv JE, Hacein-Bey L, Bruce JN. Giant cell tumors of the jugular foramen. Am J Otolaryngol. 1999; 20(3):176–9.
13. Leonetti JP, Smith PG, Anand VK, Kletzker GR, Hartman JM. Subtotal petrosectomy in the management of advanced parotid neoplasms. Otolaryngol Head Neck Surg. 1993;108(3):270–6.
14. Zanoletti E, Cazzador D, Faccioli C, Martini A, Mazzoni A. Closure of the sigmoid sinus in lateral skull base surgery. Acta Otorhinolaryngol Ital. 2014;34(3):184–8.

Infratemporal Fossa Approach

20

Paul W. Gidley, Franco DeMonte, and Randal S. Weber

Introduction

The infratemporal fossa (ITF) is involved by a variety of tumor types. Parotid, paranasal sinus, mesenchymal, nasopharyngeal, neural sheath, cutaneous, sarcomatous, and meningiomatous tumors can infiltrate or arise within the infratemporal fossa. These tumors tend to spread along preformed pathways, such as neural foramina or bony gaps, to occupy the potential space of the ITF. Given the variety of tumor types and origins, a number of different approaches to the ITF have been described including transmaxillary, transmandibular, preauricular, transtemporal, transzygomatic, and endonasal endoscopic approaches. The identification and management of important neural and vascular structures that travel adjacent to the ITF is common to each of these approaches. The management of the petrous carotid artery can be the most challenging part of these procedures. Given the bony course of the carotid in the temporal bone, the transtemporal approach gives wide exposure of the carotid along its entire petrous course. A multidisciplinary team comprised of neurotology, neurosurgery, head and neck surgery, and usually plastic and reconstructive surgery utilizes the skills of each discipline to give patients the best surgical outcome.

Anatomy

The infratemporal fossa (ITF) is roughly quadrangular in geometry [1]. Its lateral border is the zygomatic arch, parotid gland, temporalis muscle, and the medial surface of the ascending ramus and coronoid process of the mandible (Fig. 20.1). Its anterior border is the posterior wall of the maxillary sinus. Superiorly, it is bounded by the greater wing of the sphenoid and floor of the middle cranial fossa. The greater wing of the sphenoid contains the foramen rotundum, foramen spinosum, and foramen ovale. Medially, the ITF is bounded by the lateral pterygoid plate of the sphenoid, the superior constrictor muscle, and the pyramidal process of the palatine bone. Posteriorly, the ITF is bounded by the styloid process, styloid diaphragm, and the condylar process of the mandible. Inferiorly, the ITF is separated from the masticator space by the medial pterygoid muscle.

The ITF is related to two additional spaces: the parapharyngeal space and the masticator space. The medial pterygoid muscle and medial pterygoid fascia constitute the boundary between the ITF and the parapharyngeal space. The parapharyngeal space contains the internal carotid artery, internal jugular vein, and cranial nerves IX, X, XI, and XII. The masticator space contains the internal maxillary artery, pterygoid venous plexus, and pterygoid muscles.

The following foramina and fissures communicate with the ITF (Fig. 20.2). The foramen spinosum contains the middle meningeal artery. The foramen rotundum transmits the second or maxillary division of the trigeminal nerve. The foramen ovale contains the third or mandibular division of the trigeminal nerve. While not a true foramen, the internal carotid artery (ICA) courses over the foramen lacerum. The pterygomaxillary fissure is a narrow gap between the lateral pterygoid plate and infratemporal surface of the maxillary sinus. Through this fissure, the ITF communicates with the pterygopalatine fossa. The third part of the internal maxillary artery and the posterior superior alveolar arteries, veins, and nerves pass through this fissure.

Surgical Approaches

Several surgical approaches to the ITF have been described. Conley (1956) described a transmandibular approach [2]. Barbosa (1961) [3] and Honeybul et al. (1997) [4] described

P. W. Gidley, M.D., F.A.C.S. (✉) · R. S. Weber, M.D.
Department of Head and Neck Surgery, The University of Texas
M.D. Anderson Cancer Center, Houston, TX, USA
e-mail: pwgidley@mdanderson.org; rsweber@mdanderson.org

F. DeMonte, M.D.
Department of Neurosurgery, The University of Texas
M.D. Anderson Cancer Center, Houston, TX, USA
e-mail: fdemonte@mdanderson.org

P. W. Gidley, F. DeMonte (eds.), *Temporal Bone Cancer*, https://doi.org/10.1007/978-3-319-74539-8_20

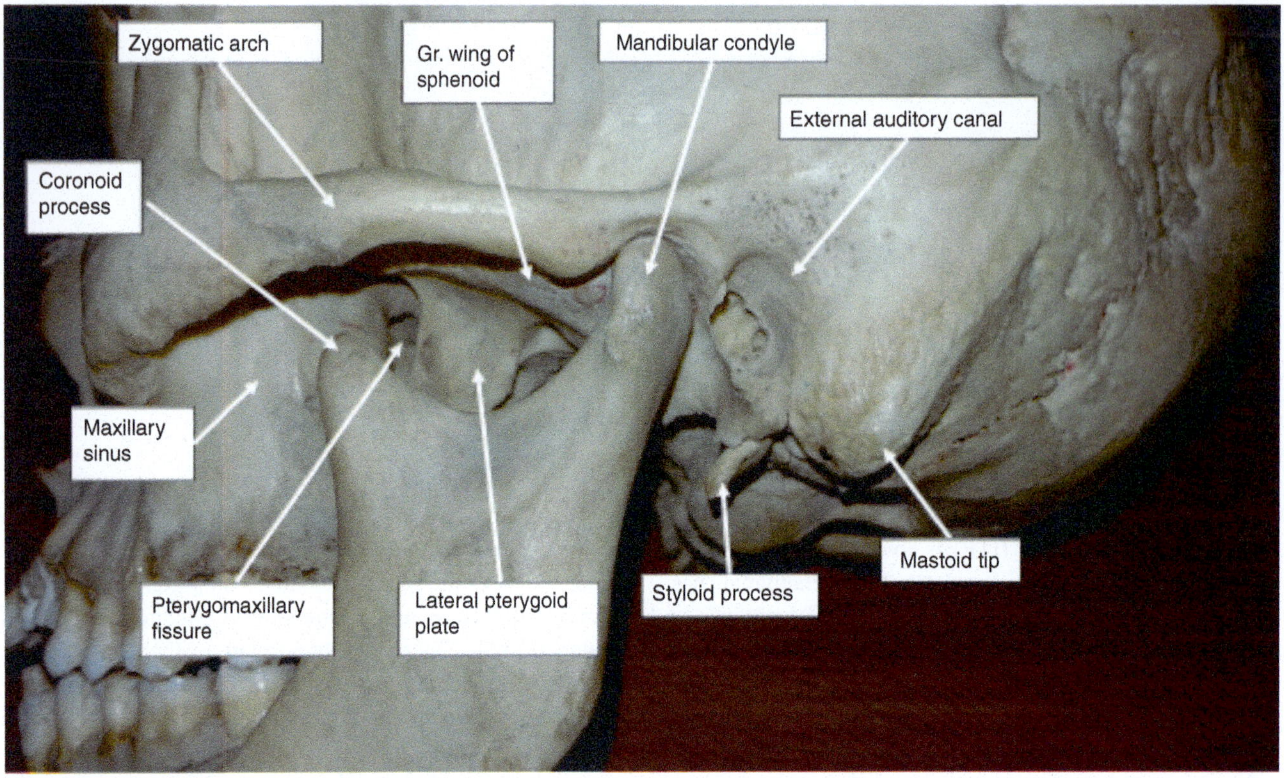

Fig. 20.1 Bone landmarks of the infratemporal fossa

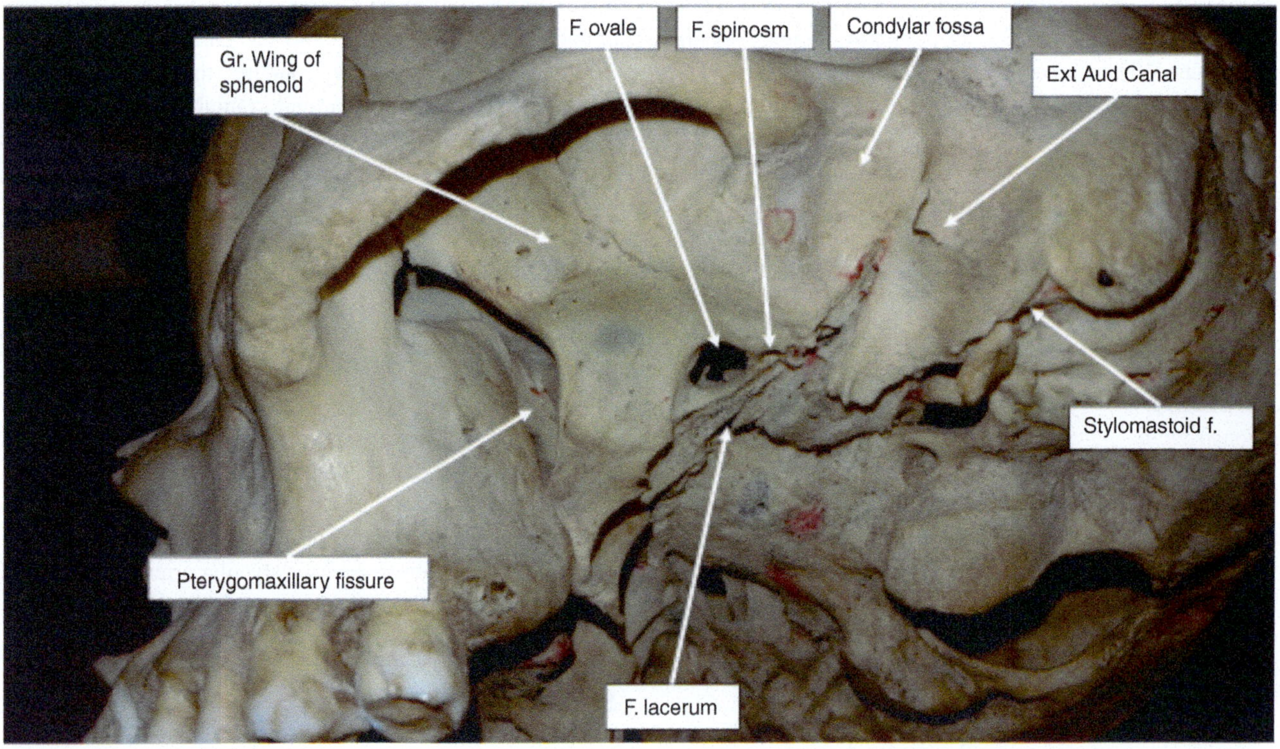

Fig. 20.2 Foramina of the ITF. The mandible has been removed (Key: *Ext Aud* external auditory, *F* foramen, *Gr* greater)

a transzygomatic approach. It was Ugo Fisch (1978) who described the transtemporal approach to the ITF [5]. He originally described three different approaches: type A which gives access to tumors of the infralabyrinthine and apical compartment of the temporal bone, type B which is used for lesions of the clivus and base of skull along the Eustachian tube, and type C for tumors in the parasellar region. These approaches were initially designed for management of paragangliomas, but indications were extended to juvenile nasopharyngeal angiofibromas and nasopharyngeal cancers [6, 7]. Obwegeser (1985) described a preauricular approach to the retromaxillary and ITF for temporomandibular joint disorders. Wetmore et al. (1986) describe a similar approach [8]. Sekhar et al. (1987) described in detail a preauricular approach to the infratemporal fossa for a variety of benign and malignant tumors, emphasizing the versatility of the approach and the management of the carotid artery [9]. Leonetti et al. (2012) used the preauricular infratemporal fossa approach for 159 parotid malignancies, concluding that this approach provided proximal identification of the facial nerve, protection of the internal carotid artery, and negative margins at the skull base [10]. While their approach is described as preauricular, the ear canal is removed and a subtotal petrosectomy is performed. Mansour et al. (2004) used a preauricular (subtemporal) ITF approach for 65 patients with both benign and malignant tumors [11].

Recent literature has concentrated on minimizing morbidity by using endoscopic endonasal approaches to the ITF [12–16]. The advantage of this approach is avoidance of facial nerve manipulation and loss of the ear canal and sequelae of maximum conductive hearing loss. These approaches are suitable for benign pathology, but they do not give adequate exposure for extirpation of malignant tumors. Other limitations include difficulty in obtaining hemostasis and lack of instruments designed for endoscopic dissection [14]. Internal carotid artery blowout has also been described with this approach [15].

A transtemporal approach to the infratemporal fossa with preservation of the conductive hearing mechanism has been described [17]. This approach uses hydroxyapatite cement to reconstruct the external ear canal.

The classic Fisch infratemporal fossa approaches have four commonalities: (1) permanent anterior displacement of the facial nerve, (2) subluxation or resection of the mandibular condyle, (3) temporary displacement of the zygomatic arch, and (4) subtotal petrosectomy with obliteration of the middle ear [5]. In his paper, subtotal petrosectomy includes exenteration of the temporal bone with the exception of the bony labyrinth and exposure of the middle and posterior fossa dura. Subtotal petrosectomy should not be confused with subtotal temporal bone resection, which includes removal of the bony labyrinth. His initial series of 51 patients included primarily paragangliomas, meningiomas, and chordomas, while squamous cell and adenoid cystic carcinomas of the nasopharynx or infratemporal fossa only totaled 12 patients [5]. It is remarkable to look back on this series and realize that it was performed without the benefit of computerized, cross-sectional imaging. While carotid angiography was performed in some cases, carotid balloon occlusion test had not yet been developed [18]. In a subsequent publication 7 years later, Fisch et al. reported an operative experience of 211 patients, with 61 patients having either squamous cell carcinoma or adenoid cystic carcinoma [19].

Since this book is dedicated to temporal bone tumors, the transtemporal approach will be discussed in detail, similar to the Fisch type C approach. However, this resection differs from the classic Fisch infratemporal fossa approach in that (1) the facial nerve is not rerouted, (2) the mandible is not displaced anteriorly but is removed, (3) parotidectomy is performed, (4) zygomatic osteotomies are performed and the zygoma occasionally resected, (5) middle fossa bone is removed, and (6) the external carotid artery distal to the facial artery is ligated.

Patient Population

Parotid, periauricular, and skull base tumors can involve the infratemporal fossa. In the MD Anderson series, 45 patients underwent a transtemporal approach to the infratemporal fossa for resection of a variety of malignant tumors. The average age was 55 (range 3–83 years). There were 31 men and 14 women. Twenty-four tumors were left-sided and 21 right-sided.

Bigelow et al. (1999) reported on 25 patients, ranging from 21 to 75 years old; and their series included 16 men and 9 women [20]. Mansour et al. (2004) described 44 patients (26 men and 18 women), ranging in age from 2 to 76 years (mean age of 49.5 years), who had malignant tumors of the infratemporal fossa treated with a preauricular approach [11]. Bilsky et al. (2005) reported a series of 25 patients with a mean age of 59 years (range, 29–82 years), 19 tumors in men and 17 tumors on the left side [21]. Leonetti et al. (2012) reported a series of 159 patients with parotid malignancies, who had a mean age of 54.2 years (range 14–92 years), involving 96 women and 63 men, with 86 right-sided to 73 left-sided tumors that were treated with an infratemporal fossa approach [10].

Several primary tumor locations were encountered with parotid and periauricular skin cancers being the most common (Table 20.1). In contrast, the series reported by Leonetti et al. was exclusively malignant parotid tumors [10]. The series by Bilsky et al. was primary maxillary sinus cancers ($N = 15$); therefore, their surgical approach was transmaxillary, and all patients underwent either partial or total maxillectomy [21]. Bigelow et al. described a series of 25 patients with a variety of primary sites including oropharynx, maxillary sinus, nasopharynx, ITF, and temporal bone.

Table 20.1 Primary tumor location in 45 patients at MD Anderson with infratemporal fossa malignancies

Primary location	No.
Parotid	11
Periauricular	10
Skull base	7
Temporal bone	7
External ear	5
Ear canal	3
Nasopharynx	1
Maxillary sinus	1

Table 20.2 Symptoms of 45 patients with infratemporal fossa malignancies

Symptom	No.
Facial nerve dysfunction	26
Hearing loss	23
Parotid swelling	19
Otalgia	18
Otorrhea	11
Facial numbness	10
Tinnitus	8
Vertigo	7
Tongue weakness	2
Hoarseness, dysphagia, and shoulder weakness	1

Of these patients, 20 underwent ITF approach for excision of the tumor [20].

In the MD Anderson series, 20 patients had previously untreated tumors, 5 with persistent disease and 20 patients with recurrent tumors. The most common symptoms were facial nerve dysfunction, hearing loss, parotid swelling, and otalgia (Table 20.2). House-Brackmann facial nerve scores were I = 19, II = 7, III = 2, IV = 3, V = 2, and VI = 12. The majority of patients (60%) had some degree of facial weakness or paralysis preoperatively. The average tumor size was 5.2 cm (range 2.5–12 cm).

Tumor histology was primary squamous cell carcinoma, followed by advanced parotid tumors and sarcoma (Table 20.3). This distribution of tumor types is similar to other reports in the literature although the group at Memorial Sloan Kettering reported more sarcomas than epithelial tumors [11, 20–22]. Perineural invasion was found in 19 patients (42.2%). Bone, cartilage, or soft tissue extension was found in 36 patients (80%). Dural invasion was found in seven patients (15.5%). Neck dissection was performed in 30 patients. Nine patients (30%) had positive lymph nodes: level 1 (one patient), II (eight patients), III (six patients), IV (four patients), and V (two patients).

Infratemporal fossa tumors in children are very rare. Cunningham et al. report on 89 children undergoing neurotologic surgery, including two who had infratemporal fossa resections [23]. Their paper does not report the tumor type for these two patients, but none of the patients in the series had malignant tumor.

Table 20.3 Histologic tumor types involving the infratemporal fossa

Tumor histology	No.
Squamous cell carcinoma	15
Sarcomas (Rhabdomyo 1, Chondro 1, Osteo 1, EWS 1)	4
Adenocarcinoma	3
Adenoid cystic carcinoma	3
Giant cell tumor	3
Sarcomatoid carcinoma	3
Basal cell carcinoma	2
Salivary duct carcinoma	2
Basosquamous carcinoma	1
Other	9

Rhabdo rhabdomyosarcoma, *Chondro* chondrosarcoma, *Osteo* osteosarcoma, *EWS* Ewing sarcoma

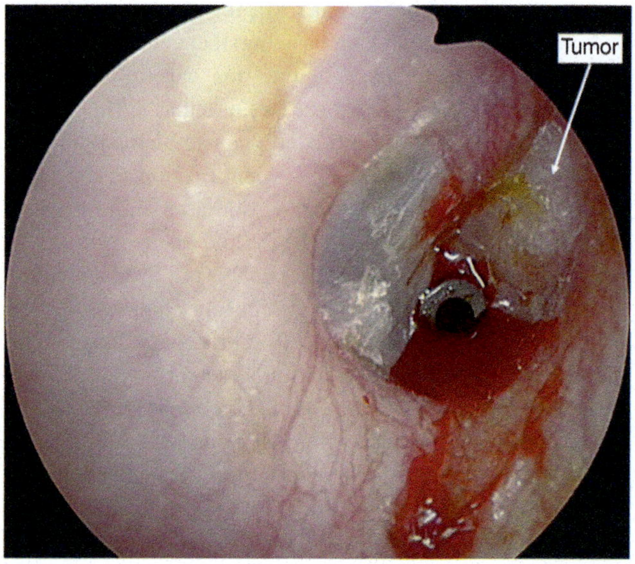

Fig. 20.3 Case #1. Giant cell tumor of ITF in a 67-year-old woman who developed right aural fullness. A PE tube was placed by the referring physician, but it did not relieve her symptoms. A CT scan was later performed revealing her tumor. Bloody otorrhea was draining through her PE tube. Tumor can clearly be seen behind the tympanic membrane, anterior to the malleus

Preoperative Evaluation

Patients with tumors of the infratemporal fossa typically have symptoms of facial numbness, facial paralysis, Eustachian tube dysfunction, and trismus or malocclusion (Fig. 20.3). As with all skull base patients, careful cranial nerve examination is important. Trigeminal and facial nerve deficits are common. Larger tumors might involve the lower cranial nerves (IX–XII), and preoperative examination of these nerves is important to verify their function. A modified barium swallow and video stroboscopy and consultation with speech pathology are warranted. Audiometry is performed to measure hearing and to decide on candidacy for an osseointegrated implant.

In the MD Anderson series, nearly half of the patients had previous radiotherapy. This fact must be borne in mind when planning incisions and reconstructive plans, since an irradiated outer ear tolerates flap elevation poorly. Many of these patients, however, have had previous surgery, and this might limit the choices for incision.

Due to involvement of the temporomandibular joint and pterygoid muscles, many of these patients have restricted mouth opening. This needs to be borne in mind for planning the anesthetic, since a fiberoptic intubation or an elective tracheostomy might be required.

These patients must be in good general physical health to undergo this procedure. Any underlying medical problem should be addressed and optimized preoperatively. Due to the extensive nature of these tumors, a multidisciplinary approach is beneficial, and consultations are sought from head and neck surgery, neurosurgery, plastic and reconstructive surgery, radiotherapy, dental oncology, and oculoplastic surgery.

Diagnostic Imaging

The extent of tumors of the ITF is not clinically evaluable by physical findings alone; therefore, CT and MRI evaluation are imperative to understand the full magnitude and scope of the tumor. Since these two imaging techniques are complimentary, both modalities are usually obtained (Fig. 20.4). CT gives superb bony anatomy definition, while contrast-enhanced MRI is useful to understand perineural invasion, dural involvement, and intracranial extension. Both imaging studies are informative regarding the state of the internal carotid artery. The CT may show destruction of the bone of the carotid canal, and MRI may show tumor abutting, narrowing, or occluding the artery.

Tumors of the infratemporal fossa usually meet the definition of stage IV disease regardless of primary site, and PET/CT is a reasonable option to rule out distant disease. If distant disease is identified, the indications for resection of the ITF tumor are severely truncated.

Carotid angiography is performed for patients with lesions involving or adjacent to the carotid artery. Temporary balloon occlusion test is performed for patients with risk of ICA injury or in those who will likely require carotid artery sacrifice. ICA occlusion is done preoperatively by the interventional endovascular team in those patients that pass the balloon occlusion test and require ICA occlusion.

Operative Procedure

Positioning and Preparation

The procedures are performed under general endotracheal anesthesia using an oral endotracheal tube or occasionally a tracheostomy. Continuous monitoring of end-tidal CO_2, oxygen saturation, and intra-arterial blood pressures is carried out throughout the procedure. A Foley catheter is placed to monitor urinary output and fluid status.

Intraoperative facial nerve monitoring is utilized, and it is important to communicate this fact to the anesthesiologist so that long-term paralytics are not given at the outset of the procedure.

These procedures are typically lengthy, especially if a microvascular free flap is required for reconstruction. The patient is padded and strapped to the operating table. Thromboembolic deterrent (TED) hose and sequential compression devices (SCDs) are placed on the legs to help prevent development of deep vein thrombosis.

The operating room table is turned so that the head is positioned 180° from the anesthesia stand. This position allows access to the head and neck and sufficient access to the lower extremities for free flap harvesting.

The head can be positioned with a horseshoe head holder or in Mayfield head holder. The latter is used when employing a surgical stereotactic navigation system. The head is turned about 45° away from the site of the lesion, and the neck is partially extended. Rigid fixation of the head also helps to prevent the head being turned during the procedure, which might cause inadvertent extubation.

An osseointegrated implant for hearing aid (OIHA) can be placed at this first procedure, and its site is marked 5.5 cm from the external auditory canal at the temporal line using methylene blue injection.

The head and neck and the lower extremities are then sterilely prepared and draped for surgery. The anterior lateral thigh flap has been very useful in reconstructing this defect, and the thighs are included in the original preparation. If facial nerve grafting is required, the lateral femoral cutaneous nerve is available as a donor, or a sural nerve graft can be obtained.

Incision and Flap Elevation

A variety of incisions can be used depending on the location and size of the tumor. If a large tumor involves the outer ear, ear canal, and preauricular skin, then a large circumferential incision is used (Fig. 20.5). This incision is taken down to the temporal squamosa above and the mastoid behind the ear and down to the sternocleidomastoid muscle and mandible below the ear.

If only the skin of the ear canal is involved, then the ear canal and tragus can be incorporated into the preauricular incision as an ellipse (Fig. 20.6).

If this skin is uninvolved, then a preauricular incision is used (Fig. 20.7). This incision includes a question-mark shape from the temporal hairline for the craniotomy, a preauricular incision for the parotidectomy and temporal bone resection, and a neck incision about 3 cm below the angle of the jaw. In this approach, the external ear is raised attached to

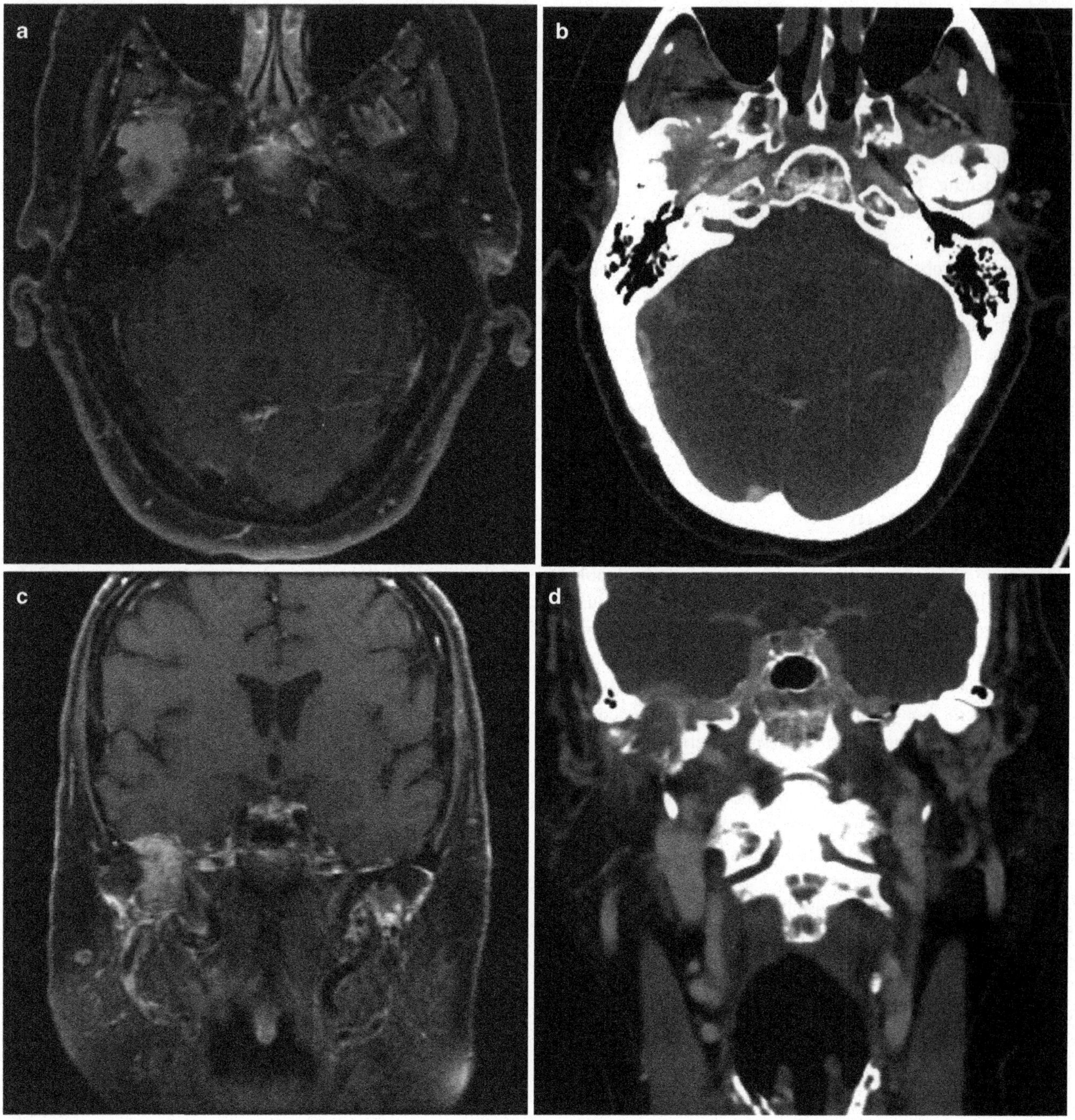

Fig. 20.4 CT and MRI of tumor of Case #1. (**a**) Axial contrast-enhanced T1-weighted MRI. (**b**) Axial contrast-enhanced CT at same level as shown in MRI. (**c**) Coronal contrast-enhanced T1-weighted MRI. (**d**) Coronal contrast-enhanced CT at same level as shown in MRI

a large posterior based flap, and the facial skin is raised anteriorly.

When a preauricular incision is made, the skin flap is raised anteriorly over the parotid and in a subplatysmal plane in the neck. The temporalis fascia is incised about two fingerbreadths above the zygoma, and the fascia is elevated down to the level of the zygomatic arch. This maneuver protects the temporal branch of the facial nerve. The skin flap is held with fishhook retractors.

The ear canal is divided at the bony-cartilaginous junction, and a plane of dissection is developed over the temporalis fascia, mastoid periosteum, and sternocleidomastoid muscle. This posterior-based flap is elevated until the methylene blue marking for OIHA is encountered. The skin of the external auditory meatus is undermined and separated from the ear canal cartilage. The skin is everted and trimmed. This trimming is the medial ear canal margin, and it can be sent for frozen section. The everted skin is sewn shut with Vicryl sutures, and the soft

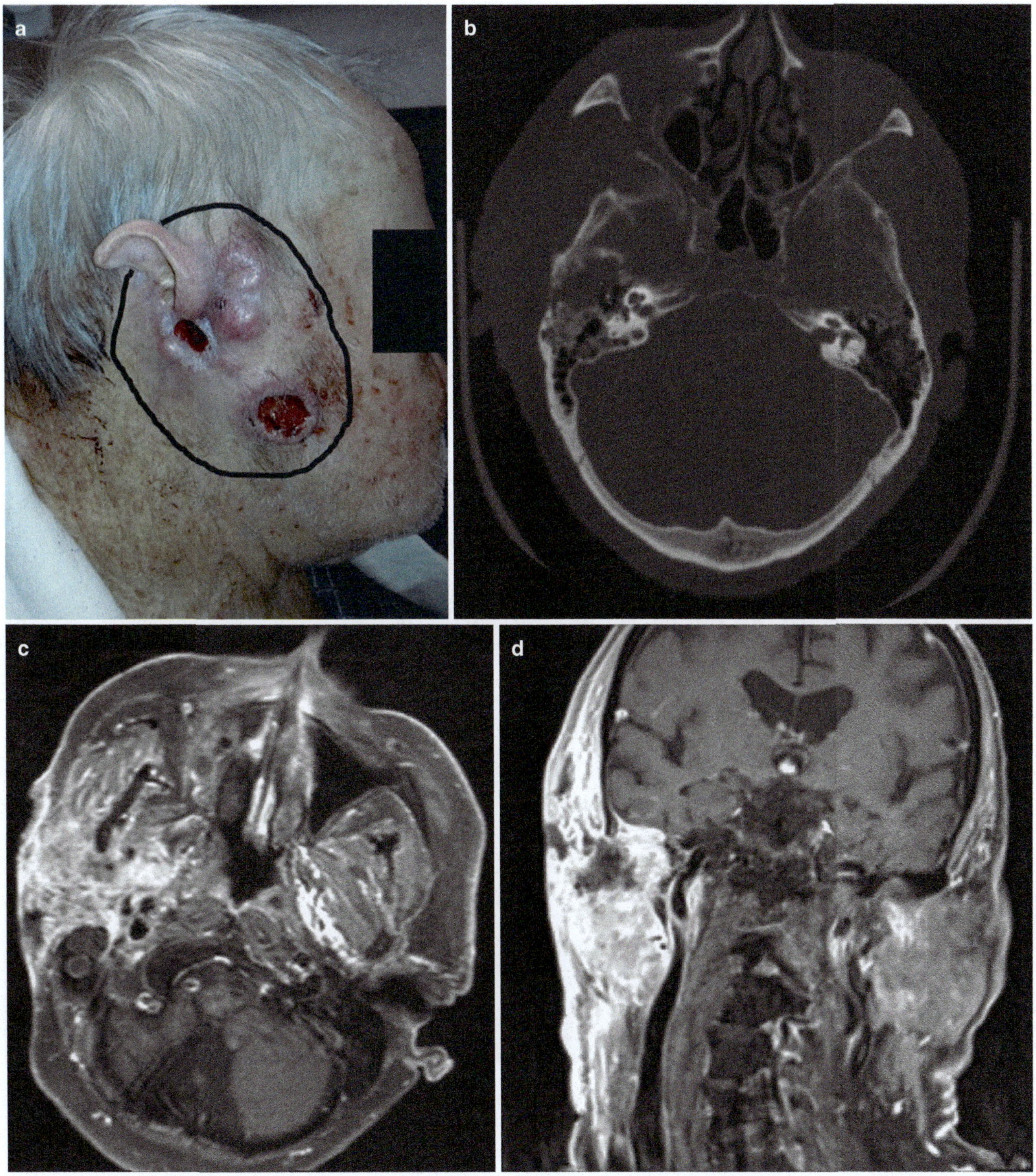

Fig. 20.5 Case #2. Extensive, recurrent squamous cell carcinoma of the right face and temporal bone in a 79-year-old man (**a**). The skin incisions are designed to include the tumor and the entire outer ear (black line). (**b**) Axial noncontrast CT at level of cochlea, showing destruction of the anterior temporal bone and glenoid fossa. (**c**) Axial contrast-enhanced T1 MRI showing enhancement around the carotid artery and jugular vein. (**d**) Coronal contrast-enhanced T1 MRI showing enhancement of middle fossa dura

tissue and cartilage on the undersurface are closed with Vicryl sutures. This creates a two-layer closure to prevent CSF leak. Fishhook retractors are used to hold the skin flap out of the way.

An alternative incision is a large C-shaped postauricular incision, where the ear is raised based on an anterior-based skin flap.

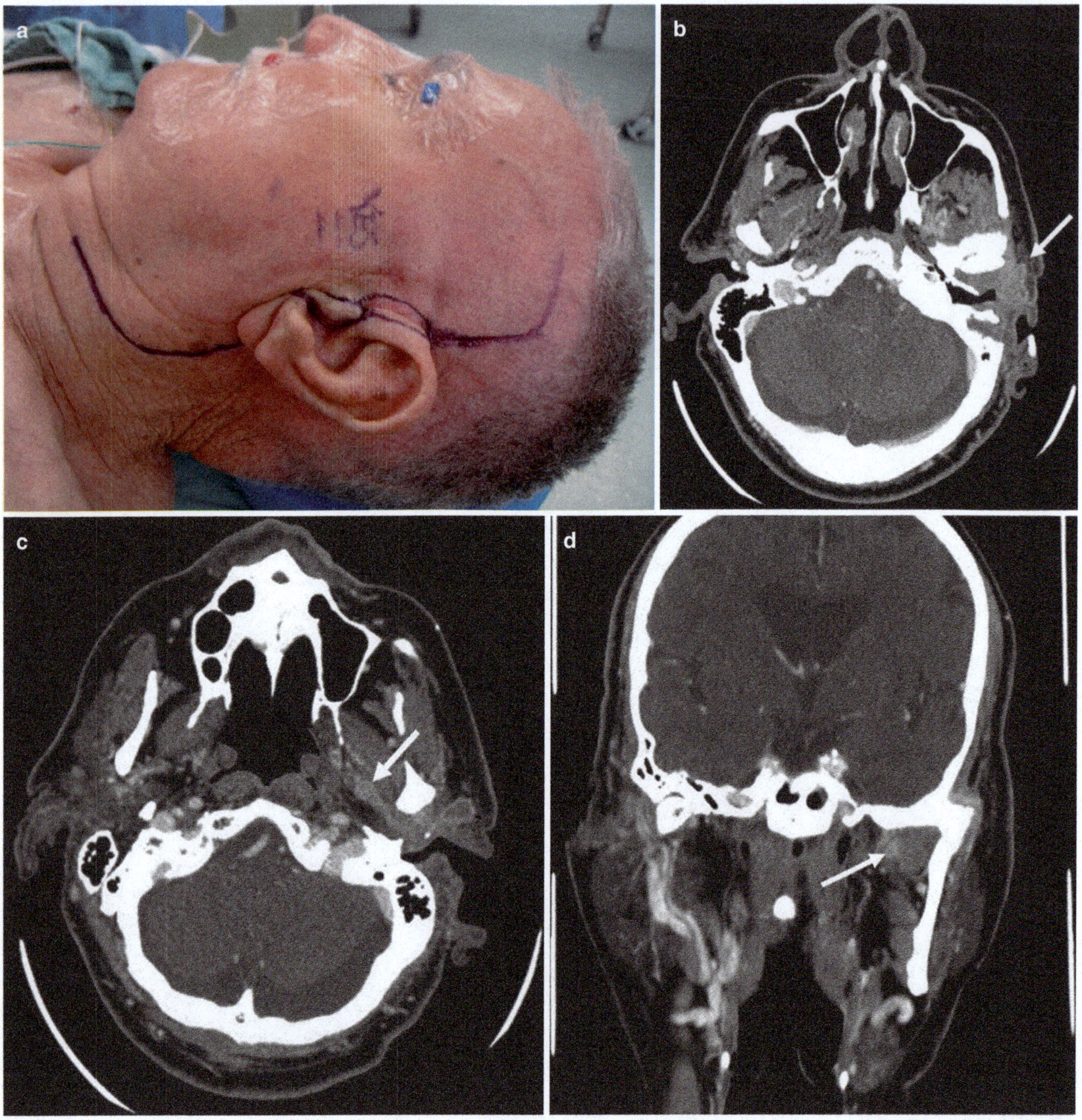

Fig. 20.6 Case #3. Squamous cell carcinoma in a 79-year-old man that presented as chronic otitis media and was biopsied through a tympanomastoidectomy prior to referral. (**a**) Preauricular incision for infratemporal fossa approach using an ellipse to excise the tragus and external auditory canal. (**b**) Axial contrast CT at level of ear canal, showing tumor at the external auditory meatus (arrow). Axial (**c**) and coronal (**d**) CT showing perineural spread along V3 (arrow)

Neck Dissection and Securing the Great Vessels

The incision is extended anteriorly and inferiorly into the neck to provide exposure for lymphadenectomy and vessel exposure. The skin flaps are elevated anteriorly and inferiorly. Level I may be included for preauricular skin cancers, as necessary. Initially the sternocleidomastoid muscle is reflected posteriorly, exposing the 11th nerve which is skeletonized. Level IIB is dissected and the packet of lymph nodes are reflected anteriorly to be kept in continuity with the level IIA lymph nodes. Next an incision is made into the deep cervical fascia approximately 4 cm posterior to the internal jugular vein down to level III or level IV as necessary to clear the lymph node basins at risk. The incision posteriorly is deepened down to the cervical rootlets, which

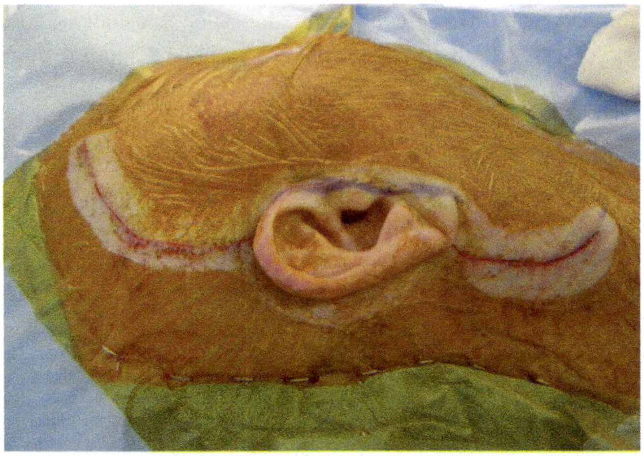

Fig. 20.7 Preauricular incision for large giant cell tumor as demonstrated in Case #1 (Fig. 20.3)

are preserved. The fibro-fatty tissues are reflected anteriorly, preserving the fascia over the levator and scalene muscles. The vagus, carotid artery, and the internal jugular vein are skeletonized as the specimen is reflected anteriorly. The dissection includes the lymph nodes lying anterior to the jugular vein, and the specimen remains in continuity. Anterior to the internal jugular vein, the 12th nerve is identified and preserved. The common facial vein is also preserved to serve as a recipient vessel for microvascular reconstruction as needed. Once the neck dissection specimen is removed, it is oriented by levels for pathologic analysis. Next the internal carotid artery is identified and encircled with a vessel loop as is the internal jugular vein. Once proximal control of the vessels is obtained, the distal external carotid artery may be ligated to diminish bleeding during the tumor resection. Arterial branches for microvascular reconstruction should be preserved to facilitate that portion of the procedure.

Temporal Bone Surgery

The goal of this portion is to remove the ear canal to allow unimpeded view of the infratemporal fossa, carotid artery, and middle fossa. The approach described is similar to a lateral temporal bone resection. A complete mastoidectomy is performed. The mastoid tegmen and sigmoid sinus are identified and skeletonized. The mastoid tip is drilled out. The antrum is opened. The horizontal semicircular canals are identified and preserved throughout the procedure.

The operating microscope is brought into place and used for the remainder of the procedure. The antrum is widened allowing identification of the incus. Drilling is continued between the ear canal and the tegmen, drilling out the zygomatic root and identifying the temporomandibular joint capsule.

If tumor is seen growing along the tegmen, then the drill is used to remove the bone along the tegmen in order to expose the dura. An assessment is made of any dural invasion, but this is addressed separately once the main tumor specimen has been removed.

Under high-power magnification, using continuous suction-irrigation and fine diamond burs, the facial recess is drilled out. The middle ear space is assessed for tumor. If tumor is found within the middle ear, it is removed, and consideration is given to subtotal temporal bone resection, removing the labyrinth and cochlea.

The facial nerve is identified in its tympanic portion and followed along the second genu and mastoid portions to the stylomastoid foramen. The stylomastoid foramen is widened with the drill. The digastric ridge is identified and drilled away. A bony cut is made inferior to the ear canal and lateral to the facial nerve; this maneuver liberates the mastoid tip. The mastoid tip is elevated away from the facial nerve, and the soft tissue attachments are divided with Bovie electrocautery.

A trough is drilled lateral to the facial nerve. The chorda tympani nerve is identified and sacrificed. Drilling continues between the facial nerve and the annulus, extending the facial recess. This dissection continues until the hypotympanic air cells are opened. The bone of the inferior tympanic ring is drilled away until soft tissue is reached anteriorly at the temporomandibular joint.

Thumb pressure on the ear canal fractures the canal anteriorly. The incus is disarticulated, and the tensor tendon is divided. A Freer elevator is used to elevate the ear canal.

The ear canal can be removed by developing a plane of dissection between the parotid and the ear canal. Alternatively, the ear canal can be left attached to the soft tissue anteriorly and removed with the main specimen en bloc (Fig. 20.8).

For carotid artery identification and dissection, the anterior tympanic ring and Eustachian tube orifice are drilled away. The petrous carotid artery is identified in the floor of the Eustachian tube. The drill is used to remove the bone covering the carotid artery, exposing 180° of the artery. The last thin shell of the bone covering the carotid is removed with Fisch instruments. This allows the artery to be mobilized. Dissection of the upper cervical ICA is limited at this point due to the presence of the mandible and temporomandibular joint contents.

The bone of the glenoid fossa is drilled away. The soft tissue of the joint capsule covering the bone is removed with the Bovie electrocautery. Bone is removed to expose the dura of the middle fossa as far medially as the superior semicircular canal and the geniculate ganglion. The tensor tympani muscle is removed.

Facial nerve decompression is then performed to help with parotidectomy. The drill is used to remove the bone of the facial canal. The last thin shell of bone on the nerve is gently removed with Fisch instruments. If only identification is required, then only 180° of the circumference of the nerve is exposed. If nerve transposition or sacrifice and grafting are required, then 270° of the circumference of the facial nerve is exposed. This larger degree of exposure is required to elevate the nerve out of its canal. For facial nerve sacrifice, the nerve is divided proximal to any area of tumoral involvement (usually identified as enlargement of the nerve), and the margin is inked and sent for frozen section (Fig. 20.9).

The osseointegrated implant for cochlear stimulation can be placed at this time. The periosteum is elevated at the site marked with methylene blue. This site is usually about 1.5–2 cm behind the posterior limit of the temporal bone resection. Standard technique is used for placing the implant. A conical cover screw is placed, and the abutment will be placed at a second stage procedure. The abutment is not placed with this first stage to avoid any skin complications from radiotherapy and to minimize the chance for CSF leakage. The second stage procedure is performed at 3 months if the patient does not receive radiotherapy or at 6 months if radiotherapy is given.

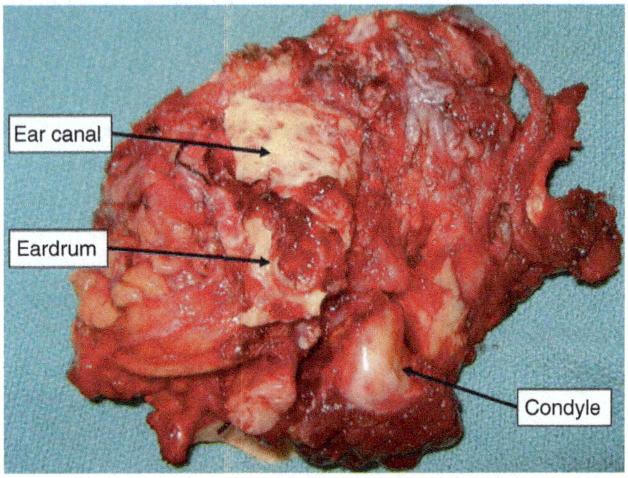

Fig. 20.8 En bloc specimen from Case #3. It includes the ear canal and mandibular condyle as well as parotid and upper neck dissection

Parotidectomy and Mandibulectomy

Given that these patients usually have facial paralysis, facial nerve sacrifice is often indicated. In the MD Anderson series, 33 patients (73.3%) required facial nerve sacrifice. In these patients, the distal branches of the facial nerve are identified and tagged for possible nerve grafting. The facial nerve trunk can be divided at the stylomastoid foramen, or a suitable location where it is free of disease, and the margin sent for frozen section. Radical parotidectomy can then be performed.

If the facial nerve is intact, then superficial or total parotidectomy is performed (Fig. 20.10). Branches are sequentially dissected and followed anteriorly until the superficial lobe is removed. The facial nerve is elevated off the mandible and the parotid deep lobe. This maneuver allows sufficient space to access the condyle and ascending ramus of the mandible. If the temporalis muscle is invaded by tumor, it is

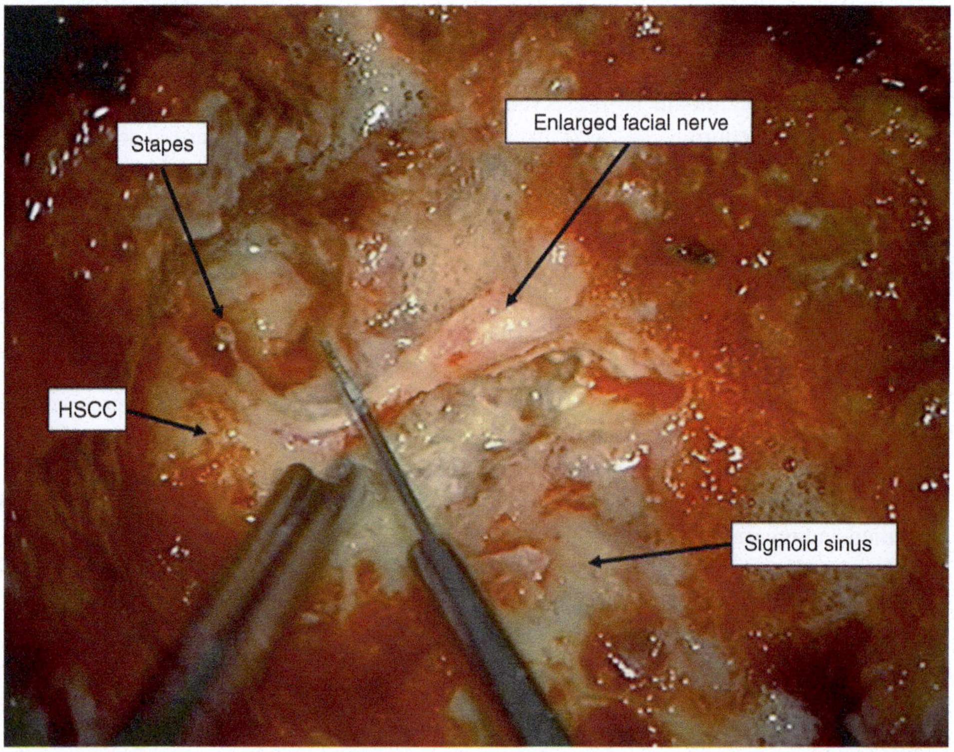

Fig. 20.9 Facial nerve sacrifice in Case #2. The nerve is divided proximal to the site of enlargement (*HSCC* horizontal semicircular canal)

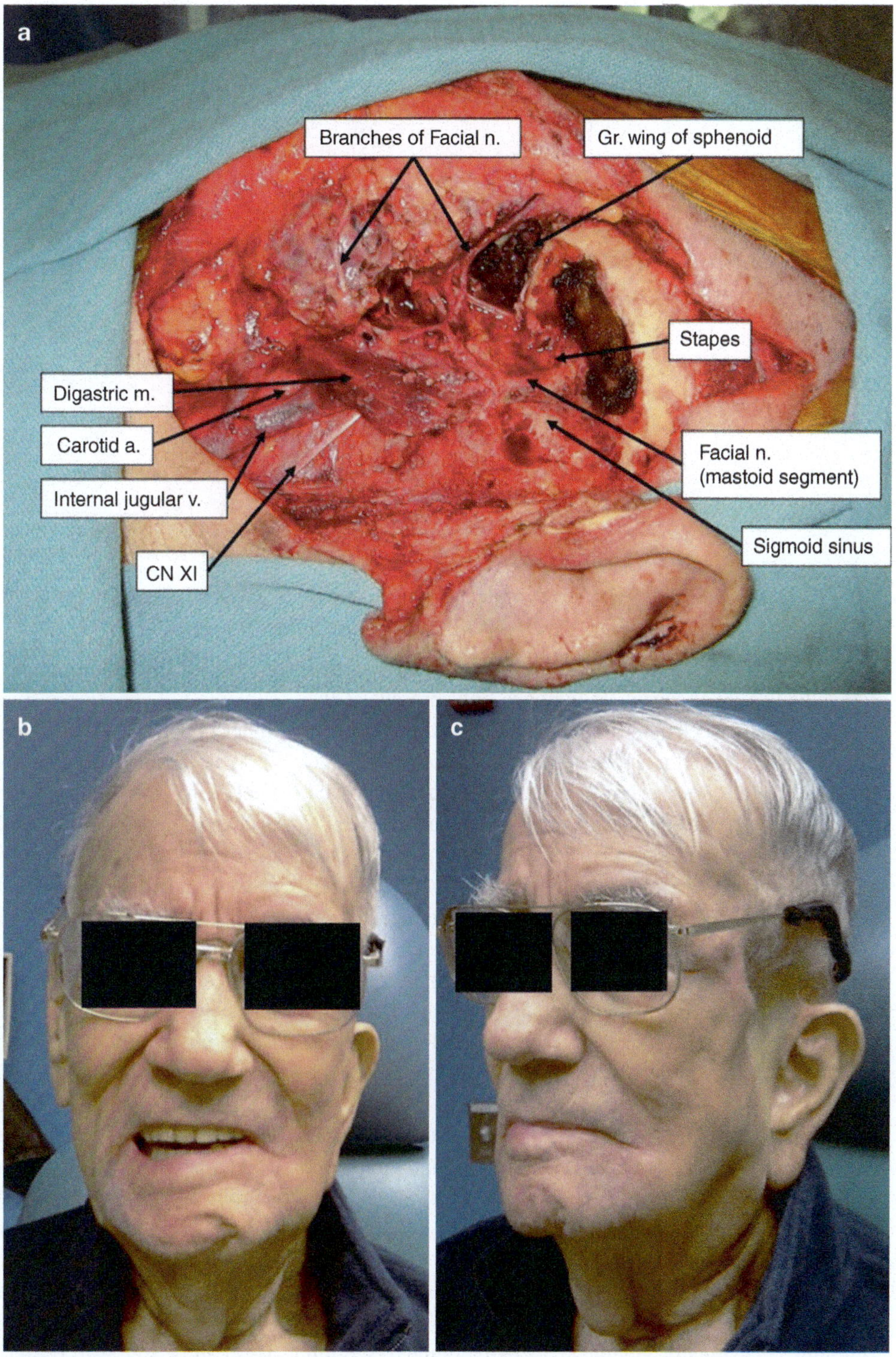

Fig. 20.10 Operative defect from Case #3. (**a**) The ascending ramus of the mandible, parotidectomy, and neck dissection were performed after lateral temporal bone resection. The facial nerve was completely preserved. In this case, no craniotomy was performed. The outer ear survived despite a small pedicle. (**b** and **c**) Postoperative result showing House-Brackmann II/VI facial function. Notice also that the left ear sags due to lack of support from missing ear canal

resected. If not, it can be reflected superiorly or inferiorly to expose the superior portion of the infratemporal fossa. The zygomatic osteotomies allow the temporalis muscle to rotate inferiorly.

If the facial nerve is already paralyzed, then no attempt is made for its preservation, and a radical parotidectomy is performed (Fig. 20.11). The distal branches of the nerve are identified and tagged for possible grafting. Anterior to the gland, the incision is deepened to the depth of the buccinator, preserving this muscle and the buccal fat pad and avoiding entry into the oral cavity.

The styloid process is removed to allow dissection along the carotid artery up to the skull base. The carotid artery can be traced from the neck superiorly to its petrous portion. Cranial nerves IX, X, XI, and XII are identified where they exit the skull base.

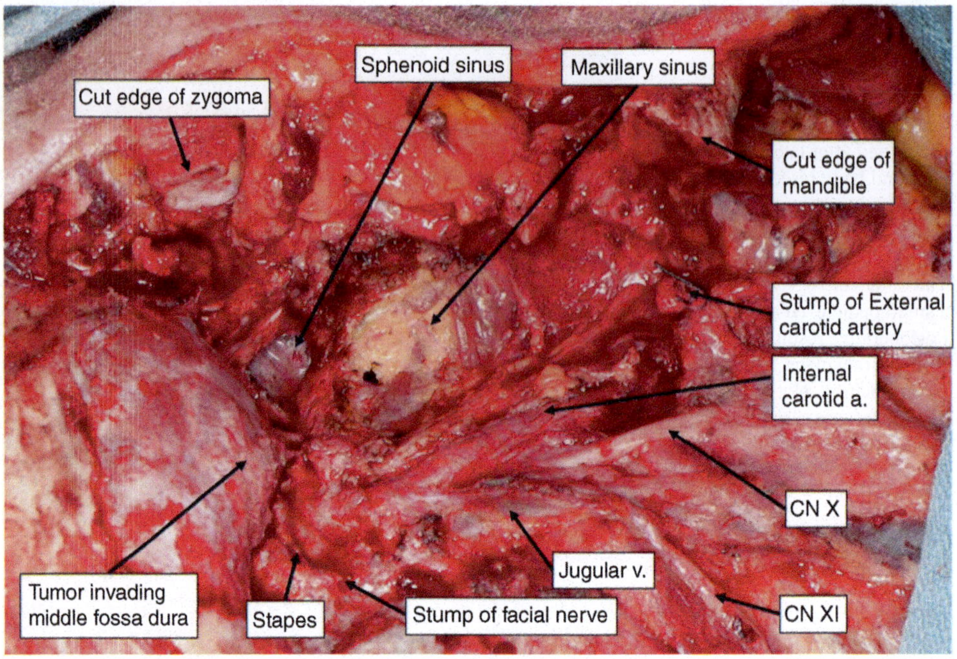

Fig. 20.11 Operative defect from Case #2. This patient had complete facial paralysis (House-Brackmann VI/VI), and no nerve grafts were performed

The level for mandibulectomy is predicated on the extent of mandibular involvement. If tumor is only present at the condyle, then the neck of the mandible is divided with double-action bone cutters. If a larger segment of the bone needs to be removed, then the posterior aspect of the mandible and angle are identified, and the masseter muscle is divided. A malleable retractor is placed underneath the mandible, and the mandible is divided with a reciprocating saw. The attachments of the temporalis, masseter, and pterygoid muscles are divided liberating the primary resection specimen.

Electrocautery is used to dissect down anterior to the parotid through the masseter muscle down to the mandible. The medial pterygoid is incised inferiorly, and a segmental mandibulectomy is performed at the angle of mandible. The mandible is mobilized so that the pterygoid muscles are exposed and their attachments are divided at the pterygoid plates. In this manner, the tumor is circumferentially freed up.

Middle Fossa and Infratemporal Fossa Dissection

Although occasionally amenable to extracranial resection alone, the majority of malignancies of the ITF will require the addition of a subtemporal craniectomy to remove potentially infiltrated bone and to assess for intracranial tumor extension. The addition of a subtemporal craniectomy and subtemporal exposure of the ITF allows management of the upper ITF under direct vision.

With the temporalis muscle reflected or resected, the bone underlying the temporal fossa is resected with the high-speed drill and rongeurs. Extradural dissection identifies the middle meningeal artery at the foramen spinosum, which is divided, as well as the foramen rotundum and ovale. Sharp division of the fibrous tissue at the junction of the temporal dura and the mandibular nerve allows access to the surgical plane between the medial temporal dura and the lateral cavernous sinus. This plane is dissected anteriorly to fully expose the maxillary nerve, posteriorly to free the mandibular nerve and to expose the lateral aspect of Meckel's cave, and medially to expose the Gasserian ganglion. Posterior to the mandibular nerve, the greater superficial petrosal nerve (GSPN) is identified. At this point, the bone can be removed to expose the horizontal petrous ICA and foramina rotundum and ovale.

Removing the bone between the maxillary and mandibular nerves will enter the lateral sphenoid sinus. Bone removal at the inferior border of the sphenoid sinus will open the Vidian canal and expose the Vidian neurovascular bundle. This can be followed posteriorly to the anterior-most aspect of the carotid canal at the entrance of the ICA into the cavernous sinus. The cartilaginous portion of the Eustachian tube is removed (Fig. 20.12).

Fig. 20.12 Case #4. A 47-year-old woman with carcinoma ex-pleomorphic adenoma, initially treated with cisplatin and radiotherapy. She developed progressive disease as pictured in (**a**) axial and (**b**) coronal MRI. She passed balloon occlusion test, and the internal carotid artery was coiled in preparation for sacrifice. (**c**) Macroscopic view of the operative defect prior to carotid artery sacrifice. (**d**) Close-up view of the operative defect, showing nerve of the Vidian canal. (**e** and **f**) Reconstruction with anterolateral thigh (ALT) flap and sural nerve graft (Reconstructive photographs **e** and **f** courtesy of Dr. Patrick Garvey)

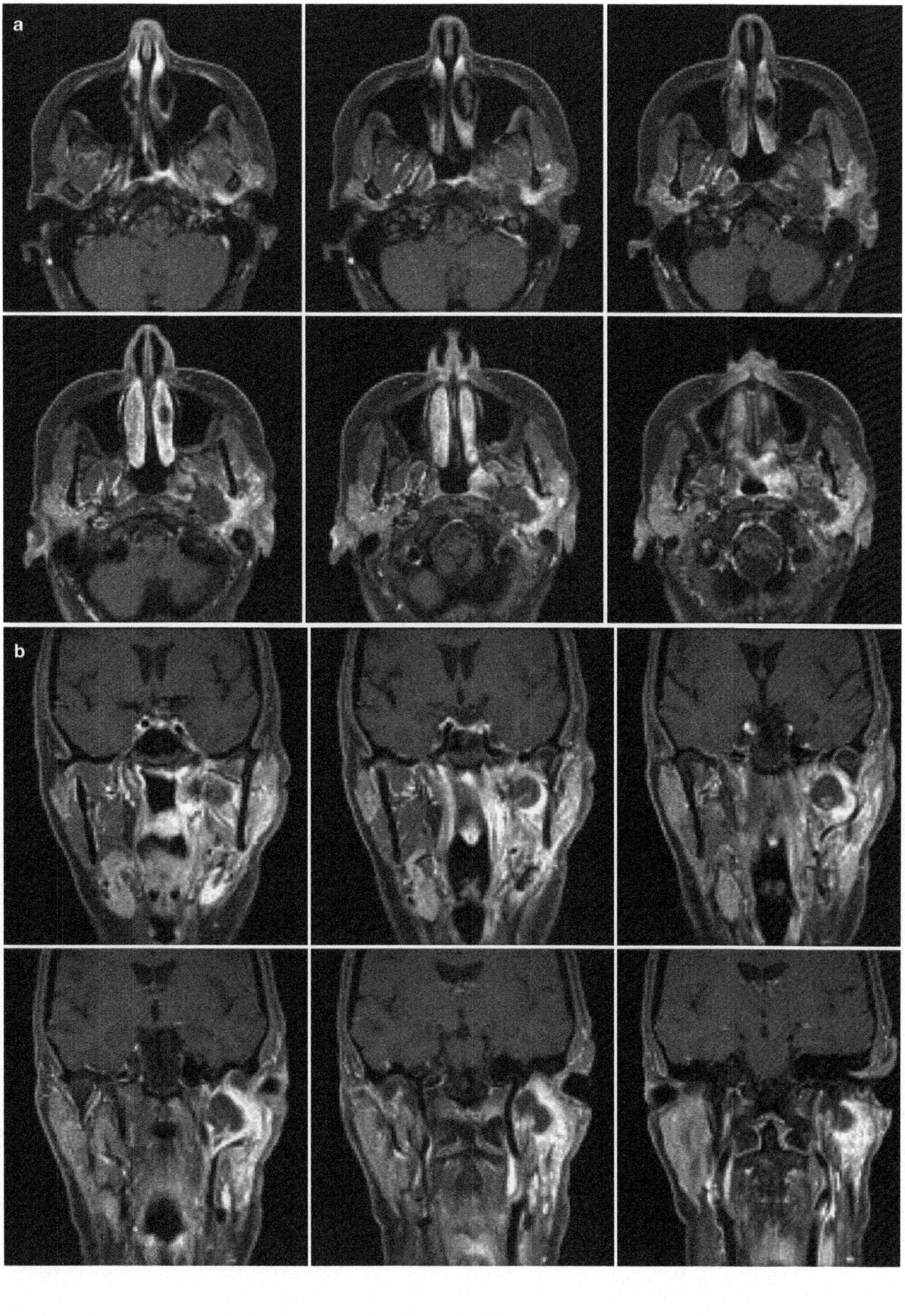
a
b

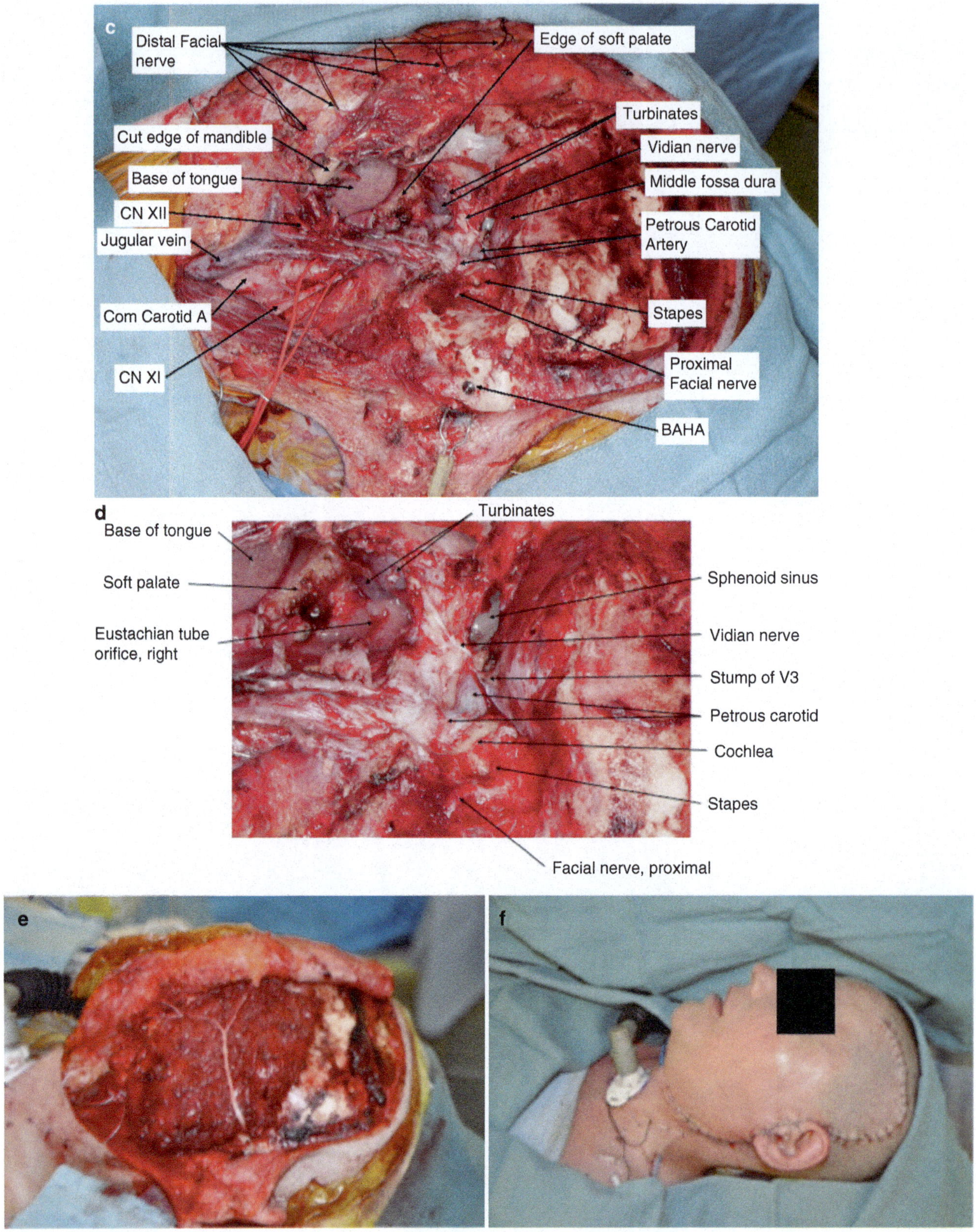

Fig. 20.12 (continued)

Combined with the transtemporal approach and neck dissection, this exposes the ICA from its origin at the carotid bifurcation to its entry into the cavernous sinus. The artery can be ligated and removed if ICA resection is intended.

The mandibular nerve is often involved by tumor and is divided intracranially. Frozen section guides the degree of nerve resection necessary. The maxillary nerve, with its anterior location and trajectory, is less commonly involved and is typically left intact. With the mandibular nerve divided, the plane between the contents of the ITF and the lateral wall of the nasopharynx can be accessed; and the tumor elevated laterally and removed.

This exposure then allows access to the lateral nasopharynx, soft palate, and oropharynx. The pterygoid plates can be removed with drill and rongeurs.

If tumor infiltrates the dura, it can be resected and reconstructed with a dural graft. Care is taken to create a watertight closure; however, dural repair becomes more difficult as the defect widens medially, i.e., over the petrous ridge. Here, the dura over the petrous ridge is thinner, and access is limited to permit suturing a dural graft. Inlay and onlay grafts are used and are reinforced with soft tissue flaps. Great care needs to be exercised if the intradural dissection extends posteriorly in order not to injure the vein of Labbe. Involvement of the vein of Labbe may require leaving residual disease since loss of the vein can result in hemorrhagic venous infarction of the temporal lobe.

If required, the bone of the jugular foramen can be drilled away to examine the contents of the foramen. Intraluminal packing can be used if resection of the jugular is required. The lateral wall of the jugular bulb can be removed, and the lower cranial nerves preserved.

Tracheostomy

The decision to perform tracheostomy is elective. If the mucosal surfaces are not violated, then tracheostomy is generally not required. In patients with upper aerodigestive tract mucosal resection, then tracheostomy is temporarily required.

Reconstruction

For tumors that lie deep to the temporalis muscle, the muscle is preserved, and it is rotated back into its anatomic position. The zygomatic arch is rigidly fixated, and soft tissues are closed in a layered fashion.

However, with tumors that involve the temporalis muscle and especially those that involve the skin, microvascular free flap reconstruction is required. In the MD Anderson series, 40 patients (88.9%) required microvascular free flap reconstruction. While much of the facial skin might remain, this surgery generally leaves a large soft tissue defect when the temporalis muscle, mandible, and zygoma are removed Microvascular free tissue transfer allows sufficient soft tissue to be placed into the defect to separate the dura and intracranial compartment from the upper aerodigestive tract and to help recreate normal facial contours (Fig. 20.12).

Postoperative Management

Patients whose resection extends intracranially are monitored closely in an intensive care unit for the first 24 h. Other patients are followed closely on the head and neck unit, with flap monitoring being performed hourly for the first 4 days.

These patients can develop a number of postoperative complications. Since facial nerve sacrifice is common for this group of patients, eye care and rehabilitation are primary concerns.

Early postoperative mobilization is important to minimize the chance of deep venous thrombosis and pulmonary embolus.

Donor site hematomas (3), wound infection (3), and CSF leak (4) were the main problems encountered in the MD Anderson series. There were no flap failures.

The use of microvascular flaps helps to minimize complications related to CSF leak and wound breakdown. Temporalis muscle flaps are usually inadequate to close these defects. This muscle is prone to necrosis due to devascularization [20]. Complication rates reported in the literature range from 24 to 64% [11, 20, 21].

Morbidity of ITF approaches includes facial nerve dysfunction, facial numbness, tongue and palatal numbness, hearing loss, Eustachian tube dysfunction, trismus, dental malocclusion, and cosmetic deformity [12, 14].

Mortality in ITF approach has been reported and is usually related to cerebrovascular accident following carotid artery sacrifice without preoperative carotid artery balloon occlusion or myocardial infarction [9, 20, 21]. The MD Anderson series did not include any perioperative deaths. The use of extracranial-intracranial bypass has been used in situations requiring carotid artery bypass, but the outcome has been relatively poor [24].

Adjuvant Therapy

Given that these tumors demonstrate aggressive features (perineural disease, lymph node metastases, bone and soft tissue invasion, and dural invasion), adjuvant therapy is indicated. Radiotherapy is the primary adjuvant therapy given. Typical dose is 60 Gy. In the MD Anderson series, postoperative radiotherapy was given in 32 (71.1%) patients. Re-irradiation was given in four patients, who had recurred after previous radiation.

Chemotherapy was given to 19 patients (42%); treatment was preoperative in 7, postoperative in 5, and pre- and postoperative in 7. A number of different protocols were used based on the underlying tumor histology.

Conclusion

The transtemporal infratemporal fossa approach can be applied to many different malignant tumor types. Patients are carefully evaluated and selected for this type of surgery. A multidisciplinary team approach is used for these procedures. The indications and preoperative evaluation are explained. The transtemporal-infratemporal fossa approach is illustrated and described. Wide exposure of the carotid artery is gained through this approach. Postoperative management and complications are mentioned. Adjuvant radiotherapy is indicated for most patients. Chemotherapy has a role in either the pre- or postoperative setting.

References

1. Woodford R, Chaudhary N, Wolf A, Lownie S, Armstrong JE. A modified retromaxillary approach to the infratemporal fossa: three case studies. J Oral Maxillofac Surg. 2015;73(4):769–80.
2. Conley JJ. The surgical approach to the pterygoid area. Ann Surg. 1956;144(1):39.
3. Barbosa JF. Surgery of extensive cancer of paranasal sinuses: presentation of a new technique. Arch Otolaryngol. 1961;73(2):129–38.
4. Honeybul S, Evans B, Lang D. The transzygomatic approach: an anatomical study. Br J Oral Maxillofac Surg. 1997;35(5):334–40.
5. Fisch U. Infratemporal fossa approach to tumours of the temporal bone and base of the skull. J Laryngol Otol. 1978;92(11):949–67.
6. Fisch U. Infratemporal fossa approach for glomus tumors of the temporal bone. Ann Otol Rhinol Laryngol. 1982;91(5):474–9.
7. Fisch U. The infratemporal fossa approach for nasopharyngeal tumors. Laryngoscope. 1983;93(1):36–44.
8. Wetmore SJ, Suen JY, Snyderman NL. Preauricular approach to infratemporal fossa. Head Neck Surg. 1986;9(2):93–103.
9. Sekhar LN, Schramm VL Jr, Jones NF. Subtemporal-preauricular infratemporal fossa approach to large lateral and posterior cranial base neoplasms. J Neurosurg. 1987;67(4):488–99.
10. Leonetti JP, Benscoter BJ, Marzo SJ, Borrowdale RW, Pontikis GC. Preauricular infratemporal fossa approach for advanced malignant parotid tumors. Laryngoscope. 2012;122(9):1949–53.
11. Mansour OI, Carrau RL, Snyderman CH, Kassam AB, Brackmann DE. Preauricular infratemporal fossa surgical approach: modifications of the technique and surgical indications. Skull Base. 2004;14(03):143–51.
12. Haidar H, Deveze A, Lavieille JP. Mini-invasive surgery of infratemporal fossa schwannomas. J Laryngol Otol. 2015;129(2):187–93.
13. Nakaya M, Kida W, Ito A, Yoshihara S, Fuchigami T. Endoscopic transoral and transmaxillary excision of the infratemporal fossa hemangioma. Auris Nasus Larynx. 2015;42(3):258–62.
14. Taylor RJ, Patel MR, Wheless SA, McKinney KA, Stadler ME, Sasaki-Adams D, et al. Endoscopic endonasal approaches to infratemporal fossa tumors: a classification system and case series. Laryngoscope. 2014;124(11):2443–50.
15. Battaglia P, Turri-Zanoni M, Dallan I, Gallo S, Sica E, Padoan G, et al. Endoscopic endonasal transpterygoid transmaxillary approach to the infratemporal and upper parapharyngeal tumors. Otolaryngol Head Neck Surg. 2014;150(4):696–702.
16. Xu F, Sun X, Hu L, Wang J, Wang D, Pasic TR, et al. Endoscopic surgical treatment of neurogenic tumor in pterygopalatine and infratemporal fossae via extended medial maxillectomy. Acta Otolaryngol. 2011;131(2):161–5.
17. Gold SR, Kamerer DB Jr. Preservation of conductive hearing in approaches to tumors of the jugular foramen. Otol Neurotol. 2006;27(8):1126–30.
18. Günther R, Süss W, Kuffner H, Meinig G, editors. Ballonokklusionstest vor Karotisligatur. RöFo-Fortschritte auf dem Gebiet der Röntgenstrahlen und der bildgebenden Verfahren. Stuttgart· New York: © Georg Thieme Verlag; 1981.
19. Fisch U, Fagan P, Valavanis A. The infratemporal fossa approach for the lateral skull base. Otolaryngol Clin North Am. 1984;17(3):513–52.
20. Bigelow DC, Smith PG, Leonetti JP, Backer RL, Grubb RL, Kotapka MJ. Treatment of malignant neoplasms of the lateral cranial base with the combined frontotemporal-anterolateral approach: five-year follow-up. Otolaryngol Head Neck Surg. 1999;120(1):17–24.
21. Bilsky MH, Bentz B, Vitaz T, Shah J, Kraus D. Craniofacial resection for cranial base malignancies involving the infratemporal fossa. Neurosurgery. 2005;57(4 Suppl):339.
22. Guo R, Guo YX, Feng Z, Guo CB. Application of a computer-aided navigation technique in surgery for recurrent malignant infratemporal fossa tumors. J Craniofac Surg. 2015;26(2):e126–32.
23. Cunningham CD 3rd, Friedman RA, Brackmann DE, Hitselberger WE, Lin HW. Neurotologic skull base surgery in pediatric patients. Otol Neurotol. 2005;26(2):231–6.
24. Feiz-Erfan I, Han PP, Spetzler RF, Lanzino G, Ferreira MA, Gonzalez LF, et al. Salvage of advanced squamous cell carcinomas of the head and neck: internal carotid artery sacrifice and extracranial-intracranial revascularization. Neurosurg Focus. 2003;14(3):1–5.

Middle Fossa Craniotomy

21

Paul W. Gidley and Franco DeMonte

Introduction

The middle fossa approach is an avenue of approach to treat many different benign tumors that primarily involve the anterior and superior petrous bone, including vestibular schwannomas, trigeminal neuromas, meningiomas, epidermoid cysts, and chordomas. The middle cranial fossa approach has been used as a means for facial nerve decompression and vestibular nerve section while preserving hearing. Very little has been written about this approach for managing malignant tumors of the middle fossa. This chapter will deal with the anatomy, clinical evaluation, and operative management of patients with malignant tumors in the middle fossa.

The middle fossa approach was popularized by Dr. William House in the 1960s. His original work described this approach for deciding if a patient had an early internal auditory canal tumor or Meniere's disease [1]. In the days prior to modern cross-sectional imaging, this decision must have been quite difficult. The middle fossa approach allowed the opportunity to remove a small tumor, if present, or to do a vestibular nerve section. This surgical approach depended on the prior development of the surgical microscope and diamond drill bits.

Dr. House then reported the usefulness of this approach for facial nerve disorders, reporting three cases operated on through the middle fossa [2]. Later that same year, he reported the results of the middle fossa approach in 50 patients with acoustic neuroma, facial nerve disorders, or Meniere's disease for vestibular nerve section.

House's approach to the IAC was expanded upon by others, most notably Michael Glasscock and Takeshi Kawase. Glasscock used the middle fossa approach to expose the Eustachian tube for tuboplasty in cases of bony or fibrous closure of the osseous segment of the tube. The landmarks for this surgical exposure, described below, carry the moniker of Glasscock's triangle. Kawase, a neurosurgeon, described the removal of the petrous apex, anterior to the IAC and medial to the ICA (Kawase's triangle or quadrangle) to pursue resection of sphenopetroclival meningiomas.

While these benign conditions remain the most common indication for these procedures, malignant tumors do occur within the middle fossa, and surgical access to these lesions usually requires extensions of House's focused middle fossa approach to the IAC.

P. W. Gidley, M.D., F.A.C.S. (✉)
Department of Head and Neck Surgery, The University of Texas
M.D. Anderson Cancer Center, Houston, TX, USA
e-mail: pwgidley@mdanderson.org

F. DeMonte, M.D.
Department of Neurosurgery, The University of Texas
M.D. Anderson Cancer Center, Houston, TX, USA
e-mail: fdemonte@mdanderson.org

Anatomy

The middle cranial fossa has a roughly ovoid shape, being bound anteriorly by the greater sphenoid wing, laterally by the squamosal portion of the temporal bone, posteriorly by the posterior petrous ridge, and medially by the basisphenoid. The temporal lobe is contained within its space. It is covered by dura, which becomes thinner and harder to elevate in patients over the age of 65 years. The middle fossa measures roughly 5.5 cm in anterior–posterior dimension and 4 cm in medial–lateral dimension. A number of important structures, foramina, nerves, and blood vessels are contained within or related to this small space (Fig. 21.1).

The bone of the middle fossa has variable thickness. The bone can be very thin over the middle ear and mastoid air cells, and dehiscences or frank herniation of dura into the mastoid and middle ear are encountered in clinical practice. The middle fossa has a highly variable topography. The arcuate eminence is generally identifiable by noting its dense, white bone compared to the thinner, darker bone of the mastoid air cell system posteriorly. The arcuate eminence marks the site of the superior semicircular canal. The canal is consistently oriented perpendicular to the petrous ridge.

P. W. Gidley, F. DeMonte (eds.), *Temporal Bone Cancer*, https://doi.org/10.1007/978-3-319-74539-8_21

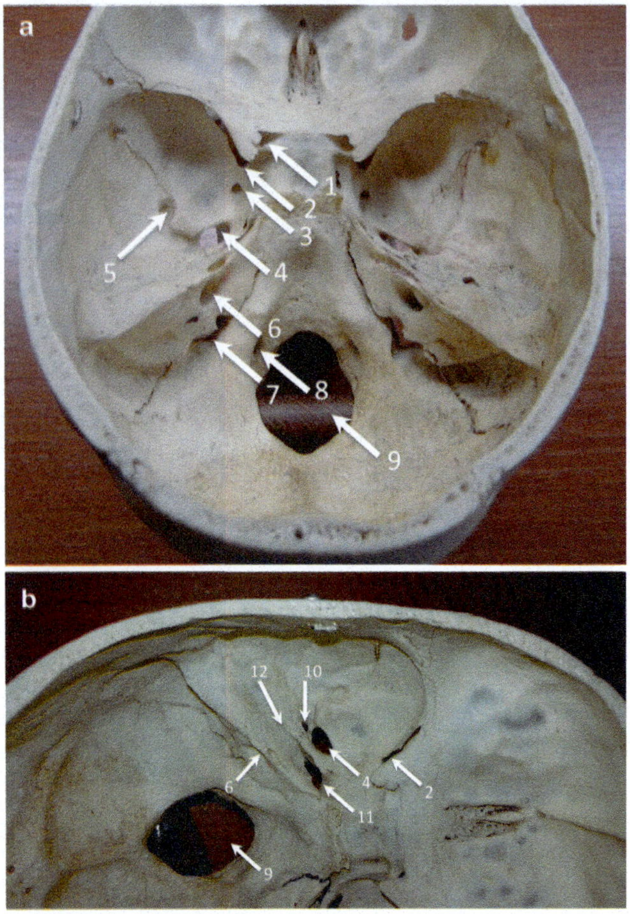

Fig. 21.1 Foramina of the middle fossa. (**a**) Skull arranged anatomically. (**b**) Detail of left middle fossa, placed in surgical position. Key: 1. optic canal, 2. superior orbital fissure, 3. foramen rotundum, 4. foramen ovale, 5. groove for middle meningeal artery, 6. internal auditory canal, 7. jugular foramen, 8. hypoglossal foramen, 9. foramen magnum, 10. foramen spinosum, 11. foramen lacerum, 12. hiatus for greater superficial petrosal nerve (GSPN)

The petrous apex is a pyramidal-shaped portion of the temporal bone. The cochlea and bony labyrinth are contained within the dense bone of the petrous apex. Aeration of the petrous apex is variable, with one-third of specimens containing some petrous apex air cells. Infection and coalescence of these air cells (petrous apicitis or Gradenigo's syndrome) can produce swelling and nerve conduction block in the abducens nerve, clinically causing abducens palsy and diplopia.

The greater superficial petrosal nerve (GSPN) emerges from a small bony hiatus just anterior to the location of the geniculate ganglion. The geniculate ganglion, a sensory ganglion of the facial nerve, is variably covered by bone, and care is necessary to avoid causing damage to the facial nerve when elevating the middle fossa dura. The GSPN carries preganglionic parasympathetic fibers and travels anteromedially along the carotid artery to meet up with postganglionic sympathetic fibers from the carotid plexus to form the nerve of the Vidian canal. These nerve fibers join up with the maxillary nerve, and the parasympathetic fibers join their postganglionic counterparts in the sphenopalatine ganglion. These autonomic nervous system fibers are sent to the lacrimal glands and nasal mucosa.

The trigeminal nerve (CN V) lies in depression at the medial aspect of the middle fossa at the petrous apex. The abducens nerve (CN VI) travels below and medial to the trigeminal nerve and at the level of the inferior petrosal sinus passes through the membranous Dorello's canal to reach the cavernous sinus.

A number of foramina perforate the floor of the middle fossa and its boundaries. The foramen spinosum admits the middle meningeal artery, one of the many foraminal branches of the internal maxillary artery. Its anterior branch is marked externally by the pterion, at the junction of the squamosal, sphenoid, and frontal bones. The mandibular branch of the trigeminal nerve passes through the large foramen ovale, a prominent foramen in the middle fossa floor. The petrous portion of the carotid artery overlays the foramen lacerum which inferiorly is bounded by cartilage. Following along the carotid artery are the branches of the sympathetic plexus. These sympathetic branches join up with the greater superficial petrosal nerve (GSPN) to form the nerve of the Vidian canal. This canal is at the most medial extent of the middle fossa. The foramen rotundum is located medial and anterior to the foramen ovale, and it allows the maxillary branch of the trigeminal nerve to pass into the pterygopalatine fossa.

A number of venous structures have important relationships to the middle fossa. The sigmoid sinus is found at the posterior lateral edge of the middle fossa floor. The superior petrosal sinus is found along the posterior petrous ridge. The inferior petrosal sinus runs along the petroclival synchondrosis and enters the cavernous sinus which is located at the anteromedial limit of the middle fossa.

The internal auditory canal is a foramen within the posterior cranial fossa. It transmits the cochlear-vestibular nerve and facial nerve to the temporal bone.

A number of "triangles" have been described within the middle fossa. Glasscock's triangle is marked by the mandibular nerve (CNV3), the GSPN, and a line from the foramen spinosum to the arcuate eminence. This triangle contains the Eustachian tube with the overlying tensor tympani muscle laterally and the anterolateral portion of the horizontal carotid canal and the horizontal petrous internal carotid artery. It forms the roof of the infratemporal fossa. Kawase's "triangle" is marked by the mandibular nerve (CNV3), the GSPN, the arcuate eminence, and the superior petrosal sinus [3]. It contains the petrous apex and the posteromedial carotid canal and horizontal IAC. The internal auditory canal is at its posterior edge. Kawase's "triangle" is an important access point for the superior anterolateral posterior fossa.

Clinical Evaluation

Given the complex and dense concentration of anatomic structures within the middle fossa, careful cranial nerve examination is required when evaluating these patients. Tumors in the petrous apex often present with multiple cranial nerve deficits, especially of CNs V and VI and occasionally of CNs VII and VIII.

Generally, the external ear and ear canal are normal, although pathology that destroys the middle fossa floor and enters the middle ear can been seen through an intact TM (Fig. 21.2).

Most approaches to the middle fossa are extradural. Given that the dura becomes more adherent and thinner with age, patients over the age of 65 years are generally not considered ideal candidates for middle fossa approaches.

Diagnostic Imaging

Cross-sectional imaging is essential in evaluating tumors that affect the petrous apex and middle fossa. Both CT and MRI provide useful information for surgical planning (Fig. 21.3).

Operative Preparation

Patients are positioned supine on the operative table. After general anesthesia is induced, the patient is endotracheally intubated, with the tube taped to the contralateral corner of the mouth. Long-term paralytic agents are not used so that facial nerve monitoring can be performed accurately.

An arterial line is placed and a Foley catheter is placed in the bladder. Continuous monitoring of end-tidal CO_2, oxygen saturation, and intra-arterial blood pressures is performed throughout the procedure. The legs are placed in anti-thromboembolic hose and sequential compression devices to prevent deep vein thrombosis. The patient is appropriately padded and strapped to the operative table, and it is turned 90° to the anesthesia stand. The patient is hyperventilated to an arterial CO_2 of 28, and mannitol may occasionally be used to optimize brain relaxation.

The head is placed in a Mayfield head holder, and the head is turned to the opposite side as dictated by the trajectory of approach to the tumor. For the extended middle fossa approach, the head is typically rotated approximately 60° and the vertex tipped slightly down toward the floor. If the neck is not supple to allow this rotation, then the patient can be positioned laterally. Once the head is secured, the stereotactic system is registered to a preoperatively acquired imaging database to allow for continuous frameless stereotactic navigation using both CT and MRI imaging. This system is used to optimize the trajectory to the tumor and to help "right size" the incision and craniotomy.

Electrodes for facial nerve and auditory brainstem response (ABR) monitoring are placed. Communication with the anesthesiologist must be clear from the outset that long-lasting paralytics should be avoided so that the facial nerve can be monitored.

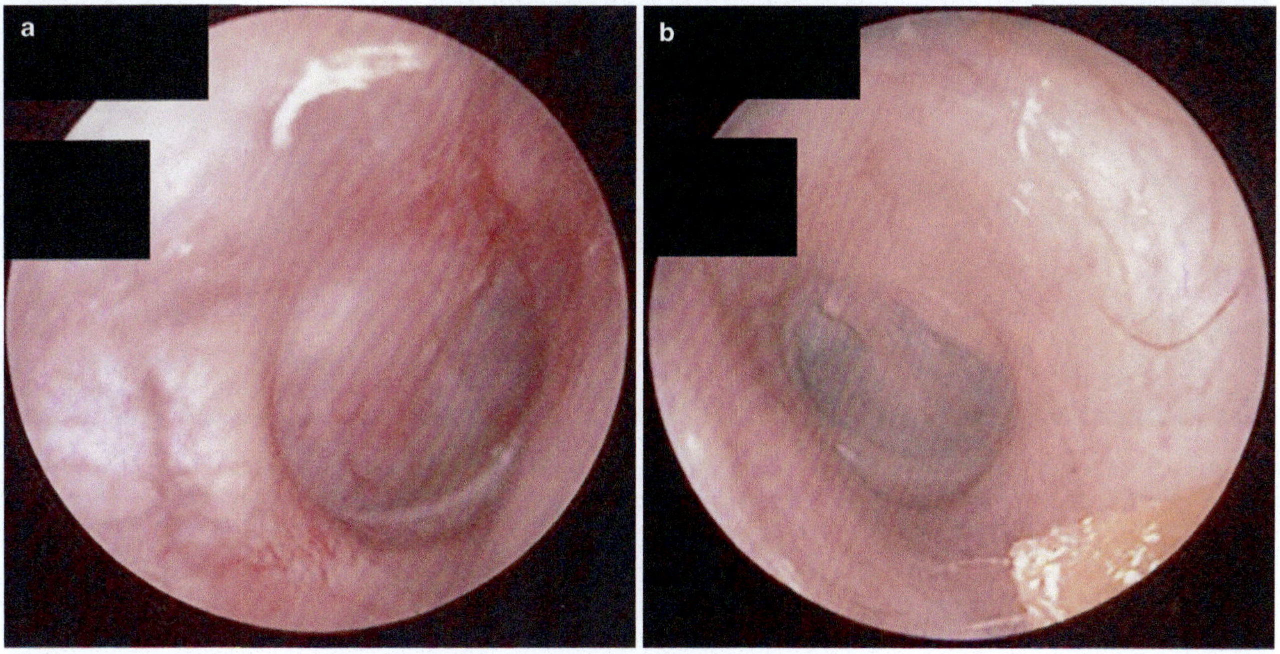

Fig. 21.2 Meningioma eroding middle fossa into the right middle ear. (**a**) Right ear, (**b**) left ear

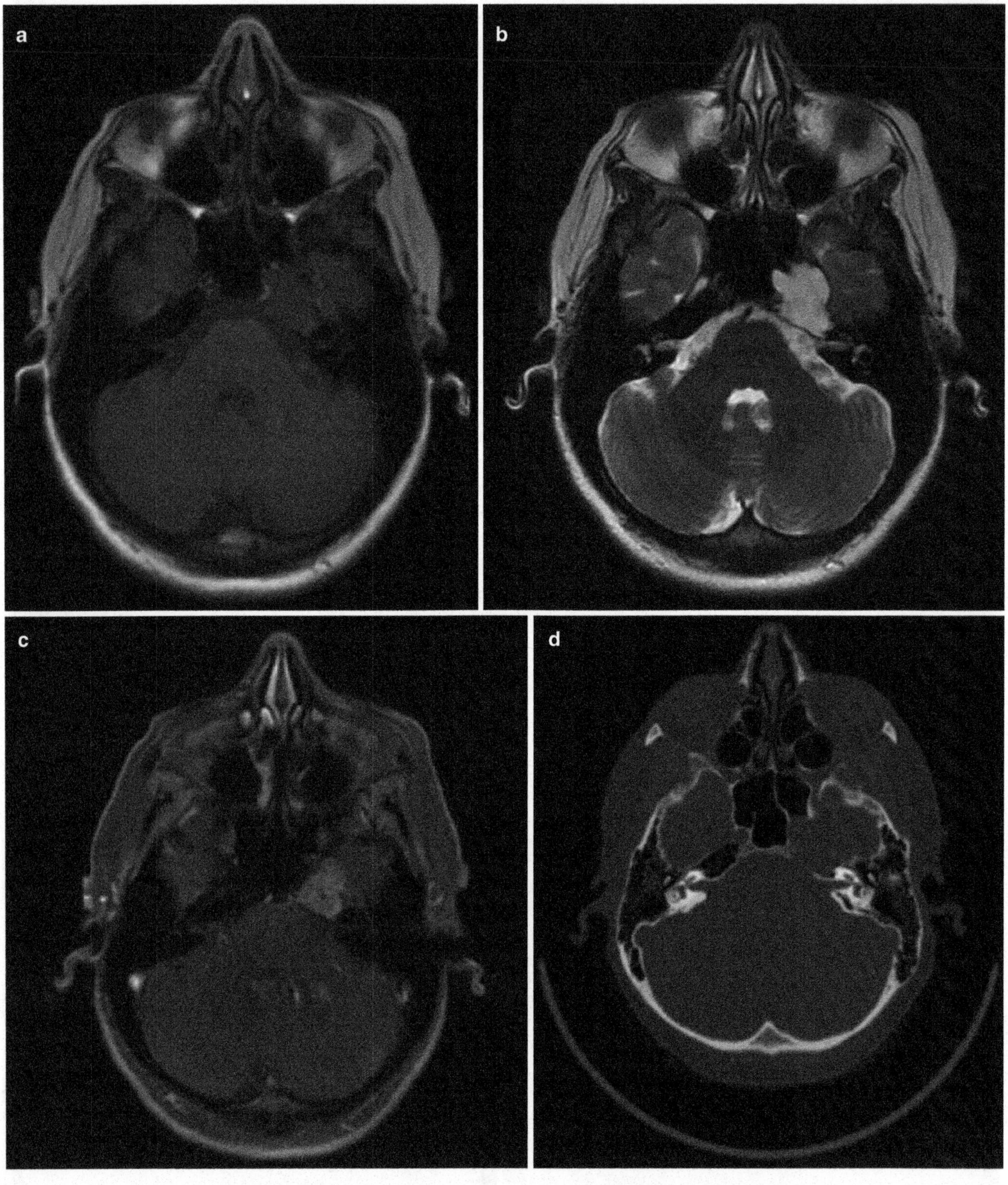

Fig. 21.3 Chondrosarcoma of the left petrous apex in a 38-year-old woman who presented with left abducens palsy. (**a**) Axial T1 non-contrast, the lesion is isointense with the brain. (**b**) Axial T2, non-contrast, the lesion is hyperintense to the brain and isointense to cerebrospinal fluid. (**c**) Axial T1 with contrast and fat suppression, the lesion is mildly enhancing with contrast. (**d**) Axial, non-contrast CT, the lesion fills petrous apex air cell but has not eroded the cochlea or internal auditory canal

Operative Procedure

A variety of incisions have been described. For small intracanalicular acoustic neuromas, an incision that follows along the temporal hairline and creates a 5-cm-wide posteriorly based skin flap is used (Fig. 21.4). An anteriorly based temporalis muscle flap is used, and the overlapping nature of soft tissues aids in closure and prevention of CSF leak. This focal approach to the IAC rarely offers enough exposure to appropriately manage malignancies which often require removal of the petrous apex.

For an extended middle fossa approach, a larger incision is required. The incision begins in the preauricular crease and extends superiorly over the parietal scalp and extended anteriorly toward the frontal scalp. Dissecting in the immediate subgaleal plane, the scalp flap is reflected anteriorly. Incisions are made in both superficial and deep layers of the temporalis fascia, approximately 1–1½ cm above the keyhole region from the superior temporal line down to the root of the zygoma.

Dissecting subfascially, in order to minimize injury to the branches of the facial nerve, the entire zygomatic arch is exposed. In patients with a high-riding arch and a bulky temporalis muscle or when the tumor extends superiorly, the zygomatic arch is divided in a wedge-shaped fashion using the reciprocating saws both anteriorly and posteriorly. The arch is left attached to the masseter and reflected inferiorly. The temporalis muscle is then elevated off the calvarium and reflected inferiorly. The soft tissues are held with self-retaining fishhook retractors (Fig. 21.5).

The navigational computer is utilized to optimize the size and position of the craniotomy. Then using a high-speed drill, an entry hole is placed in the keyhole region, entering both the anterior cranial fossa and the orbit. A second entry hole is placed just above the root of the zygoma and a third halfway between these two but remaining below the superior temporal line. The lateral greater sphenoid wing is removed, and the bone flap is elevated and set aside (Fig. 21.6).

Then using high-speed drill and rongeurs, the entire greater sphenoid wing is removed to expose the superior orbital fissure. Inferiorly, the foramen rotundum is opened and the maxillary nerve is exposed fully. Bone removal is taken down to the maxillary strut. The dura is carefully elevated, and the squamosal portion of the temporal bone is removed to make it flush with the floor of the middle cranial fossa. Any air cells that are encountered are sealed with bone wax.

Under the operative microscope, the dura is elevated off the middle cranial fossa from a posterior to anterior direction, identifying the posterior petrous ridge, the arcuate eminence, the greater superficial petrosal nerve, and the middle meningeal artery (Fig. 21.7). A self-retaining retractor is used to gently support the temporal lobe off the middle fossa floor.

The middle meningeal artery is coagulated and divided to permit visualization of the medial and anterior extent of the middle cranial fossa. The dura over the mandibular nerve is sharply incised in order to access the cleavage plane between the nerve and the medial temporal dura. Once this dissection plane is entered, blunt dissection with a dural elevator further separates the medial temporal dura from the mandibular and maxillary nerves and the Gasserian ganglion. Further sharp division of the dura posterior to the mandibular nerve allows exposure of the portion of the trigeminal root in Meckel's cave posterior to the ganglion. These maneuvers allow mobilization of the mandibular nerve, Gasserian ganglion, and trigeminal root anteriorly and give full access to the petrous apex. The meningo-orbital dural band can be divided, if

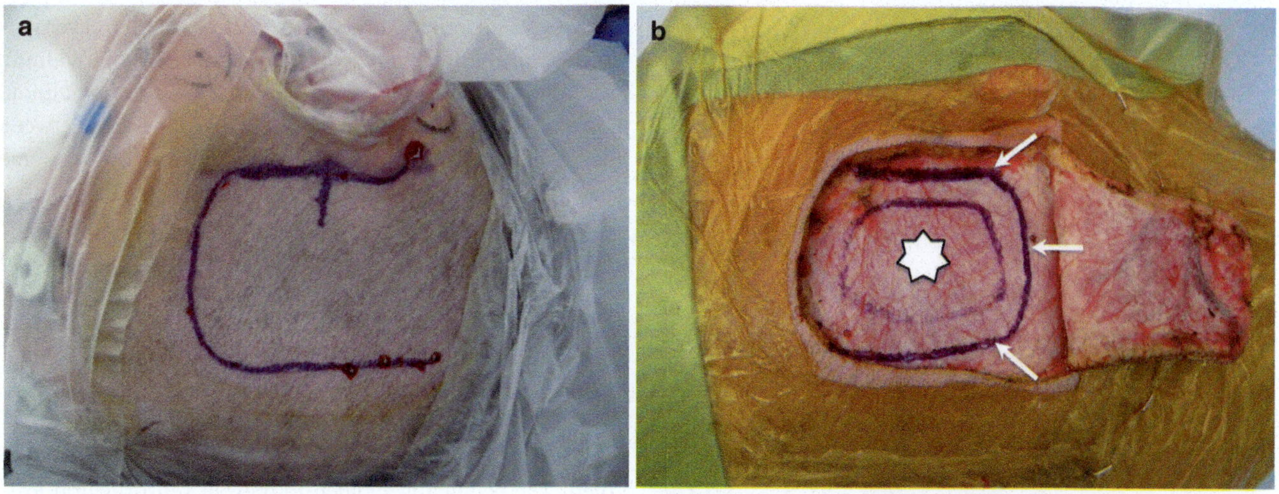

Fig. 21.4 Incision planned for middle fossa craniotomy for right acoustic neuroma. (**a**) Skin incision is marked. (**b**) Posteriorly based skin flap raised and anteriorly based temporalis muscle flap marked (arrows). Inner circle marks temporalis fascia to be harvested as a graft (star)

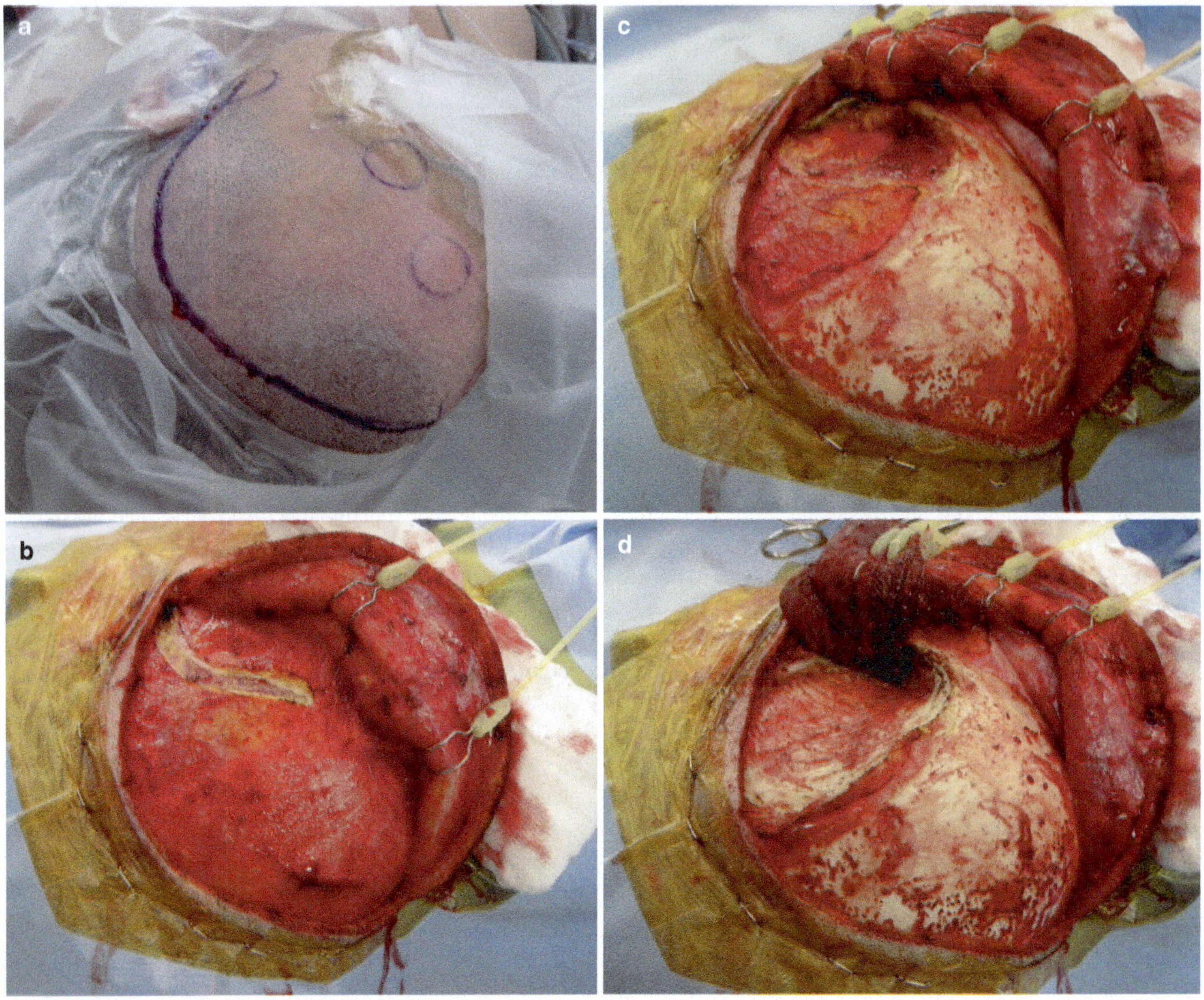

Fig. 21.5 Incision planned for left extended middle fossa. (**a**) Incision marked. (**b**) Skin flap turned and temporalis flap incised. (**c**) Periosteum elevated. (**d**) Zygoma divided and temporalis muscle elevated

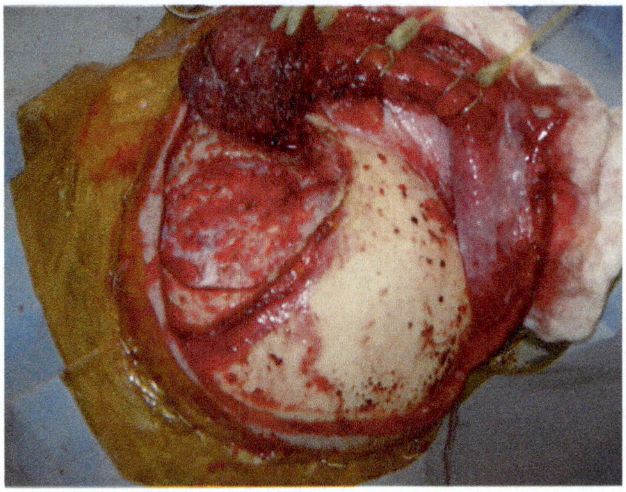

Fig. 21.6 Bone flap removed and temporal dura exposed

necessary; and the extradural dissection of the cavernous sinus can continue anteriorly to expose the ophthalmic, trochlear, and oculomotor nerves and the anterior clinoid process (Fig. 21.8). Occasionally tumor can be seen between the divisions of the trigeminal nerve, allowing for some space to remove part of the tumor anteriorly.

Stay sutures can be used to maintain elevation of the medial temporal dura. The middle fossa floor is exposed completely, permitting tumor removal (Fig. 21.9).

Bone from the middle fossa floor is removed to identify the internal auditory canal. The arcuate eminence is blue-lined, marking the site of the superior semicircular canal. Bone anterior and medial to this landmark can be safely removed until the dura of the internal auditory canal is identified. The cochlea is avoided to prevent sensorineural loss. The carotid canal is then skeletonized. The GSPN is the landmark for the carotid canal. The bone medial to the

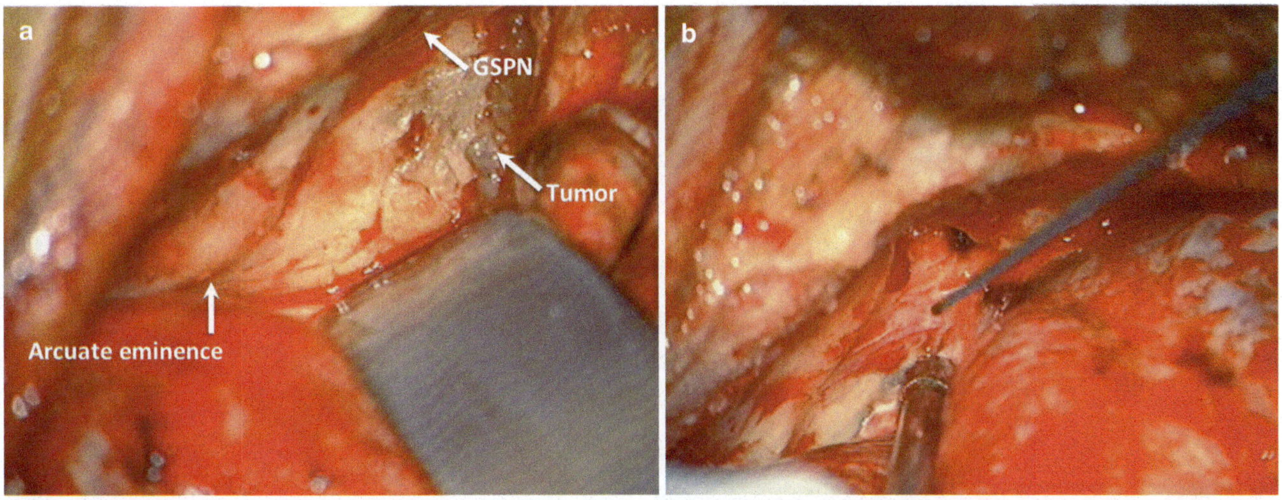

Fig. 21.7 Elevating middle fossa dura. (**a**) Dura is elevated off the middle fossa floor in a posterior to anterior direction identifying the arcuate eminence and the greater superficial petrosal nerve (GSPN). (**b**) GSPN is identified and stimulated with a Prass probe

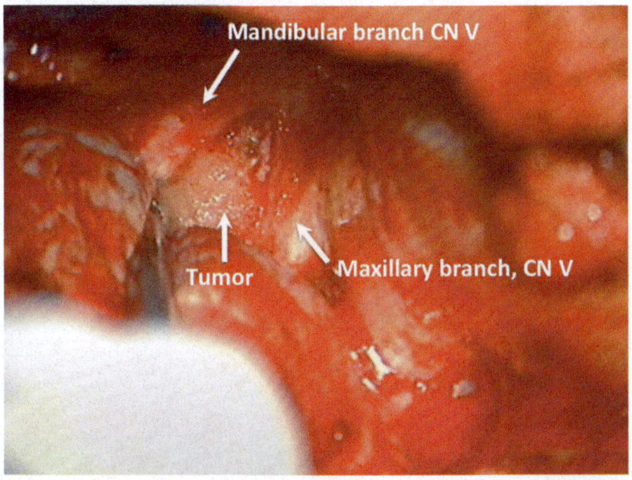

Fig. 21.8 Tumor identified between the maxillary and ophthalmic divisions of the trigeminal nerve

horizontal petrous carotid artery and posterior to the trigeminal ganglion is gradually drilled down with a diamond burr. The drilling encompasses a quadrangular area with the petrous ridge posteriorly, the trigeminal root superiorly, the trigeminal ganglion anteriorly, and the horizontal petrous ICA laterally. The dura in front of the brain stem is thus exposed down to the inferior petrosal sinus. Care must be taken at this point as the abducens nerve traverses the inferior petrosal sinus on its way to the cavernous sinus. The horizontal internal carotid artery is identified throughout its intratemporal course from its posterior genu to its precavernous segment as it turns upward deep to the mandibular nerve.

Chondrosarcomas and chordomas are primarily extradural tumors and are typically encountered by the time the petrous apex is being drilled. During tumor removal, the carotid artery is carefully protected, while surrounding diseased bone is drilled away. For these extradural tumors, the posterior fossa dura anterior to the brainstem and the dura inferior to the trigeminal ganglion and root are usually the limits of resection (Fig. 21.10).

If the tumor extends intradurally, the subtemporal dura is incised posteriorly along and above the superior petrosal sinus. The exposed posterior fossa dura anterolateral to the brainstem is incised below the superior petrosal sinus, and the sinus is thoroughly coagulated and divided. The temporal lobe is elevated, and the tentorium cerebelli is divided through to the incisura. The prepontine dura is excised down to the limits of the bony exposure (inferior petrosal sinus) to expose the caudal extent of the tumor. The tumor is progressively debulked and then dissected free from the surrounding cranial nerves (trochlear and trigeminal), vascular structures (anterior inferior and superior cerebellar arteries), and the brainstem.

Hemostasis is carefully achieved with bipolar cautery and gentle tamponade with Surgifoam. Air cells are completely occluded with bone wax. Use of a 30-degree endoscope may be useful to assess for hidden open air cells. A free fat graft can be used to obturate the dural opening into the posterior fossa. A free temporalis fascial graft is used to cover over the middle and posterior fossae to separate the middle fossa dura from the tissues in the orbit, the floor of the middle cranial fossa, and the trigeminal nerve system. The craniotomy bone flap is replaced in its anatomic position and rigidly fixated with titanium plates and screws. A pterional implant can be used to reconstruct the contour of the removed greater sphenoid wing, and titanium mesh can be used to reconstruct the squamous portion of the temporal bone. The temporalis muscle is returned to its anatomic position and sutured to the cuff of temporalis fascia. If needed, the temporalis muscle can be split sagittally and

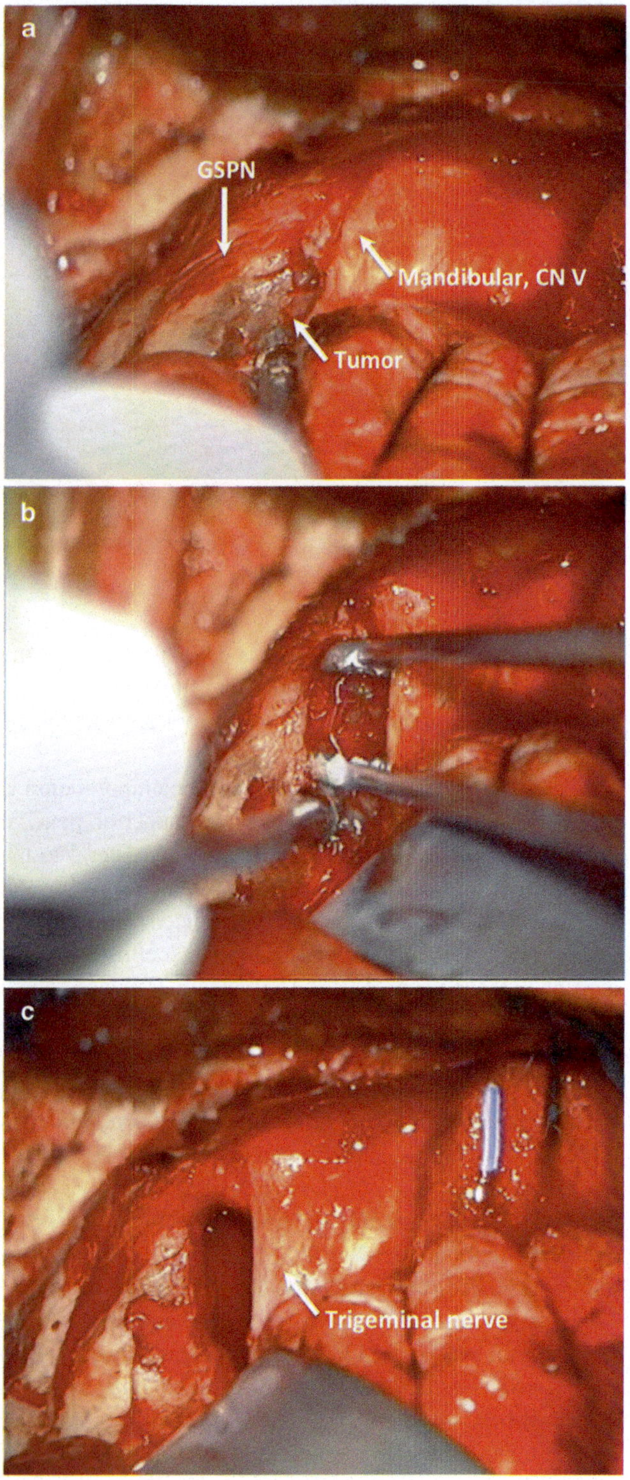

Fig. 21.9 Tumor removal. (**a**) Tumor in the petrous apex. (**b**) Tumor removal with forceps. (**c**) Trigeminal nerve exposed

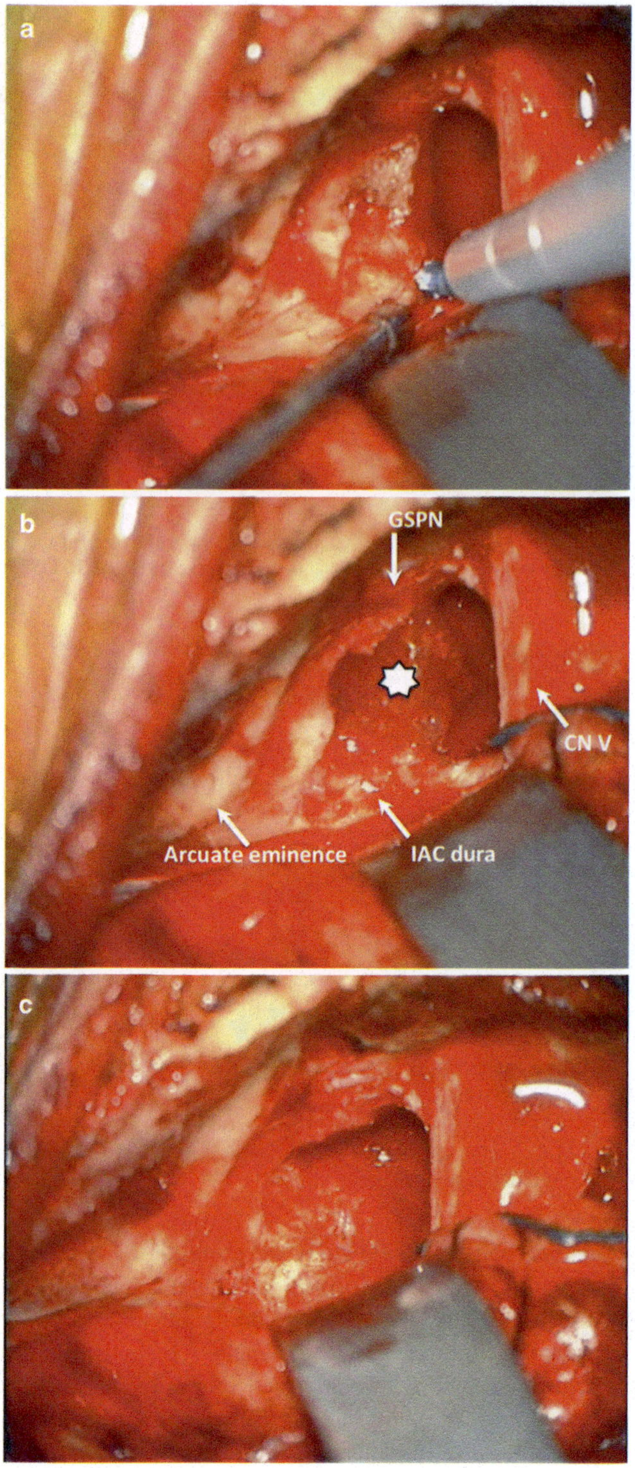

Fig. 21.10 Petrous apex exposure. (**a**) Bone of the petrous apex is removed. (**b**) Tumor (star) along the carotid canal is identified and removed. (**c**) Tumor removal complete

the inner portion turned down to cover the middle fossa floor with vascularized tissue. The zygomatic arch is placed back into its anatomic position and rigidly fixated with titanium plates and screws. The temporalis fascia is then closed over the zygomatic arch with interrupted sutures. The wound is irrigated with an antibiotic solution, and the scalp is closed in layers. The patient is taken out of the Mayfield head holder, and a mastoid dressing is applied.

Postoperative Management

These patients are observed overnight in an intensive care unit. Vital signs and neurologic function are checked frequently. Any neurological changes warrant urgent CT imaging to rule out postoperative hematoma, ischemia, or hydrocephalus.

Cranial nerve deficits need to be managed appropriately. For chondrosarcomas, cranial nerve deficits generally improve following tumor removal [4]. Cranial nerve V deficits may manifest as facial numbness or the decreased ability to chew on the ipsilateral side. Cranial nerve VI deficits produce diplopia with lateral gaze. Often this deficit will improve with time. Occasionally patients will need prismatic glasses or strabismus surgery to help with the deficit. Close cooperation with an ophthalmologist is recommended for optimal outcomes. Cranial nerve VII deficits are generally avoidable. Intraoperative facial nerve monitoring is essential for these cases. The geniculate ganglion can be dehiscent in the middle fossa, and this anatomic anomaly places the facial nerve at risk. Injury or transection of the GSPN leads to absent tear production, and patients must use daily (if not hourly) eye drops to moisturize the eye. Any facial weakness following middle fossa surgery is managed as Bell's palsy, with steroids (prednisone 1 mg/kg/day for 7 days and then taper over another 7 days) and eye care. If the facial nerve is disrupted in the procedure, facial nerve grafting can be performed using the great auricular nerve as a graft donor [5].

Prevention is the best way to manage CN VIII deficits. Intraoperative ABR monitoring should be done, if the patient has good hearing and a preoperative ABR shows reproducible waveforms. Careful intraoperative attention to sealing air cells not only prevents CSF leak, it also helps to prevent irrigation from getting into the middle ear and causing a conductive hearing loss. If the superior semicircular canal is entered while drilling the arcuate eminence, then the canal is sealed off with bone wax.

Adjuvant Therapy

Postoperative radiotherapy is indicated in patients with subtotal resection. For chondrosarcoma, grade 1 tumors are generally observed for recurrence or regrowth. For higher-grade tumors, postoperative radiotherapy with proton beam is indicated [4, 6].

Conclusion

The middle fossa approach permits access to tumor of the petrous apex, such as chondrosarcomas. A comprehension of the middle fossa anatomy is essential to navigate this approach. Careful, meticulous dissection is used to identify anatomic landmarks in order to prevent unnecessary injury and morbidity. The operative procedure is illustrated and described in detail. Postoperative management and complications are explained. Postoperative radiotherapy is indicated for subtotal resection and grade II and higher chondrosarcomas.

References

1. House WF. Surgical exposure of the internal auditory canal and its contents through the middle, cranial fossa. Laryngoscope. 1961;71:1363–85.
2. House WF. Middle cranial fossa approach to the petrous pyramid. Report of 50 cases. Arch Otolaryngol. 1963;78:460–9.
3. Kawase T, Shiobara R, Toya S. Anterior transpetrosal-transtentorial approach for sphenopetroclival meningiomas: surgical method and results in 10 patients. Neurosurgery. 1991;28(6):869–75. discussion 75–6.
4. Carlson ML, O'Connell BP, Breen JT, Wick CC, Driscoll CL, Haynes DS, et al. Petroclival chondrosarcoma: a multicenter review of 55 cases and new staging system. Otol Neurotol. 2016;37(7):940–50.
5. Gidley PW, Gantz BJ, Rubinstein JT. Facial nerve grafts: from cerebellopontine angle and beyond. Am J Otol. 1999;20(6):781–8.
6. Raza SM, Gidley PW, Meis JM, Grosshans DR, Bell D, DeMonte F. Multimodality treatment of skull base chondrosarcomas: the role of histology specific treatment protocols. Neurosurgery. 2017;81:520–30.

Parotidectomy and Neck Dissection for Temporal Bone Malignancy

22

Steven B. Chinn and Randal S. Weber

Introduction

Temporal bone malignancies have the capacity for aggressive local invasion and the potential for regional and distant metastases. Similarly, primary parotid, parapharyngeal, or cutaneous malignancies may result in temporal bone invasion via local or regional extension. Regardless of the primary location, regional control often requires addressing the lymph node basins in the parotid and neck. The drainage pattern in temporal bone malignancies is dependent on the location of the cancer. Cancers requiring lateral temporal bone resection can originate from the auricle, external auditory canal, periauricular skin, middle ear space, scalp, parotid, and temporal bone. The primary nodal basins typically involve the parotid, level II, and the posterolateral neck. The focus of this chapter will be the management of the parotid and regional nodal basins as they directly or indirectly involve the temporal bone.

Pathology

Knowledge of tumor histology is critical for determining the risk for local and regional spread. Temporal bone malignancies most commonly arise from periauricular skin, salivary (parotid) gland, cutaneous external ear, or the ear canal. Rarely, temporal bone tumors may arise from mesenchymal origins (soft tissue or osseous structures). Other than the parotid malignancies, these are typically cutaneous malignancies secondary to chronic sun exposure. Similar to other areas of the head and neck, squamous cell carcinoma and basal cell carcinoma are the most common. Tumors arising from the parotid parenchyma may directly invade the temporal bone; and conversely tumors arising from the pinna, external canal, and temporal bone can secondarily invade the parotid gland. Depending upon multiple histopathologic factors, these tumors can spread to regional nodal basins. Perineural extension from cutaneous or parotid malignancies can invade the temporal bone via the facial or auriculotemporal nerves. Common salivary gland tumors, adenoid cystic carcinoma, mucoepidermoid carcinoma, and acinic cell carcinomas may secondarily invade the temporal bone. Tumor types seen at MD Anderson are summarized in Table 22.1 [1]. The histology of these neoplasms influences the propensity to secondarily invade the temporal bone and to spread to

Table 22.1 Tumor types in this series of 157 patients [1]

Histologic type	No. of patients	% of patients
Squamous cell carcinoma	61	39.2
Basal cell carcinoma	22	13.9
Adenoid cystic carcinoma	12	7.6
Acinic cell carcinoma	9	5.7
Salivary duct carcinoma	6	3.8
Adenocarcinoma	6	3.8
Melanoma	4	2.5
Mucoepidermoid carcinoma	3	1.9
Chondrosarcoma	3	1.9
Sarcomatoid carcinoma	3	1.9
Basosquamous carcinoma	3	1.9
Pleomorphic sarcoma	3	1.9
Hemangiopericytoma	3	1.9
Mucoepidermoid carcinoma	3	1.9
Basal cell adenocarcinoma	2	1.3
Carcinoma ex pleomorphic	2	1.3
Osteosarcoma	2	1.3
Neuroendocrine carcinoma	2	1.3
Carcinoma, poorly differ	1	0.6
Clivus chordoma	1	0.6
Hidradenocarcinoma	1	0.6
Malignant mixed cancer	1	0.6
Peripheral nerve sheath tumor	1	0.6
Schneiderian carcinoma	1	0.6
Sebaceous cell carcinoma	1	0.6
Spindle cell sarcoma	1	0.6

S. B. Chinn, M.D., M.P.H.
Department of Otolaryngology — Head and Neck Surgery, University of Michigan Health System, Ann Arbor, MI, USA

R. S. Weber, M.D. (✉)
Department of Head and Neck Surgery, The University of Texas M.D. Anderson Cancer Center, Houston, TX, USA
e-mail: rweber@mdanderson.org

P. W. Gidley, F. DeMonte (eds.), *Temporal Bone Cancer*, https://doi.org/10.1007/978-3-319-74539-8_22

regional lymph nodes. Armed with this knowledge, the surgeon can make informed decisions regarding management of the parotid gland and neck.

TNM Classification and Stage

While there is no AJCC staging for temporal bone malignancy, the Pittsburgh TNM is the one most cited. The TNM classification of temporal bone and parotid gland malignancies is described in Table 22.2 [2]. Mazzoni et al. further modified the Pittsburgh staging system by stratifying T4 lesions into T4a and T4b. T4a was defined as cartilage invasion, preauricular soft tissue, or parotid invasion. Cancers invading medially, inferiorly, or posteriorly into the temporal bone or skull base were defined as T4b based on worse survival outcomes [3]. Of note, all parotid gland malignancies that invade the temporal bone are at a minimum classified as T4a (moderately advanced disease) due to ear canal invasion. Nodal classification is identical to AJCC; however, staging of temporal bone tumors differs from typical AJCC since any nodal disease, independent of T classification, upstages the tumor to at least a Stage IVA (Table 22.2). Invasion into other aspects of the temporal bone would involve the skull base and thus is classified as T4b (very advanced disease). T4b was previously described as "unresectable"; however that term is no longer routinely used as in certain instances skull base resection can be done with curative intent. Tumors classified as T4b, N+, M0 or T-I–IV, N3, and M0 are Stage IVB cancers. The presence of distant metastasis (T-I–IV, N+ any M1) is Stage IVC disease.

Table 22.2 TNM classification of the temporal bone, parotid, and skin of the head and neck

Pittsburgh temporal bone TNM classification [2, 3]	
Tumor (T) classification	
T1	Limited to the EAC without bone erosion or soft tissue involvement
T2	Limited to the EAC with bone or limited soft tissue involvement (<0.5 cm)
T3	Erosion through osseous EAC with limited soft tissue involvement (<0.5 cm) or tumor involvement of the middle ear and/or mastoid
T4	Erosion of the inner ear, petrous apex, carotid canal, jugular foremen, dura, with extensive soft tissue involvement or facial nerve paralysis
Nodal (N) classification	
N0	No regional nodes involved
N1	Single ipsilateral node, <3 cm
N2a	Single ipsilateral node, 3–6 cm
N2b	Multiple ipsilateral nodes, <6 cm
N3	Any metastatic nodes >6 cm
STAGE	
I	T1N0M0
II	T2N0M0
III	T3N0M0
IV	T4N0 and T1-4N+
Parotid gland cancer TNM classification	
Tumor (T) classification	
T1	≤2 cm in greatest dimension without extraparenchymal extension (clinical or macroscopic evidence of invasion of the soft tissues, not microscopic evidence)
T2	Tumor >2 cm but not more than 4 cm in greatest dimension without extraparenchymal extension
T3	Tumor >4 cm and/or tumor has extraparenchymal extension
T4a	Tumor invades the skin, mandible, ear canal, and/or facial nerve
T4b	Tumor invades the skull base and/or pterygoid plates and/or encases the carotid artery
Nodal (N) classification	
N0	No regional nodes involved
N1	Single ipsilateral node, <3 cm
N2a	Single ipsilateral node, 3–6 cm
N2b	Multiple ipsilateral nodes, <6 cm
N2c	Bilateral or contralateral nodes, <6 cm
N3	Any metastatic nodes >6 cm
Distant metastasis (M)	
M0	No distant metastasis
M1	Distant metastasis present

Anatomy

Knowledge of temporal bone anatomy, lymphatic drainage patterns, and histopathology is critical to understanding the spectra of neoplasia and patterns of local and regional spread of these tumors.

The external ear is made up of skin (keratinized, stratified squamous epithelium) with dermal adnexal structures, subcutaneous fibroconnective tissues, adipose tissue, and an elastic fibrocartilage for support. The external auditory canal (EAC) is divided into a cartilaginous (lateral one-third) and bony (medial two-thirds) portion. The medial limit of the EAC is the tympanic membrane which separates the middle ear from the external canal. Immediately posterior to the bony canal is the mastoid, and anterior to the canal is the temporomandibular joint. The skin of the entire canal is made up of thin keratinized stratified squamous epithelium overlying a scant fibrous stroma. The cartilaginous portion is more histologically diverse, containing ceruminous and sebaceous glands, whereas the bony portion has scant cerumen-producing glands. The cartilaginous portion offers less resistance to cancer extension than the bony portion. The bony canal is more resistant to cancer extension; however, once penetrated, it offers direct access to the mastoid, temporomandibular joint, and parotid gland.

Preformed pathways within the external ear canal facilitate local extension. In the anterior-inferior aspect of the cartilaginous canal are the fissures of Santorini. These vertically oriented clefts have been termed the "gateway" to the parotid. Similarly, the foramen tympanicum (also called the foramen of Huschke) is an anatomic defect found in the anterior-inferior aspect of the bony canal, just posteromedial to the TMJ. This defect can be identified on temporal bone CT and has a prevalence of 4.6–17.9% with one-third occurring bilaterally [4]. Thinning of the temporal bone in the region of the foramen tympanicum is seen in 35% of patients with a female predominance (Fig. 22.1) [5]. Finally the bony-cartilaginous junction represents another potential route of spread. Unlike the fissures of Santorini and the foramen tympanicum, tumor extension at the bony-cartilaginous junction can extend in all directions and provide a route of spread into the soft tissue over the mastoid, parotid, and into the infratemporal fossa. Each of these anatomic defects allows bidirectional cancer spread from the temporal bone into adjacent salivary gland tissue and from the salivary gland into the temporal bone structures.

The lymphatics of the temporal scalp, ear, and external auditory canal drain into the parotid nodal basin (preauricular) and neck (postauricular, submandibular, upper deep cervical, and retropharyngeal lymph node basins); however, aberrant drainage can occur [6] (Fig. 22.2a). The deep cervical lymphatics of the neck are divided into levels based on clinical and radiographic landmarks (Fig. 22.2b).

Cutaneous malignancies arising from the external ear has a high propensity for regional metastatic spread. In the study by Peach et al., they found that melanoma arising on the auricle drained to predominantly to sentinel lymph nodes in level II (36.4%), followed by the postauricular nodal basin (26.2%), the preauricular region (20%), and level V (11.3%). The drainage pattern in their study was highly variable. Up to 30% of all patients displayed lymphatic drainage to sentinel nodes in the preauricular and postauricular nodal basins, whereas the lobule was the only site to drain to the supraclavicular region. Levels II and V and preauricular nodes were the only areas to receive drainage from all sites on the ear, while 26% of primary melanomas of the concha, helical rim, and lobule drained to the postauricular region [7].

The lymphatics of the external auditory canal and the middle ear are less well elucidated. The drainage of the EAC, however, is similar to that of the external ear with drainage to the preauricular, postauricular, and cervical nodes. A systematic historical review of middle ear carcinomas noted that the middle ear likely has sparse lymphatics as regional spread from middle ear carcinomas is <5% [8]. In a smaller study, regional metastasis was 15% (4/27 patients), all of which were within the intraparotid nodal basin. A systematic review of squamous cell carcinoma of the temporal bone identified regional metastasis in 17.7% of patients; however, the location of regional metastasis was not cited [9].

In the classic study by Rouviére, the lymphatics of the EAC are in continuity with those of the auricle and the tympanic membrane. He described three discrete areas in the EAC that had specific lymphatic drainage: (1) the anterior aspect which drains into the parotid and preauricular nodes; (2) the inferior portion of the canal, which drains into the deep intraglandular parotid or infra-auricular nodes; and (3) the posterior aspect of the canal which drains to the deep nodes at the origin of the sternocleidomastoid muscle. The capillary network of the tympanic membrane is continuous

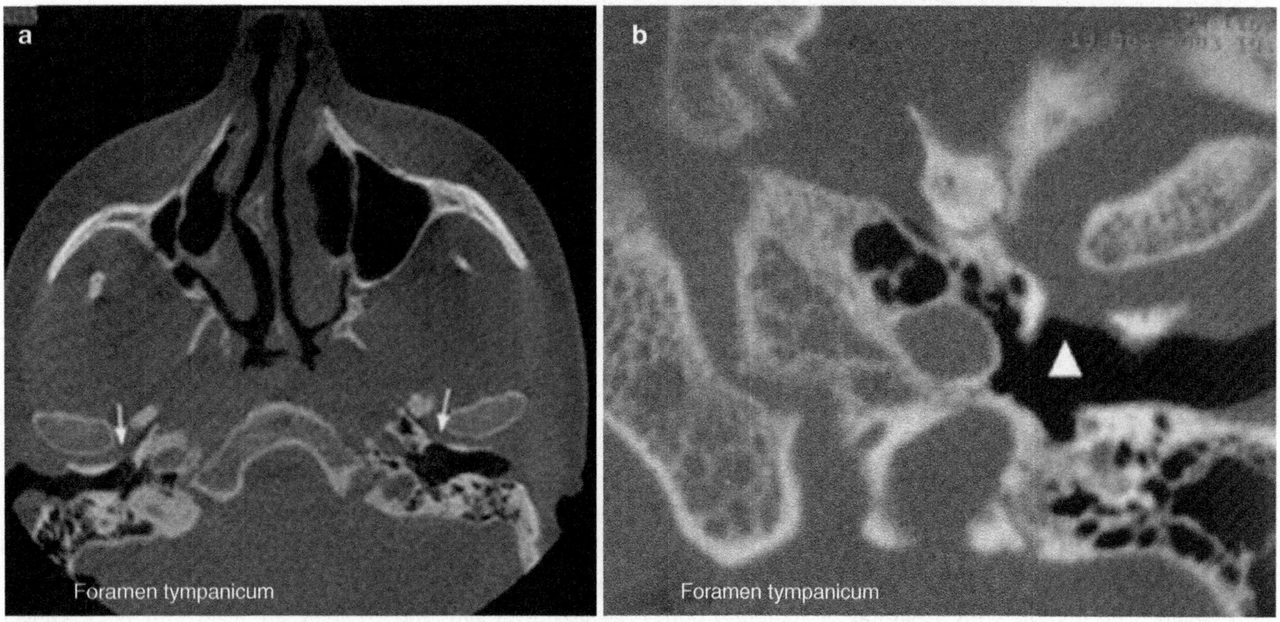

Fig. 22.1 Temporal bone CT, evaluation of foramen tympanicum. (**a**–**b**) Presence of foramen tympanicum bilateral (thin arrows). (**c**) Thinned. (**d**–**e**) No foramen tympanicum [4, 5] (Tozoglu et al. Dentomaxillofac Radiol. 2012 May; 41(4): 294–297; Lacout et al. AJNR 2005 26: 1317–1323)

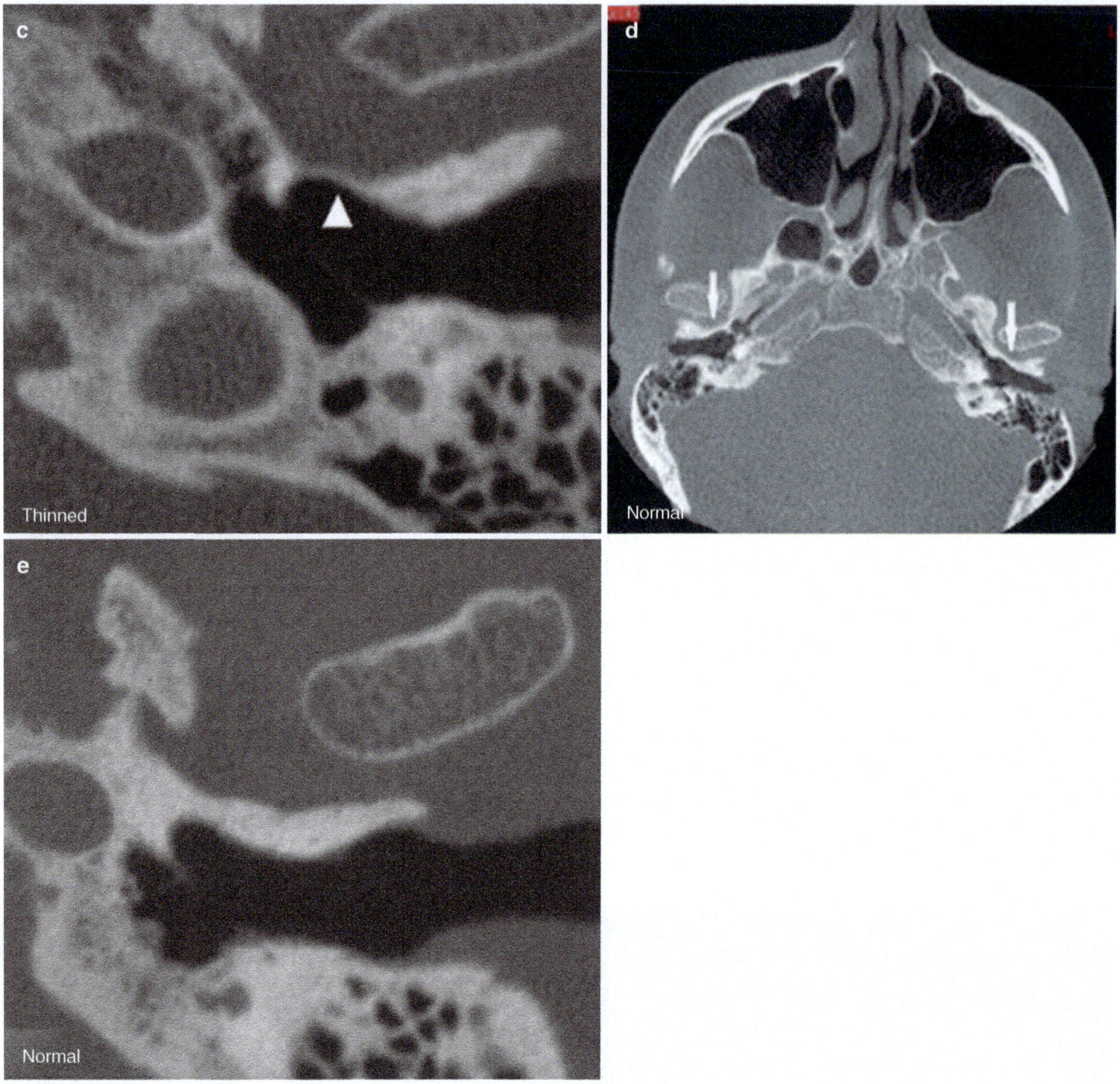

Fig. 22.1 (continued)

with that of the external auditory canal and the mucosal aspect of the middle ear [6].

Evaluation

History and Physical Exam

A thorough history and physical examination are critical for all patients who present with a parotid or temporal bone malignancy. History should focus on onset and duration of the mass, previous radiation, previous attempts at biopsy or treatment, presence of numbness in the trigeminal distribution, facial nerve weakness, hearing loss, otorrhea, otalgia, jaw pain, trismus, TMJ symptoms, pain, new onset snoring, or difficulty breathing. These symptoms suggest locally aggressive behavior, mandating imaging to delineate areas of involvement.

Many patients with temporal bone tumors are elderly, and identifying their comorbidities is important as it contributes to overall prognosis and the patient's ability to undergo what may be extensive surgery and reconstruction. Picarrillo found that 21% of all head and neck cancer patients have a moderate to severe comorbidity. Severity of comorbidities is significantly associated with poor overall survival and has an impact equal to or greater than the index

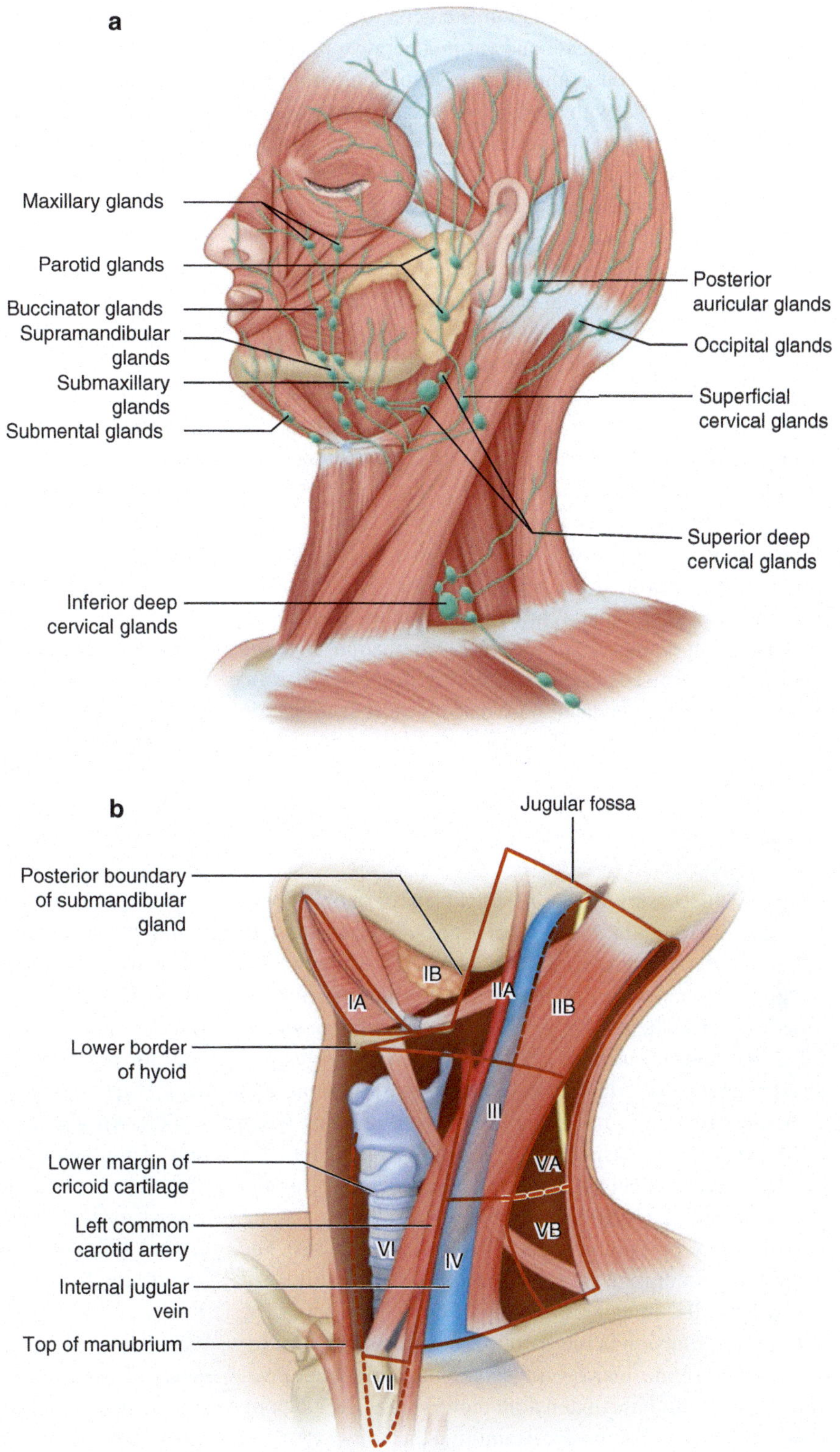

Fig. 22.2 (**a**) Lymphatic drainage from the superficial head and neck region. (**b**) Levels of the neck

malignancy in some cases. Hazard ratios for overall survival when adjusted for age, stage, gender, and race found that moderate to severe comorbidities had nearly a two- to fourfold increased risk of death [10, 11]. While these studies are based on classic head and neck cancers (oral cavity, pharynx, and laryngeal), the impact of comorbid disease has been strongly associated with survival in breast, lung, and colorectal cancers and likely has a similar implication for patients with salivary gland and temporal bone malignancies [10, 12].

The head and neck examination is crucial to understanding the extent of the disease and for preoperative planning. Otoscopic examination is important as many temporal bone malignancies present with the triad of otorrhea, otalgia, and hearing loss. Careful cranial nerve exam is essential, particularly CNs V and VII. In the senior author's experience, abnormal facial function at presentation is found in 40% of patients with a temporal bone malignancy (13% with complete paralysis), 63% of patients with a recurrent parotid malignancy (24% with complete paralysis), and 29% of patients with an aggressive skin cancer [13–15]. Palpation of the parotid will give some sense of the tumor size, but the examination must also include a thorough evaluation for trismus, indicating of temporomandibular joint invasion or extension into the masticator space. Facial numbness or weakness indicates perineural spread of tumor along CNs V and VII or direct invasion of these nerves by tumor. Noting the location of the primary tumor relative to the EAC is important to determine the need for an elective parotidectomy and neck dissection. While palpation of the parotid and neck is an important part of physical examination, imaging studies are more sensitive in identifying deep lobe parotid tumors and regional nodal disease than physical examination alone.

Imaging

Imaging is necessary for the vast majority of patients with primary or secondary temporal bone malignancies to determine the extent of disease and to plan treatment. The imaging characteristics of petrous apex malignancies are described elsewhere. For primary parotid malignancies, CT, MRI, and ultrasound (US) each have advantages and disadvantages. Ascertaining extension of parotid tumors to the temporal bone is the primary purpose of imaging when local extension is suspected. US is an excellent tool for assessing regional nodal metastasis or localizing tumors for image-guided needle or core biopsies, but it cannot identify bony invasion nor deep lobe parotid lesions. The mandible obscures deeper lesions limiting the utility of US. MRI is the imaging modality of choice for assessing soft tissue extension in the parotid, parapharyngeal, masticator space, bone marrow involvement, perineural invasion, and skull base extension; however, it lacks bony detail. CT scan is helpful for examining the bony extension of malignancy or the widening of neural foramina in the setting of perineural invasion. The sensitivity and specificity of CT are 100% and 42%, respectively, and 88% and 77% for MRI [16]. CT is equivalent to MRI for evaluating the regional nodal basins to assess for metastatic disease. CT/PET offers some anatomic imaging and can be helpful for metabolically active masses or lymph nodes, while concurrently evaluating for distant disease. McGuirt et al. compared all three imaging modalities (CT, MRI, and PET) and found that CT and MRI were each 87% accurate at identifying malignancies in the parotid gland compared to 69% for PET [17]. PET is further limited in the parotid secondary to high FDG avidity of benign Warthin's and pleomorphic adenomas. The advent of fused PET/CT allows enhanced correlative comparisons of FDG avidity while assessing the tumors' radiographic characteristics. Despite these advances, current PET/CT parameters lack the power to differentiate benign from malignant lesions with PET/CT alone [18].

Imaging characteristics, regardless of modality, for high-grade malignancy include irregular or infiltrative borders, heterogeneous/enhancing signal, and cystic or necrotic changes. If CT is the preferred imaging modality, then it should be of high quality, using thin slices (1–3 mm) and with the administration of IV contrast [19]. Likewise MRI should be contrast enhanced with gadolinium. T1-weighted images without contrast are optimal in the parotid if the tumor is well-defined relative to the fatty content of normal parotid parenchyma. Post-contrast T1-weighted sequence highlights the enhancing properties of the malignancy, and T2-weighted sequence further delineates the fluid content (Fig. 22.3). One of the major challenges in parotid imaging is low-grade carcinoma as their imaging characteristics often mimic those of their benign counterparts.

It is the authors' preference to obtain a MRI with gadolinium to assess the primary and a CT scan of the neck and chest to assess for regional and distant metastasis, respectively. The neck CT is more familiar to the head and neck surgeon, and it facilitates understanding of the vascular anatomy for potential free tissue reconstruction, particularly in the salvage setting.

Following imaging, cytologic or pathologic determination of the nature of the tumor is important for operative planning and patient counseling. Superficial parotid masses or nodal metastasis can be assessed by ultrasound-guided FNA or core needle biopsy. The sensitivity and specificity for identifying neoplastic lesions of FNA is 96% and 98%; however, these numbers drop to 80% and 97% when differentiating benign neoplasm from malignancy. Core biopsy offers a larger, histologically intact specimen with a sensitivity and specificity for identifying malignancy at 96% and 100%, respectively [20, 21]. Core needle biopsy has lowered the rate of sample inadequacy to 1.2% compared to 8.1% with FNA. The major risk for core needle biopsy is hematoma. For deeper structures, CT-guided FNA or core is helpful, especially for parapharyngeal space masses. There is no data to suggest FNA or core needle biopsy can spread or seed cancer or damage the facial nerve [21].

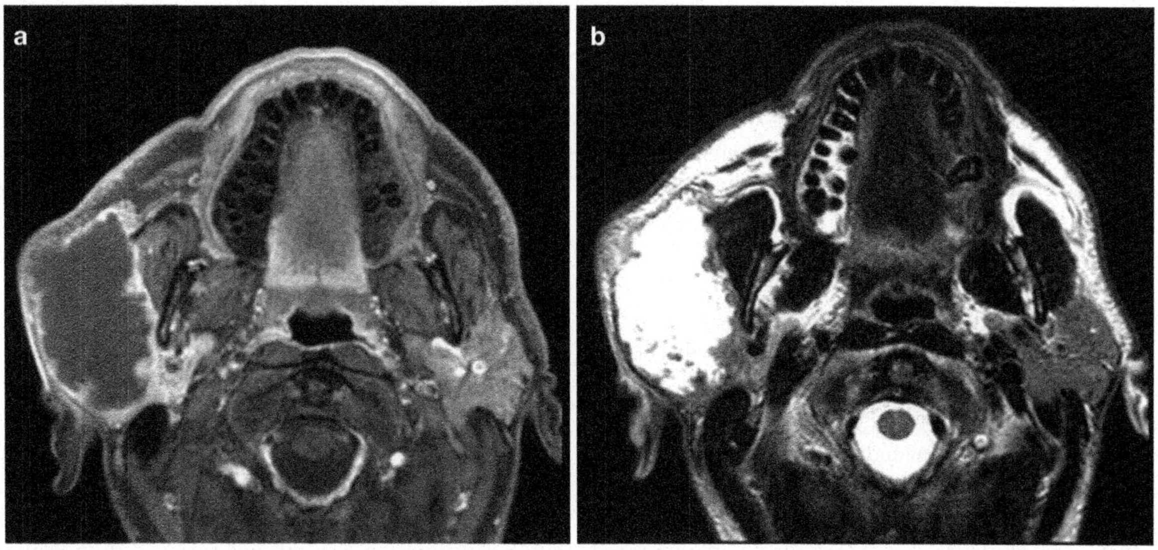

Fig. 22.3 Large parotid tumor involving facial nerve at the stylomastoid foramen

Indications for Parotidectomy and Neck Dissection

Indications for concomitant neck dissection and/or parotidectomy with temporal bone resection will vary depending upon the site of origin, local extension, histology, the presence or absence of nodal disease, and presence and extent of perineural spread. Elective parotidectomy and neck dissection are often indicated if the risk of metastasis is high. This allows accurate staging and determination of adjuvant therapy and consequently predicts survival and risk of recurrence. Absolute indications for parotidectomy and neck dissection in combination with management of the temporal bone are the presence of disease in each respective site. Less clear is when to perform elective parotidectomy or neck dissection as part of the comprehensive surgical management of temporal bone tumors. The histologic spectrum is wide, and the metastatic potential is variable. In most cases, a superficial parotidectomy is performed with lateral temporal bone resection for advanced-stage EAC and preauricular skin malignancy. Primary tumors of the EAC, middle ear, and mastoid rarely metastasize to the neck; when they do, levels II and III are the most common location [1, 15]. Extrapolation from primary parotid gland malignancy and cutaneous malignancies can help guide decision-making, particularly for elective neck dissection. Metastatic rates for temporal bone malignancies are summarized in Table 22.3.

Gidley et al. and Morris et al. have two of the largest recent series of temporal bone malignancies with 157 and 72 patients in each series, respectively. In both series, squamous cell carcinoma was the most common histology (39–54%), followed by basal cell carcinoma (14–19%) and adenoid cystic carcinoma (5.6–7.6%) [1, 22].

Gidley et al. found 60% of patients presented with facial nerve weakness. Preoperatively 67% of patients were cN0 and 18% were cN+. Neck dissection was performed in 62% of all patients. Parotidectomy was performed in 77% of patients (2/3 of which were total parotidectomy). Forty-six percent of patients required facial nerve sacrifice. Overall 34% of patients had either cervical- or intraparotid-positive adenopathy. The preauricular skin, parotid, and external ear had the highest proportion of regional metastasis (32.5%, 27.5%, and 26.9%, respectively). Tumors of the skull base and ear canal had the lowest proportion of regional metastasis (0% and 8%, respectively). The 5-year overall survival (OS) was 58%, and disease-free survival (DFS) was 55%. Stratification by subsite identified preauricular skin, temporal bone, skull base, and parotid to be associated with worse OS and DFS (OS: 42.7%, 58.0%, 34.6%, and 59.8%, respectively; DFS, 33.6%, 38.1%, 53.8%, and 64.1%, respectively) [1, 15].

In the study by Morris et al., 25% of patients presented with facial nerve weakness. The vast majority (94%) of patients were cN0 at presentation. Neck dissection was performed in 61% of patients, with 83% of these being in cT3–4 squamous cell carcinoma. Ninety-one percent of these were elective neck dissection. Parotidectomy was performed in 63% of patients, with the majority being for cT2–4 squamous cell carcinoma. The facial nerve was sacrificed in 39% of cases. On pathologic analysis, parotid invasion was identified in 36% of cases with 25% of intraparotid nodes harboring metastatic disease. Only 12.5% of patients who underwent an elective neck dissection had occult disease. Five-year OS was 62%, and DSS was 70%. The presence of parotid or cervical adenopathy had a significant impact on survival; node-negative patients had disease-specific survival

30% higher than node-positive patients. This survival difference further emphasizes the importance of parotidectomy and neck dissection as staging tools; the therapeutic effect is not entirely determined [22].

However, not all temporal bone resections are due to primary temporal bone malignancies. Understanding the risk of metastasis from other sources that directly or indirectly involve the temporal bone is crucial for decision-making.

Gidley et al. evaluated their experience with lateral temporal bone resection and mastoidectomy in the setting of salvage parotid gland malignancy [13]. The majority of these patients had a history of cutaneous malignancy followed by primary parotid gland malignancy. Nearly 20% of patients had invasion into the external auditory canal. Given this was in the salvage setting, the vast majority (88%) required a total parotidectomy and 10% required a superficial parotidectomy. Two-thirds underwent a mastoidectomy with facial nerve decompression and 30% had a lateral temporal bone resection. Over 90% of the patients underwent a neck dissection and 36% had positive nodes. It was unclear how many were found to have occult disease versus known regional disease. The most common levels of nodal positivity were II and III (22.2 and 15.6%) with levels IV and V only harboring disease in 9% and 4%, respectively. These rates of nodal metastasis are similar for primary temporal bone malignancies (Table 22.3) [1]. Seventeen patients (35%) with normal preoperative facial nerve function required facial nerve sacrifice. Postoperatively only 22% had normal or near-normal facial nerve function (I or II House-Brackman). Despite all of these being salvage cases, the 3-year overall survival was 72%. Of the recurrences, local failure was the most common (53%) followed by distant failure (50%). Regional failure was only seen in 19% of recurrences. Presence of trismus, large size (>4 cm), need for mandibulectomy or presentation with facial weakness (III–VI House-Brackman), parapharyngeal space invasion, and nodal metastasis all predicted worse survival. Each of these factors suggests an aggressive tumor or one that is in a difficult-to-access location, thus making local control more challenging [13].

Similarly, O'Connor et al. reviewed their experience with lateral temporal bone resection in the setting of metastatic cutaneous malignancies [23]. The vast majority (95%) had advanced disease. In their series, 87% underwent parotidectomy with nearly one-quarter requiring facial nerve sacrifice. Nearly all patients (94%) underwent neck dissection with 50% having positive metastatic lymph nodes. In patients still alive with recurrence, only 17% had a regional recurrence with the vast majority being distant recurrence (50%). Five- and ten-year overall survival was 40% and 23%, respectively. Five-year disease-free survival was 28%. In this study, adjuvant radiotherapy had no significant effect on survival [23].

Dean et al. reported their series of salivary (28%) and epithelial (72%) malignancies that involved the temporal bone. The vast majority presented with advanced-stage disease (94%). Sixty percent had facial nerve invasion requiring sacrifice. Seventy-two percent underwent neck dissection with regional disease present in 36.1%. Subset analysis by histologic subtype demonstrated salivary malignancies had a significantly greater risk of nodal metastasis compared to epithelial squamous cell carcinoma (71% vs 26%, respectively). Two- and five-year DFS was 68% and 50%, respectively. Similar to the study by Morris et al., regional metastasis conferred an even worse prognosis compared to pN0 patients (DFS: 34% vs 81% at 2 years and 17% vs 73% at 5 years, respectively). In cN0 patients not treated with neck dissection, 40% developed delayed regional disease [24].

In primary parotid malignancies, direct invasion or perineural involvement of the facial nerve serves as a route of spread into the temporal bone. Although rare (<1% of all parotid surgeries), occult spread into the temporal bone is a significant finding that effects management and outcomes. The Mayo Clinic Group evaluated outcomes of occult intratemporal facial nerve involvement in parotid malignancies. Direct invasion accounted for 36% of temporal bone invasion, while 74% was via perineural invasion. Local control of the facial nerve was primarily via mastoidectomy and sectioning of the nerve in the descending segment. Only 10% required lateral temporal bone resection [25].

Table 22.3 pN+ levels after neck dissection for temporal bone malignancies

	Gidley et al. [1]	Morris et al. [21]	Yin et al. [27]	Rinaldo [9]	Zannoletti [29]
Levels	N (%)	N (%)	N (%)	N (%)	N (%)
I	4 (4.1%)	–	–	–	–
II	20 (20.4)	–	–	–	–
III	13 (13.3%)	–	–	–	–
IV	6 (6.1%)	–	–	–	–
V	4 (4.1%)	–	–	–	–
Overall	47 (34%)	6 (13.6%)	13 (13.7%)	87 (17.7%)	8 (17.7%; 7.5% occult)
Intraparotid[a]	14 (11.2%)	7 (25%)	–	–	–

[a]Intraparotid were counted separately from neck dissection

Another indication for elective neck dissection is planned free flap reconstruction. Free flap reconstruction is often required for large cutaneous, parotid, and lateral skull base defects [26, 27]. Access to the neck for blood vessels often requires deep vessel exploration or selective neck dissection of levels II–III. This requirement allows a pathologic staging of the neck for potential adjuvant therapy.

As stated previously, the role of elective neck dissection (END) for temporal bone malignancies is unclear due to the rarity and heterogeneity of temporal bone malignancies. The publications discussing nodal metastasis often do not separate out the levels of involvement or the rate of clinical nodal disease versus occult nodal disease, thus making the determination to perform elective neck dissection challenging. Rinaldo et al. reviewed the largest cohort of temporal bone malignancies from 1976 to 2003 and found the incidence of positive nodal disease in temporal bone malignancies was 17.7% (87/491). Table 22.3 summarizes nodal positivity rates after neck dissections and parotidectomy [1, 9, 22, 28–30]. Typically, cancers that carry >20% risk of nodal metastasis undergo elective neck dissection. Occult nodal disease rates from temporal bone malignancies were reported in only one small study and found to be 7.5% (3/40). For temporal bone malignancies, all clinically positive necks should undergo a selective neck dissection. To determine the role of elective neck dissection, one can extrapolate from the rates of occult disease in parotid and cutaneous malignancies. Ali et al. looked at parotid gland malignancies and noted significantly higher rates of occult disease in cT3/T4 disease and high-grade malignancies. In patients who underwent an elective neck dissection, positive nodal distribution was 6.7, 28.3, 21.3, 10.8, and 6.7% for levels I–V, respectively (Fig. 22.4a). Based on this, they recommended that patients undergo END of at least levels II–IV. In patients with known regional metastasis (cN+) who underwent a therapeutic neck dissection, nodal positivity was 51.6, 77, 73, 53, and 40% for levels I–V, respectively (Fig. 22.4b). Based on this, the authors recommend a level I–V neck dissection [31]. However, this data may be biased as a therapeutic neck dissection for known disease is often targeted to known disease levels thus inflating the numbers. In the setting of cN+ disease, we recommend a therapeutic neck dissection based on the location of the primary and location of the regional metastasis to determine appropriate nodal levels to be removed. In the case of temporal bone malignancies, the posterior location of the primary puts level V at a much higher risk of regional spread and should be included in both END and TND. If the primary is in the parotid with

a

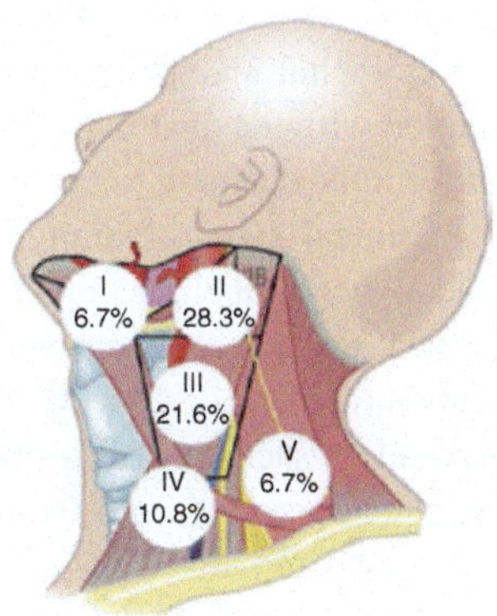

Histology	No of patients (*n* = 74)	pN+ (*n* = 26)
Acinic Cell	9	3(33%)
Adenocarcinoma	13	7(54%)
Adenoid Cystic	3	–
Anaplastic	2	1(50%)
Ca ex-Pleomorphic	16	6(37.5%)
MEC	17	4(23.5%)
Poorly Differentiated	3	1(33%)
Myoepithelial	3	–
Salivary Duct	6	3(50%)
Undifferentiated	2	1(50%)

Proportion of occult metastases stratified by histology in patients having END

b

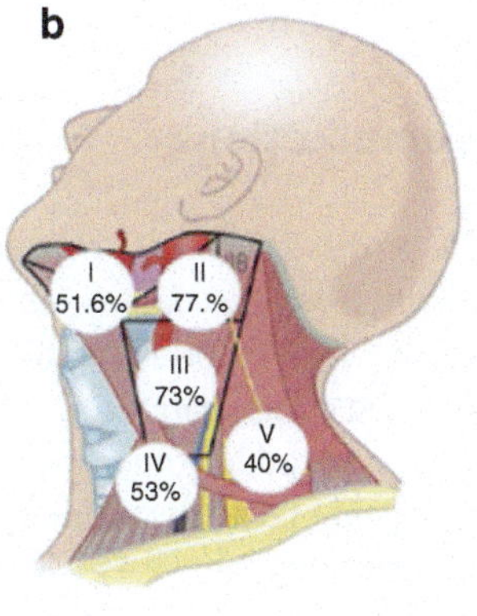

Histology	No of patients (*n* = 31)	pN+ (*n* = 27)
Adenocarcinoma	4	4(100%)
Ca ex-Pleomorphic	5	5(100%)
MEC	9	6(67%)
Poorly Differentiated	6	5(83%)
Salivary Duct	7	7(100%)

Proportion of pathological positive nodes stratified by histology in patients having TND

Fig. 22.4 Percentage of pN+ in each neck level after (**a**) elective neck dissection and (**b**)therapeutic neck dissection [30] (Ali, S et al. Treatment of neck in carcinoma of the parotid. Ann Surg Oncol 2014) extension of tumor into the temporal bone, then END may include levels II–IV.

In the case of metastatic cutaneous malignancies to the parotid, one must note the location of the primary relative to the external ear canal. The standard algorithm to determine the role of parotidectomy and neck dissection levels is based on the work by Pathak et al. in patients with melanoma (Fig. 22.5) [32]. Surgery for regional control in cutaneous malignancy of the head and neck is based upon the location of the primary. For malignancies of the anterior scalp, forehead, and face, the typical metastasis is to the parotid and neck levels I–III. For malignancies of the coronal scalp and ear, typical metastasis is to the parotid and levels I–V. Finally, for malignancies of the posterior scalp, typical metastasis is to occipital nodes and levels II–V. By using this schema, 92.3% of regional metastases were predictive. Postauricular nodal involvement was 1.5% [32].

Sentinel lymph node biopsy (SLNB) has become the gold standard for staging the neck for melanoma. SLNB helps to minimize unnecessary neck dissection. In melanoma, SLNB has been shown to have excellent positive predictive value (PPV) and negative predictive value (NPV); however, its role in temporal bone malignancy has not been studied with the exception of cutaneous malignancies and those of the external ear. For external ear melanoma, positive SLNB rate is 8–10% with drainage patterns being relatively unpredictable as described above. For cutaneous malignancies of the forehead, cheek, and scalp, SLNB identification is as high as 99.7% and SLNB positivity as high as 25%. Regional failure in SLNB-negative case occurs in 4.2% of cases [33].

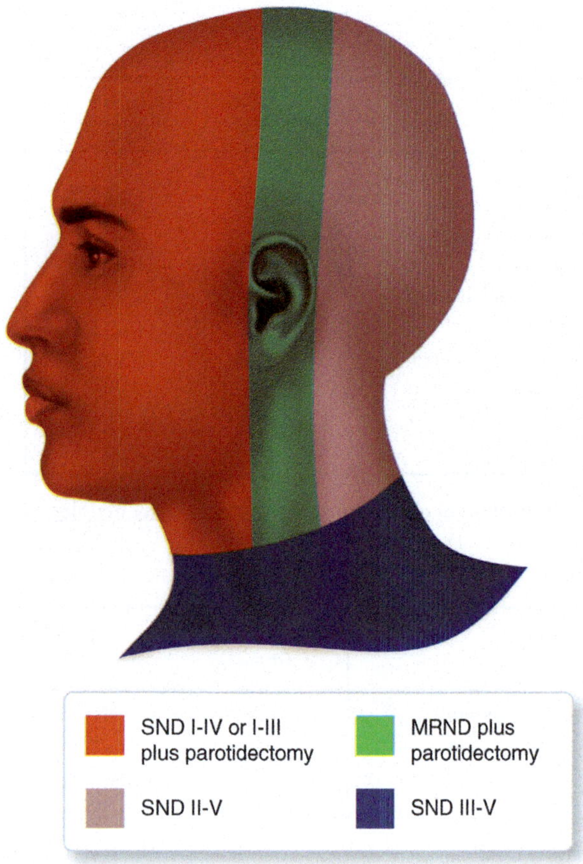

Fig. 22.5 Recommended operations for regional control in head and neck cutaneous malignancies [31] (Pathak I. et al. Head Neck 2001)

Extra-temporal Sacrifice of Facial Nerve

The decision to sacrifice the facial nerve is relatively straightforward when there is preoperative facial paralysis or obvious, gross invasion of the nerve by malignant disease. The situation is quite different when the facial nerve has completely normal function preoperatively. One of the challenges involves the uncertainty of the definitive histology at the time of the tumor resection. In differentiating benign from malignancy, FNA has a 97% specificity but only an 80% sensitivity with a 14.7% probability of indeterminate cytology [21]. FNA can help in surgical planning and preoperative patient counseling, but caution must be borne in mind.

Frozen section pathology can increase the probability of determining malignancy, but it is not 100% accurate. Sensitivity and specificity of frozen section is 98.5% and 99%, respectively, for parotid gland malignancy [34]. Thus a high probability of malignancy can be determined by frozen section. An experienced pathologist can readily differentiate an epithelial malignancy from lymphoma. This information paired with the anatomic findings at the time of surgery will inform the decision to sacrifice or preserve the facial nerve.

Clinical signs of malignancy involving or invading the facial nerve include an enlarged or erythematous nerve. When the nerve is encased and edematous and a subepineural plane of dissection cannot be established, the nerve should be sacrificed. If a plane can be developed, the nerve may be preserved with the realization that microscopic disease may remain. This microscopic disease can be effectively managed by the administration of postoperative radiation. At no time should gross disease be left behind.

Complications

Neck dissection and parotidectomy are not without risk. While these procedures are performed routinely for various causes, it is important to discuss with the patient all potential risk and complications.

For parotidectomy, the most impactful complication is iatrogenic facial nerve injury. In experienced hands, the risk of temporary paresis is 9.3–64.6% with less than 1% permanent weakness [35]. Other complications include sialocele (6–9.1%), Frey's syndrome (40–79%), cosmetic defects/

hallowing, hematoma, first bite syndrome, trismus, seroma, infection, and scar [14, 36].

The most common complication after neck dissection is infection and hematoma. Perioperative antibiotics and sterile technique are imperative. Meticulous hemostasis and attention to vascular structures are essential to avoid hematoma. Other complications include pneumothorax, cranial nerve injury (X, XI, XII), phrenic nerve injury, chyle leak, stroke, carotid injury, internal jugular vein injury/air embolus, pharyngeal injury, and paresthesia. Understanding the anatomy of the neck is critical to identifying essential structures and preserving them when possible. Neck dissection in the salvage setting increases the risk of complication due to altered anatomy and fibrosis. The risk of carotid blowout is 3–4%, especially in the salvage setting, and vessel coverage is essential to mitigate this risk [37, 38].

Operative Pearls

At the start of the procedure, the head and neck surgeon in conjunction with neurotologist and neurosurgeons discuss the planned incision to allow for adequate access for all parties. If the auricle is to be preserved, a postauricular incision is made to allow elevation of the auricle for the mastoidectomy. A preauricular incision is outlined for the parotidectomy. These two periauricular incisions can then be joined in a Y-shape below the earlobe and extended into the neck in a curvilinear fashion for the neck dissection. If the auricle is to be preserved, it is imperative to leave a superior-based blood supply to the auricle to prevent ischemia and necrosis of the ear.

If an infratemporal fossa resection or craniotomy is needed, the preauricular incision can be extended cephalad and posterior to the temporal hairline to allow for any necessary extension for a coronal or bicoronal incision.

If the skin or the auricle is involved, the necessary soft tissue/skin resection with margins can be incorporated into the abovementioned incisions.

Mastoidectomy is performed to identify the main trunk of the facial nerve as it exits the stylomastoid foramen. After the otologic surgeon has completed their aspect of the case, skin flaps are raised superficial to the parotid fascia to the anterior extent of the parotid. For superficial parotid tumors, care must be taken to leave a margin over the tumor and avoid cutting into the tumor during skin flap elevation. The flap elevation should not extend anteriorly past the parotid since careless dissection here can injure the facial nerve branches as they exit the gland.

Given the case is done in conjunction with the otologic surgeon, the descending segment of the facial nerve can be identified within the mastoid and traced as it exits the stylomastoid foramen and then anteriorly into the parotid parenchyma. A superficial or total parotidectomy is then performed followed by the neck dissection as indicated. Margins are checked via frozen section from the specimen or from the defect. If there is concern for involvement of the CN V3 nerve either by imaging (MRI) or physical examination, the buccal, lingual, inferior alveolar, and auriculotemporal nerve branches can be identified deep to the parotid, in the parapharyngeal space, masticator space, or infratemporal fossa, respectively, and traced proximally to the skull base [39]. Similarly, aggressive local invasion into the mandible may warrant a segmental mandibulectomy; typically the upper half of the ramus, condyle, and coronoid process are resected. However distal resection may be warranted as indicated by tumor extension. Removal of the mandible will also provide unfettered access to the parapharyngeal space and infratemporal fossa [13].

Reconstruction is often necessary after temporal bone and parotid resection; thus having a reconstructive team available is paramount. Local flaps can be used for small defects; however, for large defects or in the salvage setting, free flap is often required. If the facial nerve is sacrificed, immediate nerve grafting should be performed [26]. The nature of the flap will be determined by the defect and is beyond the scope of this chapter.

Conclusions

Several factors must be taken into account when deciding on the role of parotidectomy and neck dissection, specifically histology, stage, location, and extent of the primary tumor invasion and the need for reconstructive surgery. Parotidectomy is indicated for direct tumor invasion or if the parotid is within the draining nodal basin. Indication for neck dissection is clinically evident nodal disease. Elective neck dissection is based on the risk of metastasis. Temporal bone malignancy is challenging as the pathologies are heterogeneous and risk stratification is difficult. In the setting of temporal bone malignancy, the risk for nodal metastasis across all pathologies is 13–34%. We advocate elective neck dissection for advanced-stage tumors when at least a 20% risk of metastatic spread exists. Nodal levels dissected are based on the location of the primary. Overall parotidectomy and neck dissection are safe surgeries but convey risks that must be discussed with the patient.

References

1. Gidley PW, et al. The oncology of otology. Laryngoscope. 2012;122(2):393–400.
2. Arriaga M, et al. Staging proposal for external auditory meatus carcinoma based on preoperative clinical examination and computed tomography findings. Ann Otol Rhinol Laryngol. 1990;99(9 Pt 1):714–21.

3. Mazzoni A, Danesi G, Zanoletti E. Primary squamous cell carcinoma of the external auditory canal: surgical treatment and long-term outcomes. Acta Otorhinolaryngol Ital. 2014;34(2):129–37.
4. Tozoglu U, Caglayan F, Harorli A. Foramen tympanicum or foramen of Huschke: anatomical cone beam CT study. Dentomaxillofac Radiol. 2012;41(4):294–7.
5. Lacout A, et al. Foramen tympanicum, or foramen of Huschke: pathologic cases and anatomic CT study. AJNR Am J Neuroradiol. 2005;26(6):1317–23.
6. Rouvière H, Tobias MJ. Anatomy of the human lymphatic system. Ann Arbor: Edwards Brothers; 1938.
7. Peach HS, et al. The unpredictability of lymphatic drainage from the ear in melanoma patients, and its implications for management. Ann Surg Oncol. 2013;20(5):1707–13.
8. Stell PM. Carcinoma of the external auditory meatus and middle ear. Clin Otolaryngol Allied Sci. 1984;9(5):281–99.
9. Rinaldo A, et al. Nodal disease in temporal bone squamous carcinoma. Acta Otolaryngol. 2005;125(1):5–8.
10. Piccirillo JF. Importance of comorbidity in head and neck cancer. Laryngoscope. 2000;110(4):593–602.
11. Piccirillo JF, Costas I. The impact of comorbidity on outcomes. ORL J Otorhinolaryngol Relat Spec. 2004;66(4):180–5.
12. Piccirillo JF, et al. Prognostic importance of comorbidity in a hospital-based cancer registry. JAMA. 2004;291(20):2441–7.
13. Gidley PW, et al. The results of temporal bone surgery for advanced or recurrent tumors of the parotid gland. Laryngoscope. 2011;121(8):1702–7.
14. Lai SY, et al. Parotidectomy in the treatment of aggressive cutaneous malignancies. Arch Otolaryngol Head Neck Surg. 2002;128(5):521–6.
15. Gidley PW, DeMonte F. Temporal bone malignancies. Neurosurg Clin N Am. 2013;24(1):97–110.
16. Lee YY, et al. Imaging of salivary gland tumours. Eur J Radiol. 2008;66(3):419–36.
17. McGuirt WF, et al. A comparative diagnostic study of head and neck nodal metastases using positron emission tomography. Laryngoscope. 1995;105(4 Pt 1):373–5.
18. Kendi AT, et al. Is there a role for PET/CT parameters to characterize benign, malignant, and metastatic parotid tumors? AJR Am J Roentgenol. 2016;207(3):635–40.
19. Committee AASC ACR–ASNR–SPR practice parameter for the performance of computed tomography (CT) of the extracranial head and neck. 2016.
20. Witt BL, Schmidt RL. Ultrasound-guided core needle biopsy of salivary gland lesions: a systematic review and meta-analysis. Laryngoscope. 2014;124(3):695–700.
21. Douville NJ, Bradford CR. Comparison of ultrasound-guided core biopsy versus fine-needle aspiration biopsy in the evaluation of salivary gland lesions. Head Neck. 2013;35(11):1657–61.
22. Morris LG, et al. Predictors of survival and recurrence after temporal bone resection for cancer. Head Neck. 2012;34(9):1231–9.
23. O'Connor A, et al. Evaluating the outcomes of temporal bone resection in metastatic cutaneous head and neck malignancies: 13-year review. J Laryngol Otol. 2015;129(10):964–9.
24. Dean NR, et al. Outcomes following temporal bone resection. Laryngoscope. 2010;120(8):1516–22.
25. Carlson ML, et al. Occult temporal bone facial nerve involvement by parotid malignancies with perineural spread. Otolaryngol Head Neck Surg. 2015;153(3):385–91.
26. Hanasono MM, et al. Comprehensive management of temporal bone defects after oncologic resection. Laryngoscope. 2012;122(12):2663–9.
27. Hanasono MM, et al. Adipofascial perforator flaps for "aesthetic" head and neck reconstruction. Head Neck. 2011;33(10):1513–9.
28. Yin M, et al. Analysis of 95 cases of squamous cell carcinoma of the external and middle ear. Auris Nasus Larynx. 2006;33(3):251–7.
29. Mehra S, et al. Outcomes of temporal bone resection for locally advanced parotid cancer. Skull Base. 2011;21(6):389–96.
30. Zanoletti E, Danesi G. The problem of nodal disease in squamous cell carcinoma of the temporal bone. Acta Otolaryngol. 2010;130(8):913–6.
31. Ali S, et al. Treatment of the neck in carcinoma of the parotid gland. Ann Surg Oncol. 2014;21(9):3042–8.
32. Pathak I, et al. Do nodal metastases from cutaneous melanoma of the head and neck follow a clinically predictable pattern? Head Neck. 2001;23(9):785–90.
33. Erman AB, et al. Sentinel lymph node biopsy is accurate and prognostic in head and neck melanoma. Cancer. 2012;118(4):1040–7.
34. Olsen KD, Moore EJ, Lewis JE. Frozen section pathology for decision making in parotid surgery. JAMA Otolaryngol Head Neck Surg. 2013;139(12):1275–8.
35. Terrell JE, et al. Clinical outcome of continuous facial nerve monitoring during primary parotidectomy. Arch Otolaryngol Head Neck Surg. 1997;123(10):1081–7.
36. Shuman AG, Bradford CR. Ethics of Frey syndrome: ensuring that consent is truly informed. Head Neck. 2010;32(8):1125–8.
37. Chen YJ, et al. Carotid blowout in patients with head and neck cancer: associated factors and treatment outcomes. Head Neck. 2015;37(2):265–72.
38. Powitzky R, et al. Carotid blowout in patients with head and neck cancer. Ann Otol Rhinol Laryngol. 2010;119(7):476–84.
39. Chan M, et al. Imaging of auriculotemporal nerve perineural spread. Ecancermedicalscience. 2013;7:374.

Management of the Facial Nerve

23

Natalie L. Silver, Matthew L. Bush, and Jeffrey N. Myers

Introduction

Most of all facial paralyses are idiopathic and characterized by an acute onset of signs and symptoms (Bell's palsy). Neoplastic causes of facial paralysis are uncommon and only account for about 5% of paralysis cases [1]. The facial nerve can be involved with tumor along its various segments: intracranially, within the skull base, or extracranially [2]. In a recently published study of 221 patients with facial nerve paralysis caused by neoplastic disease, 17% had intracranial, 24% had intratemporal, and 59% had extratemporal involvement of the facial nerve. Malignant parotid and cutaneous tumors represented the majority of the tumors in the extratemporal group, while intratemporal and intracranial tumors were more likely to be benign [3]. In the setting of neoplasm, involvement of the nerve usually signifies advanced malignant disease. The most common malignancies affecting the facial nerve and temporal bone are skin cancers arising from the external ear and periauricular region, primary cancers of the temporal bone, and both primary and metastatic lesions involving the parotid gland. Facial nerve involvement can be through direct extension of the primary tumor to the nerve or branches of the nerve or via perineural spread of a neurotropic tumor.

N. L. Silver, M.D., M.S.
Department of Otolaryngology, University of Florida, Gainesville, FL, USA
e-mail: Natalie.silver@ent.ufl.edu

M. L. Bush, M.D., Ph.D.
Department of Otolaryngology — Head and Neck Surgery, University of Kentucky Medical Center, Lexington, KY, USA
e-mail: Matthew.bush@uky.edu

J. N. Myers, M.D., Ph.D. (✉)
Department of Head and Neck Surgery, The University of Texas M.D. Anderson Cancer Center, Houston, TX, USA
e-mail: jmyers@mdanderson.org

Tumors Affecting the Facial Nerve and Temporal Bone

Skin Cancer of the External Ear and Periauricular Region

There are more than one million new cases of nonmelanoma skin cancer reported in the United States each year, making it the most common diagnosed malignancy [4]. Basal cell carcinoma is the most common skin cancer followed by squamous cell carcinoma. Eighty to ninety percent of cutaneous squamous cell carcinomas (cSCCs) are found in the sun-exposed areas of the head and neck. The external ear is the second most common site for cSCC in the head and neck accounting for more than 20% of the disease in this location [5, 6].

Generally, most nonmelanoma skin cancers affecting the head and neck can be managed with surgery alone, and most patients have an excellent prognosis [7]. cSCCs of the head and neck that exhibit more aggressive features, such as larger size (i.e., >4 cm), recurrent disease, perineural invasion, and lymph node metastasis, require more extensive management approaches. Generally, the risk of lymph node metastasis in patients with cutaneous squamous cell carcinoma of the head and neck is approximately 3–5%. However, cutaneous SCCs of the external ear and periauricular region tend to be more aggressive with increased risk of metastatic spread to lymph nodes in up to 10–16% of cases and also have the highest death rate when compared to other cutaneous subsites [8–12]. If left untreated, these cancers can invade into local structures including the ear canal, mastoid, or stylomastoid region causing perineural invasion and facial nerve dysfunction (Fig. 23.1a and b). The lymphatic drainage patterns of the parotid lymph nodes, which drain the scalp and periauricular region, make the parotid gland a common site for skin cancer metastasis.

P. W. Gidley, F. DeMonte (eds.), *Temporal Bone Cancer*, https://doi.org/10.1007/978-3-319-74539-8_23

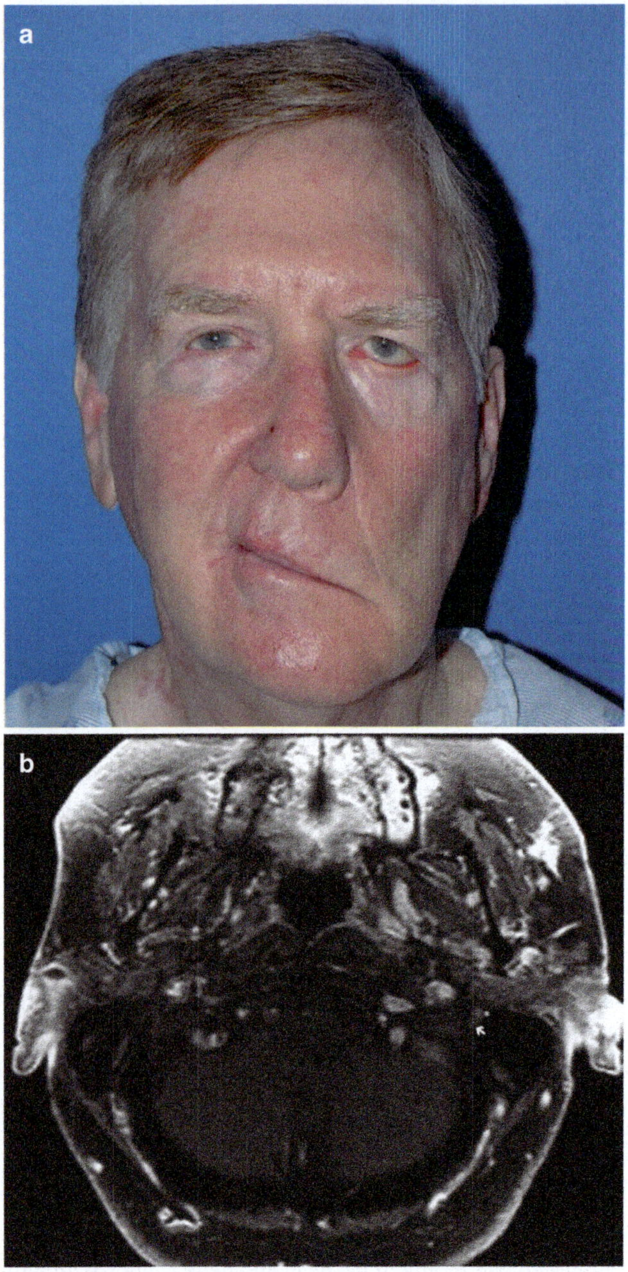

Fig. 23.1 (**a**) A patient with history of multiple facial skin cancer lesion excisions presents with a 6-month history of left-sided facial nerve dysfunction and no evidence of new skin cancer lesions. (**b**) MRI showing abnormal enhancement of the left facial nerve, the posterior genu, the descending segment into the stylomastoid foramen (arrow), and the proximal extracranial main facial trunk (asterisk). A spiculated subcutaneous mass was noted on the left cheek. Image-guided biopsy revealed poorly differentiated squamous cell carcinoma

Primary Cancer of the Temporal Bone

Primary malignant tumors of the temporal bone are exceedingly rare, are often diagnosed at late stages, and only comprise about 0.2% of all head and neck cancers [13]. Primary squamous cell carcinoma of the temporal bone accounts for about 85% of the lesions [14]. Other primary lesions are basal cell carcinoma, rhabdomyosarcoma, papillary adenocarcinoma (endolymphatic sac tumor), and adenoid cystic carcinoma [15]. In a series from MD Anderson, approximately 40% of patients with temporal bone tumors had various degrees of facial weakness or paralysis at presentation [16].

Parotid Tumors

Primary parotid gland cancers can affect the facial nerve. Facial nerve involvement can occur either in the extratemporal portion of the nerve or, more rarely, in intratemporal segments by direct extension into the fallopian canal [2]. Analyses of different histologic types of salivary gland cancers showed direct invasion of the extracranial nerve as the cause of facial paralysis, and malignant cells have been found infiltrating all microscopic components of nerves (Fig. 23.2a and b) [17–19]. In a study of 103 patients with parotid gland malignancies, facial nerve palsy at presenta-

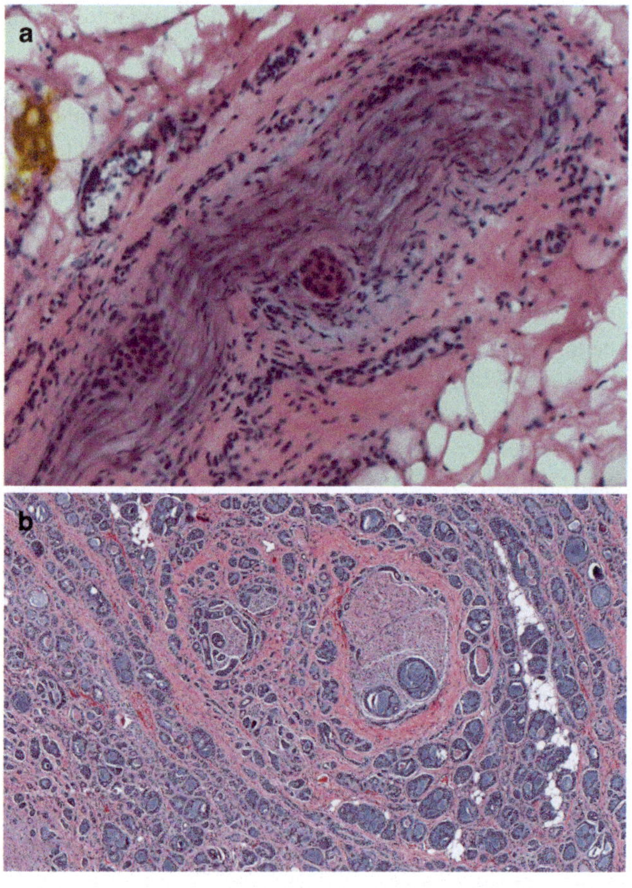

Fig. 23.2 (**a**) Hematoxylin- and eosin-stained slide showing perineural invasion of malignant squamous cell carcinoma. (**b**) Hematoxylin- and eosin-stained slide showing perineural invasion of adenoid cystic carcinoma

Table 23.1 Most common primary malignant salivary gland neoplasms of the parotid gland [20]

Mucoepidermoid carcinoma
Adenoid cystic carcinoma
Acinic cell carcinoma
Salivary duct carcinoma
Carcinoma ex-pleomorphic adenoma
Adenocarcinoma

tion was seen in 33 percent of the cases. Sixty percent of the patients with adenoid cystic carcinoma and 38% in patients with mucoepidermoid carcinoma had a facial nerve paresis or paralysis at presentation. High-grade tumors in advanced stages were more likely to present with facial nerve paresis or paralysis [17, 19]. Table 23.1 lists the most common primary malignant lesions of the parotid gland.

Presentation

Skin cancers of the auricle and periauricular region can present as an ulceration or non-healing wound or an enlarging mass. The mass can periodically bleed and may be pruritic. Primary skin cancers can metastasize to the parotid and cause enlarged lymph nodes in this region. The metastasis can invade the temporal bone and ear canal. Facial nerve weakness or facial numbness represents advanced disease [16].

In the absence of high clinical suspicion, tumors of the temporal bone can mimic chronic suppurative ear disease. The most common signs and symptoms of temporal bone malignancy are aural drainage, otalgia, hearing loss, and aural fullness. In a study of 71 patients with temporal bone squamous cell carcinoma, facial nerve weakness was present in up to 40% of patients. This finding, as well as positive lymphadenopathy, is associated with very poor prognosis [16].

Primary tumors of the parotid gland usually present as a slow-growing, painless mass or swelling of the parotid gland. The presence of a parotid mass in the setting of facial nerve paresis or paralysis indicates a malignant tumor of the gland. Benign tumors can grow quite large but do not cause functional facial nerve impairment. Associated neck lymphadenopathy may be palpable on physical exam. Metastasis from skin cancers to the parotid gland can present similarly to primary parotid tumors, and in these cases, careful examination of the surrounding skin (ear and scalp) is necessary to identify the primary lesion.

A complete head and neck physical examination is imperative, with special attention to the skin (external ear, periauricular region, and scalp), parotid gland, cervical lymph nodes, and assessment of cranial nerve function, specifically, cranial nerves V, VII, and VIII. A complete otologic examination is required including micro-otoscopy in order to assess the extent of ear canal invasion [15].

Imaging of the Facial Nerve

Perineural tumor spread along the facial nerve should be evaluated with imaging as well as physical exam findings in the treatment planning of patients with temporal bone cancers because it can influence the extent of surgery [21]. Although clinical symptoms and physical examination showing facial nerve weakness may suggest the presence of facial nerve invasion, specific imaging such as contrast-enhanced magnetic resonance imaging (MRI) with fat-suppressed T1-weighted images should be used to identify subclinical as well as clinical perineural tumor spread [21]. MRI has been reported to be 95–100% sensitive at detecting perineural spread [22, 23]. Slight enhancement of the nerve is difficult to diagnose on contrast-enhanced CT until it creates a mass lesion. However, CT scan may detect foraminal widening and bony erosion in advanced cases [22].

It is important to distinguish between perineural invasion (PNI) and perineural spread (PNS). PNI describes a microscopic finding of tumor infiltration along a nerve. It is defined by tumor cell invasion in, around, or through nerves in which tumor cells are seen within any layer of the nerve sheath. It is distinguished from PNS, which is caused by gross tumor growth along a nerve distinct from the main tumor mass on imaging [24].

General Principles in Management of Perineural Spread

Surgical management of the facial nerve in temporal bone cancer can require a multidisciplinary team involving neurotologists, head and neck surgical oncologists, plastic/reconstructive surgeons, and neurosurgeons. Cancers can travel retrograde (more commonly) toward the skull base and antegrade or distally along the branches [21].

In skin cancers that involve the temporal bone, the goal of surgery is to excise the tumor along with the affected nerve and its branches en bloc, with the goal of obtaining clear margins. Studies have shown that patients with positive margins had significantly worse overall survival when compared to patients with negative or close margins [25, 26]. The National Comprehensive Cancer Network 2016 guideline recommends a 4–6 mm margin for cSCC [27]. When the tumor extends toward the skull base, obtaining negative margins can be challenging and therefore requires careful preoperative planning and multidisciplinary consultation.

Perineural invasion is found in 5–10% of periauricular skin cancers and is associated with higher rates of both locoregional and distant metastasis [28, 29]. In a study by Goepfert et al., there was a significant increase in nodal and distant metastasis for patients with perineural invasion than in those without [29]. Standard of care in cases with perineural invasion is surgical resection followed by postoperative radiation.

With respect to primary parotid malignancies or metastasis to the parotid, if preoperative physical exam of facial nerve paralysis or paresis and imaging indicate nerve involvement, then one should be prepared to resect the facial nerve along with the primary tumor. Patients with facial nerve paresis or paralysis on presentation from a parotid malignancy have a worse overall survival than patients without facial nerve weakness. If, preoperatively, the status of facial nerve involvement is uncertain, intraoperative nerve assessment is critical in the decision-making process as to whether the nerve should be resected. Facial nerve palsy can be the clinical presentation in up to 60% of patients with adenoid cystic carcinoma and 66% of patients with squamous cell carcinoma of the parotid. Paralysis is less frequent in cancers developing from mixed tumors. Size also plays a significant role in facial palsy and occurs more often in tumors greater than 4 cm [30].

Surgical Technique: Facial Nerve Management

Management of the facial nerve is critical in the surgical treatment of advanced cSCC of the periauricular region and external ear, advanced parotid malignancies or metastases, and primary tumors of the temporal bone. In a study conducted at MD Anderson Cancer Center of 157 patients with periauricular, parotid, and temporal bone tumors, the rate of facial nerve weakness was 38.9%, and the incidence of nerve sacrifice in the cohort was 46.5%, indicating that these tumors frequently involve the nerve, and patients require preoperative counseling about the effects of facial nerve sacrifice. The patients' 5-year overall survival of 58% indicates that aggressive multidisciplinary management can offer patients with advanced disease curative treatment [16].

In patients with primary parotid malignancies or parotid metastasis, the goal is to achieve complete surgical resection with clear margins. With a fully functional nerve, preservation of the nerve is indicated without compromising oncologic principles and is done using a standard approach to parotidectomy with identification of the facial nerve and preservation.

If the tumor is in close approximation to the nerve, one should mobilize a normal-appearing nerve as much as possible in order to separate it from adjacent diseased tissue, without breaching the tumor. If the nerve cannot be separated from the tumor, frozen sections are obtained to confirm malignancy prior to nerve sacrifice. If there are positive margins on final pathology in the setting of high-grade malignancy, especially in the setting of a working facial nerve, adjuvant therapy can be planned [20].

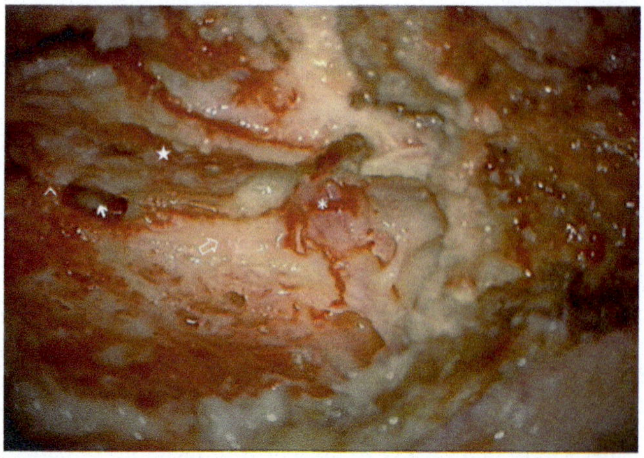

Fig. 23.3 The facial nerve is exposed in the mastoid segment (open arrow) showing involvement of the nerve with tumor (asterisk). Other anatomical landmarks include the posterior bony external auditory canal (star), incus buttress (caret), and the facial recess (solid arrow)

If the facial nerve function is significantly affected preoperatively, consideration should be given to radical parotidectomy with facial nerve sacrifice. Involved adjacent structures such as the mandible, auricular cartilage, and temporal bone may require additional resection. Branches of the nerve may be appropriately identified during surgery and cleared of tumor by using frozen sections both distally and proximally in order to perform nerve grafting. Mastoidectomy may be required to clear the proximal margin.

Mastoidectomy with decompression of the nerve is indicated for (1) parotid tumors that cause facial paralysis in order to obtain adequate margins, (2) tumors that are recurrent and the intent is to preserve facial nerve function, or (3) tumors that are bulky and involve the stylomastoid foramen or mastoid tip precluding standard preauricular surgical approaches. The mastoid segment is decompressed, and the mastoid tip is removed giving exposure to the deep lobe of the parotid [16]. The point of this step is to access the facial nerve in a previously unoperated, undisturbed area away from the main bulk of the tumor. The nerve can then be traced distally into the parotid gland to aid in parotid surgery. The nerve can also be assessed for perineural invasion in this segment. A nerve that is positive for perineural invasion may have a thicker and redder appearance (Fig. 23.3) [15].

If the nerve requires sacrifice, it is transected proximal to the lesion, and frozen section analysis is performed as a tool to assess the margins. The nerve can be followed proximally, but labyrinthectomy is generally not performed in order to achieve a negative margin. In these situations, postoperative radiation treatment is used for increased locoregional control [15]. The normal-appearing distal branches are identified in a retrograde dissection, frozen sections can be obtained as the tumor is approached, and any abnormal nerve should be sent for frozen section and excised. Large auricular cancers and large parotid tumors can be removed as a composite resection specimen involving the external ear and ear canal and parotid. Facial nerve grafting may also be performed if usable proximal and distal segments are available.

When malignant tumors involve the ear canal and do not extend into the middle ear, lateral temporal bone resection (LTBR) is required to excise the ear canal, and the facial nerve can be spared [16]. In order to remove the main bulk of the tumor and gain deeper access to the temporal bone in tumors that extend into the middle ear, LTBR is performed initially. The degree of further surgery necessary after this step is determined based on disease extent. Patients with disease extensive enough to require a subtotal temporal bone resection will often present with facial nerve dysfunction and involvement requiring facial nerve sacrifice. Labyrinthectomy is performed in these situations, and the facial nerve can then be traced proximally in order to achieve a negative margin. In some cases involving a low-grade tumor (e.g., endolymphatic sac tumor) and preoperative intact facial nerve function, the nerve can be dissected free from the tumor [15].

Reconstruction

Loss or sacrifice of the facial nerve causes significant aesthetic and functional deficits. Patients can have facial droop with oral incompetence, dry eye, and risk of corneal abrasion and irritation. It is imperative to counsel the patient on proper eye care and plan for gold weight placement. One should consider reanimation/reconstruction at the time of initial surgical procedures. The best cosmetic and functional results are provided by immediate nerve repair with direct anastomosis or placement of a cable graft [31, 32]. Static techniques for facial rehabilitation are also recommended and include gold weight placement, tarsorrhaphy, brow lift, and facial sling.

Adjuvant Treatment

Adjuvant treatment is indicated for advanced disease involving the temporal bone and with perineural invasion. Treatment consists of surgery (for resectable disease) followed by postoperative radiotherapy, which improves patient overall survival [13, 33]. The role of chemotherapy (cisplatin) in addition to postoperative radiation is less clear for PNI/PNS, and there is conflicting evidence. There have been some reports of increased locoregional control in patients with PNI who have received chemoradiotherapy and other studies that have shown no increased benefit with PNI when compared to patients without [34–36]. The role of chemotherapy continues to be investigated.

Conclusions

Due to the aggressive nature of perineural spread in the setting of temporal bone malignancy, management can be challenging and requires multidisciplinary treatment. Surgical resection to achieve negative margins is the mainstay of treatment, and careful consideration of the facial nerve in preoperative planning is essential in order to achieve this goal. Postoperative radiation improves overall survival in these patients, and the role of chemotherapy remains unclear.

References

1. May M, Schaitkin BM. History of facial nerve surgery. Facial Plast Surg. 2000;16(4):301–7.
2. Selesnick SH, Burt BM. Regional spread of nonneurogenic tumors to the skull base via the facial nerve. Otol Neurotol. 2003;24(2):326–33.
3. Leonetti JP, Marzo SJ, Anderson DA, Sappington JM. Neoplastic causes of nonacute facial paralysis: a review of 221 cases. Ear Nose Throat J. 2016;95(9):390–404.
4. Alam M, Ratner D. Cutaneous squamous-cell carcinoma. N Engl J Med. 2001;344(13):975–83.
5. Iversen T, Tretli S. Trends for invasive squamous cell neoplasia of the skin in Norway. Br J Cancer. 1999;81(3):528–31.
6. Veness MJ, Palme CE, Morgan GJ. High-risk cutaneous squamous cell carcinoma of the head and neck: results from 266 treated patients with metastatic lymph node disease. Cancer. 2006;106(11):2389–96.
7. Clayman GL, Lee JJ, Holsinger FC, et al. Mortality risk from squamous cell skin cancer. J Clin Oncol. 2005;23(4):759–65.
8. Yoon M, Chougule P, Dufresne R, Wanebo HJ. Localized carcinoma of the external ear is an unrecognized aggressive disease with a high propensity for local regional recurrence. Am J Surg. 1992;164(6):574–7.
9. Byers R, Kesler K, Redmon B, Medina J, Schwarz B. Squamous carcinoma of the external ear. Am J Surg. 1983;146(4):447–50.
10. Afzelius LE, Gunnarsson M, Nordgren H. Guidelines for prophylactic radical lymph node dissection in cases of carcinoma of the external ear. Head Neck Surg. 1980;2(5):361–5.
11. Freedlander E, Chung FF. Squamous cell carcinoma of the pinna. Br J Plast Surg. 1983;36(2):171–5.
12. Lewis KG, Weinstock MA. Nonmelanoma skin cancer mortality (1988–2000): the Rhode Island follow-back study. Arch Dermatol. 2004;140(7):837–42.
13. Moody SA, Hirsch BE, Myers EN. Squamous cell carcinoma of the external auditory canal: an evaluation of a staging system. Am J Otol. 2000;21(4):582–8.
14. Clairmont AA, Conley JJ. Primary carcinoma of the mastoid bone. Ann Otol Rhinol Laryngol. 1977;86(3 Pt 1):306–9.
15. Gidley PW. Ear and temporal bone cancer, chapter 23. In: Myers JN, Hanna EYN, Myers EN, editors. Cancer of the head and neck. 5th ed. Philadelphia: Wolters Kluwer; 2017. p. 537–60.
16. Gidley PW, Thompson CR, Roberts DB, DeMonte F, Hanna EY. The oncology of otology. Laryngoscope. 2012;122(2):393–400.
17. Vrielinck LJ, Ostyn F, van Damme B, van den Bogaert W, Fossion E. The significance of perineural spread in adenoid cystic carcinoma of the major and minor salivary glands. Int J Oral Maxillofac Surg. 1988;17(3):190–3.
18. Eneroth CM. Facial nerve paralysis. A criterion of malignancy in parotid tumors. Arch Otolaryngol. 1972;95(4):300–4.

19. Frankenthaler RA, Luna MA, Lee SS, et al. Prognostic variables in parotid gland cancer. Arch Otolaryngol Head Neck Surg. 1991;117(11):1251–6.
20. Deschler DG, Eisele DW. Surgery for primary malignant parotid neoplasms. Adv Otorhinolaryngol. 2016;78:83–94.
21. Amit M, Eran A, Billan S, et al. Perineural spread in noncutaneous head and neck cancer: new insights into an old problem. J Neurol Surg B Skull Base. 2016;77(2):86–95.
22. Gandhi MR, Panizza B, Kennedy D. Detecting and defining the anatomic extent of large nerve perineural spread of malignancy: comparing "targeted" MRI with the histologic findings following surgery. Head Neck. 2011;33(4):469–75.
23. Baulch J, Gandhi M, Sommerville J, Panizza B. 3T MRI evaluation of large nerve perineural spread of head and neck cancers. J Med Imaging Radiat Oncol. 2015;59(5):578–85.
24. Ginsberg LE. Imaging of perineural tumor spread in head and neck cancer. Semin Ultrasound CT MR. 1999;20(3):175–86.
25. Solares CA, Lee K, Parmar P, O'Rourke P, Panizza B. Epidemiology of clinical perineural invasion in cutaneous squamous cell carcinoma of the head and neck. Otolaryngol Head Neck Surg. 2012;146(5):746–51.
26. Solares CA, Mason E, Panizza BJ. Surgical management of perineural spread of head and neck cancers. J Neurol Surg B Skull Base. 2016;77(2):140–9.
27. NCCN Practice Guidelines in Oncology: Squamous Cell Skin Cancer. 2016.; https://www.nccn.org/professionals/physician_gls/pdf/squamous.pdf.
28. Cherpelis BS, Marcusen C, Lang PG. Prognostic factors for metastasis in squamous cell carcinoma of the skin. Dermatol Surg. 2002;28(3):268–73.
29. Goepfert H, Dichtel WJ, Medina JE, Lindberg RD, Luna MD. Perineural invasion in squamous cell skin carcinoma of the head and neck. Am J Surg. 1984;148(4):542–7.
30. Wierzbicka M, Kopec T, Szyfter W, Kereiakes T, Bem G. The presence of facial nerve weakness on diagnosis of a parotid gland malignant process. Eur Arch Otorhinolaryngol. 2012;269(4):1177–82.
31. Gullane PJ, Havas TJ. Facial nerve grafts: effects of postoperative irradiation. J Otolaryngol. 1987;16(2):112–5.
32. DeRubeis DA, Woulfe J, Rosso D, et al. Case of the month: June 1997—a 42 year old man with left facial weakness. Brain Pathol. 1998;8(1):233–4.
33. Gidley PW, Roberts DB, Sturgis EM. Squamous cell carcinoma of the temporal bone. Laryngoscope. 2010;120(6):1144–51.
34. Langendijk JA, Slotman BJ, van der Waal I, Doornaert P, Berkof J, Leemans CR. Risk-group definition by recursive partitioning analysis of patients with squamous cell head and neck carcinoma treated with surgery and postoperative radiotherapy. Cancer. 2005;104(7):1408–17.
35. Bernier J, Cooper JS, Pajak TF, et al. Defining risk levels in locally advanced head and neck cancers: a comparative analysis of concurrent postoperative radiation plus chemotherapy trials of the EORTC (#22931) and RTOG (# 9501). Head Neck. 2005;27(10):843–50.
36. Cooper JS, Zhang Q, Pajak TF, et al. Long-term follow-up of the RTOG 9501/intergroup phase III trial: postoperative concurrent radiation therapy and chemotherapy in high-risk squamous cell carcinoma of the head and neck. Int J Radiat Oncol Biol Phys. 2012;84(5):1198–205.

Facial Reanimation for Temporal Bone Cancer

24

Matthew M. Hanasono

Introduction

The facial nerve is frequently at risk during the surgical treatment of cancers that involve the temporal bone, either from planned resection due to tumor invasion or from inadvertent injury. Division or resection of the facial nerve results in an inability to contract the superficial musculature of the face. Functionally, this condition is associated with an inability to close and protect the eye, show expression, and maintain oral competence, which can interfere with drinking, eating, and speech. Therefore, facial reanimation is a topic that should be discussed with virtually every patient being evaluated for temporal bone surgery.

Anatomy

After crossing the tympanic cavity, the facial nerve travels through the mastoid bone from the pyramidal eminence to the stylomastoid foramen, from which it emerges anterior to the styloid process. The posterior belly of the digastric muscle is a surgical landmark, with the facial nerve lying approximately 1 cm deep to the insertion of the digastric muscle into the mastoid bone. Within the parotid gland, the facial nerve divides into two main trunks, supplying the upper and lower facial muscles, respectively. As the facial nerve exits the gland, there are between 8 and 15 branches making up the 5 named divisions of the facial nerve, temporal, zygomatic, buccal, marginal mandibular, and cervical, which control various muscles of facial expression. Beyond the parotid gland, there is significant arborization with multiple internuncial branches.

M. M. Hanasono, M.D.
Department of Plastic Surgery, The University of Texas
M.D. Anderson Cancer Center, Houston, TX, USA
e-mail: mhanasono@mdanderson.org

Preoperative Assessment

The cause and time course of paralysis must be elucidated during the preoperative evaluation as they have bearing on the outcome and help to determine what procedures are indicated. In cases where the facial nerve remains in continuity following surgery, neuropraxia may occur that can take up to a year to recover. Even in the setting of expected recovery, however, some temporary static procedures, mostly involving eye protection, can be considered. Beyond 12 months, spontaneous recovery is usually unlikely, and surgical intervention is usually indicated. In other cases, the patient presents with paresis or paralysis prior to tumor resection, or radiologic findings suggesting invasion of the facial nerve, and must be counseled about the need for facial nerve repair or static and dynamic procedures for reanimation. Occasionally, facial nerve division or resection is unplanned prior to oncologic surgery, but reconstruction becomes indicated intraoperatively due to unexpected tumor involvement or unanticipated iatrogenic injury.

During the preoperative consultation, the patient is examined for facial muscular tone and volitional movement. If the level of a facial nerve lesion is not known, the exam can also help in pinpointing the site of injury. If the facial nerve is affected within the temporal bone or intracranially, there may be a deficit in taste due to loss of chorda tympani function or hyperacusis due to loss of stapedius muscle function. A lesion of the facial nerve within the temporal bone would be expected to result in global dysfunction, while distal lesions, such as those within the parotid gland, may present with more focal deficits of one or more facial regions or branches of the facial nerve.

During the exam, the patient is asked to raise the eyebrows, close the eyes, smile, pucker the lips, and show the lower teeth to assess function of each of the major facial nerve branches. Brow ptosis and superior visual field obstruction are noted if

P. W. Gidley, F. DeMonte (eds.), *Temporal Bone Cancer*, https://doi.org/10.1007/978-3-319-74539-8_24

present. The eye on the paralyzed side is assessed for degree of closure; the presence of Bell's phenomenon, which aids in corneal protection; and signs of corneal exposure or abrasions. A "snap test" is performed to assess lower lid tone, and the presence of epiphora is noted. Loss of the nasolabial crease, deviation of the philtrum, commissure depression, and deviation of the lips and nose toward the normal side are signs of lack of facial muscular tone. The vector of mouth movement on the unaffected side is also recorded in preparation for static suspension or dynamic smile reconstruction.

Because the House-Brackmann [1] grading system (Table 24.1), which rates facial nerve function from I (normal) to VI (complete paralysis), was designed to assess global facial nerve dysfunction rather than function of individual branches, its usefulness in extracranial nerve injury, beyond the point into which it begins to arborize into divisions and branches, can be limited. However, it remains a popular means of communicating facial nerve dysfunction, so it is often recorded in the medical record. Recording the specific degree of function (either descriptively or using a percentage of normal) for each of the facial regions is more useful and accurate when there is differential injury to the temporal, zygomatic, buccal, and marginal mandibular nerve branches.

Table 24.1 House-Brackmann facial nerve grading system

Grade	Function
I (normal)	Normal facial function in all areas
II (slight dysfunction)	Gross: slight weakness noticeable on close inspection; may have very slight synkinesis At rest: normal symmetry and tone Motion: forehead, moderate to good function; eye, complete closure with minimum effort; mouth, slight asymmetry
III (moderate dysfunction)	Gross: obvious but not disfiguring difference between two sides; noticeable but not severe synkinesis, contracture, and/or hemi-facial spasm At rest: normal symmetry and tone Motion: forehead, slight to moderate movement; eye, complete closure with effort; mouth, slightly weak with maximum effort
IV (moderate severe dysfunction)	Gross: obvious weakness and/or disfiguring asymmetry At rest: normal symmetry and tone Motion: forehead, none; eye, incomplete closure; mouth, asymmetric with maximum effort
V (severe dysfunction)	Gross: only barely perceptible motion At rest: asymmetry Motion: forehead, none; eye, incomplete closure; mouth, slight movement
VI (total paralysis)	No movement

Adapted from: House, J.W., Brackmann, D.E. Facial nerve grading system. Otolaryngol. Head Neck Surg, [93] 146–147. 1985

The more distal the facial nerve injury, the more arborization of the nerve branches makes it unnecessary to repair the nerve. A rough guide is that division of a nerve branch distal to the lateral orbit does not usually need to be repaired. Proximal transection of the nerve should be repaired, although the risk for synkinesis is higher. Repair within 72 h of the injury, if not recognized and repaired immediately during extirpative surgery, takes advantage of the fact that the distal nerve stump can still be stimulated resulting in muscular contraction if the distal nerve is not easily identified.

Imaging studies, such as computed tomography (CT) and magnetic resonance imaging (MRI), can be useful in cases where the diagnosis is uncertain or to predict the extent of facial nerve resection so that the appropriate procedures can be planned. Electromyographic studies can be useful in predicting whether spontaneous recovery will occur as well as in assessing whether viable motor end plates exist if a delayed nerve repair or nerve transfer is being considered.

Facial Nerve Repair

For nerve transections and resection of small segments, immediate direct nerve repair is indicated to provide the best results in terms of motor function. When resections are larger and the nerve cannot be repaired directly, interposition or "cable" nerve grafting is indicated (Fig. 24.1). Cable nerve grafts can be obtained by sacrifice of the great auricular nerve, branches of the cervical plexus at the C3 and C4 levels, or the sural nerve (Fig. 24.2). When concomitant soft tissue reconstruction with an anterolateral thigh free flap is being performed, it is also convenient to harvest the lateral femoral cutaneous nerve as a graft.

Results of facial nerve repair following treatment for malignancy have only been documented in a few studies [2–5]. We observed at least some facial nerve recovery in 75% of patients (with <12 months of facial nerve paralysis and in whom the proximal and distal ends of the facial nerve could be located) that underwent nerve graft repair occurring at a mean time of 7.7 months postoperatively. Recovery was observed even in patients with prior weakness or paralysis, postoperative radiation, and advanced age (Fig. 24.3) [5]. Iseli et al. [3] reported at least some facial nerve recovery at a median time of 6.2 months postoperatively in 97% of their series of 33 patients who underwent facial nerve grafting, although their patient population contained a different mix of follow-up time, preoperative function, age, and radiation history. These results argue for performing facial nerve repair in all patients who have not undergone motor end plate degeneration regardless of the presence of risk factors for poor reinnervation whenever feasible, based on the premise that even partial recovery results in improved appearance and function.

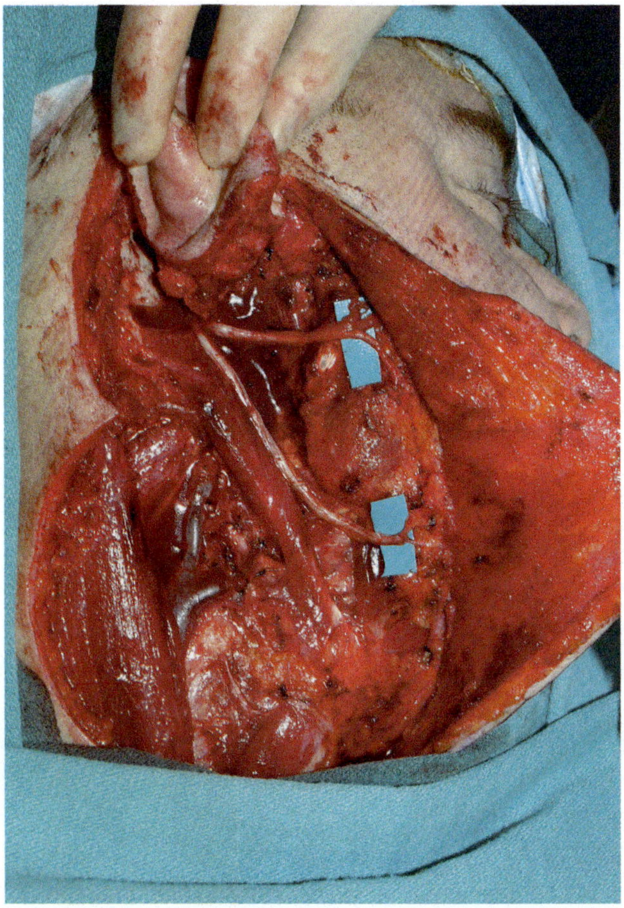

Fig. 24.1 Repair of the facial nerve following temporal bone and parotidectomy. Multiple nerve graft strands or single nerve graft strands that branch can be utilized as interpositional or "cable" nerve grafts to guide axonal regrowth for reinnervation of the facial muscles

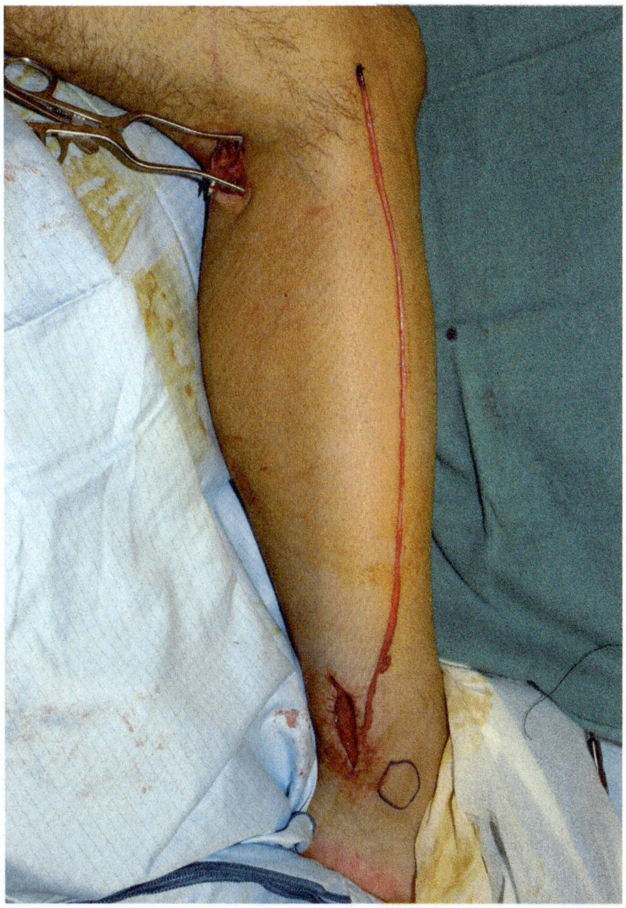

Fig. 24.2 The sural nerve located in the posterolateral lower leg is a common donor site for facial nerve grafts that provides an ample amount of nerve with minimal donor site morbidity

Nerve Transfer

When there is no proximal facial stump, immediate dynamic reanimation can be performed by coapting the distal facial nerve to the hypoglossal or masseteric nerves. This may serve as the definitive procedure for facial reanimation or may act as a "babysitter" procedure to keep the facial muscles from atrophying while awaiting axonal growth through cross facial nerve graft(s). When the hypoglossal or masseteric nerve is used as a "babysitter," the nerve anastomosis is later taken down and replaced with a cross facial nerve graft in about 6–12 months.

Hypoglossal-Facial Nerve Transfer

The hypoglossal-facial nerve transfer has been used to restore resting tone to the face [6–8]. The hypoglossal nerve is readily found running deep and parallel to the posterior belly of the digastric muscle and superficial to the external carotid artery (Fig. 24.4). An end-to-end anastomosis has the disadvantage of causing unilateral tongue paralysis with concomitant impairment of speech and swallowing function. An end-to-side anastomosis decreases the morbidity of this procedure. In end-to-side grafting, the epineurium is locally removed, and some (25–30%) of the hypoglossal nerve axons are transected so that they may grow into the distal facial nerve. An interposition never graft is usually needed to reach the hypoglossal nerve. Speech and swallowing morbidity and synkinesis and mass motion with tongue movement have been shown to be greatly reduced using an end-to-side technique. In general, the innervation produced by this technique is not robust, and it is used as a babysitter or as an adjunct to other techniques.

Masseteric Nerve Transfer

A procedure that has more recently become popular is the use of the masseteric branch of the trigeminal nerve for dynamic facial reanimation [9–12]. This nerve exits the intracranial cavity via the foramen ovale and passes over the lateral pterygoid

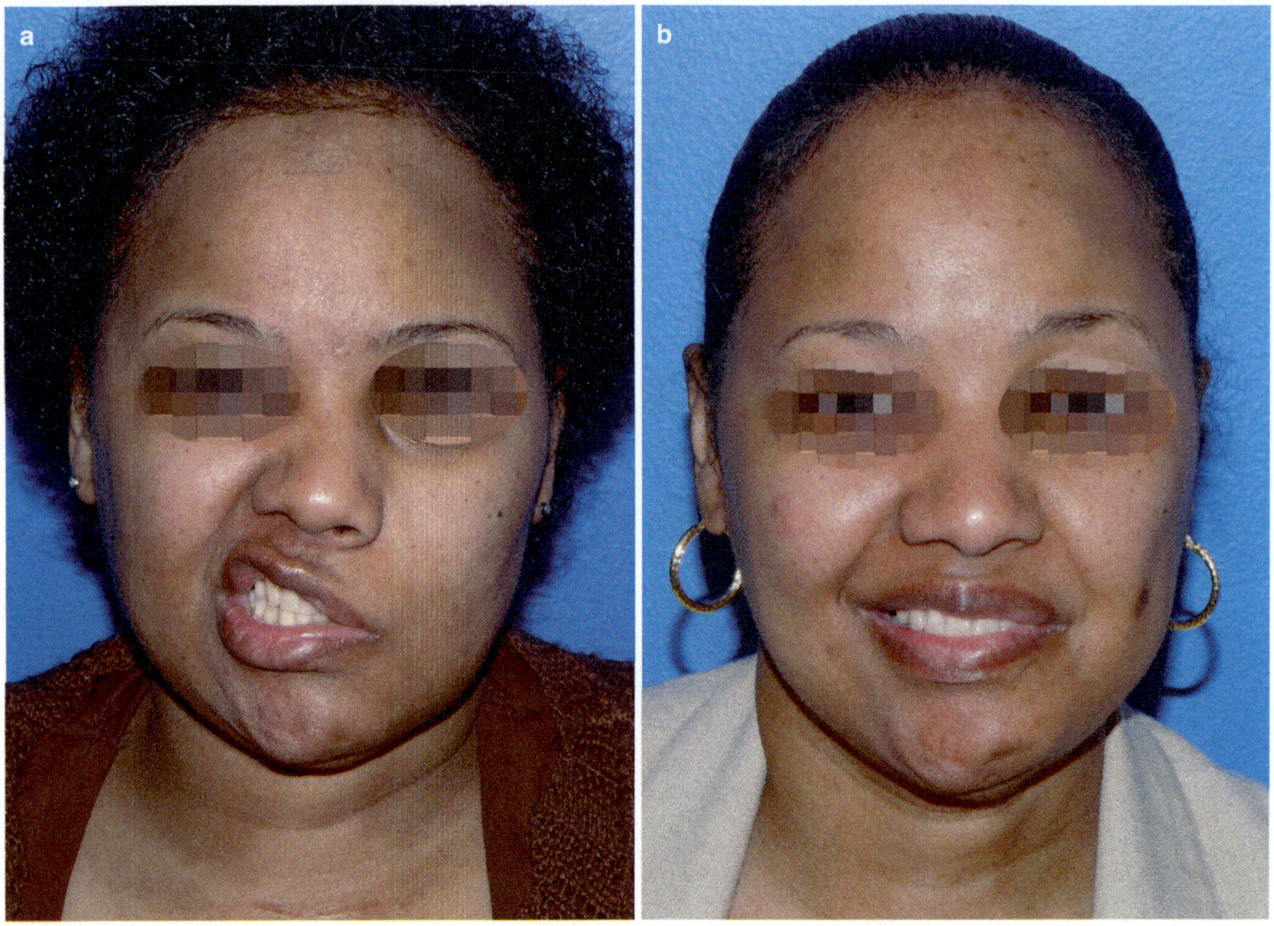

Fig. 24.3 Patient following parotidectomy with facial nerve resection at the main trunk (**a**). The facial nerve was reconstructed with a cable nerve graft. By 12 months, the patient had near-normal facial movement (House-Brackmann Grade 2) (**b**)

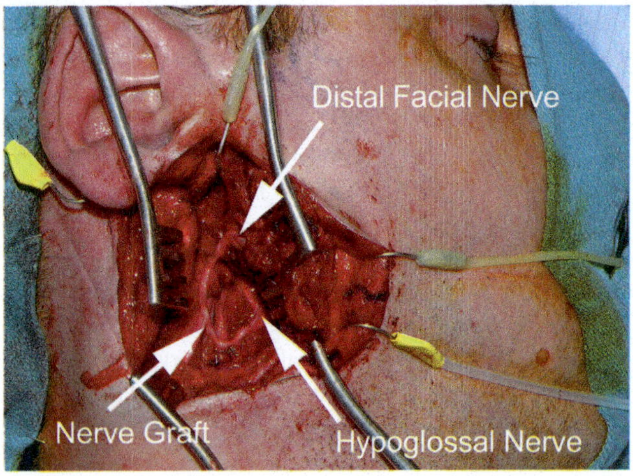

Fig. 24.4 A nerve graft has been used to connect the hypoglossal nerve, which lies deep to the posterior belly of the digastric muscle, to the distal cut end of the facial nerve

muscle and through the coronoid notch of the mandible to enter the posterior surface of the masseter muscle near its origin beneath the zygomatic arch. It is found by careful lysis of the masseteric muscle fibers beginning at the posterior border of the mandible. The nerve usually takes an oblique course within the deep substance of the muscle, traveling from posterior superior to anterior inferior. Following the nerve distally allows adequate length to be gained for direct anastomosis to either the main facial nerve trunk when intact or to the zygomatic and buccal branches, which are usually preferentially selected for reinnervation due to their important expressive and sphincteric functions.

Sacrifice of the masseteric nerve does not result in functional problems with mastication, probably owing both to the sparing of proximal masseteric nerve fibers and to the redundant function of the masseter and temporalis muscles. The masseteric nerve has a strong motor impulse, which provides strong muscular activation and a fast reinnervation time, usually within 3 months. Unlike the hypoglossal nerve, the location of the masseteric nerve close to the route of the facial nerve usually means that interpositional nerve grafting is unnecessary. Because of these advantages, masseteric nerve transfer had replaced hypoglossal nerve transfer as the preferred technique in many practices.

Patients can learn to activate the facial muscles by focusing on tongue or jaw contraction following hypoglossal or masseteric nerve transfer, respectively. With either procedure, synkinesis can occur, as can unwanted activation during mastication and speech. Cerebral cortical adaptation is often possible after rehabilitation with masseteric nerve transfer, and emotional nerve activation has been reported [10–12]. The spinal accessory nerve has also been described as a donor nerve, but its use is uncommon due to the high degree of morbidity associated with the loss of motor function that accompanies its sacrifice, resulting in shoulder drop and pain. Additionally, control of facial movement independent of neck and shoulder function appears to be very difficult. The phrenic nerve has also been used for facial reanimation but can cause marked contraction with coughing, laughing, and deep inspiration and is contraindicated in patients with pulmonary disease.

Cross Facial Nerve Grafting

Cross facial nerve grafting has the advantage of providing natural emotional activation without retraining [13–15]. In cross facial nerve grafting, motor axons from the contralateral normal facial nerve grow through interpositional nerve grafts to reinnervate sectioned nerves on the paralyzed side. In this procedure, one or more nerves on the normal side are sacrificed and connected to a nerve graft, which is tunneled subcutaneously to the affected side of the face. Exposure of the contralateral normal nerve is usually performed through a facelift incision, elevating a skin flap, and nerve branches are identified and mapped as they exit the parotid gland and travel toward the muscles of facial expression. The sural nerve is the most commonly used donor nerve for cross facial nerve grafting owing to its length, availability, minimal donor site morbidity, and ease of harvest.

Intraoperative mapping of the contralateral normal side is performed using a nerve stimulator to identify redundant branches of the facial nerve that innervate the same groups of muscles. Grafting of zygomatic and buccal nerve branches has been described most frequently, again because of their relatively more valuable functions and contribution to symmetry in repose. If a dominant nerve is identified, it is spared, and secondary branches that produce weaker amplitude contractions when stimulated are preferred as donor nerves, in order to minimize the risk of dennervating the donor site. The course of the interposition nerve grafts is usually within the upper lip or lower lip soft tissue. Some authors advocate reversing the orientation of the sural nerve graft so that the direction of axonal growth is orthotopic.

Cross facial nerve grafting has been described as either a one-stage or a two-stage procedure. Single-stage procedures reduce the number of surgeries required, and patients may benefit from faster reinnervation. In a two-stage procedure, nerve graft(s) are sutured to the donor nerve branch on the normal side and tunneled to the affected side and left there. Axonal growth is typically estimated to be approximately 1 mm per day as a rough guide for the amount of time needed before the second stage is performed. Nerve growth can sometimes be followed clinically by the presence of Tinel's sign along the nerve graft. For practical purposes, usually 6–12 months elapse before the second stage is performed. In the second stage, the distal end of the nerve graft is exposed, and the nerve is trimmed sharply to remove any neuroma and sutured to the distal portion of the severed facial nerve on the paralyzed side. An advantage of two-stage procedures is that the severed facial nerve can be grafted to the masseteric or hypoglossal nerves as babysitter nerves while waiting for cross facial axonal growth [16]. This at least theoretically serves to keep the facial motor units viable due to earlier reinnervation from the babysitter nerves.

The main disadvantage of cross facial nerve grafting is that results are inconsistent, not only between surgeons but by single surgeons using the same technique. Undesirable weakening of the normal contralateral side is a potential risk that can be avoided by locating and using non-dominant branches as donor nerves. Grafting of distal nerve branches, rather than of the proximal facial nerve trunk, minimizes the risk for synkinesis and facilitates spontaneous emotional facial movement without the need for retraining. Muscle excursion is also usually less strong than with masseteric or hypoglossal nerve transfer. Because the regenerating axons must cross two suture lines and travel longer distances than ipsilateral donor nerves, reinnervation is slow and usually only partial. Best results for cross facial nerve grafting are usually when the nerve injury is recent (<6 months), to limit motor end plate degeneration and muscle atrophy.

Free Muscle Transfer

In many situations, facial nerve repair or nerve transfers are not feasible, either because the ends of the facial nerve cannot be located or too much time has elapsed since facial nerve injury or sacrifice during which the motor end plates of the affected facial muscles have degenerated and the muscles have undergone atrophy and fibrosis, generally around 12–18 months. In such cases, the best option is functional muscle transplantation, which involves performing free tissue transfer of a given donor muscle and performing a motor neurorrhaphy either to a branch of the contralateral facial nerve or to the ipsilateral masseteric nerve. The most commonly transferred muscles include the pectoralis minor as described by Terzis and Manktelow [17], the latissimus dorsi as described by Dellon and Mackinnon [18], and the gracilis as described by Harii et al. [19]. Generally, 10–12 cm of muscle

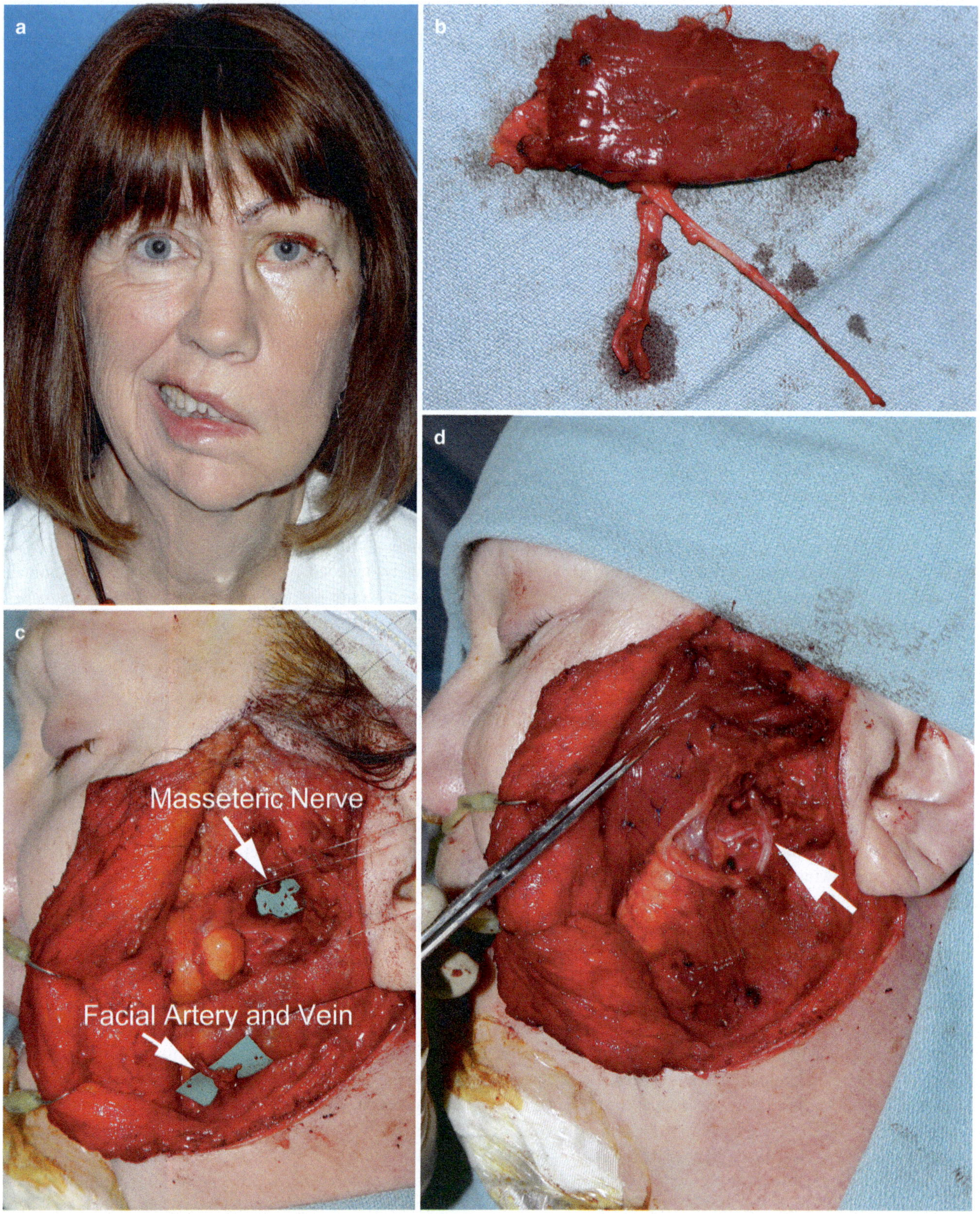

Fig. 24.5 Patient who presents with facial nerve paralysis following resection for cancer (a direct browlift, lateral canthoplasty, and upper eyelid gold weight placement have already been performed) (**a**). A partial thickness portion of the gracilis muscle with the vascular pedicle and motor nerve (**b**). The masseteric nerve and facial blood vessels are prepared at the recipient site (**c**). The vascular pedicle is anastomosed to the facial artery and vein, and a neurorrhaphy was performed to the masseteric nerve, as indicated by the arrow (**d**). Postoperative result, approximately 1 year after surgery (**e**)

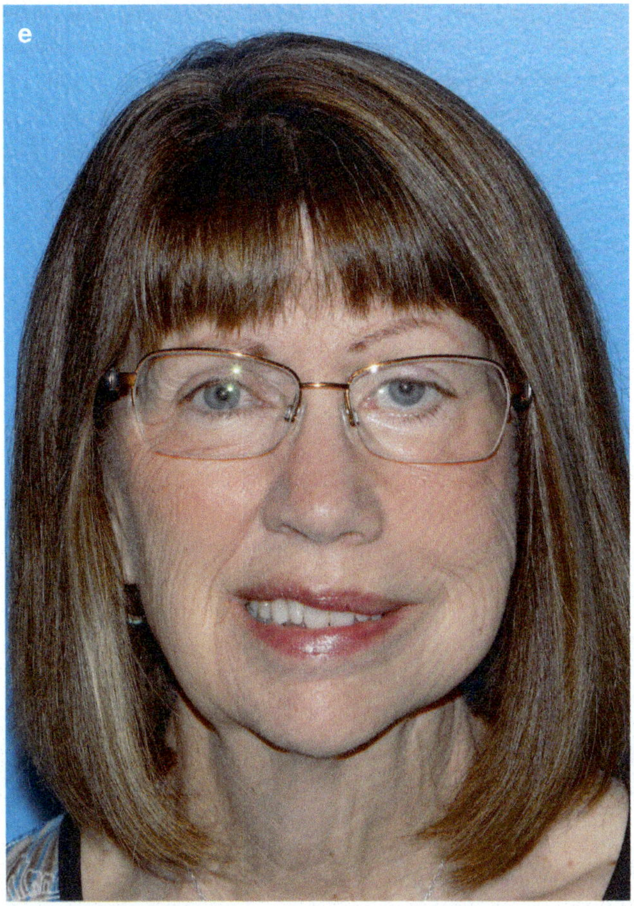

Fig. 24.5 (continued)

length is needed, and the muscle should provide adequate excursion without being too thick so as to not create an unappealing bulge in the side of the face it is used.

The gracilis muscle is the author's preference due to its predictable anatomy, thinness, and minimal donor site morbidity (Fig. 24.5). The gracilis muscle is located between the adductor longus (anterior) and adductor magnus (posterior) muscles. It originates at the anterior margin of the pubic symphysis and ramus of the ischium and inserts on the medial surface of the tibia. The vascular pedicle, which is a branch of the medial circumflex femoral artery, is located about 10 cm inferior to the pubic symphysis. The motor nerve (anterior branch of the obturator nerve) is usually about 8–10 cm in length. It is located parallel to the vascular pedicle and arborizes into many branches.

The muscle is harvested with the patient in the "frog leg" position. The adductor longus can be palpated with the thigh abducted. A longitudinal incision is made two to three fingerbreadths posterior to the adductor longus muscle, and the gracilis muscle should be readily identified. The pedicle and nerve lie deep to the adductor longus muscle, which is retracted anteriorly. The muscle is split longitudinally as the entire circumference of the muscle will be too bulky and is unnecessary to reestablish facial movement. The segment of muscle should be dissected with an intact motor nerve supply. Before dividing the muscle proximally and distally, temporary sutures are placed at 2 cm intervals to mark the length of muscle at resting stretch so that it can be inset in the face under the same amount of tension.

The muscle is transferred to the face, which is exposed via a preauricular incision. Distally, it is secured to the oral commissure and orbicularis oris of the upper and lower lips and the nasolabial crease. The facial artery and vein are used as recipient vessels when they are available. The obturator nerve is connected either to a previously placed cross facial nerve graft or the nerve to the masseter muscle, depending on the reconstructive approach. The muscle is then attached proximally to the zygomatic arch periosteum along a vector of pull that mimics the natural vector of movement in the contralateral face, which is marked preoperatively.

The advantages and disadvantages of cross facial versus masseteric nerve innervation for free muscle transfer are the same as those discussed above for nerve transfer for facial nerve repair [20]. The masseteric nerve has the advantages of not requiring a two-stage procedure and providing stronger contraction with essentially no donor site morbidity. The disadvantage is that muscle contraction will not be spontaneous with facial movement of the contralateral side and that undesirable contraction can occur with chewing. However, many patients are able to train themselves to smile and limit unintended muscle contraction over time, some even without conscious thought.

Cross facial nerve grafting has the advantage of being spontaneous without need for retraining. Its disadvantages are that it is a two-stage procedure with risk of contralateral face denervation and it generally results in weaker muscle contraction than that associated with using the masseteric nerve as the donor nerve. When cross facial nerve grafting is performed, the author usually makes a small incision lateral to the nasolabial crease and spreads in the subcutaneous tissues until two branches of the facial nerve are located (Fig. 24.6). The incision can also be hidden in the nasolabial crease for cosmesis, and the tissues lateral to the incision are explored for the buccal nerve branches. Nerves are stimulated with a handheld stimulator to confirm that they innervate the lip elevator muscles and that they are redundant so that division of one will not result in deanimation of the normal side of the face. One of the branches is cut, and a sural nerve graft is coapted to the proximal end with an epineural suture repair.

The nerve graft is then tunneled across the upper lip to the contralateral side. The free end of the graft is marked with a colored suture and banked in the preauricular region of the contralateral face, accessed via a preauricular incision, which

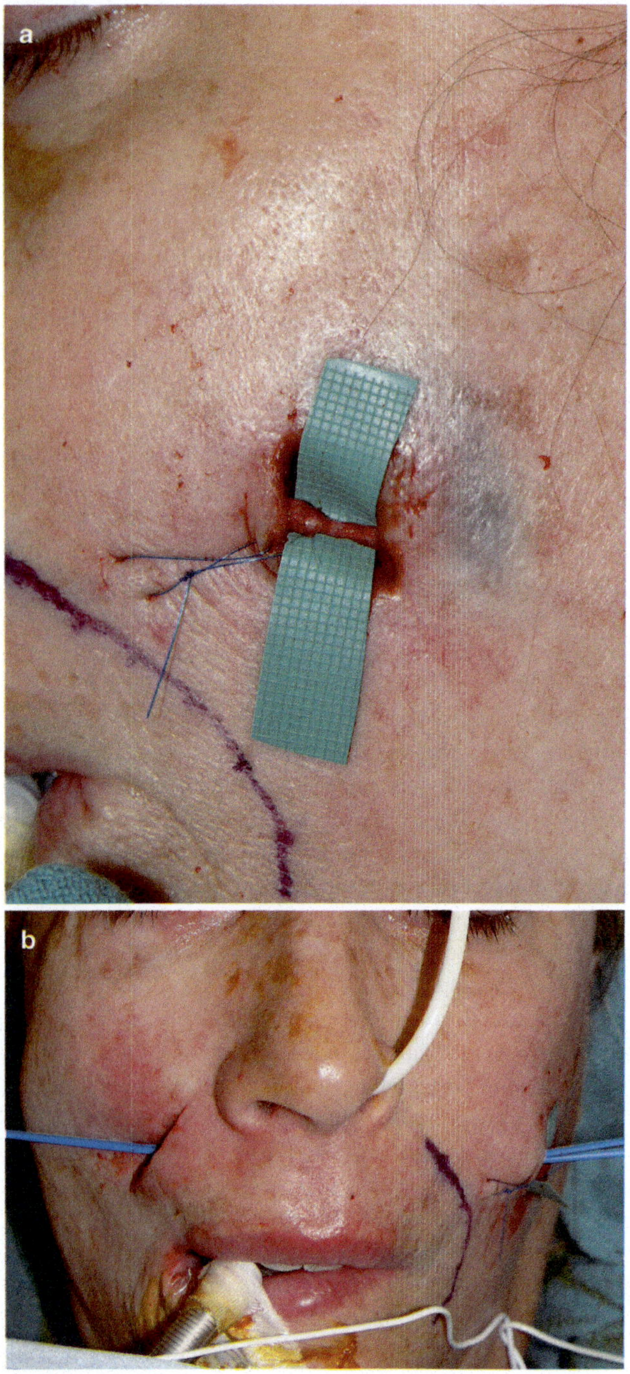

Fig. 24.6 A buccal branch of the normally functioning facial nerve is divided, and a neurorrhaphy is performed to a sural nerve graft (**a**). The nerve graft is tunneled subcutaneously to the affected side of the face (**b**). Prior to sacrifice of the buccal branch, a second branch is identified and stimulated to ensure that the lip elevator muscles are still innervated

will be reused for the muscle free flap transfer. At the time of second-stage surgery, the distal end of the graft can be biopsied to insure that axonal growth has occurred. Single-stage muscle transfer with cross facial innervation has been described with encouraging results, although there is a theoretic risk of muscle atrophy and motor end plate degeneration occurring during the long time period that elapses while axonal regrowth into the muscle flap is occurring [21]. Microvascular anastomoses are to the facial artery and vein as they cross the lower border of the mandible. The preauricular incision is usually curved anteriorly into a transverse neck skin crease to provide adequate exposure of the facial vessels.

Static Facial Reanimation

Facial nerve rehabilitative procedures can also be of great help to patients. They have a low rate of complications and typically do not require revision surgery. Immediate rehabilitation has the advantage of sparing the patient some of the morbidity of facial paralysis, especially during and immediately after adjuvant therapy when further surgery may be risky. Rose [22] and Deleyiannis et al. [23] have shown that facial nerve recovery is not prevented by facial paralysis rehabilitative procedures performed at the time of the initial surgery and believe static procedures complement nerve repair. Golio et al. [24] also did not find a higher rate of complications nor an effect on symptomatic improvement in eye exposure in patients who had early periocular surgeries for facial nerve rehabilitation, before radiation therapy was administered, compared to patients who had the same procedures in a delayed setting.

Brow/Forehead

Eyebrow symmetry can be attained by disabling the intact contralateral normal temporal branch with a neurectomy. The problem with this approach is that the brows may become too ptotic and create a tired or stern appearance and, in some individuals, result in superior visual field obstruction. Chemodenervation with botulinum toxin of the contralateral nonparalyzed side of the frontalis and other facial muscles is a temporary procedure that can also be attempted to improve symmetry. If favorable results in appearance and function are achieved, then permanent denervation with neurectomy can be performed.

A browlift procedure is more commonly performed in the cancer population, where the mean age and, consequently, the incidence of natural brow ptosis are relatively high. An endoscopic or pretrichial browlift may be sufficient in mild cases of asymmetry, but a direct (just above the brow), or indirect (within a mid-forehead rhytid), browlift generally results in a

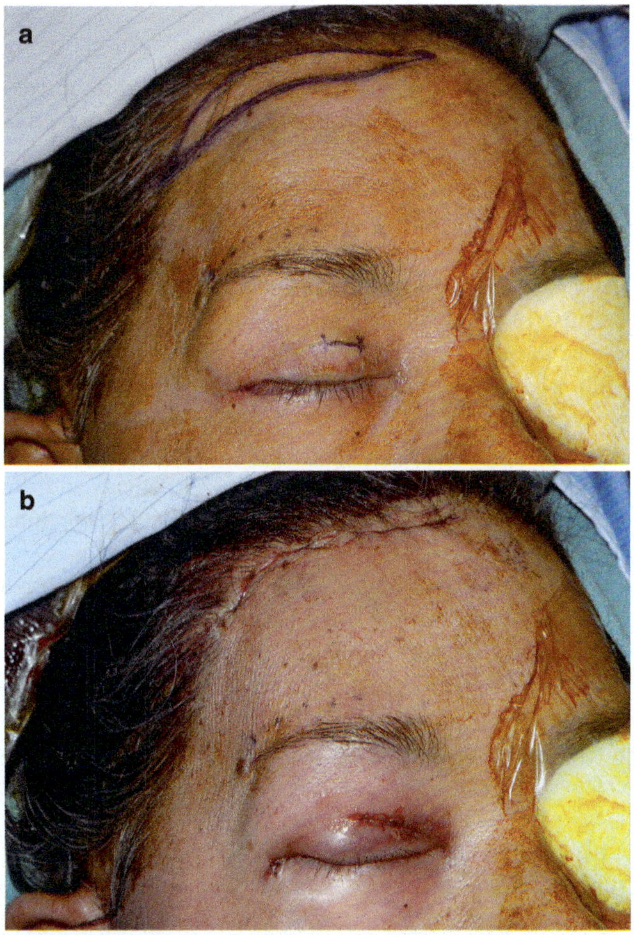

Fig. 24.7 A pretrichial browlift is performed for brow ptosis following facial nerve resection. Skin markings for the browlift as well as for upper eyelid gold weight placement (**a**). Immediate result (**b**)

much greater degree of correction (Fig. 24.7). A skin excision is performed to elevate the skin as appropriate for symmetry with the contralateral side as measured when the patient is awake with their eyes open. Overcorrection is sometimes needed if the patient tends to have a hyperactive contralateral frontalis muscle (due to natural senile brow ptosis), or a bilateral procedure can be performed. The frontalis muscle is also suspended to the frontal periosteum before the skin is closed with long-acting absorbable or permanent sutures.

Upper Eyelid

Patients with facial nerve paralysis have difficulty closing the affected upper eyelid but can open normally because the levator palpebrae superioris, which is innervated by the oculomotor nerve (cranial nerve III), is still intact. Gold eyelid weights can be very reliable with low rates of exposure

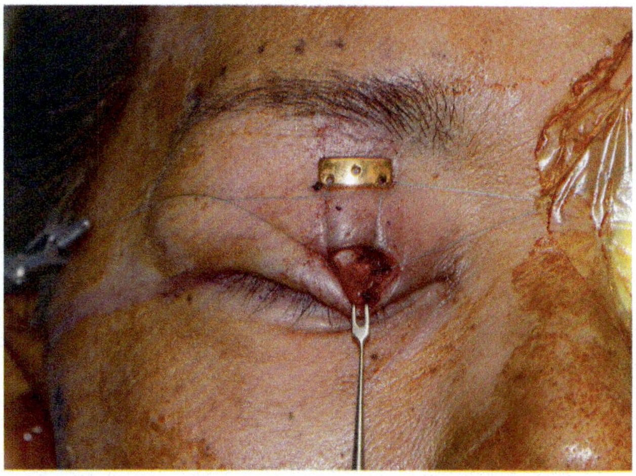

Fig. 24.8 A gold upper eyelid weight is about to be inserted superficial to the tarsal plate through a small incision made in the upper eyelid crease. It is secured with three fine, nonabsorbable sutures to the perichondrium of the tarsal plate

(under 10% in a series of 104 weights reported by Rofagha and Seiff) [25]. Such weights are available in weights ranging from 0.6 to 1.8 g in 0.2 g increments. Ideally, the appropriate weight is chosen preoperatively in the office by taping sample implants to the upper lid and observing for complete eye closure.

Most commonly, a 1.0 g weight is the appropriate starting point and is also chosen when facial paralysis does not exist at the time of preoperative evaluation. If the weight turns out to be inappropriate, it can easily be exchanged for another weight at a later date, under local anesthesia in the office if need be, to avoid delaying adjuvant treatment. Alternatively, gold eyelid weight placement can be performed in a delayed manner, and eye closure can be managed with nonsurgical methods such as lubrication and lid taping. Also, as facial nerve function improves following nerve repair or nerve transfer, eyelid weights can be removed or downsized. Platinum weights are also available and have the advantage of being thinner because of the increased density of platinum compared to gold.

Placement is via a small incision made in the supratarsal crease. A precise pocket is dissected superficial to the tarsal plate as close as possible to the lid margin. The gold weight is secured to the perichondrium using 7-0 polypropylene sutures (Fig. 24.8). The incision is closed with a 6-0 absorbable running suture.

Lower Eyelid

Lower lid laxity resulting in ectropion is most frequently treated with lid tightening procedures, such as lateral canthoplasty using a tarsal strip technique (Fig. 24.9). In this procedure, a

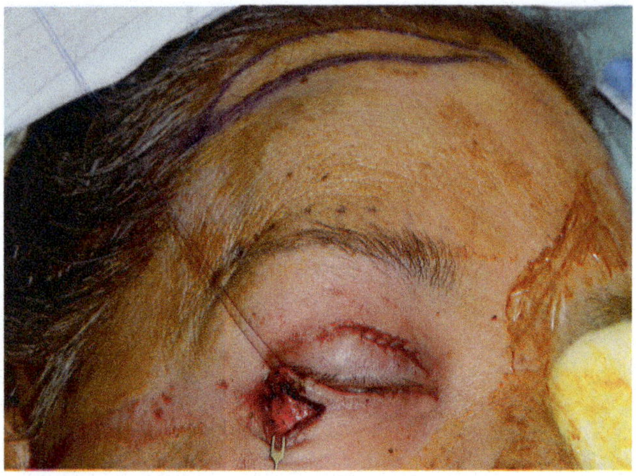

Fig. 24.9 A lateral canthoplasty (tarsal strip procedure). The denuded tarsal strip is suspended to the upper, inner lateral orbital rim periosteum with permanent suture

lateral canthotomy is made with scissors, and then a lower lid cantholysis is performed by cutting the lower lid canthal tendon. This should free the lower eyelid. A subciliary incision is made, and a short skin flap is elevated. The amount of canthal suspension is estimated by pulling on the canthal tendon in a lateral-superior vector. The lid margin is excised and the conjunctiva removed based on the amount of advancement anticipated. A horizontal mattress suture with long-lasting absorbable suture or permanent suture is used to suspend the denuded "tarsal strip" to the inner, upper lateral orbital periosteum. The suture is tied so that the knot faces superficially, away from the globe surface. Excess skin is conservatively trimmed, and then the subciliary incision and lateral canthotomy are closed with fine absorbable suture.

The lateral canthoplasty occasionally needs to be repeated for recurrent ectropion, particularly in elderly patients. Combining the lateral canthoplasty with a lateral tarsorrhaphy in which a few millimeters of both upper and lower lid margins are denuded and sutured to create a lid adhesion (tying the knot laterally, away from the cornea) can be used to treat severe ectropion and lagophthalmos, but horizontally narrows the lid aperture, which can be cosmetically unappealing. In some cases, even after fairly aggressive lid tightening with a lateral canthoplasty, there is residual medial lagophthalmos. A medial canthoplasty can augment the lateral canthoplasty by using sutures to plicate or suspend the lax medial canthal tendon to the medial orbital periosteum. Care needs to be taken not to constrict or suture through the upper and lower tear duct canaliculi when performing a medial canthoplasty.

Cheek and Mouth

A flaccid cheek and downturned lower face with an adynamic commissure can interfere with speech and oral competence, as well as nasal breathing due to nasal alar collapse. Both static and dynamic (described above) procedures have been designed to address the lower face. Static procedures consist of subcutaneous fascia or tendon graft suspension. The author prefers to use fascia lata of the thigh because of its abundance and the fact that it can be harvested through the same donor site incision simultaneously with preparation of the anterolateral thigh free flap, which is often used for concurrent soft tissue reconstruction (Fig. 24.10) [26]. Others have described using the plantaris tendon, which is present in about 85% of patients and can be obtained through a short transverse incision just behind the medial malleolus.

The author usually uses either several grafts or splits a single graft into several slips distally to suspend the oral commissure, the upper lip at the nasolabial crease, and the nasal ala. The graft is tunneled from a preauricular incision to each of these target areas. Slips of fascia are cut to differing lengths to achieve the desired amount of pull needed to create symmetry with the contralateral side. A small counter-incision at each site is made, and the distal slips of the graft are secured to the deep fascia and dermis with permanent suture. The slip that goes to the oral commissure is further split so that it attaches to the orbicularis muscles of the upper and lower lips and the modiolus at the commissure. The counter-incisions are closed first, and then the proximal fascia graft(s) are secured to the zygomatic arch periosteum under tension in the appropriate vector needed to match the contralateral direction of muscular movement. Overcorrection is desirable as the amount of suspension rapidly decreases over the first 2 weeks following surgery, after which it usually stabilizes.

In unilateral facial paralysis, the paralyzed lower lip is higher than the contralateral side due to absence of lower lip depressor function supplied by the marginal mandibular branch of the facial nerve. The contralateral normally functioning lower lip depressors can be temporarily paralyzed with botulinum toxin to restore symmetry to the smile. If permanent correction is desired, a marginal mandibular neurectomy can be performed through a direct incision about one fingerbreadth below the lower mandibular border. The marginal mandibular nerve can be reliably located beneath the platysma muscle running transversely across the superficial surface of the facial vein.

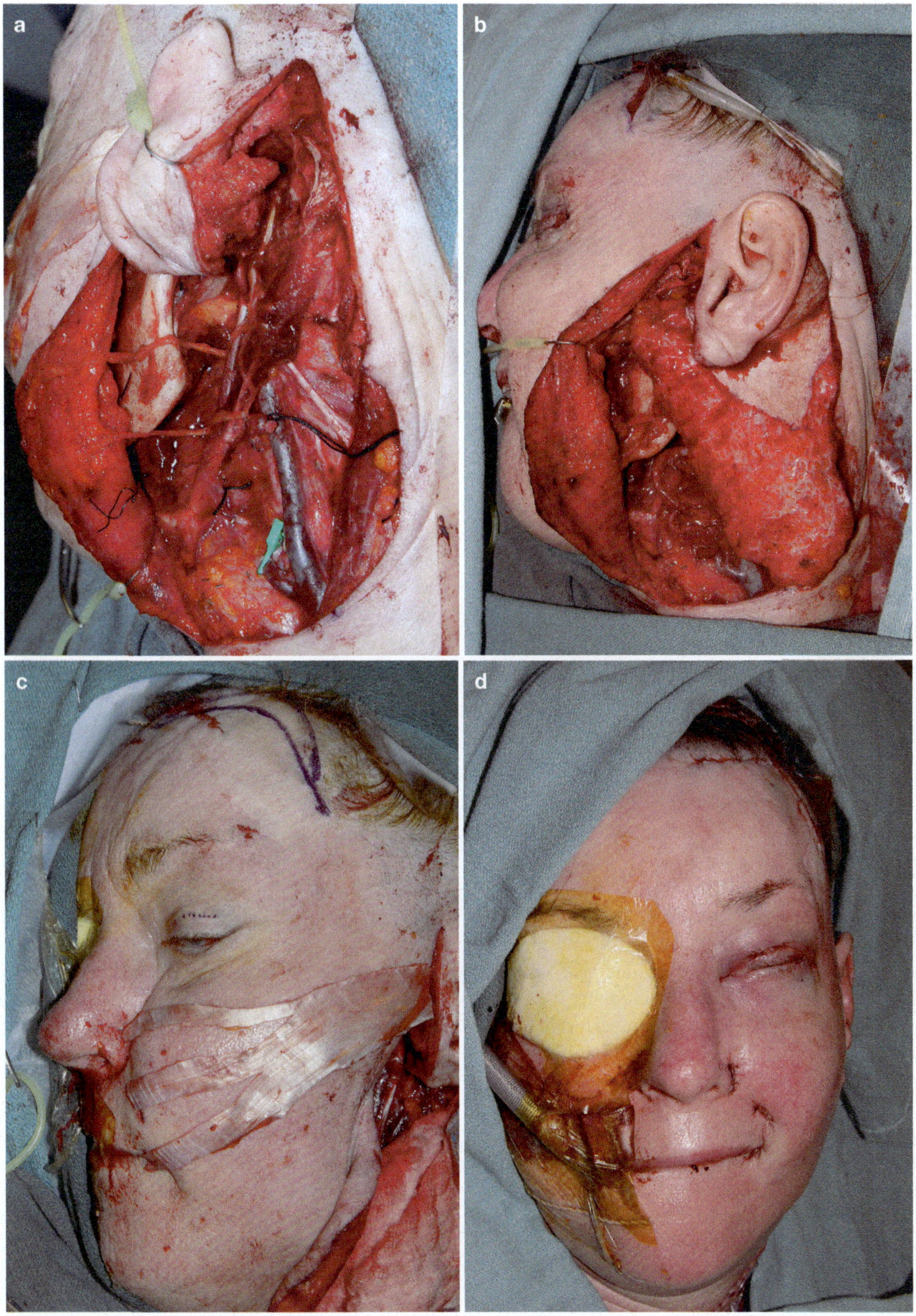

Fig. 24.10 Example of a temporal bone and parotidectomy reconstruction, including cable nerve grafting with the lateral femoral cutaneous nerve (**a**), anterolateral thigh free flap soft tissue reconstruction (**b**), and a fascia lata graft from the thigh which is used for static reanimation of the lower face (**c**). The graft is split into separate slips to suspend the nasal ala, nasolabial fold, and the corner of the mouth to the periosteum of the zygoma. Immediate postoperative appearance (**d**). In addition, a gold upper eyelid weight was placed, and a pretrichial browlift was performed. Postoperative result (**e**)

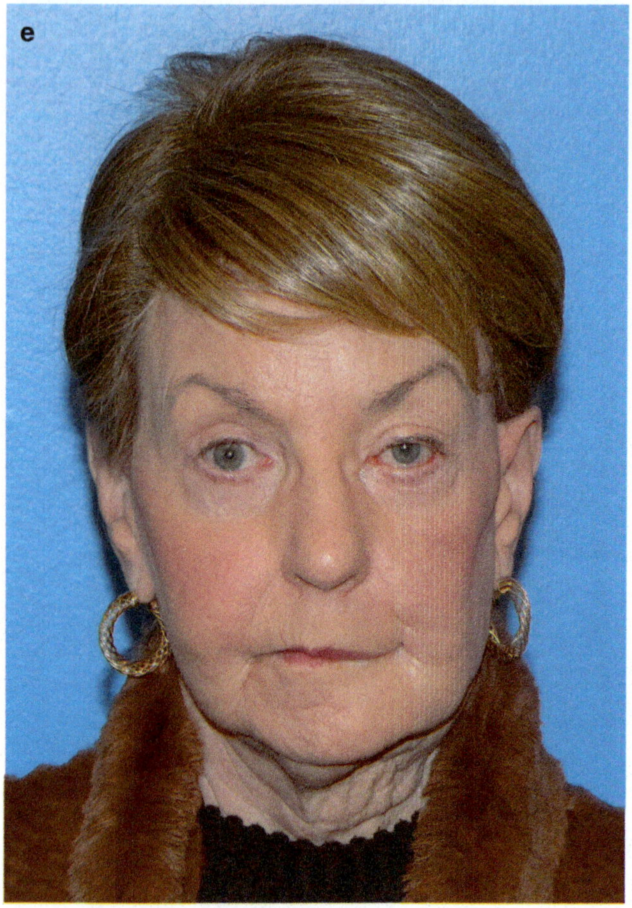

Fig. 24.10 (continued)

Reconstructive Algorithm

A reconstructive algorithm is summarized in Fig. 24.11. In the author's practice, all patients are considered for static procedures, regardless of whether dynamic procedures are planned. If the outcome of dynamic procedures is expected to be favorable, static procedures are not performed. If the outcome is felt to be unpredictable or only partial return of function after a relatively long delay is expected, static procedures are discussed with the patient. Static procedures can be performed secondarily if the degree of dysfunction and disfigurement is unknown or hard to predict preoperatively. However, in the cancer population, the author frequently performs static procedures immediately following tumor resection because the opportunity for secondary procedures is limited by the need to proceed with adjuvant therapy [5]. Performing simultaneous static procedures even if dynamic procedures are also performed can spare the patient much of the morbidity of facial nerve paralysis, including superior visual field obstruction, corneal exposure, epiphora, nasal obstruction secondary to alar collapse, speech impairment, and oral incompetence, during recovery from surgery and while undergoing adjuvant therapy. Static procedures are especially indicated in the elderly population because of skin and ligamentous laxity associated with senescence, and many patients may even benefit from bilateral procedures to correct problems with the contralateral, nonparalyzed side. Eyelid weight placement is often reversed or the weight downsized if facial nerve function returns following successful nerve repair, grafting, or transfer. Often, elderly or infirm patients may not desire or be good candidates for additional surgery with a motorized muscle free flap, and immediate static procedures are the best option.

With regard to dynamic procedures, nerve repair and cable nerve grafting are performed whenever the proximal and distal facial nerve stumps can be identified. If not, nerve transfer is considered. Free muscle transfer has usually been performed as a secondary procedure, mainly due to the long length of skull base resection and soft and bony tissue flap reconstruction. Also, the effect of postoperative radiation therapy to a motorized muscle free flap has not been well studied. However, in selected cases, immediate dynamic reconstruction with a muscle free flap innervated by nerve coaptation to the masseteric nerve can be considered, particularly when radiation therapy is not planned.

Postoperative Care

Patients should be counseled about wearing eye protection when blinking is impaired. The eyes should be lubricated frequently with hydroxypropyl methylcellulose eye drops during the day and a more viscous ointment during the night. When passive eye closure is incomplete, the eye can be taped laterally (rather than over the cornea) or a moisture chamber can be obtained. Patients especially at risk for exposure keratitis and corneal ulceration are those with combined cranial nerve V and VII deficits with an absent corneal reflex and decreased corneal sensation.

The benefit of physical therapy in facial nerve recovery following repair has not been well studied. There are significant variations in technique and limited outcome data using validated quantitative measurements. Retraining following nerve transfer or motorized free muscle flap reconstruction is likely of benefit. When the masseteric nerve is used to supply either the facial muscles or a muscle free flap, the patient must learn to create facial movement by biting down on the ipsilateral side of the jaw. Eventually, many patients can learn to move their face even without clenching the teeth, and some can develop a spontaneous smile.

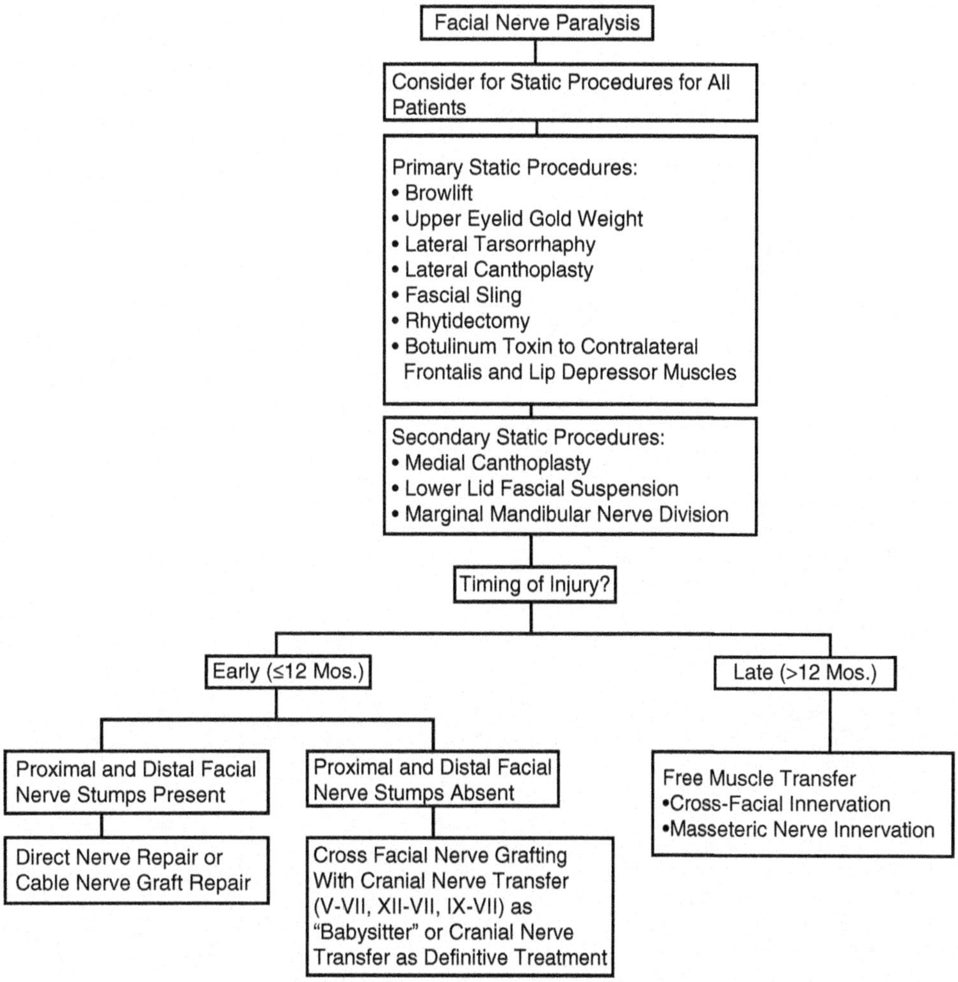

Fig. 24.11 Algorithm for addressing facial nerve defects in head and neck cancer patients

References

1. House JW, Brackmann DE. Facial nerve grading system. Otolaryngol Head Neck Surg. 1985;93:146–7.
2. Brown PD, Eshleman JS, Foote RL, Strome SE. An analysis of facial nerve function in irradiated and unirradiated facial nerve grafts. Int J Radiat Oncol Biol Phys. 2000;48:737–43.
3. Iseli TA, Harris G, Dean NR, Iseli CE, Rosenthal EL. Outcomes of static and dynamic facial nerve repair in head and neck cancer. Laryngoscope. 2010;120:478–83.
4. Gidley PW, Herrera SJ, Hanasono MM, et al. The impact of radiotherapy on facial nerve repair. Laryngoscope. 2010;120:1985–9.
5. Hanasono MM, Silva AK, Yu P, Skoracki RJ, Sturgis EM, Gidley PW. Comprehensive management of temporal bone defects after oncologic resection. Laryngoscope. 2012;122:2663–9.
6. Korte W. Nerve grafting: facial nerve on hypoglossal. Dtsch Med Wochenschr. 1903;29:293–5.
7. Conley J. Hypoglossal crossover: 122 cases. Trans Sect Otolaryngol Am Acad Ophtalmol Otolaryngol. 1977;84:ORL 763–8.
8. Koh KS, Kim JK, Kim CJ, et al. Hypoglossal–facial crossover in facial-nerve palsy: pure end-to-side anastomosis technique. Br J Plast Surg. 2002;55:25–31.
9. Spira M. Anastomosis of masseteric nerve to lower division of facial nerve for correction of lower facial paralysis. Plast Reconstr Surg. 1978;61:330–4.
10. Matketlow RT, Tomat LR, Zuker RM, Chang M. Smile reconstruction adults with free muscle transfer innervated by the masseter motor nerve: effectiveness and cerebral adaptation. Plast Reconstr Surg. 2006;118:885–9.
11. Coombs CJ, Ek EW, Wu T, Cleland H, Leung MK. Masseteric-facial coaptation: an alternative technique for facial nerve reinnervation. J Plast Reconstr Aesthet Surg. 2008;62:1580–8.
12. Klebuc MJ. Facial reanimation using the masseter-to-facial nerve transfer. Plast Reconstr Surg. 2011;1127:1909–15.
13. Anderl H. Reconstruction of the face through cross-face nerve transplantation in facial paralysis. Eur J Plast Surg. 1973;2:17–45.
14. Scaramella LF. Anastomosis between the two facial nerves. Laryngoscope. 1975;85:1359–66.
15. Baker DC, Conley J. Facial nerve grafting: a thirty-year retrospective review. Clin Plast Surg. 1979;6:343–60.
16. Terzis JK, Tzaffetta K. The 'babysitter' procedure: minihypoglossal to facial nerve transfer and cross-facial nerve grafting. Plast Reconstr Surg. 2009;123:865–76.
17. Terzis JK, Manktelow RT. Pectoralis minor: a new concept in facial reanimation. Plast. Surg Forum. 1982;5:106–10.
18. Dellon AL, Mackinnon SE. Segmentally innervated latissimus dorsi muscle. Microsurgical transfer for facial animation. J Reconstr Microsurg. 1985;2:7–12.
19. Harii K, Ohmori K, Torii S. Free gracilis muscle transplantation with microneurovascular anastomoses for the treatment of facial paralysis. A preliminary report. Plast Reconstr Surg. 1976;57:133–43.

20. Birgfeld C, Neligan P. Surgical approaches to facial nerve deficits. Skull Base. 2011;21:177–84.
21. Kumar PA, Hassan KM. Cross-face nerve graft with free-muscle transfer for reanimation of the paralyzed face: a comparative study of the single-stage and two-stage procedures. Plast Reconstr Surg. 2002;109:441–62.
22. Rose EH. Autogenous fascia lata grafts: clinical applications in reanimation of the totally or partially paralyzed face. Plast Reconstr Surg. 2005;116:20–32.
23. Deleyiannis FWB, Askari M, Schmidt KL, et al. Muscle activity in the partially paralyzed face after placement of a fascial sling: a preliminary report. Ann Plast Surg. 2005;55:449–55.
24. Golio D, De Matelaere S, Anderson J, et al. Outcomes of periocular reconstruction for facial nerve paralysis in cancer patients. Plast Reconstr Surg. 2007;119:1233–7.
25. Rofagha S, Seiff SR. Long-term results for the use of gold eyelid load weights in the management of facial paralysis. Plast Reconstr Surg. 2010;125:142–9.
26. Hanasono MM, Sacks JM, Goel N, Ayad M, Skoracki RJ. The anterolateral thigh free flap for skull base reconstruction. Otolaryngol Head Neck Surg. 2009;140:855–60.

Reconstructive Techniques for Temporal Bone Cancer

25

Albert H. Chao and Matthew M. Hanasono

Introduction

Reconstruction of defects resulting from oncologic temporal bone resection can be challenging for the reconstructive surgeon. Temporal bone resections may include substantial cutaneous defects as well as exposed cranial nerves, major blood vessels, and dura mater or the brain. In addition to skin deficits, there can be substantial contour abnormalities, partial or total loss of the auricle, and transection of the facial nerve. Furthermore, there is the potential for major, life-threatening complications that may occur should the reconstruction fail, such as dural or brain exposure, pneumocephalus, cerebrospinal fluid (CSF) leak, meningitis, and osteomyelitis [1, 2]. Reconstructive techniques that minimize the risk of these complications and restore facial appearance and function have become a critical part of the management of patients undergoing resections for temporal bone cancer. Advances in reconstruction and oncologic treatment have substantially decreased the morbidity and increased the efficacy of skull base tumor treatment, as they minimize wound healing complications, restore function, and correct disfigurement.

Surgical Anatomy

The temporal bone is closely associated with a number of important underlying structures, including the cranial nerves (facial, glossopharyngeal, vagus, spinal accessory, hypoglossal), the internal jugular vein, the internal carotid artery, and the brain. Following tumor extirpation, exposure of these structures requires soft tissue coverage or functional reconstruction as in cases involving facial nerve transection.

A. H. Chao, M.D. (✉)
The Ohio State University Plastic Surgery, Columbus, OH, USA
e-mail: Albert.Chao@osumc.edu

M. M. Hanasono, M.D.
Department of Plastic Surgery, The University of Texas
M.D. Anderson Cancer Center, Houston, TX, USA
e-mail: mhanasono@mdanderson.org

Preoperative Considerations

A detailed preoperative history, physical exam, and work-up including imaging should be undertaken in order to identify the specific reconstructive needs for each individual case. The goals of reconstruction following temporal bone resection depend on the extent of the defect and may include providing cutaneous wound closure, coverage of dura and neurovascular structures, prevention of cerebrospinal fluid leaks, restoring facial contour, compensating for loss of facial nerve function, and supporting an auricular prosthesis. Identifying these goals, in turn, allows for the appropriate selection and design of reconstructive technique. The exam together with preoperative imaging (i.e., CT or MRI) allows the reconstructive surgeon to predict the extent of resection and counsel the patient appropriately on the procedures required for reconstruction.

A variety of potential functional deficits may result from resections of temporal bone cancers, including those related to loss of the facial, glossopharyngeal, vagus, spinal accessory, and hypoglossal nerves. In any case where transection of the facial nerve is a possibility, related reconstructive procedures and rehabilitation should be discussed with the patient preoperatively (Chap. 24). Resection of the vagus nerve can result in uncoordinated swallowing and aspiration, which may be addressed with temporary or permanent gastrostomy tube placement as well as postoperative speech and swallowing therapy. Unilateral hypoglossal nerve deficits are generally well tolerated but may also require speech and swallowing therapy. Vocal cord paralysis can be addressed by an otolaryngologist postoperatively with vocal cord injection of various filler materials and/or medialization thyroplasty. Transection of the spinal accessory nerve results in shoulder drop that is best addressed with physical therapy.

A discussion of the patient's desire for an auricular prosthesis should take place preoperatively since the desire for a prosthesis may influence flap selection, and consultation with an anaplastologist may be beneficial. Auricular prostheses may require osseointegrated implants for stable fixation, and consideration may be given to immediate placement,

P. W. Gidley, F. DeMonte (eds.), *Temporal Bone Cancer*, https://doi.org/10.1007/978-3-319-74539-8_25

particularly when postoperative radiation is anticipated since implants may be less reliable when placed after radiation. In many cases, placement of osseointegrated implants may be challenging after substantial resection of bone, since there must be fairly thick bone stock (about 3 mm around the implant on all sides) in order for the implant to be stable. In such cases, adhesive-retained rather than implant-retained prostheses may be the only option.

Reconstructive Techniques

General Considerations

All rungs of the reconstructive ladder should be considered in patients who may require reconstructive surgery for temporal bone cancers, ranging from simpler techniques such as primary closure and skin grafting to more complex microvascular free tissue transfers (Fig. 25.1). However, many defects will require local or regional flaps at a minimum, given the nature of resections, which often result in exposed critical structures, large cutaneous defects, and significant dead space. More recently, microvascular free flap reconstructions have been favored, given their greater versatility in achieving the various reconstructive goals in these patients and low rates of flap loss in the current era of microsurgery. Furthermore, these procedures can be effective even in the setting of advanced age, chemotherapy, tobacco use, and medical comorbidities [1, 2]. Although bone is commonly removed during tumor ablation, the focus of temporal bone reconstructions is generally on replacement of skin and soft tissue.

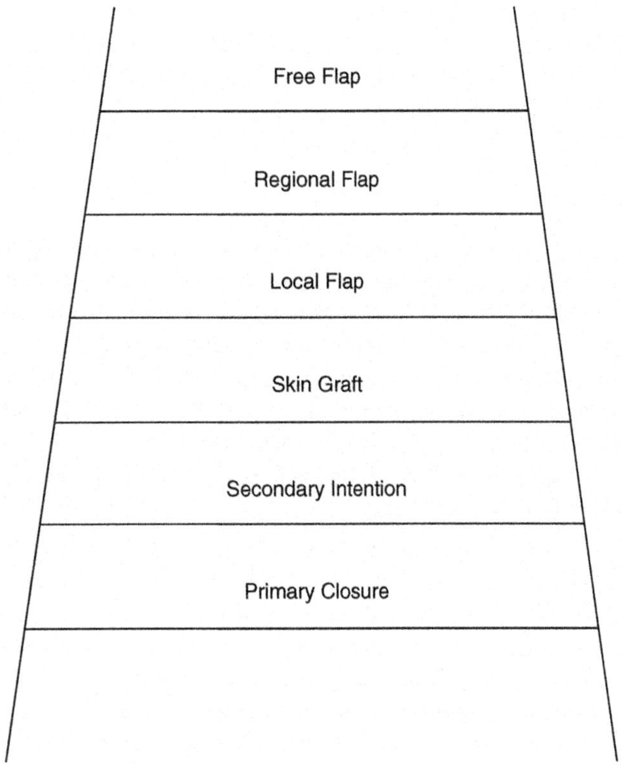

Fig. 25.1 The classic reconstructive ladder in which the simplest option is considered first and increasingly complex options are considered in succession only if the simpler options are not feasible. In skull base reconstruction, the reconstructive ladder concept still applies, with the understanding that the method chosen should produce the most reliable results as well as the best functional and cosmetic outcome provided the morbidity of that method is acceptable

Adjacent Tissue Transfer

The skin and subcutaneous tissues directly adjacent to the defect can sometimes be used to reconstruct temporal bone defects. The chief advantages of these techniques are the shorter operative times and lesser donor site morbidity involved compared to flap reconstructions. However, they have a number of disadvantages that limit their use in the reconstruction of temporal bone defects. These tissues are based on a random pattern blood supply; and therefore, their vascularity may be unreliable or compromised in patients who have been previously irradiated or operated. In addition, adjacent tissues in the temporal region are relatively limited in thickness and amount; and thus they are not able to fill dead space nor provide durable coverage over critical structures nor address contour abnormalities. Therefore, adjacent tissue rearrangement techniques tend to be most useful for small defects in nonirradiated and unoperated beds.

The most commonly described types of adjacent tissue rearrangement for temporal bone reconstruction include cervicofacial and scalp flaps [3, 4]. Cervicofacial flaps utilize adjacent cheek and neck tissues that are transposed from an inferior to superior direction and involve incisions that extend into the neck and sometimes to the shoulder and chest, depending on the amount of tissue needed. Additional advancement can be gained by making back cuts or skin grafting of the donor site. Scalp tissues may also be used to reconstruct temporal bone defects and are designed in a similar fashion to those used for the reconstruction of scalp defects, typically as large rotation-advancement flaps. Galeal scoring of scalp flaps and skin grafting of their donor sites can allow for further flap transposition.

Local Flaps

Local flaps are most useful for limited defects of the temporal bone region or for reinforcing dural repairs. Those that have been described for use in temporal bone reconstruction include temporalis muscle flaps, pericranial flaps, and temporoparietal fascia flaps [5–7]. The most useful of these options is the temporalis muscle flap due to its greater bulk and size. The temporalis muscle is supplied by the anterior and posterior deep temporal arteries that are located on its deep aspect. During harvest, the flap is first elevated along its superficial aspect in a suprafascial plane. Anteriorly, prior to reaching the superficial temporal fat pad, the deep temporal fascia should then be entered to expose the temporalis muscle, and further anterior to this, the temporal branch of the facial nerve has a superficial course [8]. The temporalis muscle flap can then be incised along its anterior, superior, and posterior margins and then elevated on its deep aspect off of the bone of the temporal fossa. A split temporalis muscle flap can also be used based on either the anterior or posterior deep temporal arteries. Donor site morbidity is minimal with the temporalis flap, although patients may develop temporal hollowing when the entire muscle is used.

Regional Flaps

Traditionally, the most commonly described regional pedicled flaps for temporal bone reconstruction have been the pectoralis major and trapezius myocutaneous flaps [9, 10]. However, their use is typically restricted to modest defects, as the arc of rotation of flaps from the torso is limited for the head and neck region, which often barely reaches the superior-most extent of temporal bone defects. Furthermore, postoperative contracture of regional pedicled muscle flaps over time can restrict neck movement. More recently, other pedicled regional flaps have been reported for use in temporal bone reconstruction, including the submental and supraclavicular flaps. The submental flap can be performed as a musculocutaneous flap based off of the submental branch of the facial artery and can include the bilateral mylohyoid and bilateral anterior bellies of the digastric muscles in a unilateral flap reconstruction [11, 12]. The supraclavicular flap is a fasciocutaneous flap based off of the supraclavicular artery. When used for temporal bone reconstruction, the distal skin paddle is typically extended laterally over the deltoid muscle to increase its extent [13, 14]. Both flaps are associated with minimal donor site morbidity.

Free Flaps

Microvascular free flap reconstruction may be required for a number of commonly encountered clinical scenarios in patients with temporal bone cancers. Free flaps are preferred when extensive resections have resulted in large cutaneous defects or significant dead space, since local and regional flaps are limited in the quantity of tissue they are able to provide. Free flaps are also often advisable in previously irradiated or operated fields where local tissues have been compromised. Lastly, free flaps provide more reliable coverage when critical structures, such as dura or the carotid system, are exposed.

A variety of different free flaps have been described for use in the reconstruction of temporal bone defects including the anterolateral thigh, gracilis, lateral arm, latissimus dorsi, omental, scapular, radial forearm, and rectus abdominis flaps [15–19]. The ideal donor site is one that provides a sufficient amount of skin and muscle tissue, allows for a two-team approach (i.e., does not require repositioning or re-prepping), has minimal associated morbidity, and confers a long pedicle length. Historically, the rectus abdominis myocutaneous (RAM) flap has been favored for microsurgical reconstruction of temporal bone defects (Fig. 25.2) [15, 18]. The RAM flap can provide a large skin paddle, up to 8 cm in width that extends from the costal margin to the pubis if needed. It is supplied by the deep inferior epigastric artery and its paired venae comitantes, which arise from the external iliac artery and vein, respectively. Multiple cutaneous perforating vessels pierce the rectus abdominis muscle and supply the overlying skin. However, although the RAM flap allows for simultaneous harvest and resection, as well as consistent anatomy with a long vascular pedicle, the tissue can sometimes be excessively thick or bulky and carries a potential risk of an abdominal donor site hernia.

More recently, the anterolateral thigh (ALT) flap has become a more favored option for temporal bone reconstruction. The ALT flap possesses all of the advantages of the RAM flap but has minimal donor site morbidity and a more suitable thickness, which is supported by lower revision rates when compared to the RAM flap (Fig. 25.3) [1, 17, 20]. The ALT flap can be harvested with similar dimensions to the RAM flap and is based on the descending branch of the lateral circumflex femoral artery and its paired venae comitantes, which can be found along the axis of an imaginary line drawn between the anterior superior iliac spine (ASIS) and the upper lateral border of the patella. Another advantage of this flap is that the associated nerve, the lateral femoral cutaneous nerve, which arises within a few centimeters of the ASIS and travels toward the knee along the mid-patellar line, can be sacrificed with minimal morbidity and used as a nerve graft in those cases where facial nerve grafting is indicated (see Chap. 24). Additionally, fascia associated with the tensor fascia lata muscle, which forms the iliotibial band, can be harvested and used as a graft in static facial reanimation.

With regard to recipient artery choice for microvascular free flaps, the facial and distal external carotid arteries are most commonly used. Free flap inset is typically configured such that the muscle component fills the deep portion of the wound and the skin paddle resurfaces the cutaneous defect, if present (Fig. 25.4). If there is no cutaneous defect, the skin paddle can be de-epithelialized and buried (Fig. 25.5). When composite defects exist where other adjacent structures have

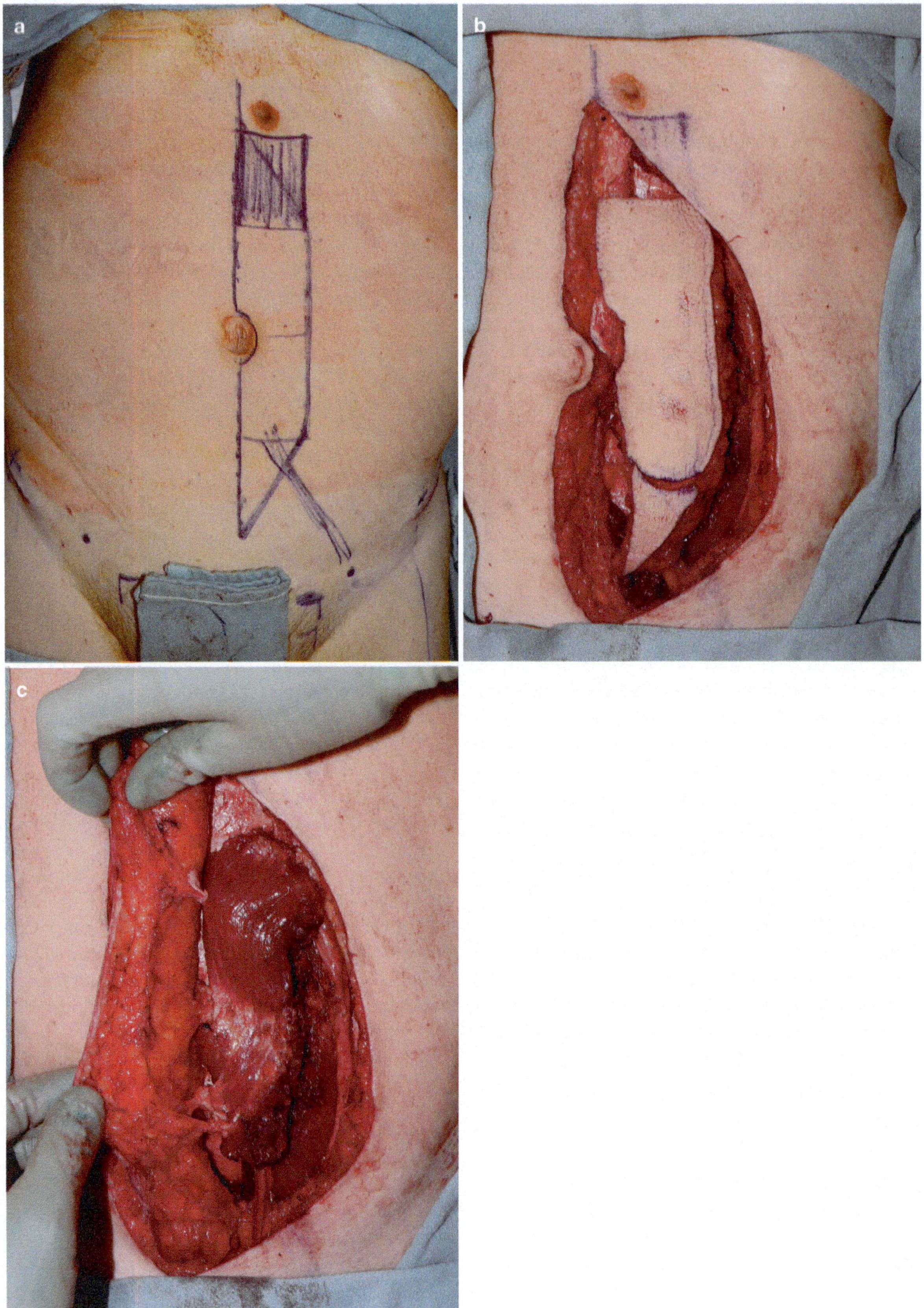

Fig. 25.2 The rectus abdominis myocutaneous (RAM) free flap is one of the primary flap choices for temporal bone reconstruction. Skin markings for left RAM free flap (**a**). After flap elevation (**b**). View of the musculocutaneous perforators that supply blood to the skin paddle (**c**). The amount of muscle and skin with subcutaneous fat is tailored to the size of the defect

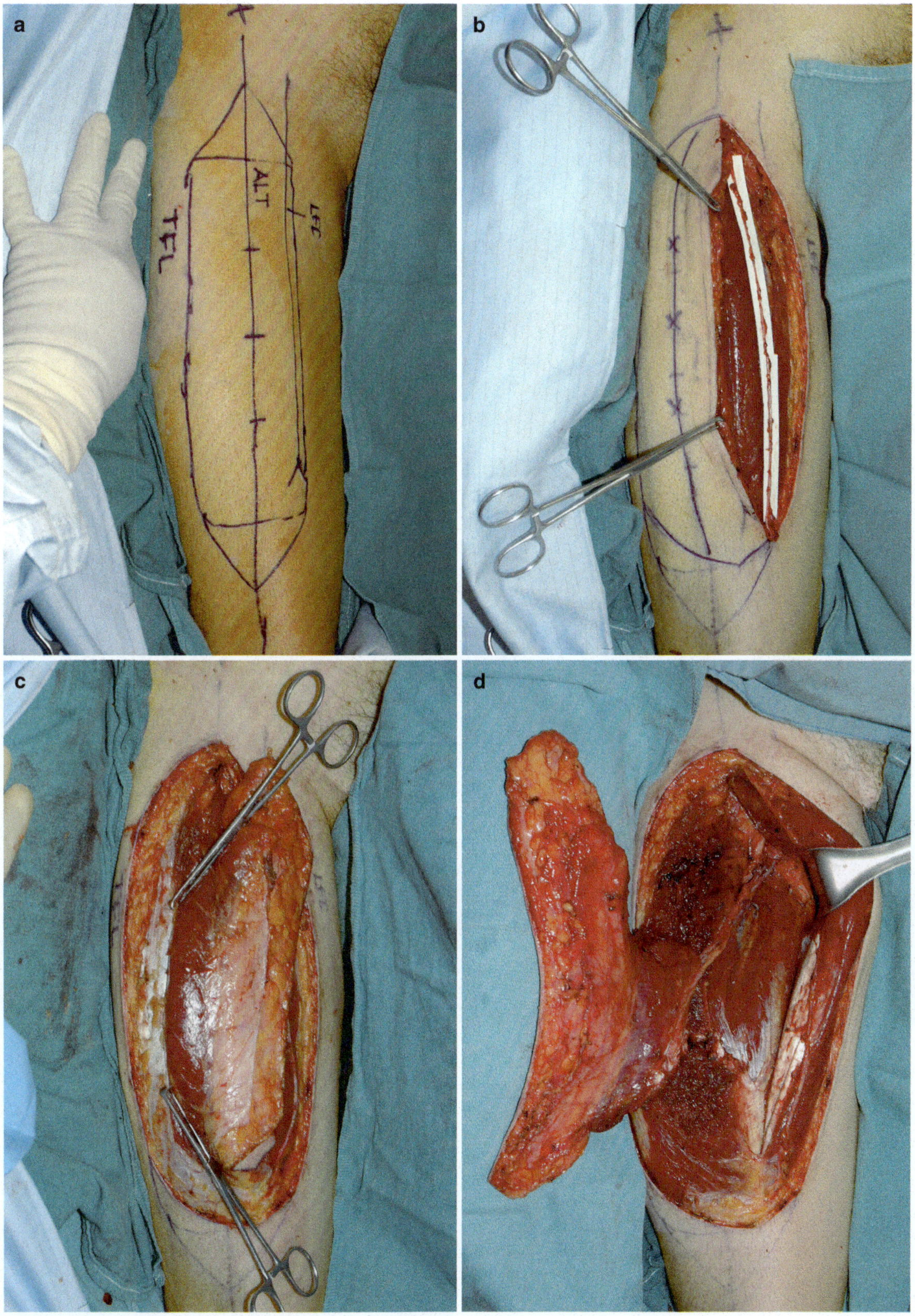

Fig. 25.3 The anterolateral thigh (ALT) free flap is our preferred flap for temporal bone reconstruction as it is usually intermediate in thickness between the RAM free flap and the radial forearm fasciocutaneous (RFF) free flap, which is often too thin to fill the dead space following temporal bone resection. Skin markings (**a**). The lateral femoral cutaneous (LFC) nerve can also be harvested as a nerve graft (**b**), and a fascial graft from the tensor fascia lata (TFL) can be harvested for static facial reanimation (**c**) from the same donor site when the facial nerve is paralyzed or needs to be sacrificed. The ALT free flap can be designed to include a portion of the vastus lateralis muscle depending on the size of the defect (**d**)

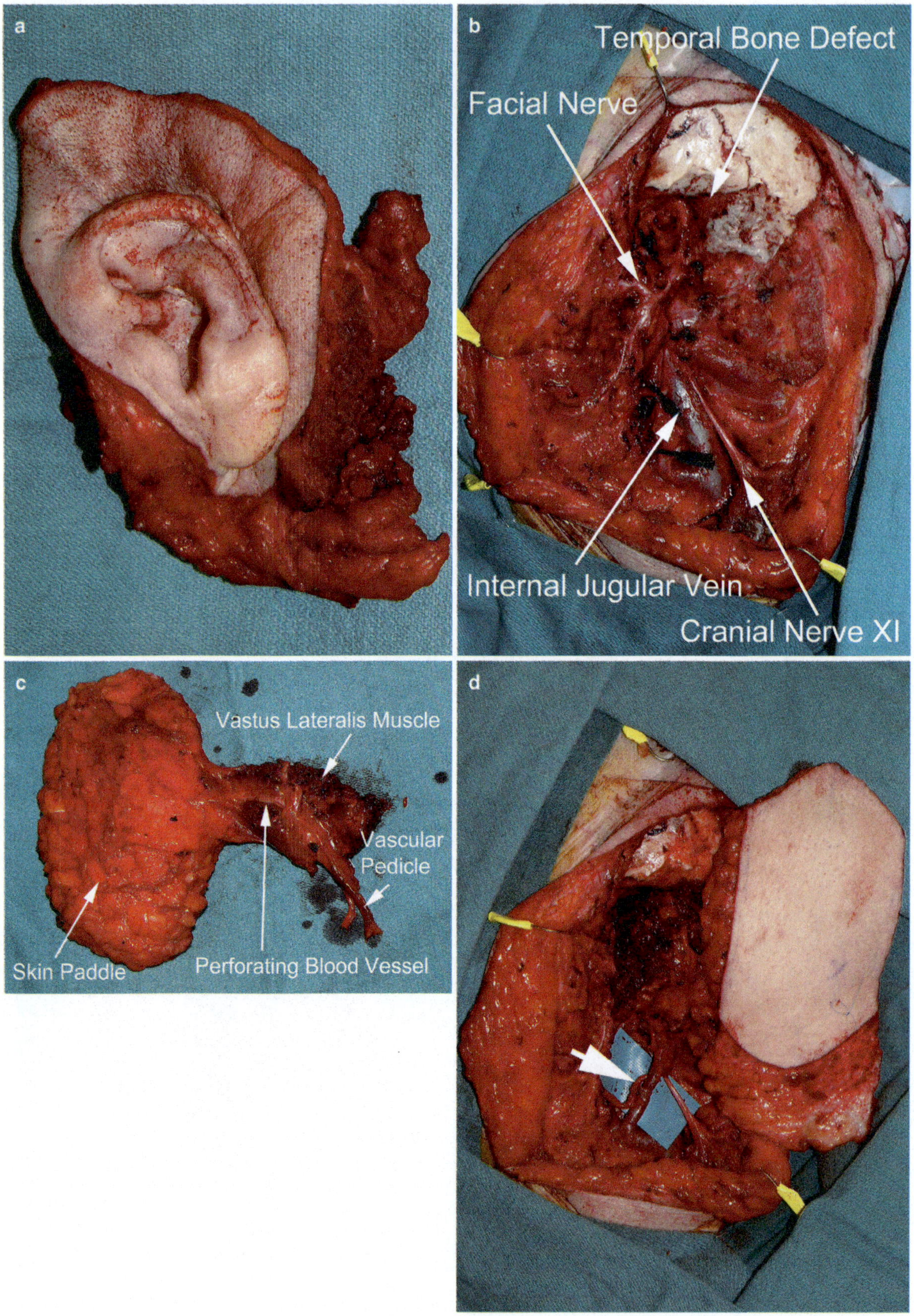

Fig. 25.4 Specimen from a lateral temporal bone resection and total auriculectomy for a recurrent postauricular skin cancer (**a**). The surgical defect following left temporal bone resection (**b**). An ALT free flap is used to reconstruct the defect (**c**). The vastus lateralis muscle component is placed into the deep portion of the wound and is used to occlude the Eustachian tube orifice (**d**). Postoperative appearance (**e**)

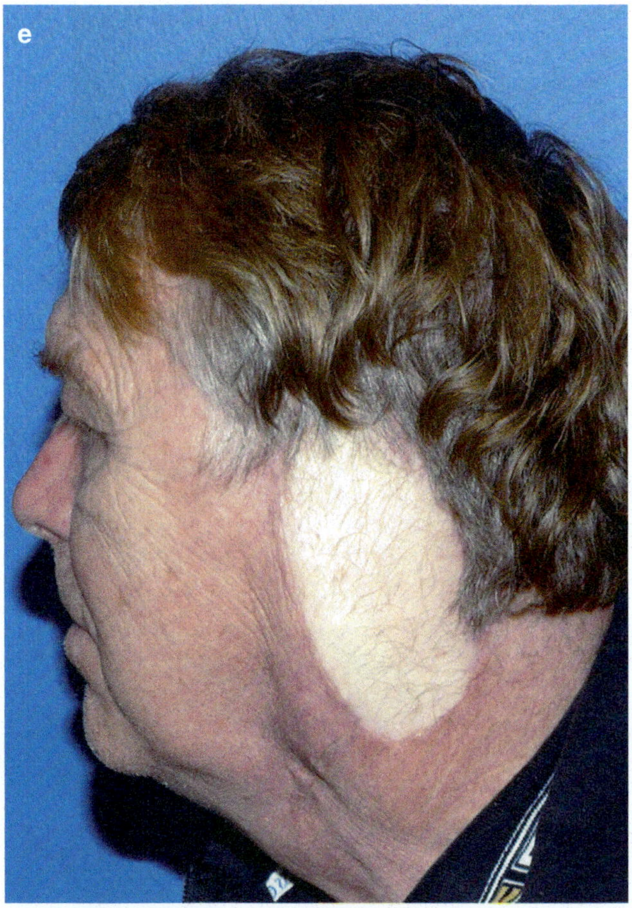

Fig. 25.4 (continued)

been resected such as the parotid gland, posterior mandible, or posterolateral maxilla, the ALT and RAM free flaps can be designed to include multiple skin paddles based on separate perforators, in order to address all defects. Microvascular anastomoses are performed to upper cervical blood vessels. If the facial artery and distal external carotid artery have been ligated and divided during the resection, then one of them is preferentially used as a recipient. Venous anastomoses are typically performed end-to-side to the internal jugular vein. Vein grafts are rarely, if ever, needed to reach the recipient blood vessels.

Other Reconstructive Considerations

The external ear, if resected, is usually best reconstructed at a separate stage in a delayed manner if postoperative radiation is anticipated. Prosthetic rehabilitation for total auricular reconstruction is usually the mainstay in oncologic surgery due to the lack of thin, pliable cutaneous tissue to cover a cartilaginous framework carved from costochondral grafts or alloplasts such as porous polyethylene. Partial defects of the auricle can be reconstructed with local tissue flaps or incorporated into the design of free flaps used for skull base reconstruction. If the facial nerve must be transected during tumor extirpation, a variety of different reconstructive techniques may be indicated, as discussed in Chap. 22.

Postoperative Care

Postoperative monitoring of both pedicled and free flaps is essential in patients who undergo temporal bone reconstruction. Flap color and capillary refill should be evaluated, as well as cutaneous Doppler signals in free flaps. Free flap monitoring is typically performed hourly for 48 h, followed by every 2 h for 48 h, and then every 4 h thereafter until discharge. For both pedicled and free flaps, attention should be paid to the neck position both during and after the procedure ensuring that there is no excessive tension, kinking, or compression of the vascular pedicle. Our preference is to use a closed suction drain beneath the flap as long as the risk for creating a CSF leak is low. Care is taken to place the drain at some distance from any dural repairs.

In addition to flap monitoring, routine cardiovascular and neurologic monitoring should also be performed. Postoperative computed tomography or magnetic resonance scans may be necessary, and great care must be exercised with patient movement in and out of the scanners. MRI may not be possible if implanted Dopplers are utilized. While it is not uncommon for there to be a small amount of intracranial air on imaging in the early postoperative period, clinical neurologic abnormalities and evidence of increasing pneumocephalus on serial imaging represent indications for prompt operative reexploration. Prophylactic antibiotics with good CSF penetration should be used to prevent perioperative infection, especially in patients with preexisting CSF leaks or in those who undergo dural reconstruction. Because placement of either a regional or free flap may inhibit the ability to detect a local recurrence by physical examination, serial imaging is mandatory for disease surveillance.

Patients typically stay at least 5 days in the hospital for monitoring when a free flap is performed as the rate of free flap loss drops precipitously following this time period. Patients with pedicled flaps need only stay in the hospital for the amount of time necessary for recovery from the skull base resection, since pedicled flap compromise is usually evident within the first 24 h. Drains are left in place until draining less than 30 ml of serous fluid per day, especially for the flap donor site since donor site seromas are relatively common. For most free flaps (i.e., ALT and RAM flaps), full weight-bearing ambulation is initiated as soon as cleared from a neurosurgical standpoint. Prophylactic antibiotics are used while the recipient site drain is in place, but not necessary for the donor site drain.

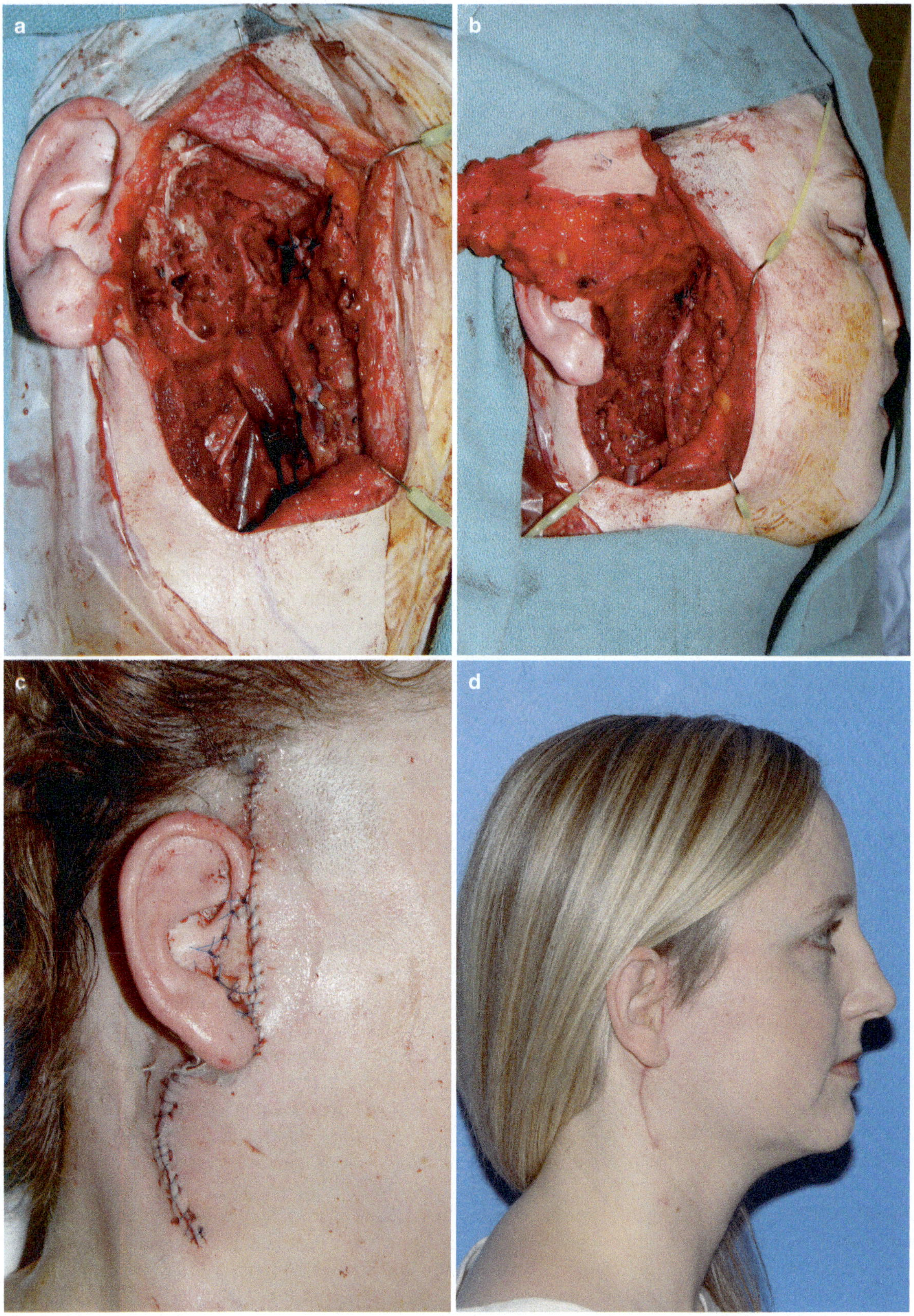

Fig. 25.5 Surgical defect following temporal bone resection in which the auricle has been preserved (**a**). An ALT free flap with vastus lateralis muscle is used to fill the dead space and restore facial contour (**b**). Most of the skin paddle is de-epithelialized except for a very small skin island that is used to close the external auditory canal wound (**c**). Postoperative appearance showing good contour and facial symmetry (**d**, **e**)

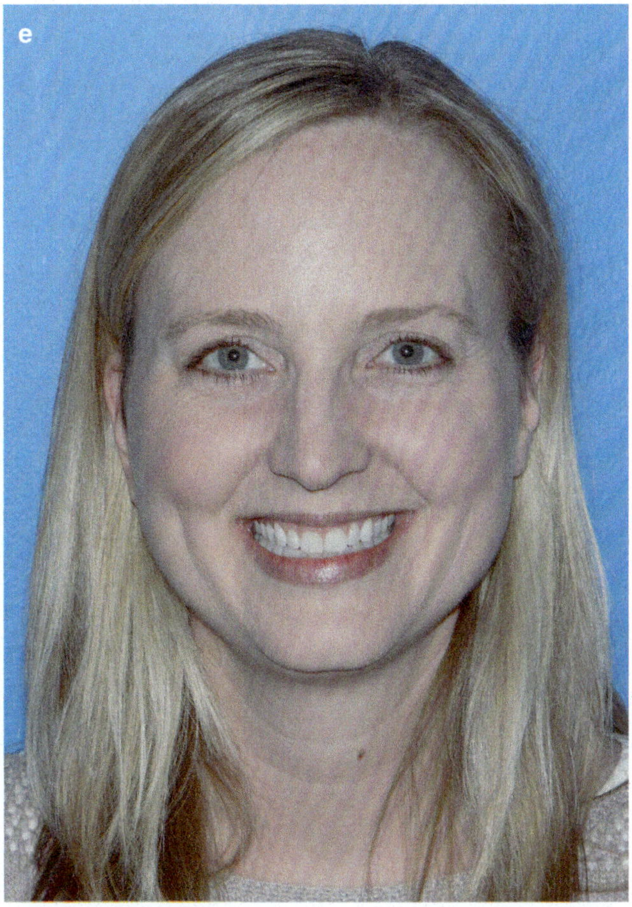

Fig. 25.5 (continued)

Complications

Patients undergoing skull base surgery are at risk for neurologic complications, including cerebrovascular accident, meningeal or brain infections, pneumocephalus, and CSF leak. Such complications should be managed with a neurosurgeon. Dural repairs and the likelihood of CSF leaks should be discussed intraoperatively at the commencement of the reconstruction. Inset of soft tissue flaps to completely cover sites of durotomy can help prevent CSF leaks. A judicious amount of volume overcorrection in these areas can be beneficial to ensure reinforcement of dural repairs, though not so much as to adversely affect intracranial pressure. Minor CSF leaks can sometimes be observed or treated with a lumbar drain, while recalcitrant or major CSF leaks may require further surgery.

Partial or total loss of local pedicled flaps, such as pericranial, temporoparietal fascia, and temporalis muscle flaps, can result if their vascular supply has been injured or ligated as a part of the resection, and this event can be avoided by confirming an intact vascular supply prior to flap harvest. These flaps may also be unreliable in previously irradiated patients. Although free flap loss will always remain a potential risk with microvascular reconstructions, the rates of this complication remain low (less than 2%) and do not appear to be increased in the skull base when compared to other sites in head and neck region [16]. Flap losses can rarely be managed with conservative measures in skull base reconstruction. Loss of a pedicled flap or a free flap usually necessitates attempt of an additional free flap because of the presence of dura and other critical neurovascular structures at the base of resection cavity. In most cases, a secondary free flap can be expected to have a success rate approaching that of an initial free flap [21].

Conclusions

Reconstructive surgery is often necessary in patients undergoing resections for temporal bone cancers. A number of different techniques of soft tissue reconstruction may be indicated, ranging from adjacent tissue transfer to microvascular free flaps. However, in many cases, pedicled and free flap reconstructions are required given the nature of defects that result from temporal bone resections. Preoperative evaluation and planning, including coordination with the otolaryngologist and neurosurgeon, as well as the intraoperative execution and postoperative care are all essential to the success of these often complex reconstructions.

References

1. Hanasono MM, Silva AK, Yu P, Skoracki RJ, Sturgis EM, Gidley PW. Comprehensive management of temporal bone defects after oncologic resection. Laryngoscope. 2012;122(12):2663–9.
2. Marzo SJ, Benscoter B, Leonetti JP. Contemporary options for lateral skull base reconstruction following tumor extirpation. Curr Opin Otolaryngol Head Neck Surg. 2011;19(5):330–4.
3. Moffat DA, Grey P, Ballagh RH, Hardy DG. Extended temporal bone resection for squamous cell carcinoma. Otolaryngol Head Neck Surg. 1997;116:158–60.
4. Moore BA, Wine T, Netterville JL. Cervicofacial and cervicothoracic rotation flaps in head and neck reconstruction. Head Neck. 2005;27:1092–101.
5. Patel R, Buchmann LO, Hunt J. The use of the temporoparietal fascial flap in preventing CSF leak after lateral skull base surgery. J Neurol Surg B Skull Base. 2013;74(5):311–6.
6. Smith JE, Ducic Y, Adelson RT. Temporalis muscle flap for reconstruction of skull base defects. Head Neck. 2010;32(2):199–203.
7. Stow NW, Gordon DH, Eisenberg R. Technique of temporoparietal fascia flap in ear and lateral skull base surgery. Otol Neurotol. 2010;31(6):964–7.
8. Hanasono MM, Utley DS, Goode RL. The temporalis muscle flap for reconstruction after head and neck oncologic surgery. Laryngoscope. 2001;111:1719–25.
9. Gal TJ, Kerschner JE, Futran ND, Bartels LJ, Farrior JB, Ridley MB, Klotch DW, Endicott JN. Reconstruction after temporal bone resection. Laryngoscope. 1998;108(4 Pt 1):476–81.

10. McLean JN, Carlson GW, Losken A. The pectoralis major myocutaneous flap revisited: a reliable technique for head and neck reconstruction. Ann Plast Surg. 2010;64(5):570–3.
11. Howard BE, Nagel TH, Barrs DM, Donald CB, Hayden RE. Reconstruction of lateral skull base defects: a comparison of the submental flap to free and regional flaps. Otolaryngol Head Neck Surg. 2016;154:1014–8.
12. Miller C, Hanley JC, Gernon TJ, Erman A, Jacob A. The submental island flap for reconstruction of temporal bone defects. Otol Neurotol. 2015;36(5):879–85.
13. Hunt JP, Buchmann LO. The supraclavicular artery flap for lateral skull and scalp defects: effective and efficient alternative to free tissue transfer. J Neurol Surg Rep. 2014;75(1):e5–10.
14. Kokot N, Mazhar K, Reder LS, Peng GL, Sinha UK. Use of the supraclavicular artery island flap for reconstruction of cervicofacial defects. Otolaryngol Head Neck Surg. 2014;150(2):222–8.
15. Disa JJ, Rodriguez VM, Cordeiro PG. Reconstruction of lateral skull base oncological defects: the role of free tissue transfer. Ann Plast Surg. 1998;41(6):633–9.
16. Hanasono MM, Silva A, Skoracki RJ, Gidley PW, DeMonte F, Hanna EY, Chang DW, Yu P. Skull base reconstruction: an updated approach. Plast Reconstr Surg. 2011;128(3):675–86.
17. Rosenthal EL, King T, McGrew BM, Carroll W, Magnuson JS, Wax MK. Evolution of a paradigm for free tissue transfer reconstruction of lateral temporal bone defects. Head Neck. 2008;30(5):589–94.
18. Teknos TN, Smith JC, Day TA, Netterville JL, Burkey BB. Microvascular free tissue transfer in reconstructing skull base defects: lessons learned. Laryngoscope. 2002;112:1871–6.
19. O'Connell DA, Teng MS, Mendez E, Futran ND. Microvascular free tissue transfer in the reconstruction of scalp and lateral temporal bone defects. J Craniofac Surg. 2011;22(3):801–4.
20. Hanasono MM, Skoracki RJ, Yu P. A prospective study of donor-site morbidity after anterolateral thigh fasciocutaneous and myocutaneous free flap harvest in 220 patients. Plast Reconstr Surg. 2010;125(1):209–14.
21. Corbitt C, Skoracki RJ, Yu P, Hanasono MM. Free flap failure in head and neck reconstruction. Head Neck. 2014;36:1440–5.

Management of the Eye in the Setting of Facial Nerve Paralysis

26

Richard C. Allen

Involvement of an ophthalmologist in the care of a patient with facial paralysis is mandatory to ensure adequate protection of the eye [1, 2]. Although the sequelae of facial paralysis are, in general, nonurgent, the health of the eye may be acutely compromised. The most acute issue is corneal dryness, which potentially may lead to corneal infection and could progress to sight-threatening situations. Nonurgent issues include eyelid malpositions, midface descent, brow ptosis, and epiphora, which may significantly affect the quality of life of the patient [3]. The purpose of this chapter is to aid the physician in the evaluation and management of the eye in patients with facial paralysis.

History

An adequate history, emphasizing issues which may affect the eye, is necessary in the evaluation and management of the patient with a facial nerve palsy. The etiology of the paralysis must be discerned to plan care accordingly. If the paralysis is expected to be temporary and improve, often conservative management will suffice. If the palsy is thought to be permanent, or if the palsy will worsen with an upcoming surgery, longer-term and more invasive care may need to be planned.

Previous ocular history should be queried. Is the patient on any ocular medications? Does the patient have any previous ocular disease? Has the patient undergone any previous ocular or eyelid surgery? Use of ocular medications may worsen keratopathy in the setting of a facial nerve palsy. Patients who are on chronic ocular medications (e.g., glaucoma drops, intravitreal injections for macular degeneration) will need to continue these medications; and therefore, some tarsorrhaphy procedures may be contraindicated as they would not allow the patient to have the medications placed. If the patient has any ongoing ocular conditions that need to be monitored, a tarsorrhaphy may also be contraindicated. If the patient has a poorly seeing eye on the contralateral side to the palsy, this should be considered. Previous dry eye will worsen keratopathy as well as previous corneal surgery (e.g., LASIK, corneal transplants) which decreases corneal sensation. Any previous eyelid surgery may contribute a cicatricial etiology to the paralytic condition. Previous cosmetic procedures including blepharoplasty, rhytidectomy, botulinum toxin, and filler injection may affect the outcome of treatment and planning. Medical conditions such as diabetes and Sjogren syndrome should be elicited as they may affect the health of the cornea.

Examination

A full eye examination should be performed in all new patients to exclude any coexisting ocular condition. Visual acuity, pupil examination, extraocular motility, Bell's phenomenon, visual field, external and slit-lamp exam, corneal sensation, intraocular pressure, and optic nerve and fundus examination are the basic components of an ocular examination in a patient presenting with a facial nerve palsy. Visual acuity may be compromised if the patient has any keratopathy. If the patient has a pupil abnormality, visual field defect, and/or extraocular motility defect, additional cranial nerves may be involved which must be investigated with imaging if not previously performed.

External examination includes evaluation of the brows, eyelids, and midface. Brow paralysis may result in a visual field defect, and midface descent may worsen lower lid malposition. Eyelid measurements include palpebral fissure height, margin reflex distance (MRD) 1 and 2, and lagophthalmos. Palpebral fissure height is the distance between the upper eyelid margin and lower eyelid margin with the eyes in

All videos in this chapter are available at http://webeye.ophth.uiowa.edu/eyeforum/video/plastics/

R. C. Allen, M.D., Ph.D., F.A.C.S.
Section of Ophthalmology, Department of Head and Neck Surgery, The University of Texas M.D. Anderson Cancer Center, Houston, TX, USA
e-mail: rcallen1@mdanderson.org

P. W. Gidley, F. DeMonte (eds.), *Temporal Bone Cancer*, https://doi.org/10.1007/978-3-319-74539-8_26

primary position (looking straight ahead). MRD1 is the distance between the upper eyelid margin and the central corneal light reflex with the eyes in primary position fixating on a penlight, while MRD2 is the distance between the lower eyelid margin and the central corneal light reflex. Lagophthalmos is the distance between the upper eyelid margin and lower eyelid margin with the eyes gently closed; the presence of lagophthalmos is defined as any incomplete closure of the eyelids. Bell's phenomenon (palpebral-oculogyric reflex) is the protective mechanism of supraduction of the eyes with eye closure. Some patients will have a good Bell's phenomenon in which the eye supraducts well, which will protect the cornea under the upper lid especially with coexisting lagophthalmos. Some patients may have poor or even a reverse Bell's phenomenon (infraduction of the eye with closure) which will predispose the cornea to dryness with coexisting lagophthalmos. Upper eyelid skin contracture has been described in patients with long-term facial nerve palsy as well as upper eyelid entropion [4]. Axial position of the eye should also be noted as patients with prominent/proptotic eyes may have more significant lagophthalmos than those that are relatively enophthalmic.

Slit lamp examination is performed to evaluate the health of the cornea, conjunctiva, and anterior chamber of the eye. Keratopathy should be documented, and any corneal defect should be measured. White blood cell infiltration of the cornea should also be documented as this is a hallmark of infection. Inflammation within the anterior chamber indicates significant corneal inflammation, which is concerning for an ongoing infectious process. Prior to placing any drops in the eye, corneal sensation is critical to check since sensation is one of the greatest prognosticators of ocular morbidity. Good sensation of the cornea portends a good prognosis, as the patient will be able to monitor their dryness by noting any ongoing or worsening foreign body sensation or pain. The patient with the anesthetic cornea is unable to monitor the effectiveness of the treatment of their dryness reliably. Causes of decreased corneal sensation include a coexisting trigeminal nerve defect, previous corneal surgery, advanced age, previous herpes zoster or simplex infection, and diabetes. Sensation can be evaluated with an esthesiometer (Cochet-Bonnet); however, the simplest evaluation is to use fibers from a cotton-tipped applicator and run the fibers across the cornea to see if the patient feels it. This should be performed on both eyes to assess any asymmetry. In addition, it is useful to ask the patient directly if they can "feel" when their eye gets dry.

Fluorescein staining is mandatory to determine the presence or absence of corneal dryness. Fluorescein will stain an exposed basement membrane of the epithelium of the cornea, and when visualized under blue light with the slit lamp, the staining will be highlighted. Tear production measurement using Schirmer strips can be difficult in patients with a facial nerve palsy; the testing may not be accurate with lagophthalmos and lower lid malposition. Intraocular pressure and a dilated fundus examination complete the full ocular exam to rule out any coexisting or preexisting conditions.

Grading Systems

Facial nerve grading instruments for ophthalmic involvement of facial nerve palsy have been described [5, 6]. The CADS grading scale is based on four aspects of periorbital involvement: cornea, asymmetry, dynamic function, and synkinesis [5]. Although not yet adopted routinely, their use would be of benefit [6].

Treatment

Treatment of the eye in the patient with a facial nerve palsy depends on the severity of the ocular findings, the presence or absence of an anesthetic cornea, and the expected duration of the palsy. Severe dryness in a patient with a temporary palsy may be best treated with a temporizing tarsorrhaphy, while mild dryness in the patient who is not expected to recover can be addressed with artificial tears. In general, treatment is usually stepped up from conservative to invasive unless the eye is acutely at risk.

Medical Treatment

Initial medical treatment of the patient with or predisposed to keratopathy secondary to a facial nerve palsy consists of ocular lubrication. The goal of lubrication is to prevent keratopathy, and this should be instituted if possible prior to initiation of the palsy and ocular signs or symptoms. The patient should understand that the lubrication should ideally be used, prior to their noticing any symptoms. Often, patients will admit that they use the drops when they "feel" that the eye is dry; by definition, they are using the drops too late in the process. A basic initial regimen is to use artificial tears four times per day and lubricating ointment at night. Lubrication is over-the-counter and comes in three different types, depending on the viscosity of the medication. Drops are available in a thinner and thicker consistency, while ointment is the most viscous. If drops four times per day with ointment at night do not effectively treat the dryness, then the patient can increase the frequency of the drops or use a more viscous modality during the day. The disadvantage of a viscous drop or ointment during the day is that it will blur the patient's vision. If the frequency of the drop is greater than six times per day, then a preservative-free artificial tear should be used due to potential sensitivity to the preservative with frequent use. There are multiple different brands of artificial tears and ointment, all of which are essentially equivalent. Cyclosporine drops (Restasis) are not effective for dry eye secondary to exposure from facial paresis. Rarely, patients will use drops made from autologous serum for intractable keratopathy not amenable to other treatments.

The tear film is made of three layers: an outer oil layer made by the Meibomian glands, a middle aqueous layer made by the main and accessory lacrimal glands, and an inner mucous layer made by the goblet cells of the conjunctiva. Artificial tears are formulated to replace the outer oil layer. The Meibomian glands are situated in the tarsus of the upper and lower lids and exit at the eyelid margin. Anatomical studies have shown that the act of blinking results in contraction of muscles adjacent to the glands that aid in emptying of the glands [7]. In facial paralysis, the emptying of the Meibomian glands is compromised, resulting in an inadequate oil layer of the tears. Infrared examination of patients with a unilateral facial nerve palsy shows blockage and dropout of Meibomian glands on the side of the paralysis compared to the contralateral side [8–10]. Due to these findings, patients can optimize the health and emptying of the Meibomian glands by using warm compresses as well as digital compression of the glands.

Punctal plugs occlude the tear drainage system and may help in improving dryness. There are many types of plugs, but the use of intracanalicular plugs is discouraged [11]. Plugs may be placed in the upper and/or lower puncta. If there is lower lid ectropion, placement of a plug in the lower punctum is not helpful. Patients should be aware that placement of plugs may worsen epiphora.

Although patching and taping of the eye at night is a frequent recommendation, some in the ophthalmic community discourage this practice due to the risk of causing a corneal abrasion if the eye opens and rubs on the abrasive surface [12]. Taping the lower eyelid upward toward the lateral canthus can provide temporary improvement in closure. In addition, a moisture chamber using cellophane or even swim goggles is helpful.

Tarsorrhaphy

The prudent placement of a tarsorrhaphy can be sight-saving in a patient with a facial nerve palsy. A tarsorrhaphy works by facilitating epithelialization of the cornea by closing the eyelids. A multitude of factors go into the decision to place a tarsorrhaphy, and there are numerous tarsorrhaphy procedures. A tarsorrhaphy will usually be placed in one of two situations: (1) The patient has significant corneal compromise and medication alone will likely not improve the situation. (2) The patient has corneal compromise and is to embark on a prolonged treatment course (e.g., surgery, chemotherapy, radiation); closing the eye until a later date will allow concentration on the other treatments. Tarsorrhaphy procedures are categorized into whether they are temporary or permanent. Although labeled "permanent," these tarsorrhaphies are always reversible.

Temporary tarsorrhaphies include the use of suture (with or without bolsters), glue, and botulinum toxin. A suture tarsorrhaphy without a bolster can be performed with either 5-0 chromic or 5-0 Vicryl suture. The chromic suture will last about 3 weeks, while the Vicryl can last 5 weeks or even longer. The disadvantage of using Vicryl is the associated inflammatory response to the suture. The procedure is performed after anesthetizing the upper and lower lids with local anesthetic. In patients with a trigeminal nerve compromise, the procedure can often be performed without anesthesia. Two to three horizontal mattress sutures are placed along the eyelid margin to close the eyelids (video available at https://vimeo.com/143472037). This tarsorrhaphy is especially useful in those instances in which the patient has not been using lubrication and needs the eye closed temporarily, so that when it opens, lubrication alone will be adequate to control the dryness. It is essentially a "catch-up" procedure.

Placement of a tarsorrhaphy with bolsters has similar advantages to the suture tarsorrhaphy without bolsters. The additional advantage to using bolsters is that the bolsters can be loosened to allow examination of the cornea, while using sutures alone does not allow this. This is especially useful in those situations in which a corneal infection is suspected and the cornea needs to be periodically examined and in the patient who needs medications placed. In this procedure, a 5-0 Prolene or nylon suture is used with bolster material (catheter tubing) (video available at https://vimeo.com/132967652). It is difficult for these bolsters to be effective for longer than about 3 weeks, and they can be somewhat uncomfortable for the patient due to their bulk.

A glue tarsorrhaphy can be placed quickly and easily in the clinic or the bedside [13]. Cyanoacrylate glue is placed over the closed eyelids (video available at https://vimeo.com/132966666). This tarsorrhaphy has a duration of 2–3 weeks. The advantage of this procedure is that it is easy to perform and does not require anesthesia. The glue does tend to cause some "stinging" when it is initially placed. The disadvantage of this tarsorrhaphy is that it is somewhat cumbersome to remove; and there is a risk of causing a corneal abrasion with the glue, which can go undetected in patients with a neurotrophic cornea. In patients with poor sensation, it is likely more appropriate to place a suture tarsorrhaphy.

Botulinum toxin can be used to induce a complete, paralytic ptosis. In this procedure, a single injection of 10 units of botulinum toxin A (Botox) is placed in the vicinity of the levator palpebrae muscle. This can be placed transcutaneously or transconjunctivally. The procedure is useful in situations in which a "strong" tarsorrhaphy is not needed. Patients with a poor Bell's phenomenon and lower lid retraction/ectropion may not be completely protected with this procedure. An advantage to the botulinum tarsorrhaphy is that the eye can be easily examined by lifting the upper eyelid. The toxin will often affect the superior rectus muscle as well, and patients may note diplopia when the eyelid is lifted, which almost always resolves. The effect of the induced ptosis has been found to last for a mean of 46 days following an onset 4 days after the injection [14, 15].

Permanent tarsorrhaphies include medial, lateral, and pillar procedures. A permanent lateral tarsorrhaphy is the gold standard tarsorrhaphy for effectively protecting the eye. The procedure creates a permanent adhesion between the upper and lower eyelids. The extent of the tarsorrhaphy is defined by the percentage of the eyelid closure from the lateral canthus. Preoperatively, the amount of tarsorrhaphy needed is determined; it is better to overcorrect as the tarsorrhaphy can be opened easily after the surgery. The upper and lower lids are anesthetized with local anesthetic with epinephrine. A #15 blade is used to make an incision along the gray line on the upper and lower eyelid margin to separate the anterior and posterior lamella. Westcott scissors are used to dissect the pretarsal orbicularis muscle from the anterior surface of the tarsus. The mucocutaneous junction of the posterior lamella is excised. The posterior lamellae of the upper and lower eyelids are sutured together with interrupted 5-0 Vicryl sutures. The anterior lamella can be sutured together with a 7-0 Vicryl suture (video available at https://vimeo.com/132967645). The advantages of this procedure are its permanence and its effectiveness in closure of the eyelids. Disadvantages of the procedure include the inability to examine the eye when the extent of the tarsorrhaphy is significant. The tarsorrhaphy can be easily opened with scissors (video available at https://vimeo.com/138019892); however, the eyelid margin may be irregular after opening the lids and result in misdirected lashes (trichiasis). In opening the tarsorrhaphy, it is useful to open it in stages to determine the amount that is needed to prevent dryness. Usually, patients will want the tarsorrhaphy eventually opened, due to the cosmetically objectionable nature of the procedure and the occlusion of the vision. In the patient with facial paralysis, rehabilitation will then need to be planned. In some instances, it may be in the patient's best interest to keep the tarsorrhaphy in long term: (1) patients who may undergo additional surgery or radiation in the area, (2) patients whose health is compromised, (3) patients who may have difficulty making frequent visits for evaluation of the eye, (4) eyes which have a poor prognosis for vision, etc.

A medial tarsorrhaphy is a relatively weak procedure in which the upper and lower lids are sutured together medial to the puncta. This procedure is usually performed in conjunction with other eyelid procedures to provide medial support. It can be performed as a stand-alone procedure when a mild amount of medial lower lid elevation (1–2 mm) is needed. Cosmetically, the procedure is well tolerated. The medial eyelids are anesthetized, and a V-shaped incision is made just anterior to the eyelid margin extending from the level of the lower punctum to the upper punctum. Care is taken not to compromise the canalicular system. The anterior lamella is dissected from the posterior lamella along the incision. The posterior lamella is sutured together with 6-0 Vicryl suture with one or two interrupted sutures. The anterior lamella is sutured together with 7-0 Vicryl sutures (video available at https://vimeo.com/132967647).

A pillar tarsorrhaphy uses small tarso-conjunctival flaps from the upper lid that are sutured to the lower lid to close the eye (Fig. 26.1) [16]. This procedure will result in complete, permanent closure of the eyelids, has the advantage of allowing examination of the eye, and can be easily opened. For the procedure, the eyelids are anesthetized, and the upper eyelid is everted over a shoehorn speculum. Two small tarso-conjunctival flaps are raised corresponding the level of the medial and lateral limbus. On the lower lid, the posterior lamella is excised at the eyelid margin at the level of the flaps. The flaps are transposed to the lower lid and sutured into position with 5-0 Vicryl sutures (video available at https://vimeo.com/132967649). This results in an adhesion of the posterior lamella between the upper and lower eyelids. The advantages of the procedure are that the eye is permanently closed and that the eye can be examined easily. In addition, the tarsorrhaphy can be opened in stages with topical anesthetic. The procedure, however, is not as strong as the permanent lateral tarsorrhaphy. A variation of the pillar tarsorrhaphy is the use of a larger lateral tarso-conjunctival flap for lateral support [17].

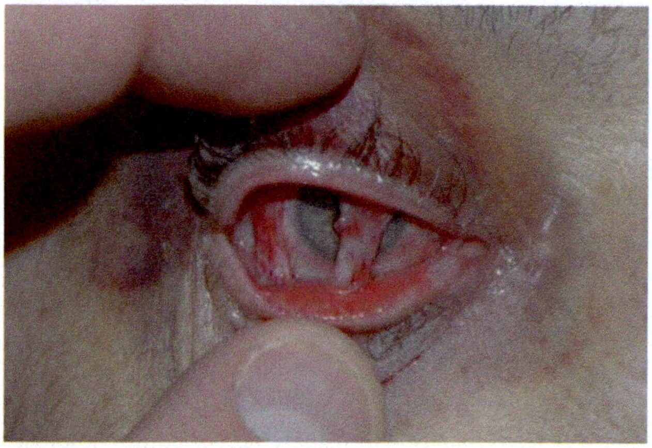

Fig. 26.1 Pillar tarsorrhaphy in a patient with a history of exposure keratopathy. Two tarso-conjunctival pillars have been advanced from the upper eyelid to the lower eyelid

Scleral Contact Lens

The use of scleral contact lenses in the management of exposure keratopathy has proven to be very effective in some situations [18, 19]. A scleral lens is a large, gas-permeable contact lens which creates a precorneal fluid reservoir beneath the lens allowing protection of the entire cornea (Fig. 26.2). In addition, the lens optimizes visual acuity. The greatest promise of this lens is in the treatment of patients with coexisting fifth and seventh nerve palsies. Recent studies have shown that a significant number of patients have been salvaged with the use of a scleral lens after undergoing multiple surgical interventions for corneal protection. Disadvantages of the scleral lens include cost; many insurance plans in the United States do not reimburse for this device. The lens is removed each night, and, due to the size of the lens, insertion and removal can be difficult for some patients.

Periocular Rehabilitation

Periocular rehabilitation should be undertaken when the eye is not acutely at risk. Acute corneal compromise should be addressed completely with lubrication and/or tarsorrhaphy. In general, rehabilitation will address chronic non-vision-threatening dryness, upper and lower lid malposition, epiphora, or visual field concerns.

Upper Eyelid Procedures

Exposure keratopathy can be improved by decreasing the palpebral fissure height and decreasing lagophthalmos. Palpebral fissure height can be improved with a lateral tarsorrhaphy, but this procedure is objectionable to many patients due to the appearance and decrease in temporal visual field. In patients undergoing rehabilitation, static and dynamic upper eyelid procedures are most effective in decreasing lagophthalmos.

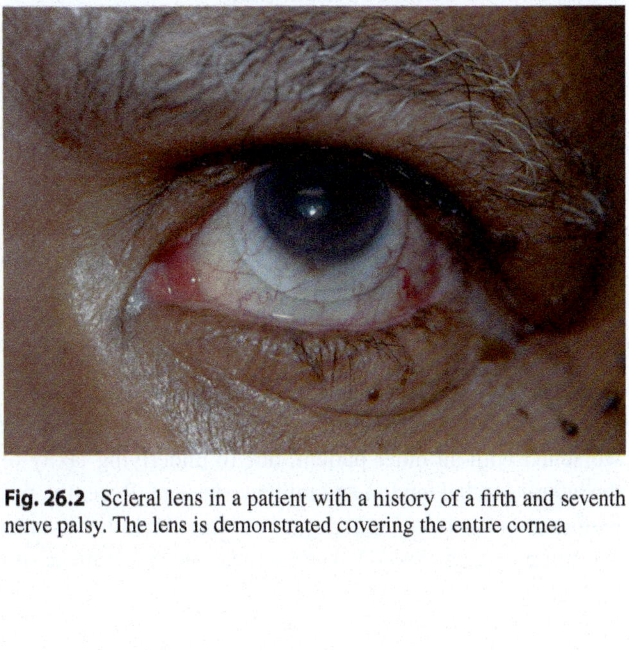

Fig. 26.2 Scleral lens in a patient with a history of a fifth and seventh nerve palsy. The lens is demonstrated covering the entire cornea

Mechanical loading of the upper eyelid is the most effective static procedure. The main disadvantage of upper eyelid loading is the dependence on gravity for its effect; closure will be less effective with the patient in a supine position. In addition, the weights have limited effectiveness in providing a dynamic blink [20]. Preoperatively, the amount of weight needed is determined with sizing weights of 0.2 g increments. The amount of weight needed should close the eyelid without inducing mechanical ptosis (Fig. 26.3). In general, this weight will range from 0.8 g to 1.2 g. Materials used include gold, platinum, and dermal fillers. Previously, gold had a cost advantage over platinum. The disadvantage of gold is that as high as 5% of the population has a gold sensitivity [21, 22]. Current weights are made in thinner profile than previously which helps make them less apparent [23]. In addition, platinum chains are available which are less apparent [24, 25]. Upper lid loads can be removed if facial nerve function improves. The use of dermal fillers has also been described to load the upper lid which has the advantage of being non-incisional and the possibility of a temporary load in patients who will recover function [26].

In placing an upper lid weight, two positions can be used. Traditionally, a pretarsal position has been preferred (Fig. 26.4). An incision is made through the eyelid crease, and the pretarsal orbicularis muscle is dissected from the underlying tarsus. The weight is placed in the pocket and sutured to the anterior surface of the tarsus with 6-0 Prolene suture. The weight should be placed somewhat medially, centered over the medial border of the pupil. A double layer closure is performed suturing the orbicularis together with interrupted buried 7-0 Vicryl suture followed by the skin with a running 6-0 Prolene suture (video available at https://vimeo.com/132966668). The advantage of this position is the ease of the surgery. Disadvantages include visibility of the load in the eyelid and possible extrusion of the weight. Use of barrier materials over the weight has been described to decrease exposure/extrusion of the weight [27, 28]. In addition, placement of the weight in this position has been shown to induce corneal astigmatism [29].

The weight can be placed higher in the eyelid at the superior border of the tarsus [30]. In this procedure, an incision is made at the eyelid crease. The orbital septum is opened, and the levator aponeurosis is disinserted from the anterior surface of the tarsus. Dissection is performed between the levator aponeurosis and the underlying Muller's muscle. The weight is placed with its inferior border at the superior border of the tarsus on top of Muller's muscle. The levator aponeurosis can cover the weight. The orbicularis muscle is closed with 7-0 Vicryl suture, incorporating the levator aponeurosis into the closure, and the skin is closed with a

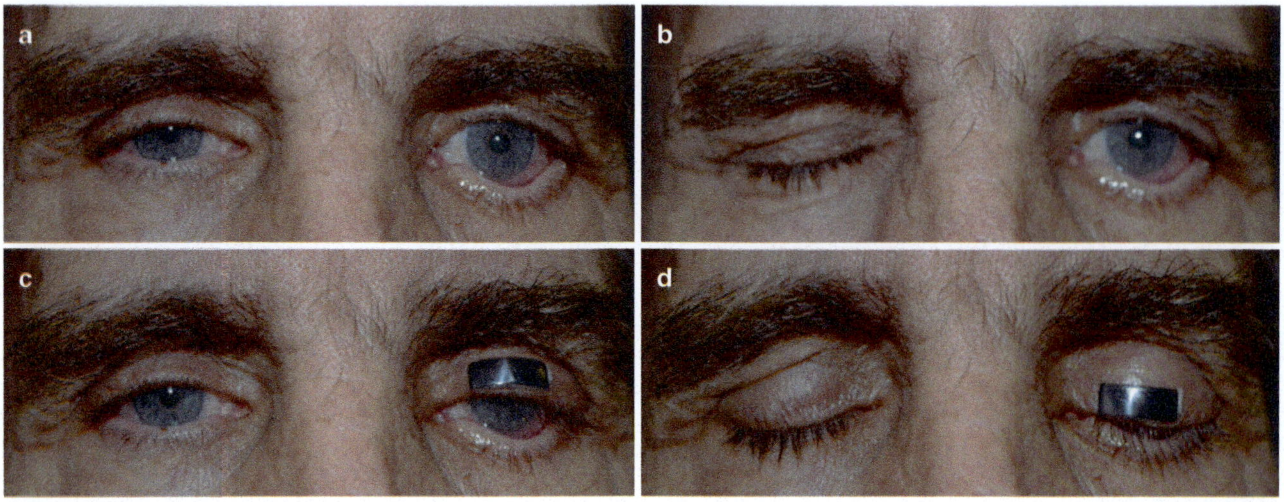

Fig. 26.3 Trial weight in a patient with a left facial nerve palsy. Appearance with eyes open (**a**) and closed (**b**). Note the poor Bell's phenomenon. Appearance after placement of 1.2 g trial weight with eyes open (**c**) and closed (**d**)

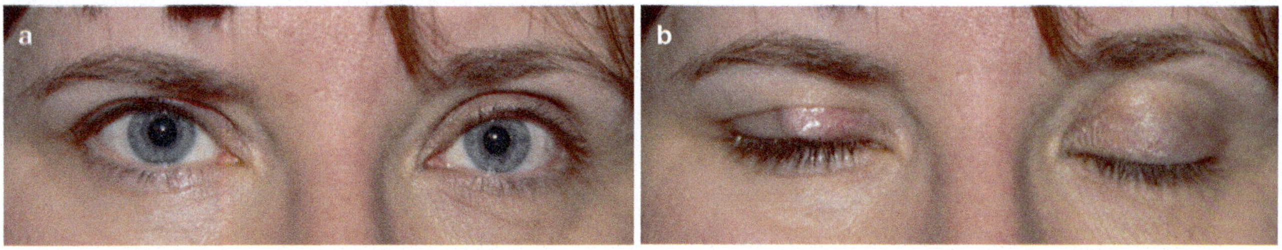

Fig. 26.4 Patient with a right facial nerve palsy after placement of a pretarsal gold weight with eyes open (**a**) and closed (**b**)

running 6-0 Prolene suture (video available at https://vimeo.com/138019890). The advantage of this procedure is that the weight is above the superior border of the tarsus, and the load is not externally visible. In addition, the weight has an extra layer of tissue (levator aponeurosis) over the weight which may decrease extrusion. With the weight being higher, less corneal astigmatism is also induced [31]. Incorporation of the levator aponeurosis into the eyelid crease closure also provides the establishment of a strong lid crease with upward traction on the pretarsal anterior lamella, which may decrease entropion which can be observed long term in these patients.

Dynamic procedures for the upper eyelid include placing a palpebral spring. In experienced hands, this procedure has the potential of giving a good closure to the upper eyelid without depending on gravity and gives a greater degree of reflex blinking [32, 33]. The procedure is used less than upper lid loading due to the difficulty and length of the surgery. Complications associated with springs include extrusion, breakage, metal fatigue, overcorrection, and under-correction. The Arion silicone sling provides sphincter-like action but has not been widely adopted by surgeons [34]. Authors have also described the use of magnets to aid in eyelid closure. Magnets can be implanted into the upper and lower eyelid near the lid margin or placed in the upper lid and on the inferior aspect of spectacles [35–37]. In patients who would be under surveillance with magnetic resonance imaging (MRI), palpebral springs or placement of a magnet would not be advisable.

External weights (Blinkeze External Lid Weights, MedDev Corporation, Sunnyvale, CA) are useful in situations of a temporary paralysis to aid in eye closure and decrease the dependence on drops. Some patients have found them useful for extended periods [38].

Residual upper eyelid retraction can be addressed with upper eyelid recession procedures. Usually, an upper eyelid load will improve upper eyelid retraction. In the rare patient with upper eyelid retraction alone without the need for an upper eyelid load, various eyelid retraction correction procedures have been described [39, 40]. In patients with relatively prominent eyes or proptosis in the setting of a facial nerve palsy, orbital decompression can be considered in recalcitrant cases to improve lagophthalmos.

Lower Lid Malposition

Lower eyelid malposition in facial nerve palsy has traditionally been classified as an ectropion. This malposition is worsened with an older patient, due to underlying laxity of the lateral canthal tendon and midface descent. Recently, this malposition has been argued to be a retraction rather than an ectropion (Fig. 26.5) [41]. The implication of this reclassifi-

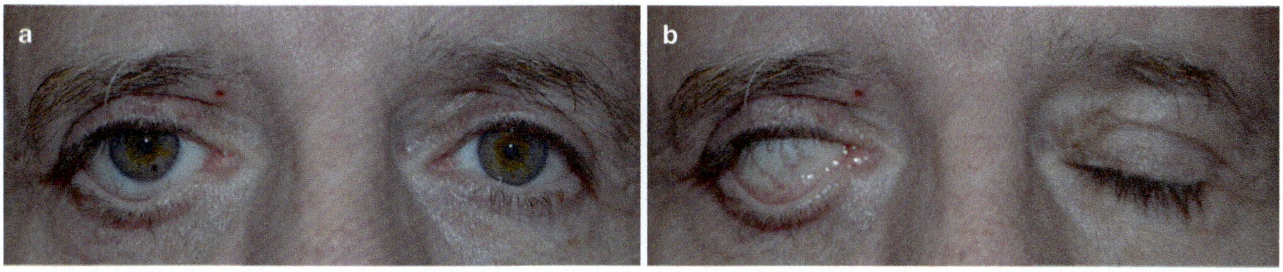

Fig. 26.5 Patient with a right facial nerve palsy with lower eyelid retraction with eyes open (**a**) and closed (**b**). Note the good Bell's phenomenon

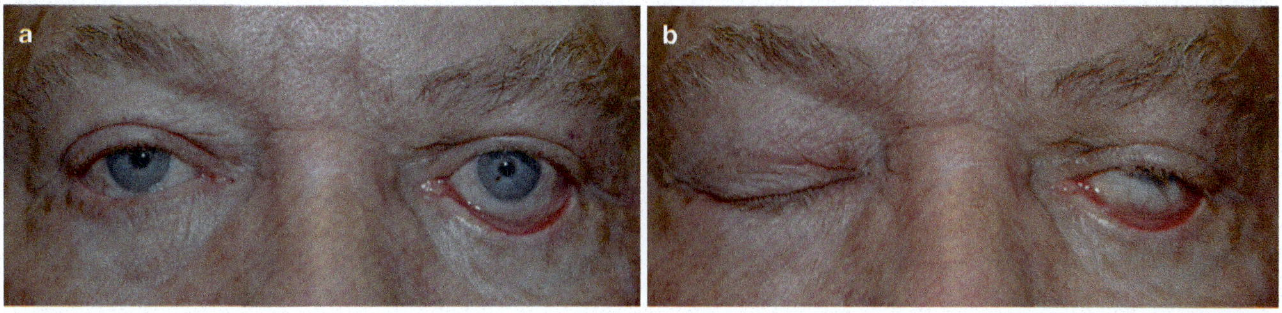

Fig. 26.6 Patient with a left facial nerve palsy with lower lid retraction and ectropion worsened by a relatively heavy cheek and actinic, cicatricial changes with eyes open (**a**) and closed (**b**)

cation affects surgical planning. If thought of as an ectropion, the malposition would be treated with horizontal lower lid-tightening procedures. Treating lower lid paralytic malposition as an ectropion has led to high recurrence rates of the malposition.

Paralytic lower lid malposition results in unopposed action of the lower lid retractors due to protractor (orbicularis) paralysis. Thus, treatment of this malposition should also address weakening the unopposed lower lid retractors. Evaluation of the lower lid in patients with facial paralysis should include horizontal lower lid laxity, lower lid retraction, and midface descent. In younger patients, the absence of lower lid laxity and midface descent often results in minimal lower lid malposition in the setting of facial paralysis. In the older patient, malposition is exacerbated by involutional horizontal lower lid laxity and midface descent. Horizontal eyelid tightening is addressed by tightening the lateral canthal tendon. Although there is often a component of medial canthal tendon laxity, techniques to tighten the medial canthal tendon are difficult with significant risk to the lacrimal outflow system [42].

In treating patients with paralytic lower lid retraction without significant midface descent, the preferred surgery is horizontal tightening with a lateral tarsal strip, retractor recession with placement of a spacer, and medial tarsorrhaphy. For the procedure, a lateral canthotomy and inferior cantholysis are performed. A 4-0 Silk suture is placed through the lower lid margin at the level of the tarsus to provide traction and also to act as a Frost suture postoperatively. The needle tip cautery is used to make a transconjunctival incision inferior to the inferior border of the tarsus, extending from the level of the punctum medially to the lateral canthus laterally. Dissection is carried out between the orbicularis muscle and the orbital septum to the inferior orbital rim. The conjunctiva is dissected from the lower lid retractor/orbital septum complex. A spacer is placed between the inferior border of the tarsus and the lower lid retractor/orbital septum complex. In general, approximately 6–8 mm of vertical height from the spacer is needed. The conjunctiva is closed over the spacer and sutured to the inferior border of the tarsus with 7-0 Vicryl suture. Attention is directed to horizontal lower lid tightening where a lateral tarsal strip procedure is performed. If the periosteum is poor at the lateral orbital rim, two drill holes can be placed in order to fixate the lateral tarsal strip to the lateral orbital rim. A medial tarsorrhaphy is performed, and the 4-0 Silk suture is taped to the forehead to keep the eyelid on upward traction for 1 week (video available at https://vimeo.com/133680716).

There are different types of spacers to use; each has advantages and disadvantages. An acellular porcine dermal matrix is a very useful graft for paralytic retraction [43]. Ear cartilage can be harvested if needed. If the patient has failed previous surgery, a hard palate graft is very effective as a spacer.

If the patient has significant midface descent, midface elevation should be performed at the time of lower lid retraction repair (Fig. 26.6). Depending on the extent of the descent, a preperiosteal or subperiosteal lift can be performed. Preperiosteal lifts are effective for mild amounts of descent. If there are cicatricial changes present, then a stronger subperiosteal lift should be performed [44, 45]. Placement of inverting sutures is helpful in preventing postoperative ectropion by stabilizing the inferior border of the tarsus.

Brow Ptosis

Similar to midface descent, brow ptosis is greater in older patients due to involutional changes, which are exacerbated by the paralysis. In younger patients, brow descent is less noticeable unless there is dynamic movement of the contralateral forehead. In younger patients, the asymmetry from movement can effectively be treated with the application of botulinum toxin to the frontalis muscle on the side contralateral to the paralysis.

Paralytic brow ptosis may encroach on the visual field of the patient, resulting in a functional defect (Fig. 26.7). The decrease in visual field should be documented with an examination of the superior visual field with the brow taped and untaped. Surgical correction of brow ptosis will depend on the extent of the ptosis and the wishes of the patient. One must be cognizant of the "natural" upper lid load that brow ptosis provides; correction of this may worsen or cause lagophthalmos. There are many brow ptosis correction procedures, each with advantages and disadvantages. The most effective, least invasive procedure is a direct browplasty. For this procedure, an incision is made above the brow cilia, and a flap of skin and subcutaneous fat are removed. Closure of the defect results in elevation of the brow. Preoperatively, the amount of resection should be marked. The vertical height of the resection usually is between 10 and 15 mm. The advantage of the procedure is that it is effective and predictable; it can be performed under minimal anesthesia. The disadvantage is that it may leave a cosmetically objectionable scar and it is difficult to get effective elevation of the medial portion of the brow. A small "up-slant" to the incision can be performed medially to improve the medial brow incision (video available at https://vimeo.com/132966661). In closure of the defect, some surgeons will incorporate the periosteum to fixate the brow in place postoperatively.

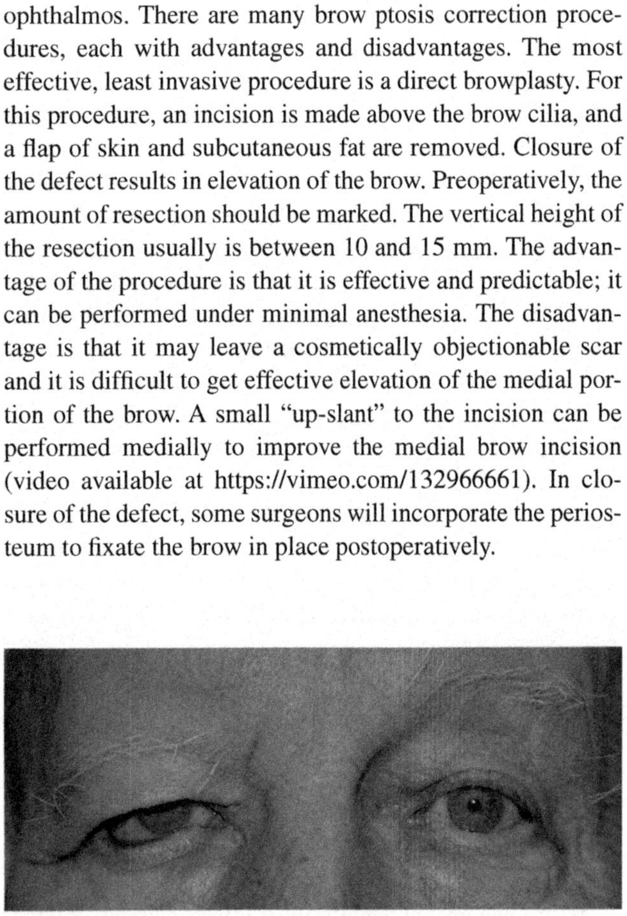

Fig. 26.7 Patient with a right seventh nerve palsy and visually significant paralytic brow ptosis

Other brow elevation procedures to consider include a mid-forehead, pretrichial, endoscopic, or coronal procedure. The endoscopic approach is the least effective of the procedures but may be appropriate for the younger patient with mild asymmetry. The mid-forehead, pretrichial, and coronal procedures are all essentially equal in their effectiveness and can lift the medial brow. The disadvantages of these procedures compared to the direct browplasty are their invasiveness and the fact that they are less effective for millimeter of tissue removed for millimeter of brow elevation. A browpexy procedure should not be performed for any significant paralytic brow ptosis as this procedure results in minimal elevation.

Tearing

Epiphora (tearing) in the setting of facial paralysis is multifactorial. Corneal irritation secondary to dryness or keratopathy will result in reflex tearing. Lower lid malposition may result in lacrimal punctal malposition. Incomplete closure of the eyelids also results in tear stasis with poor transfer of the tears toward the puncta. Lastly, orbicularis weakness results in a poor lacrimal pump—the mechanism whereby tears are propelled through the puncta, canaliculus, and nasolacrimal duct.

Prior to any surgical intervention for epiphora, lubrication of the ocular surface must be optimized. The eyelids can be in optimal position, but if the eye is still dry, there may continue to be reflex tearing. The cornea must be examined under a slit lamp with fluorescein staining to ensure that the ocular surface is healthy. Lower lid malposition can be addressed using the procedures noted above, and apposition of the eyelids can be optimized with upper lid loading and lower lid retraction repair. However, even with the ocular surface and eyelid position optimized, the patient may continue to tear due to a poor lacrimal pump. For patients who are debilitated by tearing secondary to a poor lacrimal pump, treatment options are limited. Authors have described success with placement of a Jones tube; however, the tear outflow may be so efficient that a dry eye can be induced [46, 47]. Small lumen Jones tubes are available which may obviate this problem. Conservative injection of botulinum toxin into the lacrimal gland can also be considered.

Other etiologies of tearing can be related to aberrant reinnervation. Parasympathetic stimulation of the lacrimal gland is responsible for tear production, which originates from fibers conveyed in the facial nerve. After synapse in the pterygopalatine ganglion, postsynaptic parasympathetic fibers travel within the zygomatic and zygomaticotemporal nerves into the orbit. The zygomaticotemporal nerve communicates with the lacrimal nerve, and then secretomotor fibers enter the gland [48]. Gustatory lacrimation is a result of misdirected innervation of the efferent fibers from the superior salivary nucleus to the lacrimal gland. This can be effectively treated with botulinum toxin to the lacrimal gland [49, 50].

Timing of Procedures

When to perform particular procedures and in what sequence is controversial. Protection of the cornea is paramount; and, as noted previously, a prudent tarsorrhaphy can be sight-saving. The benefits of a tarsorrhaphy usually far outweigh the risks or inconvenience of the procedure.

Gold weight placement should be considered when accurate estimation of the size of the weight needed can be performed. However, the argument can be made for placing a weight at the time of a predicted sacrifice of the facial nerve, for example, at the time of tumor excision and before clinical facial paralysis is evident [51–53]. The main disadvantage is the potential inaccuracy of the size of the weight needed. A 1.2 g weight is a good estimate. Placing the weight will also be beneficial in the early postoperative period to protect the eye. In addition, it may save the patient a subsequent surgical session. If the weight is not needed or if the facial nerve recovers, it can be removed under minimal anesthesia (video available at https://vimeo.com/138016656).

Soft tissue repositioning of the brow, lower lid, and midface should likely be delayed until the patient is stable in their treatment. In patients who will undergo radiation therapy, surgery should be delayed at least a month after finishing radiation. For patients undergoing chemotherapy, discussion with the medical oncologist regarding the possibility of discontinuing the chemotherapy perioperatively should be undertaken. For some patients on long-term chemotherapy, the medication may not be able to be discontinued, and the risks of continuing the chemotherapy perioperatively should be discussed with the patient.

For patients who have had a tarsorrhaphy placed, rehabilitation can be somewhat more difficult since accurate measurements cannot be made without first opening the tarsorrhaphy. Opening the tarsorrhaphy is usually necessary to obtain an accurate estimate of the amount of weight needed in the upper lid or the degree of lower eyelid malposition. This assessment can be performed intraoperatively; however, the local anesthesia needed to open the tarsorrhaphy can affect measurements. In patients with trigeminal nerve compromise, the opening can be performed without anesthesia. For patients with a functioning trigeminal nerve, the tarsorrhaphy can be opened the week before the planned surgery, and then measurements can be performed on the day of surgery. Patients need to be reminded to use copious lubrication between the time of opening the tarsorrhaphy and planned rehabilitation.

The author prefers to separate upper eyelid and lower eyelid surgery into two sessions, separated by at least a month. With the lower eyelid being placed on upward traction for a week postoperatively with a Frost suture, the author has noted unpredictable outcomes of the upper eyelid position if it is performed concurrently with the lower eyelid, presumably due to the upper eyelid creating unfavorable scar due to its limited movement postoperatively. Repositioning of the brow can be performed with either surgery.

Situations with Multiple Cranial Neuropathies

Patients who have multiple cranial neuropathies should be approached cautiously. As noted previously, any patient with evidence of multiple cranial neuropathies should be imaged completely to discern the etiology, if not already performed.

Patients with optic nerve compromise and a facial nerve palsy should be evaluated closely, even though the eye may have poor vision. These patients can have significant dryness which can lead to eye-threatening infection and have minimal symptoms.

Patients with ocular motility issues secondary to a third, fourth, or sixth nerve palsy will complain of diplopia in addition to the symptoms from their facial nerve palsy. A temporizing tarsorrhaphy has the added benefit of occluding the eye and eliminating the diplopia. In patients with a sixth nerve palsy, the resulting esotropia may make a lateral tarsorrhaphy ineffective in closing the eye over the cornea.

The most worrisome cranial neuropathy in addition to a facial nerve palsy is trigeminal nerve compromise. An ophthalmologist should be involved in these cases immediately. Due to the cornea being anesthetic/neurotrophic, patients can have significant corneal damage and be entirely asymptomatic. In addition, repositioning of the eyelid effectively often still results in corneal decompensation and a suboptimal outcome. Early tarsorrhaphy is recommended in patients who will undergo a prolonged treatment course or hospitalization. The most effective current treatment of these patients is placement of a scleral lens.

Synkinesis/Pseudoptosis

Periocular issues related to synkinesis or aberrant reinnervation of the facial nerve include a decrease in palpebral fissure height and changes in eyelid position with movement of the face. With the resting tone of the orbicularis muscle increased, patients notice a decrease in the palpebral fissure height [54]. In addition, aberrant reinnervation often results in narrowing of the palpebral fissure with movement of the mouth during smiling or eating. The pseudoptosis related to aberrant reinnervation should not be addressed by tightening the eyelid retractors, as is performed with traditional ptosis repair. Rather, weakening of the protractors (orbicularis muscle) can be effectively achieved with application of botulinum toxin. Periocular placement of 2.5–5 units of botulinum toxin type A per site to the medial and lateral upper and lower pretarsal orbicularis muscle is performed. For initial injection, starting with 2.5 units per sites will allow assessment. Weakening the orbicularis muscle may result in worsening dryness of the eye, and patients should prophylactically start artificial tears after the injections [55–57].

Pediatric Patients

Care of pediatric patients with facial nerve palsy should involve a pediatric ophthalmologist to evaluate the patient for any associated ocular abnormalities and strabismus. Pediatric patients with facial nerve palsy may have an associated abduction deficit secondary to Moebius syndrome or Duane's syndrome. Treatment of amblyopia is mandatory to prevent permanent visual loss [58]. Authors have also described associated entropion of the lower lid in pediatric patients with isolated peripheral facial nerve paresis [59, 60].

Future Directions and Conclusions

There are a number of potential future therapies for the management of ocular concerns in patients with a facial nerve palsy. Repositioning of adjacent muscle groups to aid in eyelid closure has been reported as well as the use of other functioning cranial nerves [61–63]. Electrical stimulation of existing, but denervated, muscle groups has interesting appeal; transcutaneous facial nerve stimulation has been demonstrated to artificially elicit eyelid closure [64]. Neurotization of the cornea has also been described with impressive results in patients with a neurotrophic cornea [65–67]. Unfortunately, most of the references in this chapter correspond to retrospective studies or case series. Prospective, randomized, case-controlled studies are in desperate need to effectively evaluate our treatment of ocular issues in patients with a facial nerve palsy.

References

1. Bhama P, Bhrany AD. Ocular protection in facial paralysis. Curr Opin Otolaryngol Head Neck Surg. 2013;21:353–7.
2. Lee V, Currie Z, Collin JRO. Ophthalmic management of facial nerve palsy. Eye (Lond). 2004;18:1225–34.
3. Henstrom DK, Lindsay RW, Cheney ML, Hadlock TA. Surgical treatment of the periocular complex and improvement of quality of life in patients with facial paralysis. Arch Facial Plast Surg. 2011;13:125–8.
4. Ziahosseini K, Venables V, Neville C, Nduka C, Patel B, Malhotra R. Occurrence and severity of upper eyelid skin contracture in facial nerve palsy. Eye. 2016;30:713–7.
5. Malhotra R, Ziahosseini K, Litwin A, Nduka C, El-Shammah N. CADS grading scale: toward better grading of ophthalmic involvement in facial nerve paralysis. Br J Ophthalmol. 2016;100:866–70.
6. Ziahosseini K, Nduka C, Malhotra R. Ophthalmic grading of facial paralysis: need for a closer look. Br J Ophthalmol. 2015;99:1171–5.
7. Lipham WJ, Tawfik HA, Dutton JJ. A histologic analysis and three-dimensional reconstruction of the muscle of Riolan. Ophthal Plast Reconstr Surg. 2002;18:93–8.
8. Takahashi Y, Dadizaki H. Meibomian gland dysfunction and cranial nerve VII palsy. Ophthal Plast Reconstr Surg. 2015;31:179–81.
9. Call CB, Wise RJ, Hansen MR, Carter KD, Allen RC. In vivo examination of Meibomian gland morphology in patients with facial nerve palsy using infrared meibography. Ophthal Plast Reconstr Surg. 2012;28:396–400.
10. Shah CT, Blount AL, Nguyen EV, Hassan AS. Cranial nerve seven palsy and its influence on Meibomian gland function. Ophthal Plast Reconstr Surg. 2012;28:166–8.
11. Marcet MM, Shtein RM, Bradley EA, et al. Safety and efficacy of lacrimal drainage system plugs for dry eye syndrome: a report by the American Academy of Ophthalmology. Ophthalmology. 2015;122:1681–7.
12. Seiff SR. Surgical management of seventh nerve paralysis and floppy eyelid syndrome. Curr Opin Ophthalmol. 1999;10:242–6.
13. Diamond JP. Temporary tarsorrhaphy with cyanoacrylate adhesive for seventh-nerve palsy. Lancet. 1990;335:1039.
14. Ellis MF, Daniell M. An evaluation of the safety and efficacy of botulinum toxin type A (BOTOX) when used to produce a protective ptosis. Clin Experiment Ophthalmol. 2001;29:394–9.
15. Naik MN, Gangopadhyay N, Fernandes M, Murthy R, Honavar SG. Anterior chemodenervation of levator palpebrae superioris with botulinum toxin type-A (Botox) to induce temporary ptosis for corneal protection. Eye (Lond). 2008;22:1132–6.
16. Tanenbaum M, Gossman MD, Bergin DJ, Friedman HI, Lett D, Haines P, McCord CD Jr. The tarsal pillar technique for narrowing and maintenance of the interpalpebral fissure. Ophthalmic Surg. 1992;23:418–25.
17. Tao JP, Vemuri S, Patel AD, Compton C, Nunery WR. Lateral tarsoconjunctival onlay flap lower eyelid suspension in facial nerve paresis. Ophthal Plast Reconstr Surg. 2014;30:342–5.
18. Weyns M, Koppen C, Tassignon MJ. Scleral contact lenses as an alternative to tarsorrhaphy for the long-term management of combined exposure and neurotrophic keratopathy. Cornea. 2013;32:359–61.
19. Gire A, Kwok A, Marx DP. PROSE treatment for lagophthalmos and exposure keratopathy. Ophthal Plast Reconstr Surg. 2013;29:e38–40.
20. Abell KM, Baker RS, Cowen DE, Porter JD. Efficacy of gold weight implants in facial nerve palsy: quantitative alterations in blinking. Vision Res. 1998;38:3019–23.
21. Bair RL, Harris GJ, Lyon DB, Komorowski RA. Noninfectious inflammatory response to gold weight eyelid implants. Ophthal Plast Reconstr Surg. 1995;11:209–14.
22. Fowler J Jr, Tahlor J, Storrs F, et al. Gold allergy in North America. Am J Contact Dermat. 2001;12:3–5.
23. Silver AL, Lindsay RW, Cheney ML, Hadlock TA. Thin-profile platinum eyelid weighting: a superior option in the paralyzed eye. Plast Reconstr Surg. 2009;123:1697–703.
24. Berghaus A, Neumann K, Schrom T. The platinum chain: a new upper-lid implant for facial palsy. Arch Facial Plast Surg. 2003;5:166–70.
25. Bladen JC, Norris JH, Malhotra R. Cosmetic comparison of gold weight and platinum chain insertion in primary upper eyelid loading for lagophthalmos. Ophthal Plast Reconstr Surg. 2012;28:171–5.

26. Mancini R, Taban M, Lowinger A, Nakra T, Tsirbas A, Douglas RS, et al. Use of hyaluronic acid gel in the management of paralytic lagophthalmos: the hyaluronic acid gel 'gold weight'. Ophthal Plast Reconstr Surg. 2009;25:23–6.
27. Singh M, Kruse C, Eriksson E, Caterson EJ. Deep temporal fascia coverage of the loading weight in paralytic lagophthalmos patients. J Craniofac Surg. 2015;26:1631–3.
28. Foster JA, Perry JD, Cahill KV, Holck DE, Dugler L. Processed human pericardium barrier for gold weight implantation. Ophthal Plast Reconstr Surg. 2004;20:107–9.
29. Mavrikakis I, Beckingsale P, Lee E, Riaz Y, Brittain P. Changes in corneal topography with upper eyelid gold weight implants. Ophthal Plast Reconstr Surg. 2006;22:331–4.
30. Rozen S, Lehrman C. Upper eyelid postseptal weight placement for the treatment of paralytic lagophthalmos. Plast Reconstr Surg. 2013;131:1253–65.
31. Saleh GM, Mavrikakis I, de Sousa JL, Xing W, Malhotra R. Corneal astigmatism with upper eyelid gold weight implantation using the combined high pretarsal and levator fixation technique. Ophthal Plast Reconstr Surg. 2007;23:381–3.
32. Demirci H, Frueh BR. Palpebral spring in the management of lagophthalmos and exposure keratopathy secondary to facial nerve palsy. Ophthal Plast Reconstr Surg. 2009;25:270–5.
33. Levine RE, Shapiro JP. Reanimation of the paralyzed eyelid with the enhanced palpebral spring or gold weight: modern replacements for tarsorrhaphy. Facial Plast Surg. 2001;16:325–36.
34. Arion HG. Dynamic closure of the lids in paralysis of the orbicularis muscle. Int Surg. 1972;57:48–50.
35. Hasmat S, Lovell NH, Eviston T, Ekmejian R, Suaning GJ, Clark J. Creating eye closure in patient with facial nerve paralysis using an implantable solenoid actuator. Conf Proc IEEE Eng Med Biol Soc. 2015;2015:1357–60.
36. Barmettler A, Nissanka N, Rosenblatt MI, Rao R, Lipson D, Lelli GJ Jr. Magnetic systems for tarsorrhaphy. Ophthal Plast Reconstr Surg. 2014;30:305–8.
37. Hinzpeter EN, Riehm E. Preliminary experience with lid magnets for paralytic lagophthalmos. Trans Ophthalmol Soc UK. 1976;96:73–8.
38. Seiff SR, Boerner M, Carter SR. Treatment of facial palsies with external eyelid weights. Am J Ophthalmol. 1995;120:652–7.
39. Demirci H, Hassan AS, Reck SD, Frueh BR, Elner VM. Graded full-thickness anterior blepharotomy for correction of upper eyelid retraction not associated with thyroid eye disease. Ophthal Plast Reconstr Surg. 2007;23:39–45.
40. Hassan AS, Frueh BR, Elner VM. Mullerectomy for upper eyelid retraction and lagophthalmos due to facial nerve palsy. Arch Ophthalmol. 2005;123:1221–5.
41. Compton CJ, Clark JD, Nunery WR, Lee HB. Recession and extirpation of the lower eyelid retractors for paralytic lagophthalmos. Ophthal Plast Reconstr Surg. 2015;31(4):323.
42. Sira M, Norris JH, Nduka C, Malhotra R. Transcaruncular medial canthal tendon plication with lower eyelid suture sling in facial nerve palsy. Orbit. 2014;33:159–63.
43. Dailey RA, Marx DP, Ahn ES. Porcine dermal collagen in lower eyelid retraction repair. Ophthal Plast Reconstr Surg. 2015;31:233–41.
44. Graziani C, Panico C, Botti G, Collin RJ. Subperiosteal midface lift: its role in static lower eyelid reconstruction after chronic facial nerve palsy. Orbit. 2011;30:140–4.
45. Olver JM. Raising the suborbicularis oculi fat (SOOF): its role in chronic facial palsy. Br J Ophthalmol. 2000;84:1401–6.
46. Madge SN, Malhotra R, Desousa J, et al. The lacrimal bypass tube for lacrimal pump failure attributable to facial palsy. Am J Opthalmol. 2010;149:155–9.
47. Lim C, Martin P, Benger R, Kourt G, Ghabrial R. Lacrimal canalicular bypass surgery with the Lester Jones tube. Am J Ophthalmol. 2004;137:101–8.
48. Scott G, Balsiger H, Kluckman M, Fan J, Gest T. Patterns of innervation of the lacrimal gland with clinical application. Clin Anat. 2014;27:1174–7.
49. Falzon K, Galea M, Cunniffe G, Logan P. Transconjunctival botulinum toxin offers an effective, safe and repeatable method to treat gustatory lacrimation. Br J Ophthalmol. 2010;94:379–80.
50. Montoya FJ, Riddell CE, Caesar R, Hague S. Treatment of gustatory hyperlacrimation (crocodile tears) with injection of botulinum toxin into the lacrimal gland. Eye (Lond). 2002;16:705–9.
51. Razfar A, Branstetter BF, Christopoulos A, et al. Ocular outcomes after gold weight placement and facial nerve resection. Otolaryngol Head Neck Surg. 2009;140:82.
52. Watts TL, Chard R, Weber SM, Wax MK. Immediate eye rehabilitation at the time of facial nerve sacrifice. Otolaryngol Head Neck Surg. 2011;144:353.
53. Maas CS, Benecke JE, Holds JB, Schoenrock LD, Simo F. Primary surgical management for rehabilitation of the paralyzed eye. Otolaryngol Head Neck Surg. 1994;110:288–95.
54. Chen C, Malhotra R, Muecke J, Davis G, Selva D. Aberrant facial nerve regeneration (AFR): an under-recognized cause of ptosis. Eye (Lond). 2004;18:159–62.
55. Couch SM, Chundury RV, Holds JB. Subjective and objective outcome measures in the treatment of facial nerve synkinesis with onabotulinumtoxinA (Botox). Ophthal Plast Reconstr Surg. 2014;30:246–50.
56. Cecini M, Pavese C, Comelli M, et al. Quantitative measurement of evolution of postparetic ocular synkinesis treated with botulinum toxin type A. Plast Reconstr Surg. 2013;132:1255–64.
57. Chua CN, Quhill F, Jones E, Voon LW, Ahad M, Rowson N. Treatment of aberrant facial nerve regeneration with botulinum toxin A. Orbit. 2004;23:213–8.
58. Patil-Chhablani P, Murthy S, Swaminathan M. Ophthalmic profile and systemic features of pediatric facial nerve palsy. Eye Sci. 2015;30:147–50.
59. Alsuhaibani AH, Bosley TM, Goldberg RA, Al-Faky YH. Entropion in children with isolated peripheral facial nerve paresis. Eye (Lond). 2012;26:1095–8.
60. Pasco NY, Kikkawa DO, Korn BS, Punja KG, Jones MC. Facial nerve paralysis: an unrecognized cause of lower eyelid entropion in the pediatric population. Ophthal Plast Reconstr Surg. 2007;23:126–9.
61. Terzis JK, Karypidis D. Blink restoration in adult facial paralysis. Plast Reconstr Surg. 2010;126:126–39.
62. Terzis JK, Karypidis D. The outcomes of dynamic procedures for blink restoration in pediatric facial paralysis. Plast Reconstr Surg. 2010;125:629–44.
63. Sadiq SA, Kharmasena A. Dynamic muscle transfer in facial nerve palsy: the use of contralateral orbicularis oculi muscle. Facial Plast Surg. 2015;31:145–51.
64. Frigerio A, heaton JT, Cavallari P, Knox C, Hohman MH, Hadlock TA. Electrical stimulation of eye blink in individuals with acute facial palsy: progress toward a bionic blink. Plast Recontr Surg. 2015;136:515e–23e.
65. Bains RD, Elbaz U, Zuker RM, Ali A, Borschel HG. Corneal neurotization from the supratrochlear nerve with sural nerve grafts: a minimally invasive approach. Plast Reconstr Surg. 2015;135:397e–400e.
66. Elbaz U, Bains R, Zuker RM, Borschel GH, Ali A. Restoration of corneal sensation with regional nerve transfers and nerve grafts: a new approach to a difficult problem. JAMA Ophthalmol. 2014;132:1289–95.
67. Terzis JK, Dryer MM, Bodner BI. Corneal neurotization: a novel solution to neurotrophic keratopathy. Plast Reconstr Surg. 2009;123:112–20.

Auditory Rehabilitation for Temporal Bone Cancer

27

Badr Ibrahim, Owen Woods, Issam Saliba, and Marc-Elie Nader

Abbreviations

ABR	Auditory brainstem response
AC	Air conduction
BC	Bone conduction
CROS	Contralateral routing of signal
EAC	External auditory canal
HBO	Hyperbaric oxygen
N-cm	Newton centimeter
OAEs	Otoacoustic emissions
OIHA	Osseointegrated hearing aid
RT	Radiation therapy
SNHL	Sensorineural hearing loss

Introduction

The treatment of temporal bone cancer almost invariably leads to some degree of hearing loss. Surgical approaches to temporal bone tumors predictably produce unilateral conductive hearing loss and, depending on the tumor's spread and extent of the resection, may lead to sacrifice of inner ear structures resulting in sensorineural hearing loss (SNHL). Radiation therapy (RT) directed at the temporal bone can cause additional SNHL. While T1 and T2 tumors of the temporal bone have excellent 5-year survival rates, the survival for T3 and T4 tumors is significantly less favorable [1]. Still, a significant subset of patients live long enough to experience the morbidities associated with their treatments. One of the most significant functional morbidities associated with the treatment of such cancers is hearing loss, which must be addressed in a comprehensive treatment plan to improve quality of life. Due to partial or total sacrifice of external ear structures, conventional hearing aids may not be suitable for hearing rehabilitation.

Osseointegrated hearing aids (OIHAs) have emerged as the most efficient method for hearing rehabilitation in the setting of temporal bone cancers. When it is possible to preserve the inner ear anatomy during oncological resection, OIHAs allow for ipsilateral cochlear stimulation and restoration of binaural hearing in the setting of maximal conductive hearing loss. If, on the other hand, significant SNHL exists on the ipsilateral side, then OIHAs can be used to stimulate the contralateral cochlea provided it is functional.

As OIHAs are the mainstay of hearing rehabilitation following the treatment of temporal bone cancer, this chapter will focus on OIHAs and explore various issues related to their use in the oncologic setting.

Historical Perspective

The concept of osseointegration was defined and described by Branemark et al. in the 1960s [2]. It relies on the unique properties of titanium in its relation to the bone and soft tissue. Specifically, an implanted titanium screw has the ability to become anchored in the host bone by directly contacting remodeling bone and serving as a surface for osteoblast proliferation without intervening the soft tissue. This concept was later put to use by Tjellstrom in the 1980s for development of a bone-anchored hearing aid and the further demonstration that when osseointegration has happened adequately,

B. Ibrahim, M.D. · I. Saliba, M.D., F.R.C.S.C.
Division of Otolaryngology — Head and Neck Surgery, Université de Montréal, Centre Hospitalier de l'Université de Montréal (CHUM), Montreal, QC, Canada

O. Woods, M.D., M.Sc.
Division of Otolaryngology — Head and Neck Surgery, Université de Montréal, Hôpital Maisonneuve-Rosemont, Montreal, QC, Canada

M.-E. Nader, M.D., M.Sc. (✉)
Division of Otolaryngology — Head and Neck Surgery, Université de Montréal, Centre Hospitalier de l'Université de Montréal (CHUM), Montreal, QC, Canada

Department of Head and Neck Surgery, The University of Texas M.D. Anderson Cancer Center, Houston, TX, USA
e-mail: mnader@mdanderson.org

P. W. Gidley, F. DeMonte (eds.), *Temporal Bone Cancer*, https://doi.org/10.1007/978-3-319-74539-8_27

the titanium screw may extend through the skin with minimal soft tissue reaction [3].

Indications of OIHA

OIHA is indicated in patients with temporal bone malignancies who cannot use conventional hearing aids for conductive or mixed hearing loss that occurs following surgical treatment. In patients who undergo temporal bone resections, the external auditory canal (EAC), tympanic membrane, and ossicles are usually sacrificed. The loss of these structures renders conventional hearing aids an inadequate rehabilitation option as these devices rely on the conducting mechanisms of the ear. OIHAs become the next best choice in order to restore hearing. Their design and function are fundamentally different than those of conventional hearing aids. Whereas conventional hearing aids use the existing external and middle ear anatomy to transmit sound waves to the inner ear, OIHA acts as a prosthetic device and replaces the missing sound-conducting parts of hearing. Sound is sensed directly in the cochlea, which may explain the improved sound quality patients perceive with OIHA when compared to conventional aids [4] OIHA can be used when the average bone conduction (BC) in the affected ear is 45 dB HL or better. An improvement in hearing can be expected independently of conductive hearing loss on the OIHA-fitted side; however, conductive hearing loss should not be greater than 65 dB HL [5].

OIHA may also be considered in the context of unilateral SNHL when contralateral hearing is preserved. OIHA becomes particularly useful when contralateral routing of signal (CROS) hearing aids cannot be used, such as when the auricle is sacrificed. In the case of unilateral SNHL, OIHA should be considered when the affected ear shows profound SNHL *and* contralateral hearing is normal with a hearing threshold of 20 dB HL or better [5].

Audiometric Evaluation

Audiometric evaluation of patients with temporal bone cancers poses specific challenges. These patients are often difficult to test when they have tumors blocking the ear canal. Air conduction (AC) thresholds may not be obtained, and only BC thresholds can sometimes be evaluated. The protocol for speech audiometry must also be changed accordingly because it is usually performed by AC. Speech audiometry using BC is feasible and correlates well with BC pure tone thresholds between 500 and 2000 Hz [6]. The role of otoacoustic emissions (OAEs) and auditory brainstem responses (ABRs) is also limited in this patient population. OAEs may be difficult to assess if the probe cannot be fitted in the ear canal. Although ABRs can be performed using bone-conducted stimuli [7], they are rare, if ever tested in patients with temporal bone cancers. Additionally, we usually do not rely on acoustic reflex testing for the evaluation of facial paralysis.

OIHA Systems

A variety of OIHA systems are currently commercially available (Table 27.1). They either rely on percutaneous attachment of a sound processor to an osseointegrated implant or on transcutaneous transmission of sound waves to a bone conduction implant. Newer prostheses like the Baha® Attract and Sophono systems have been developed to facilitate the use of the device and facilitate postimplantation care. They rely on the transcutaneous conduction of vibration to the implant via magnets holding the processor in place on either side of the skin and soft tissue layer. Transcutaneous OIHA systems have yet to be evaluated in the context of temporal bone cancer reconstructions; the remainder of this chapter will focus on the percutaneous OIHA systems. Furthermore, concerns regarding possible pressure-induced wounds at the site of the magnet fixture in fragile irradiated tissues lead us to favor percutaneous implants for the time being.

While differences exist in the shape and make of percutaneous implants and vibrating sound processors, they are invariably composed of (1) an external vibrating sound processor, (2) a skin abutment component, and (3) an osseointegrated implant (Fig. 27.1).

All osseointegrated devices use titanium screws of variable diameter and length. Titanium is an inert material that has been demonstrated to be ideal for proper osseointegration [8]. Over the years, changes in width as well as microtopography of the implant have led to wider implants with modification of the screw to create a rougher surface than

Table 27.1 Commercially available osseointegrate hearing aids

Company	Brand	Attachment type	Number of microphones	Directional listening	Programmability
Cochlear™	Baha®	Abutment and magnet	2	Omnidirectional, manual, and automatic adjustments	Customizable gain, output, and frequency response
Oticon Medical	Ponto™	Abutment	2	Manual adjustments and four automatic modes	Four different programs
Medtronic	Sophono®	Magnet	2	Omni and adaptive directional programs available	Four different programs

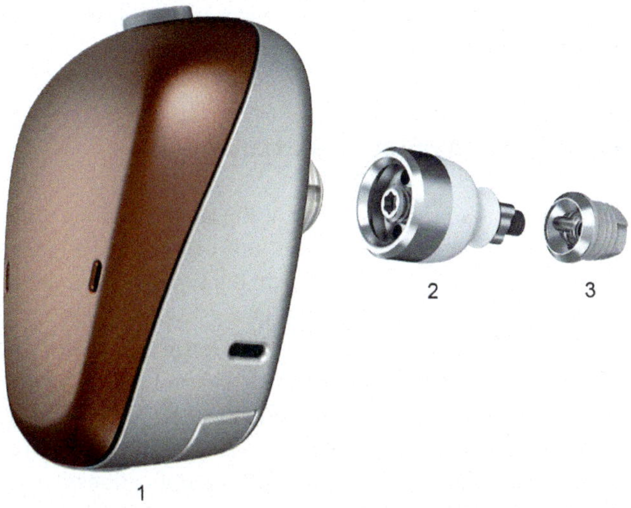

Fig. 27.1 Basic component of a percutaneous OIHA system. (Images provided courtesy of Cochlear Americas, © 2017 Cochlear Americas. 1, sound processor; 2, skin abutment; 3 osseointegrated implant)

initially described by Branemark. These changes seem to have improved the osseointegration process.

The abutment component serves as a link between the vibrating processor and the osseointegrated implant and, as such, must be attached to both while extruding through the skin and soft tissue. Abutments vary in coating material and in length, depending on the thickness of the soft tissue present at the implant site. They are the most common site of infection and local reaction in the entire OIHA system. Hydroxyapatite concave abutment components have been developed and have shown to cause less adverse soft tissue and skin reaction than the traditional titanium abutment component [9].

Percutaneous OIHA processors are marketed by Cochlear Ltd. as the Baha® family of processors (Cochlear Baha® hearing system; Cochlear, Lane Cove, NSW, Australia) and Oticon Medical as the Ponto™ family of processors (Oticon Medical AB, Datavägen, Sweden). The sound processor is composed of one or multiple microphones receiving sound waves. These are then interpreted by the internal processor and converted to vibrations, which in turn are transmitted via the abutment to the osseointegrated implant. Variations in the number of microphones, their sensitivity, capacity to detect ambient sounds and directional listening, as well as programmability of the processor exist within the same family of processors and between brands.

Physiology of Bone Conduction Hearing

The EAC, the middle ear, and the inner ear all play crucial roles in BC hearing. While each of these structures is essential, the results of extensive experimental and clinical research summarized by Stenfelt et al. [10] indicate that fluid inertia in the inner ear would be the most influential factor contributing to BC hearing in lower frequencies. The inertia of the inner ear's incompressible fluid causes it to vibrate as one compartment in phase with the surrounding bone. The presence of the highly compliant oval and round windows allows for a longitudinal wave to travel through the cochlea generating a stimulus to the basilar membrane. A contribution of inner ear compression and distension with vibration of the skull is thought to contribute to BC hearing in higher frequencies.

Mechanisms of Hearing Loss in Temporal Bone Cancer

Hearing loss may occur as a conductive hearing loss with or without added sensorineural loss in the context of temporal bone cancer treatment.

The most common cause of hearing loss in the treatment of temporal bone cancers results from the sacrifice of the EAC and the ossicles. Furthermore, since RT is often part of the treatment regimen of more advanced tumors, its effects on the potential for reconstruction of the EAC must be taken into consideration. External auditory canal defects are best managed by obliteration rather than canalplasty in the setting of RT [11]. Hence, a persistent conductive hearing loss can be expected in all cases of temporal bone cancer resections.

Sensorineural hearing loss may result from different mechanisms in patients with temporal bone tumors. First, resection of inner ear structures, which may be necessary to obtain negative margins, invariably leads to SNHL. Additionally, RT and chemotherapy can both cause SNHL. Platinum-based chemotherapeutic regimens have showed promising results in the treatment of squamous cell carcinoma of the temporal bone [12]. However, ototoxicity is a well-established side effect of this class of chemotherapeutic drugs, especially cisplatin and to a lesser extent carboplatin [13]. Ototoxicity from RT may further exacerbate SNHL in cancer patients. It is dose dependent and rarely seen with cochlear radiation levels of 30 Gy or less [14] However, cisplatin and RT have synergistic effects on the cochlea, and inner ear toxicity may occur at lower RT levels in patients treated concurrently with these two modalities [14]

There are therefore multiple pathways inherent to the treatment of temporal bone cancers that can lead to both conductive and SNHL, hence the need for appropriate hearing rehabilitation options tailored to each patient.

Effect of Radiation Therapy on OIHA

While it is clear that RT increases the risk of complications in the process of osseointegration in the postradiation setting, there is conflicting data regarding the dose-related impact on the survival of implants and very limited temporal bone-specific data. It is advisable to exercise greater caution in soft tissue handling and surgical method with rising RT doses.

The effects of radiation on bony tissues were highlighted in a series of experiments conducted by Marx et al. [15]. Radiation-induced inflammation and loss of vascularization of tissues over time were found to ultimately lead to increased fibrosis. The loss of microvascular content appeared initially at 6 months after RT and worsened over time [15]. In a parallel series of investigations, histologic assessments of osseointegrated implants in an animal model demonstrated a decreased contact area between postradiation bone and implant [16]. These factors may explain higher rates of implant extrusion and failures in this patient population.

A review of the literature by Ihde et al. [17] showed that the risk of implant failure in irradiated bone was 12 times higher than in non-irradiated bone for all craniofacial implants. No details pertaining to dosage or site-specific data were available to interpret these findings in the context of radiation to the lateral skull base for temporal bone tumors. Similarly, Granstrom et al. [18] have shown in a large series of more than 600 implants, more than 100 of them being in the temporoparietal region, that osseointegration failure rate was 6.6 times higher in irradiated temporoparietal bones.

In contrast, when looking at implantation in irradiated mastoid bones specifically, around 55 cases were reported in the literature [19–21]. Their survival rates range from 90 to 100% (with the exception of one study reporting the failure of 2/2 irradiated mastoid implants). Despite the increased risk of postradiation implant failure, it seems that the mastoid bone is a more favorable site for implantation post-RT than other craniofacial subsites like the nasal or orbital bones [19].

A relationship between RT doses and implant survival could not be established in a study by Nader et al. [20] nor was it verified in a prospective study of implants in other irradiated craniofacial sites [22]. Granstrom et al., however, observed a dose-dependent effect of radiation on implant failure in their large retrospective review [18] with a cumulative radiation effect higher than 30 Gy strongly associated with implant failure.

Implantation Method

General Principles

The following guiding principles should be observed when placing OIHA, especially in patients receiving RT to the temporal bone: (1) gentle handling of soft tissues, (2) use of a high-torque drill at slow speeds (2000 RPM), (3) use of lower torque of 30 N/cm for implant insertion in irradiated bone, (4) use of sharp drill bits to avoid undesired damage to the implant bed, and (5) use of proper irrigation to prevent bone heating.

Timing of Implantation and Loading

Implantation is best performed at the time of initial oncological resection. Perhaps the most probing evidence regarding the outcomes of OIHA in relation to the sequence of treatment in temporal bone tumors is provided by a series from Nader et al. [20]. In this retrospective review, 51 implants were analyzed based on the timing of implantation to primary oncological resection and RT. Interestingly, implantation performed at the time of primary oncological resection yielded significantly fewer complications than if it was delayed in a secondary procedure. The only two instances of implant extrusion in that series occurred in patients implanted following radiation during a second surgical procedure. This prompted the author to define the group of most favorable outcomes as those patients being implanted at the time of primary oncological resection prior to RT.

There is no consensus on optimal processor loading time when OIHAs are implanted in irradiated temporal bones. In our practice, we recommend that patients wait at least 6 months before using their processor. In non-irradiated bones, loading can be performed 3 months following implantation (as per the manufacturers' instructions, Cochlear™ and Oticon Medical).

Recent advances in implant technology and the experience derived from the dental implant literature have led some authors to suggest early loading at 2–4 weeks postimplantation with various implantation methods [23–25]. However, the patient populations in these studies were comprised of healthy adults with no evidence of traumatized or poor quality bone, thus making these findings less applicable to the oncologic setting. We do not recommend loading in such a short time frame following implantation in patients with temporal bone cancer.

Surgical Technique

We currently favor a two-stage procedure when implanting OIHA in patients being treated for temporal bone cancers.

Implants should be placed 50–60 mm from the EAC along the temporal line. Given these anatomical landmarks may not be present following excision of the tumor, marking of the optimal implantation site should be done prior to incision by marking the future site of implantation with methylene blue using a fine needle tip. Following resection and before soft tissue reconstruction, implantation is performed in the bony area marked by the methylene blue.

At the targeted site, a 3 mm hole is drilled at slow speed (2000 RPM) staying perpendicular to the bone surface. A drill indicator may be used to facilitate orientation. The depth of the hole is palpated with a blunt instrument. If sufficient cortical bone is present, the hole is deepened with a 4 mm drill bit. The implant bed is then widened with a 4 mm countersink drill bit in order to create a countersink halo, which increases the contact surface area with the implant and helps to prevent skin cells from undermining the implant.

The implant is inserted in place very slowly with a torque-controlled drill. When RT is planned, a lower torque setting of 30 Newton centimeter (N-cm) should be employed. In the experience at the UT MD Anderson Cancer Center, one implant extruded after being screwed in at 40 N-cm leading the group to change their practice and implant OIHA at 30 N-cm [20]. Very soft bone might require only 20 N-cm torque force. Abundant irrigation should be used throughout these steps. Care must be exercised that the implant is fully inserted. If the implant is not fully inserted, then the drill should be reversed and the implant removed and placed again.

Once the implant is properly secured, a cover screw may be placed to protect the internal threads of the implant. Soft tissue closure with a temporalis muscle flap or microvascular free flap, as dictated by the deficit, protects the implant and allows for healing and proper osseointegration. Postoperative radiation is dictated by the stage and pathologic findings. When no radiation is given, then second-stage procedure can be performed at 3 months postoperatively.

The abutment is placed during a second-stage procedure after waiting at least 6 months following implantation and completion of RT. Up until recently, abutments came in a fixed length. In patients with thicker subcutaneous layers, soft tissue reduction was required to obtain a proper cutaneous implant junction and to avoid skin overgrowth. Abutments are now available in variable lengths, allowing their placement without the need to thin the subcutaneous tissue. In a recent study, soft tissue preservation was associated with less numbness at the site of implantation, improved esthetics, fewer peri-implant infections, and less abutment removal [26].

Placement of the abutment may be done under local or general anesthesia. The implant is first located by palpation. Preoperative CT scan may offer additional guidance. The thickness of the subcutaneous layer is estimated using a needle and a clamp, and an abutment of adequate length is chosen. A curvilinear incision is made, and subcutaneous tissues are dissected to the level of the implant. After removal of the cover screw, the abutment is connected to the implant.

The wound is closed in two layers with interrupted sutures around the abutment. The latter is left to extrude between two sutures at the skin. Alternatively, the incision may be performed off-center, and a 4 mm punch biopsy may be used to create a hole through which the abutment extrudes. A protective cap is then placed on the abutment, and a gauze dressing is applied between the skin and the healing cap, followed by a mastoid dressing.

An even less invasive punch technique has been described recently. A 6 mm skin biopsy punch is used to remove the skin, subcutaneous tissue, and periosteum overlying the site of implantation. According to the authors, this method was shown to decrease surgical time when compared to the linear incision methods with soft tissue reduction without increasing soft tissue complications [27]. However, this technique has not been verified in previously irradiated temporal bones.

When OIHAs are placed in a secondary procedure following temporal bone resection, a single-stage approach is used. The steps essentially follow the same ones as described above. Preoperative CT scan, usually done in the context of tumor surveillance, can help determine an appropriate implantation site.

Complications of OIHA Implantation

Complications of OIHA placement can be categorized as minor or major. Minor complications include local inflammation, soft tissue overgrowth not necessitating surgery, or friction between the processor and the skin. Major complications are composed of bone exposure, implant extrusion, or any soft tissue reaction requiring surgical treatment [20]. Radionecrosis can also occur in the context of radiotherapy.

Soft tissue reactions were classified by Holgers et al. in 1988 [28], which allow standardization of assessment of complications. It was later modified in 2008 by Wazen et al. [29] to account for granulation tissue, skin overgrowth, and keloid formation successfully treated in the office. Both classifications are presented in Tables 27.2 and 27.3.

Complications are treated according to the severity of the reaction using a scale of different modalities ranging from topical ointments to free flap covering. Local skin reactions and granulation tissue can be treated by a combination of topical steroids and antibiotics as well as systemic antibiotics. Injection of medium potency steroids, such as triamcinolone, can be helpful in more stubborn cases. If, however, the granulation tissue is too extensive or unresponsive to conservative treatment, surgical excision can be performed under local or general anesthesia with appropriate

Table 27.2 Holgers classifications of skin reaction at implant site

Grade	Clinical description
Grade 0	No irritation
Grade 1	Slight redness
Grade 2	Red and moist tissue
Grade 3	Granulation tissue
Grade 4	Infection leading to removal of the abutment

Table 27.3 Modified Holgers classifications of skin reaction at implant site

Grade	Clinical description
Grade 0	No irritation: epithelial debris removed if present
Grade 1	Slight redness: temporary local treatment indicated
Grade 2	Red and slightly moist; no granulation tissue present
Grade 3	Red and moist with granulation tissue, skin overgrowth, or scar formation: local treatment indicated
Grade 4	Extensive granulation, skin overgrowth, or scar formation requiring revision surgery
Grade 5	Removal of skin-penetrating abutment necessary to control infection

From: Wazen et al. Successes and complications of the Baha system. Otol Neurotol. 2008 Dec;29 [8]:1115–9. (http://journals.lww.com/otology-neurotology/)

topical and systemic antibiotics and/or steroids to help healing and prevent recurrence.

In the case of bone exposure, various reconstructive methods may be employed such as skin grafting, local advancement flaps, or even free flaps if healthy, non-irradiated tissue is needed to close the deficit. In our experience, our one patient who had a free flap to save the implant lost his implant a few months later. Anecdotally, twice daily application of antibiotic ointment has also helped encourage skin growth to cover exposed bone. Fortunately, none of the patients who lost their implants developed persistent exposed bone or osteomyelitis at the implant site.

Radiation therapy can induce radionecrosis following OIHA placement. The effect of hyperbaric oxygen (HBO) therapy preimplantation has been studied to evaluate ways to decrease the failure rate of osseointegration following RT. While there is evidence to support the use of HBO therapy for most craniofacial subsites [18, 30, 31], the benefit of HBO therapy for temporoparietal implantation specifically has yet to be demonstrated [18]. In addition, when considering osseointegration in the temporal bone specifically, failure rates following RT have been very variable ranging from 0 to 17% [19–21, 31]. These numbers are extrapolated from studies with great variability in treatment regimens and patient characteristics. In light of the high success rate of osseointegration in temporal bone and the controversy regarding the benefit of HBO therapy in cases of mastoid irradiation, we cannot yet conclude on the routine use of HBO at the present time, though it appears to be unnecessary.

It seems that patients receiving RT and fitted with an OIHA are at a higher risk of developing major complications including implant loss. The largest series of temporal bone cancer patients fitted with OIHA showed a 31.6 % ($n = 8/19$) overall complication rate in irradiated patients as opposed to 24.1% ($n = 7/29$) in the non-irradiated group [20]. Only one major complication was recorded in the non-irradiated group consisting of tissue overgrowth over the abutment necessitating surgical excision. No implant extrusion was recorded. However, in the irradiated group, five major complications occurred: (1) instance of tissue overgrowth needing surgical excision, (2) two instances of bone exposure and two implant extrusions. The remainder of minor complications in both groups consisted of limited soft tissue reactions (19% in non-irradiated and 21% in irradiated patients).

Furthermore, studies on the timing of OIHA placement showed that patients fitted with OIHA following RT had more complications than patients fitted prior to RT. In the series by Nader et al., no minor or major complications occurred in patients implanted before RT, while 38% of patients in the postirradiation group suffered a major complication. The complication rate was even higher in the postirradiation group when stratifying according to timing of the implantation to the primary oncological resection: no major complications were noted in patients implanted at the time of primary oncologic resection, while those implanted during a second-stage procedure had a 45% rate of major complications.

In comparison, patients fitted with OIHA in a non-oncological setting have highly variable rates of minor and major complications. The main complications of percutaneous OIHA implantation were assessed in a meta-analysis by Kiringoda et al. [32]. This meta-analysis identified 2134 patients (mixed adult and pediatric) who underwent 2310 implantation procedures across 45 studies for non-oncological indications. The most frequent complication was a Holgers grade 2–4 skin reaction at the abutment site in 16.1–38.1% of cases. The remainder of complications noted was infection with clinical signs in 1–21.4% of cases, soft tissue overgrowth requiring surgical excision in 8.4–9.4% of cases, and failure of osseointegration in 0–18% of cases. Overall, the rates of complications of OIHA implantation in the oncological setting are within the upper limit of the reported range in this larger, heterogonous, non-oncological patient pool.

Alternative to Implantation

An alternative exists for patients who want to use the OIHA sound processor independently of its abutment. All three OIHA companies offer the option to use the sound processors with soft headbands. These bands are made of elastic materials worn around the head that secure the processor in place. This option can be offered right after surgery to implanted patients while they are waiting for osseointegration to occur. However, care must be exercised so that pressure is not exerted on a fresh microvascular free flap. Soft bands can also be used in patients who do not want to undergo the second-stage procedure or in those who lose their implant.

Patient Satisfaction and Quality of Life

The impact of OIHA systems on quality of life and patient satisfaction has been reported in multiple regional OIHA programs to assess the efficacy of the intervention. Collectively, these studies demonstrated a benefit in quality of life and patient satisfaction as well as cosmesis, quality of sound, and face-to-face conversation [33–35]. Notably, 78–90% of respondents in these various studies used their OIHA system more than 8 h per day, and usage patterns did not vary between recently fitted patients and those who had been fitted for years [33]. Seventy percent of respondents in various studies reported an improvement of their quality of life following OIHA [33, 34], and 75% favored their OIHA over their previous conventional aid [33]. The main drawback reported in multiple studies was a drop in patient satisfaction when using the OIHA in noisy environment or group discussion settings [33, 34, 36]. Moreover, patients fitted with an OIHA after having used a conventional hearing aid have reported significantly higher satisfaction with sound quality, speech recognition, and feedback problems and handling as well as a decreased rate of ear infections [4]. As well, OIHA provides better sound quality than a traditional conduction hearing aid with a contralateral routing of the sound signal with no occlusion effect or connecting cable [37]. Of note however, these data reflect patient satisfaction and quality of life assessment in patients fitted in a non-oncologic context. No data presently assess the quality of life benefit of OIHA in temporal bone cancer patients. In light of the importance of hearing rehabilitation for the improvement of quality of life in temporal bone cancer patients, it is safe to extrapolate data from such studies to guide practice for the time being, until more precise data becomes available.

Chapter Highlights

- Conductive hearing loss and SNHL are common consequences of temporal bone cancer treatments.
- OIHA is presently the best available option for hearing rehabilitation in the context of temporal bone cancer.
- Radiation induces bony and soft tissue damage that increases the risk of implant failure.
- OIHA implantation is best performed at the time of the primary oncological resection prior to tissue irradiation if possible.
- Great care must be exercised in handling the soft tissue during OIHA implantation to decrease the risk of complications and allow for proper osseointegration.
- Processor loading should not be performed earlier than 3 months postimplantation in non-irradiated patients and 6 months in irradiated patients.
- The most frequent complication of OIHA implantation is soft tissue reaction at the site of the abutment.
- Radiation therapy may increase the risk of major complications and implant failures, especially when OIHAs are placed following irradiation.
- Auditory rehabilitation with OIHA improves patients' quality of life.

References

1. Chi FL, Gu FM, Dai CF, Chen B, Li HW. Survival outcomes in surgical treatment of 72 cases of squamous cell carcinoma of the temporal bone. Otol Neurotol. 2011;32(4):665–9.
2. Branemark PI, Adell R, Breine U, Hansson BO, Lindstrom J, Ohlsson A. Intra-osseous anchorage of dental prostheses. I. Experimental studies. Scand J Plast Reconstr Surg. 1969;3(2):81–100.
3. Tjellstrom A, Hakansson B, Lindstrom J, Branemark PI, Hallen O, Rosenhall U, et al. Analysis of the mechanical impedance of bone-anchored hearing aids. Acta Otolaryngol. 1980;89(1-2):85–92.
4. McDermott AL, Dutt SN, Reid AP, Proops DW. An intra-individual comparison of the previous conventional hearing aid with the bone-anchored hearing aid: The Nijmegen group questionnaire. J Laryngol Otol Suppl. 2002;28:15–9.
5. Johnson JT, Rosen CA, Bailey BJ. Bailey's head and neck surgery—otolaryngology. Philadelphia, PA: Wolters Kluwer Health/Lippincott Williams & Wilkins; 2013.
6. Goetzinger C, Proud G. Speech audiometry by bone conduction. AMA Arch Otolaryngol. 1955;62(6):632–5.
7. Kramer SJ. Frequency-specific auditory brainstem responses to bone-conducted stimuli. Audiology. 1992;31(2):61–71.
8. Albrektsson T, Branemark PI, Hansson HA, Lindstrom J. Osseointegrated titanium implants. Requirements for ensuring a long-lasting, direct bone-to-implant anchorage in man. Acta Orthop Scand. 1981;52(2):155–70.
9. Wilkie MD, Chakravarthy KM, Mamais C, Temple RH. Osseointegrated hearing implant surgery using a novel hydroxyapatite-coated concave abutment design. Otolaryngol Head Neck Surg. 2014;151(6):1014–9.
10. Stenfelt S, Goode RL. Bone-conducted sound: physiological and clinical aspects. Otol Neurotol. 2005;26(6):1245–61.
11. Gal TJ, Kerschner JE, Futran ND, Bartels LJ, Farrior JB, Ridley MB, et al. Reconstruction after temporal bone resection. Laryngoscope. 1998;108(4 Pt 1):476–81.
12. Zanoletti E, Lovato A, Stritoni P, Martini A, Mazzoni A, Marioni G. A critical look at persistent problems in the diagnosis, staging and treatment of temporal bone carcinoma. Cancer Treat Rev. 2015;41(10):821–6.
13. Landier W. Ototoxicity and cancer therapy. Cancer. 2016;122(11):1647–58.
14. Paulino AC, Lobo M, Teh BS, Okcu MF, South M, Butler EB, et al. Ototoxicity after intensity-modulated radiation therapy and cisplatin-based chemotherapy in children with medulloblastoma. Int J Radiat Oncol Biol Phys. 2010;78(5):1445–50.
15. Marx RE, Johnson RP. Studies in the radiobiology of osteoradionecrosis and their clinical significance. Oral Surg Oral Med Oral Pathol. 1987;64(4):379–90.
16. Brogniez V, D'Hoore W, Gregoire V, Munting E, Reychler H. Implants placed in an irradiated dog mandible: a morphometric analysis. Int J Oral Maxillofac Implants. 2000;15(4):511–8.
17. Ihde S, Kopp S, Gundlach K, Konstantinovic VS. Effects of radiation therapy on craniofacial and dental implants: a review of the

literature. Oral Surg Oral Med Oral Pathol Oral Radiol Endod. 2009;107(1):56–65.
18. Granstrom G. Osseointegration in irradiated cancer patients: an analysis with respect to implant failures. J Oral Maxillofac Surg. 2005;63(5):579–85.
19. Abu-Serriah MM, McGowan DA, Moos KF, Bagg J. Extra-oral craniofacial endosseous implants and radiotherapy. Int J Oral Maxillofac Surg. 2003;32(6):585–92.
20. Nader ME, Beadle BM, Roberts DB, Gidley PW. Outcomes and complications of osseointegrated hearing aids in irradiated temporal bones. Laryngoscope. 2016;126:1187–92.
21. Wilkie MD, Lightbody KA, Salamat AA, Chakravarthy KM, Luff DA, Temple RH. Stability and survival of bone-anchored hearing aid implant systems in post-irradiated patients. Eur Arch Otorhinolaryngol. 2015;272(6):1371–6.
22. Tolman DE, Taylor PF. Bone-anchored craniofacial prosthesis study: irradiated patients. Int J Oral Maxillofac Implants. 1996;11(5):612–9.
23. McLarnon CM, Johnson I, Davison T, Hill J, Henderson B, Leese D, et al. Evidence for early loading of osseointegrated implants for bone conduction at 4 weeks. Otol Neurotol. 2012;33(9):1578–82.
24. Faber HT, Dun CA, Nelissen RC, Mylanus EA, Cremers CW, Hol MK. Bone-anchored hearing implant loading at 3 weeks: stability and tolerability after 6 months. Otol Neurotol. 2013;34(1):104–10.
25. Hogsbro M, Agger A, Johansen LV. Successful loading of a bone-anchored hearing implant at two weeks after surgery: randomized trial of two surgical methods and detailed stability measurements. Otol Neurotol. 2015;36(2):e51–7.
26. Hultcrantz M, Lanis A. A five-year follow-up on the osseointegration of bone-anchored hearing device implantation without tissue reduction. Otol Neurotol. 2014;35(8):1480–5.
27. Gordon SA, Coelho DH. Minimally invasive surgery for osseointegrated auditory implants: a comparison of linear versus punch techniques. Otolaryngol Head Neck Surg. 2015;152(6):1089–93.
28. Holgers KM, Tjellstrom A, Bjursten LM, Erlandsson BE. Soft tissue reactions around percutaneous implants: a clinical study of soft tissue conditions around skin-penetrating titanium implants for bone-anchored hearing aids. Am J Otol. 1988;9(1):56–9.
29. Wazen JJ, Young DL, Farrugia MC, Chandrasekhar SS, Ghossaini SN, Borik J, et al. Successes and complications of the Baha system. Otol Neurotol. 2008;29(8):1115–9.
30. Granstrom G, Tjellstrom A, Branemark PI. Osseointegrated implants in irradiated bone: a case-controlled study using adjunctive hyperbaric oxygen therapy. J Oral Maxillofac Surg. 1999;57(5):493–9.
31. Granstrom G. Radiotherapy, osseointegration and hyperbaric oxygen therapy. Periodontol 2000. 2003;33:145–62.
32. Kiringoda R, Lustig LR. A meta-analysis of the complications associated with osseointegrated hearing aids. Otol Neurotol. 2013;34(5):790–4.
33. Mace AT, Isa A, Cooke LD. Patient quality of life with bone-anchored hearing aid: 10-year experience in Glasgow, Scotland. J Laryngol Otol. 2009;123(9):964–8.
34. Badran K, Bunstone D, Arya AK, Suryanarayanan R, Mackinnon N. Patient satisfaction with the bone-anchored hearing aid: a 14-year experience. Otol Neurotol. 2006;27(5):659–66.
35. Dutt SN, McDermott AL, Jelbert A, Reid AP, Proops DW. Day to day use and service-related issues with the bone-anchored hearing aid: the Entific Medical Systems questionnaire. J Laryngol Otol Suppl 2002;(28):20–28.
36. Dutt SN, McDermott AL, Burrell SP, Cooper HR, Reid AP, Proops DW. Patient satisfaction with bilateral bone-anchored hearing aids: the Birmingham experience. J Laryngol Otol Suppl. 2002;28:37–46.
37. Niparko JK, Cox KM, Lustig LR. Comparison of the bone anchored hearing aid implantable hearing device with contralateral routing of offside signal amplification in the rehabilitation of unilateral deafness. Otol Neurotol. 2003;24(1):73–8.

28 Auricular Prosthetic Rehabilitation

Patricia C. Montgomery, Theresa M. Hofstede, and Mark S. Chambers

Introduction

Facial prosthetic rehabilitation is a reliable alternative to autograft reconstruction in cases that may not be able to achieve satisfactory cosmetic results surgically. Prosthetic rehabilitation of the auricle is performed by a specialty service, maxillofacial prosthodontists and anaplastologists (Fig. 28.1). To obtain the best esthetic outcome for prosthetic rehabilitation, a presurgical evaluation of the patient is necessary and should include all team members involved in the plan of care. Prosthetic reconstruction of the auricle has multiple main goals: noninvasive reconstruction of an esthetically pleasing auricle, effective retention, repeatable placement, and reduction of the psychological distress associated with the disfigurement [1, 2] [*Case example 1: Female patient with total auriculectomy distress*] (Fig. 28.2a, b, c, d).

Auricular reconstruction from native soft tissues is a substantial challenge for surgeons. Issues due to vascular compromise, available soft tissue, cartilaginous and osseous support, as well as revision of failed grafts and flaps, may lead to inconsistent results producing an unsatisfactory outcome. Patient expectation and acceptance of the reconstruction may compromise a successful outcome [3]. An unsuccessful reconstruction may also compromise a successful prosthetic outcome (Fig. 28.3).

Prosthetic rehabilitation has become a functional and esthetic alternative to tissue reconstruction. Since the introduction of percutaneous endosseous implants for use with bone conduction hearing devices in 1977, titanium implants have had an important role in the rehabilitation of patients with craniofacial defects. Specific implants and retentive components are designed exclusively for auricular prostheses to create a reliable, reproducible, and effective retention. Osseointegration biotechnology has revolutionized auricular prosthetic retention, and its retentive benefits have been well studied. However, not every patient is a candidate for implant placement since adequate bone stock might not be available for the implants. While the ultimate goal of cancer surgery is the eradication of the cancer, patients should be informed preoperatively about the options available for prosthetic replacement of the outer ear. This chapter is devoted to the alternative of autograft technique and will cover prosthetic rehabilitation of the auricle, including retention and fabrication.

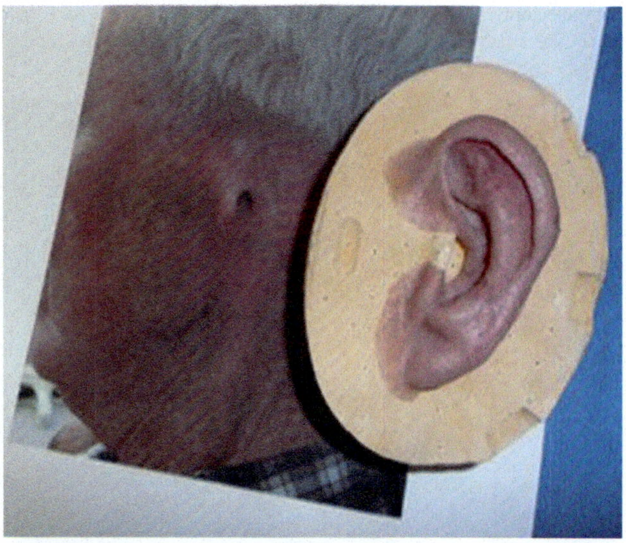

Fig. 28.1 Total auricular prosthetic rehabilitation

Total Versus Partial Auricular Prosthesis

A total auricular prosthesis is a restoration alternative when a complete auriculectomy (pinnectomy) is done. A partial auricular prosthesis can be fabricated when a subtotal auriculectomy is performed and partial preservation of the external

P. C. Montgomery · T. M. Hofstede, D.D.S., F.A.C.P.
M. S. Chambers, D.M.D., M.S. (✉)
Section of Oral Oncology and Maxillofacial Prosthodontics, Department of Head and Neck Surgery, The University of Texas M.D. Anderson Cancer Center, Houston, TX, USA
e-mail: pmontgo@mdanderson.org; thofstede@mdanderson.org; mchamber@mdanderson.org

P. W. Gidley, F. DeMonte (eds.), *Temporal Bone Cancer*, https://doi.org/10.1007/978-3-319-74539-8_28

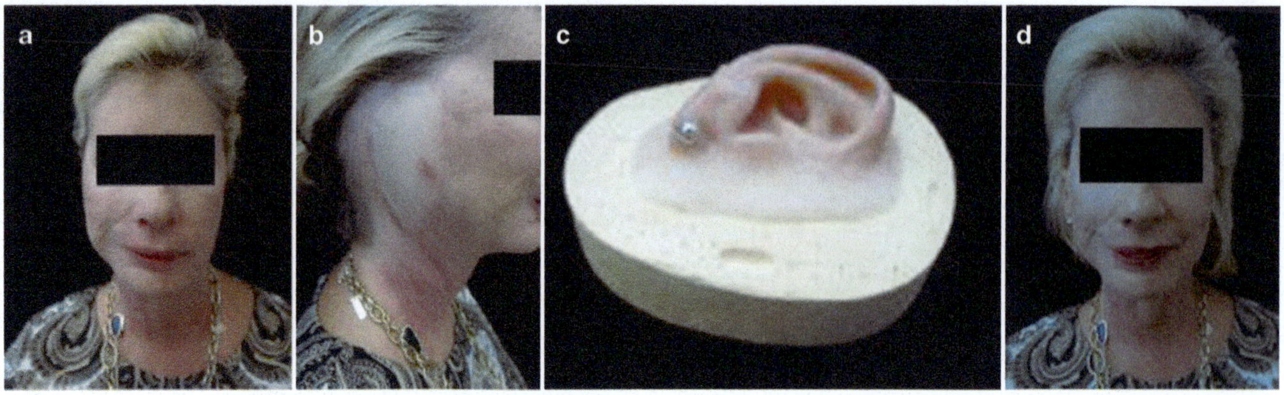

Fig. 28.2 (**a**) Invasive squamous cell carcinoma necessitating total auriculectomy. (**b**) Full auriculectomy with small skin paddle. (**c**) Patient desires to wear earrings again, and the silicone prosthesis allows for customization. (**d**) Final prosthesis in position using water-based adhesive. Lobule is more visible on prosthesis to allow for visibility of earring as requested by patient. Patient can now wear all her earrings again

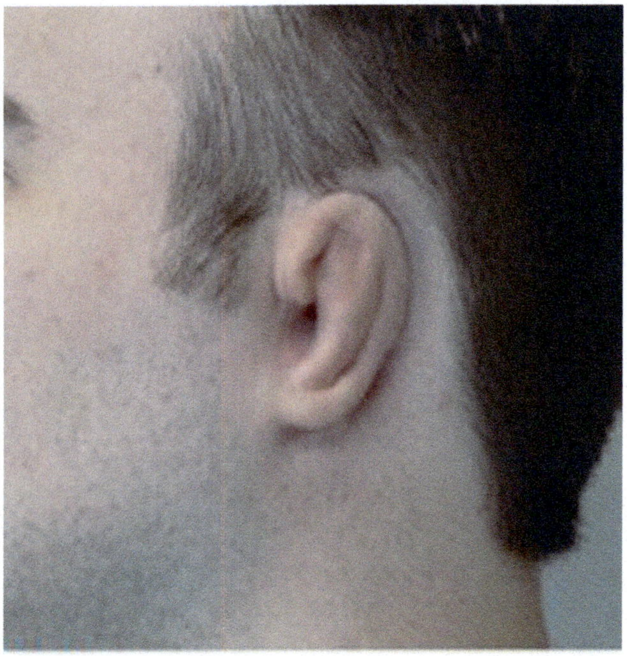

Fig. 28.3 An example of multiple reconstructions without patient satisfaction in esthetic outcome. Successful prosthetic rehabilitation would necessitate surgical ablation of reconstructed tissue replacing with a split-thickness skin graft. Osseointegrated implants may be a consideration

ear is possible without distortion or displacement of the remaining ear. Microvascular reconstruction of a complete or subtotal auriculectomy is usually multistage and complex with current techniques rarely offering the esthetics that can be achieved by a prosthesis. Auricular defects present several challenging elements to the design and fabrication of an acceptable prosthesis that should be easy to position, should have repeatable orientation, and is stable [4].

The total auriculectomy defect is less complicated to restore prosthetically than that of a subtotal defect. With that being said, successful prosthetic rehabilitation depends upon the foundation provided following surgery. Ideally, the defect site should resemble the contours of the contralateral side and not be completely flat. Bulky reconstruction flaps, hair follicles, bone exposure, and distorted tissue remnants all compromise prosthetic rehabilitation (Fig. 28.4a, b, c, d). A smooth, well-contoured skin flap provides a stable foundation and allows for an adheophilic surface necessary for retention of a prosthesis (Fig. 28.5a, b, c, d, e) [4].

The subtotal auriculectomy defect is a challenge for prosthetic rehabilitation. The superior helical rim can be used to support eyeglasses as long as a cartilaginous scaffold remains and if it is not displaced or distorted (Fig. 28.6). In most cases, a small remnant of earlobe is too mobile and not helpful for prosthetic rehabilitation and should be removed. The tragus, however, is an important anatomic structure to maintain. If possible, the tragus should be spared to hide the anterior margin of the prosthesis and to decrease the surface needed for retention to the underlying tissue. This will provide for a more seamless, esthetically pleasing prosthesis. Additionally, the tragus can help guide the placement of the prosthesis.

Patients who undergo postoperative radiation following tumor ablation present additional challenges. Their prosthetic rehabilitation must be delayed for 6–12 months (post-radiation) due to dermatitis, pain, desquamation of the skin, and monitoring/restaging priorities. Radiotherapy may also negatively affect osseointegration of implants. Irradiated skin is less resilient than normal skin.

Retention

A successful auricular prosthesis is more than just a beautifully sculpted and colored silicone ear (Fig. 28.7). The retention of the prosthesis is the patient's number one concern, since inadvertent and untimely loss of the prosthesis can be very embarrassing. There are multiple proven methods of retention: osseointegrated implants, medical grade water-based adhesive, medical grade silicone-based adhesive, surgical double-sided tape, anatomical topography assisted, and eyeglass assisted (Fig. 28.8a, b, c) [5–7].

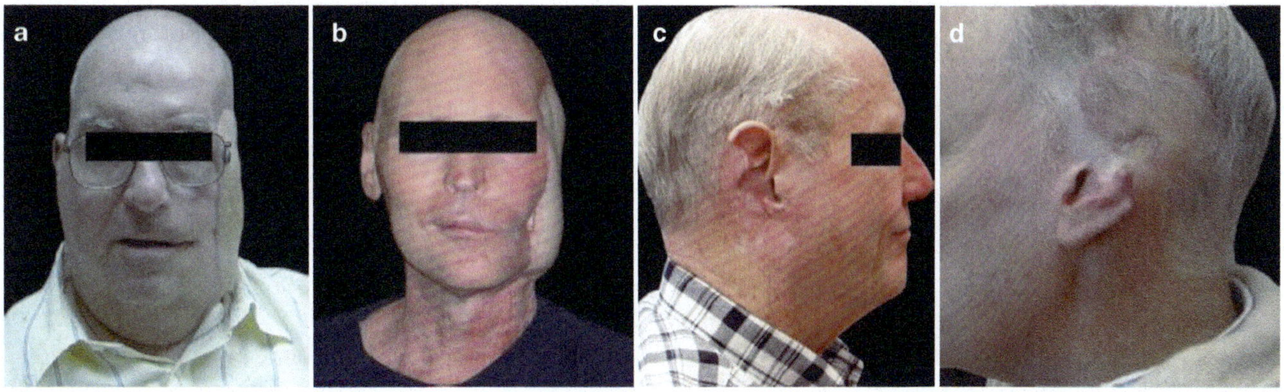

Fig. 28.4 (**a**, **b**, **c**, **d**) It is very difficult to contour large flaps to match the contours of the contralateral side

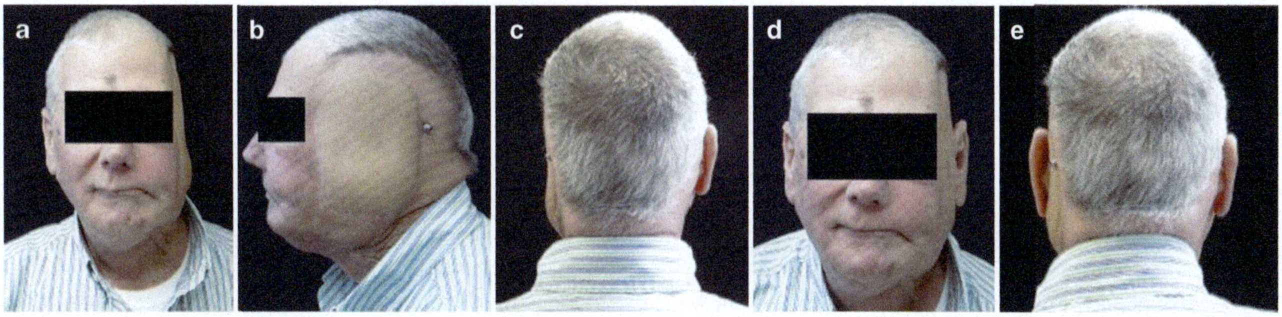

Fig. 28.5 (**a**) Full auriculectomy with large skin paddle. Facial symmetry has been compromised by the contour of the large skin paddle. (**b**, **c**) Large skin paddle without landmarks to aid in placement of an adhesive retained left auricular prosthesis. (**d**, **e**) Final prosthesis matching contralateral ear. Retention of prosthesis is obtained by using double-sided surgical tape

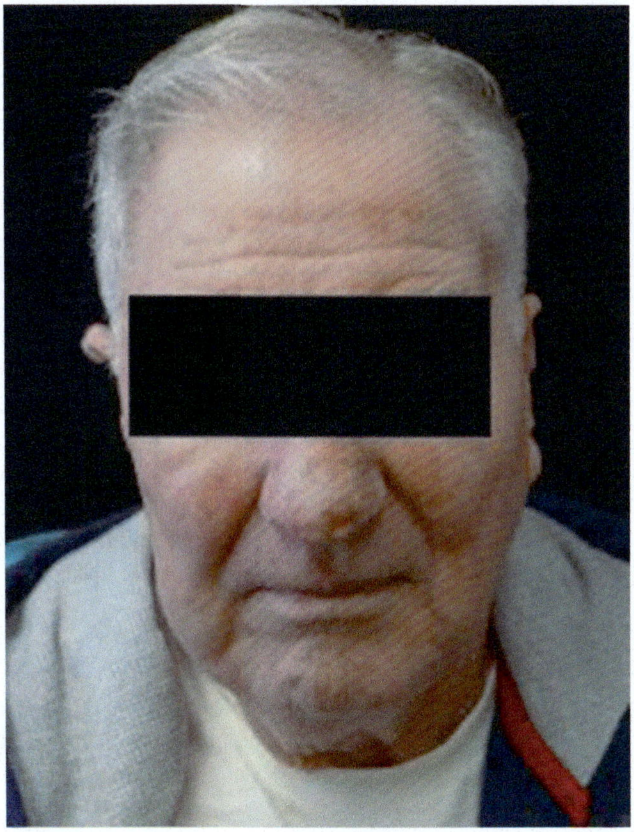

Fig. 28.6 Displaced partial helix remnant making prosthetic rehabilitation challenging

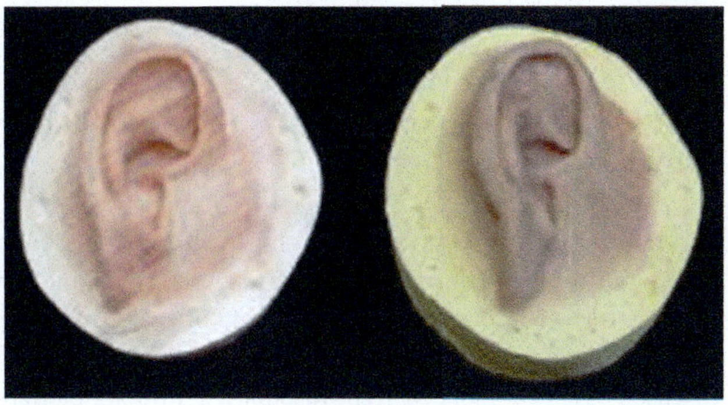

Fig. 28.7 Sculpted wax pattern and final skin tone matched silicone prosthesis

A preoperative evaluation with the prosthetic rehabilitation team is essential to determine how the future auricular prosthesis will be designed and retained to the defect site. At this initial appointment, photographs are taken, and virtual software applications are used to simulate from the contralateral ear what prosthetic rehabilitation can accomplish. Additionally, it will allow for discussion of limitations of a prosthesis and set realistic expectations.

The mobility of tissue associated with the movement of the temporomandibular joint in front of each ear will vary from person to person and can compromise the retention of some prostheses. Direct adhesive fixation (commercially available skin adhesives) requires a daily

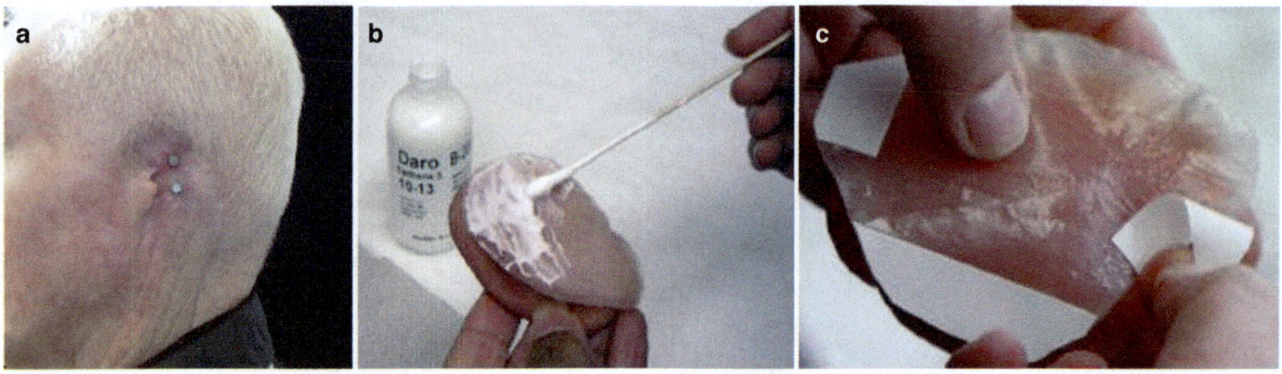

Fig. 28.8 (**a**) Size of the ear and available bone determines number of implants to be placed. Magnetic retention has gained favor over bar/clip retention. For optimum retention and stability, two or three implants are needed. (**b**) Medical grade water-based adhesives rarely irritate tissue and are easier to remove from the prosthesis eliminating adhesive buildup. Adhesion is diminished in hot climates and wet climates; therefore, silicone-based adhesives are preferred for optimum retention when perspiration or moisture is present. Silicone adhesives are difficult to completely remove from the prosthesis causing tearing of thin margins and adhesive buildup which compromise the longevity of the silicone material. (**c**) Surgical double-sided tape offers easier positioning for the patient with a split-thickness skin graft without anatomical landmarks for placement. The surface should be absent of hair growth. An auricular prosthesis fabricated with a polyurethane liner allows for a smooth adheophilic surface

application and removal of adhesive that often leads to early deterioration of the thin margins of the silicone prosthesis [8].

The size of an auricular defect, availability of viable bone for implant placement, patient manual dexterity, and tissue bulkiness and mobility govern the choice of retention for an auricular prosthesis [*Case example 2: Patient with mid-ear defect presents a challenge to the placement of a prosthesis using liquid adhesive*] (Fig. 28.9a–i).

Osseointegrated Implant-Retained Auricular Prosthesis

The most secure of all retentive possibilities are endosseous implants for a total auricular prosthesis. When deciding to place extraoral implants in an auriculectomy site, multiple considerations must be taken into account: no evidence of disease, radiation-induced hypovascularity, fibrosis or dermatitis, skin quality, presence of hair, mobility of tissue, and quality of bone and thickness [*Case example 3: Presurgical evaluation of patient*] (Fig. 28.10a–e).

Other considerations are the location and the method of retention associated with auricular implants: bar-clip attachment or magnet retention. Before implant placement, the prosthetic rehabilitation team will aid in determining the number of implants, position of implants, and the retentive components to be used in the future auricular prosthesis. A surgical template can be designed and fabricated to confirm proper implant placement (Fig. 28.11a–e). All of the planning is necessary to ensure the implant abutments and retentive components will be hidden under the prosthesis, ideally deep to the antihelix of the ear. Implants placed without presurgical planning may not be positioned for usefulness, and thus, patient acceptance is diminished.

Literature supports the use of different types of surgical templates for the optimal placement of extraoral endosseous implants [9–13]. To enhance precision in planning and positioning of implants, a three-dimensional surgical template that closely resembles the future prosthetic ear is an effective method. Currently, advances in intraoperative three-dimensional technology can offer a digital workflow in virtual surgical planning and prosthetic reconstruction with three-dimensional printed surgical placement guides for craniofacial implant placement [14–16].

Patients requiring temporal bone resection may not benefit from implant placement for an auricular prosthesis due to lack of or density of viable bone and/or bulky skin grafts that cannot be altered or contoured. The inability to hide the retentive components within the auricular prosthesis if the implant(s) is placed too high in the temporal bone is contradictive to an esthetically pleasing prosthetic rehabilitation. In some large skin paddle cases, a single implant placed in the temporal bone region with magnetic retention component relieves the prosthesis placement difficulty for the patient (Fig. 28.12a, b, c). Patients with extensive disease who have undergone a resection followed by radiation therapy may not be a candidate for implants due to compromised bone, poor wound healing, and risk of recurrence of disease.

Technique

Design and fabrication of an auricular prosthesis begins with an accurate impression of a well-healed defect and surrounding tissue. In the case of a subtotal resection, attention must be

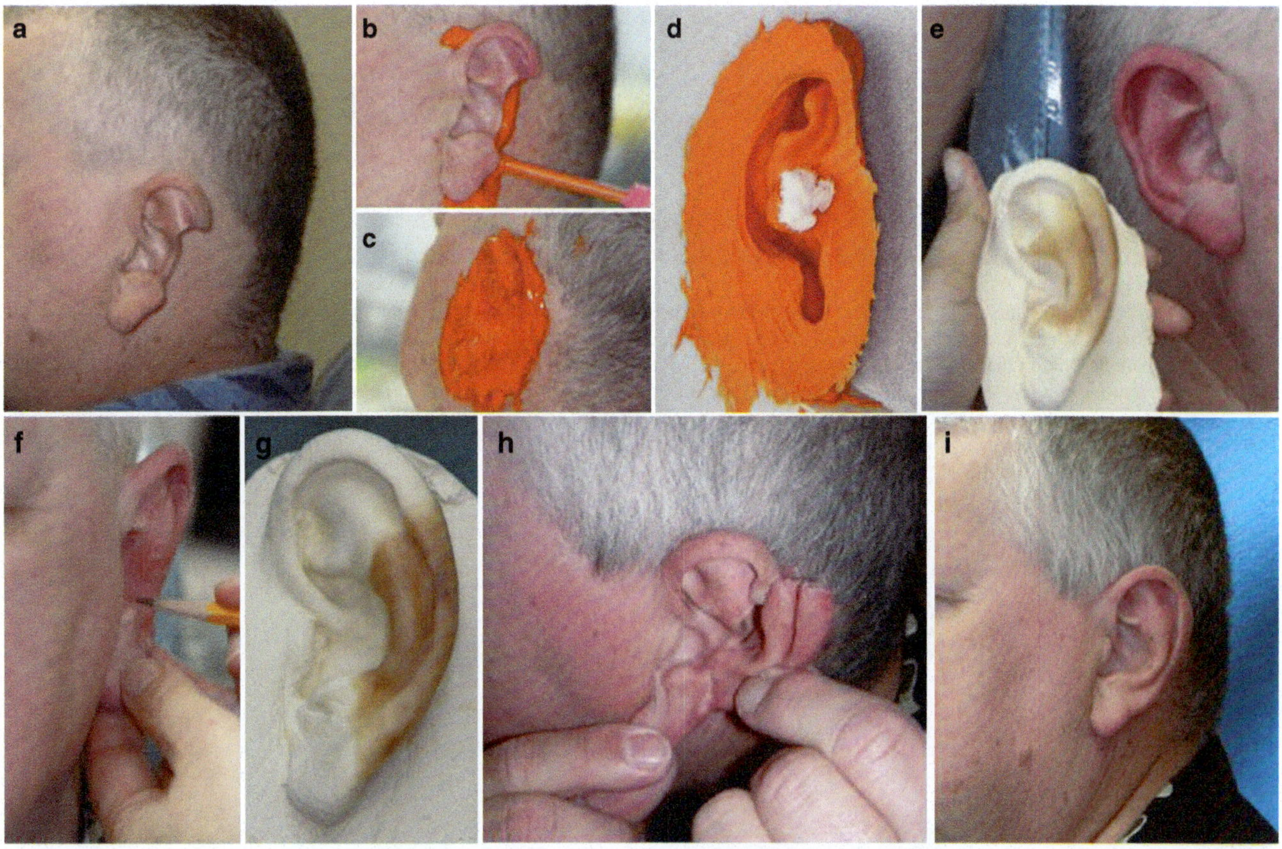

Fig. 28.9 (**a**) Patient with mid-ear defect presents a challenge to the placement of a prosthesis using liquid adhesives. Anatomical retention utilizing undercuts was possible but may not be esthetically acceptable to the patient. Options and limitations of retention were discussed with the patient, and he desired anatomical retention over adhesives. (**b**) Defect site and surrounding tissue were very lightly coated with petroleum jelly to allow for easy removal of the impression material. A small amount of cotton gauze was inserted in the ear canal. An initial impression was made of the ear using a light body polyvinyl siloxane (PVS) material dispensed in small increments, starting with the posterior surface. (**c**) PVS light body material was dispensed until it covered the entire ear with a thickness that would not tear when twisted to remove from the ear. Heavy body PVS was not added to back the light body in this case because it would make the material too stiff to remove easily. (**d**) Impression was carefully removed, and a stone mold master cast was poured from the impression. (**e**) The ear on the master cast was slightly reduced by using sandpaper. This reduction allowed for a tighter adaptation of the substructure to the ear tag. The substructure was designed in wax on the master cast to capture the desired undercuts needed for retention while creating the proper anatomy. A mold was made of the wax pattern and then processed with heat cure acrylic resin. (**f**) Processed acrylic resin substructure was adapted to the patient defect, trimmed, and thinned as needed until a secure adaptation was achieved. The patient was asked to place the substructure onto his defect to assure proper placement could be achieved. (**g**) Second impression was made with the reduced substructure in position. The impression was poured up in stone with the substructure embedded in the stone mold. The wax sculpting of the partial ear was done directly on the substructure on the master cast. Once acceptable, molds were made of the wax sculpting, and a color-matched silicone ear with substructure was processed. (**h**) Additional extrinsic coloration was added until a skin tone match was achieved. Patient was able to achieve proper position of the prosthesis by pulling, turning, and stretching the tissue until retention was secured. (**i**) Final prosthesis in position secured without adhesive

taken to capture the residual tissue as accurately as possible without distorting the remnant [*Case example 4: Patient with partial auriculectomy*] (Fig. 28.13a–g). When implants for an auricular prosthesis are present, special lab components are needed to achieve an accurate impression of the position of the implant abutments and the method of attachment being utilized. On average it takes five daily outpatient appointments from impression to final silicone prosthesis delivery. A stone cast is made from the impression to be used as the base for a wax sculpting of the missing anatomy. A contralateral ear impression is made and poured up in stone to be used as a guide in carving a mirror-image wax pattern. Current technology allows for the use of computer-aided design and manufacturing (CAD/CAM) techniques to enhance the reproduction accuracy of a mirror-image pattern [17, 18].

Anatomically, when the auditory meatus or tragus remains and has not been displaced during surgery, these structures can be used as landmarks to begin sculpting of the ear prosthesis. With the patient present, orientation marks can be made onto a master stone cast to indicate the junction of the anterior helix and earlobe with the side of the head. Such measurements can be obtained from the contralateral ear and help the prosthodontist or anaplastologist with accuracy in determining the details of the ear prosthesis: shape and

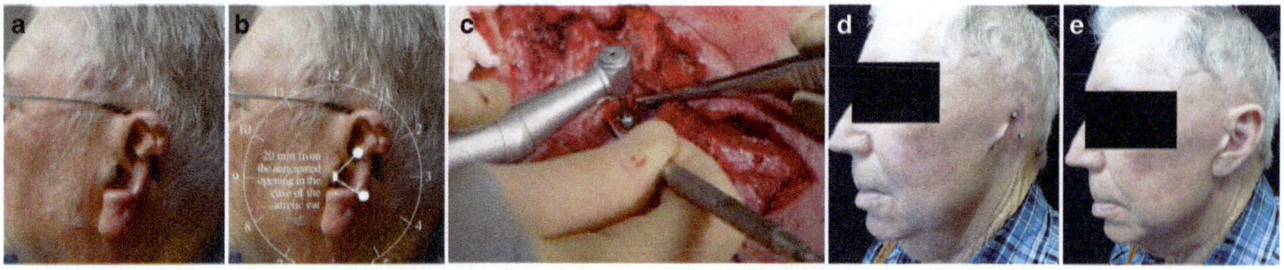

Fig. 28.10 (**a**) Patient presented for a presurgical evaluation for future auricular prosthesis where methods of retention were discussed. Dexterity of patient was evaluated. Patient expressed concerns with applying and removing liquid adhesive daily. (**b**) Implant placement was agreed upon depending on extent of surgery. Recommendations were made to salvage the tragus, if possible. Guidelines for implant placement were discussed with the surgeon to determine placement of two extraoral implants 18 mm from the ear canal at the 1:30 and 4:00 o'clock position based on the size of the patients' ear. (**c**) Interoperative photo of implant placement. (**d**) Magnetic retention components added to implant abutments. (**e**) Final prosthesis with extrinsic coloration added to match skin tones. While a seamless transition to the skin is desirable, the silicone margins are not thinned to add longevity to the prosthesis

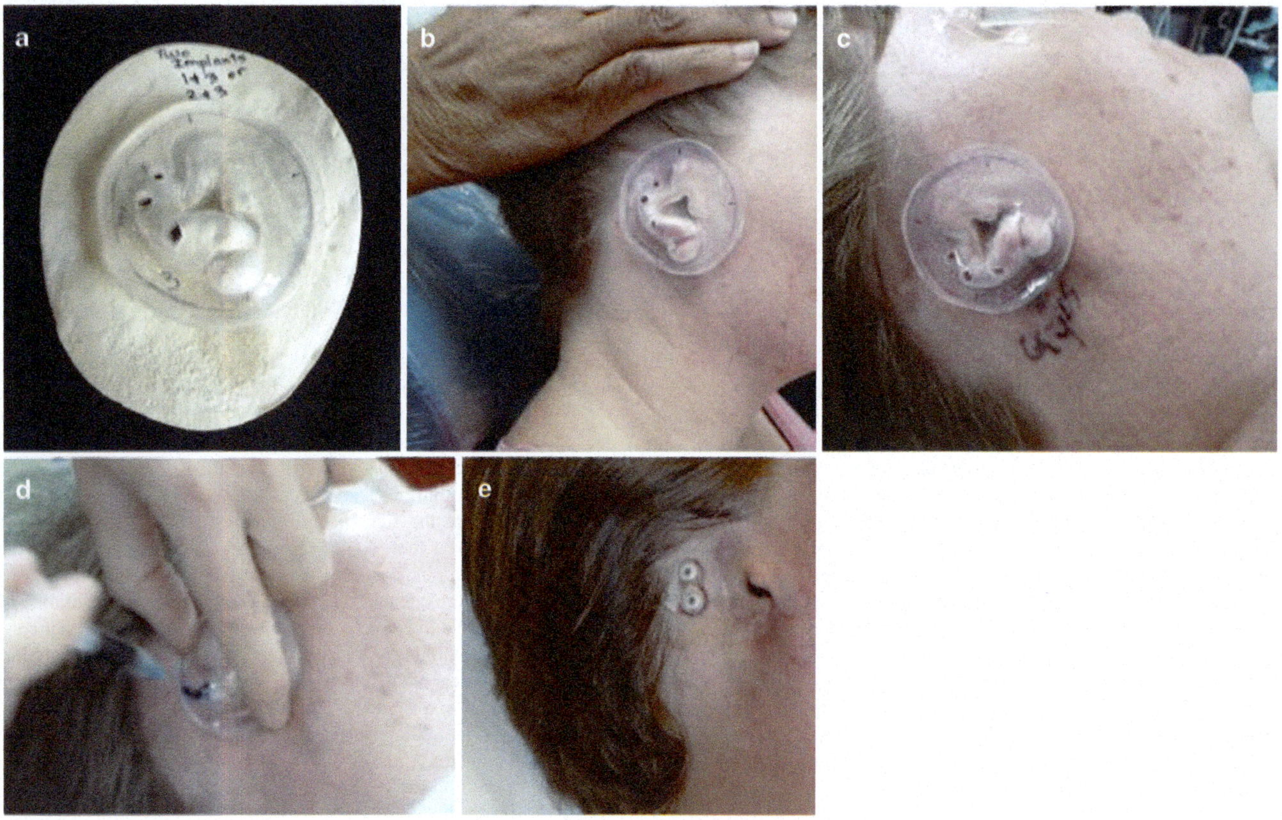

Fig. 28.11 (**a**) An example of a surgical template to guide in the accurate placement of osseointegrated implants in a one-stage surgery procedure. A pre-op impression was made of the patients' ear remnant and then poured up in stone to produce a master cast. A clear thermoplastic material was used on a vacuum forming machine to produce a replica of the remnant. A presurgical planning session with the surgeon and maxillofacial prosthodontist is necessary to determine the number, type, and positioning of implants in the defect. (**b**) Adaptation of template was verified on patient followed by sterilization prior to surgery. (**c**) Patient in supine position with template securely in position. (**d**) Methylene blue dye was injected through the tissue to the bone using the predetermined spots marked on the template before the ear remnant was surgically removed. (**e**) Patient with surgical dressing wrapped around the healing caps

length of the ear, tragus and antitragus location, lobe measurement, tragus to inner concha rim details, superior helical rim dimension, etc. [9].

Sculpting and designing a complete prosthesis requires artistic skill due to the absence or lack of anatomical landmarks. The goal of reproducing a mirror image of the contralateral ear with a realistic outcome is dependent on the skill of the practitioner. Sculpting of the total auricular prosthesis starts with a baseplate made of thin wax adapted to the stone cast. This will be tried onto the patient to check the accuracy

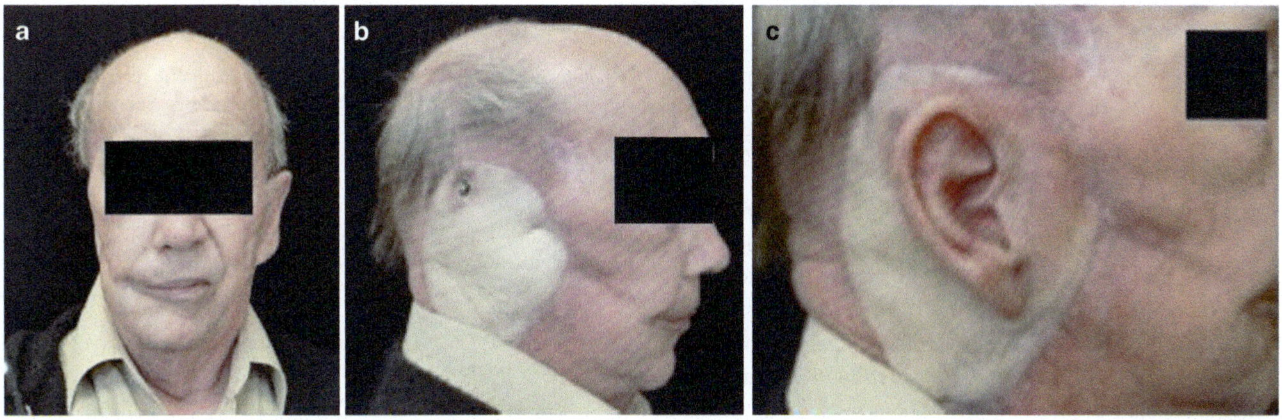

Fig. 28.12 (**a**) Total auriculectomy with large skin paddle and postsurgical facial paralysis on ipsilateral side. (**b**) BAHA implant in temporal bone. Larger skin paddles make eventual prosthesis orientation and retention more complicated for older patients. (**c**) The magnet component is slightly visible through silicone material behind the helix. Esthetic demands and placement difficulty with realistic expectations should be discussed with the patient for acceptance prior to implant placement

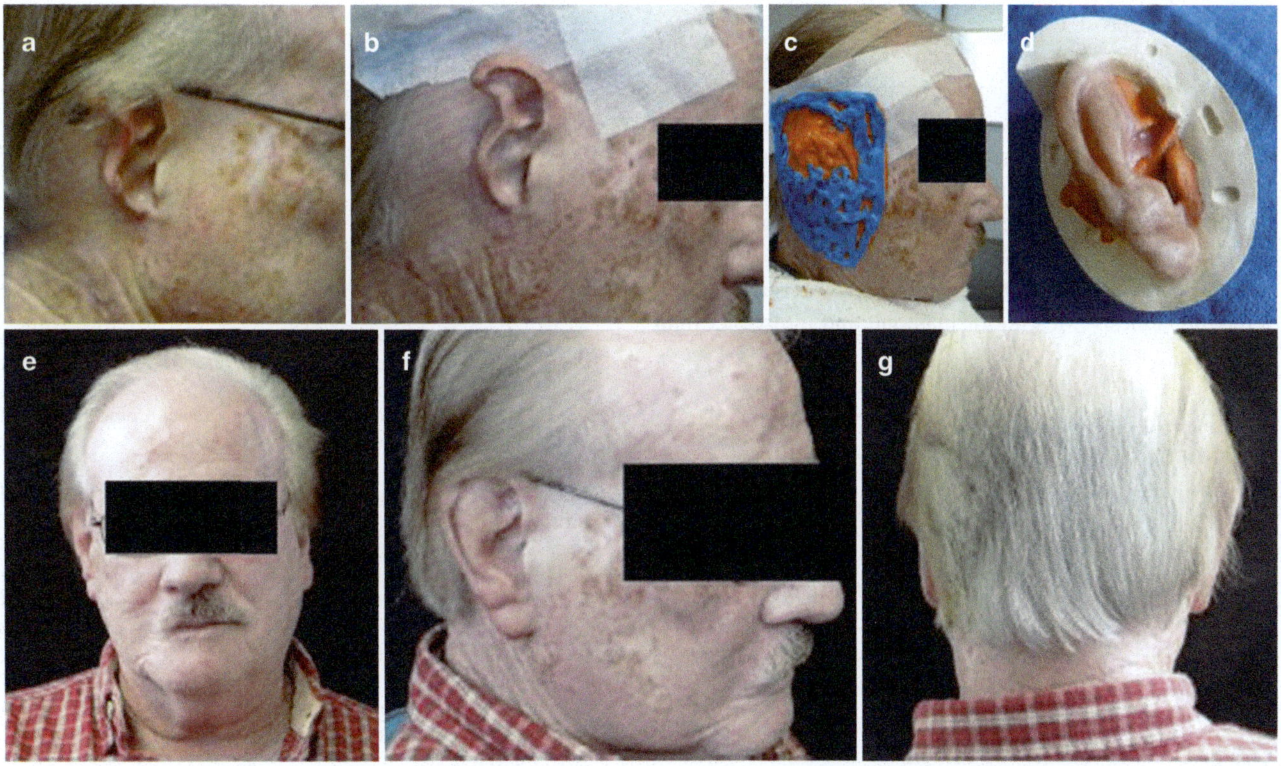

Fig. 28.13 (**a**) Partial right ear defect with helix tag displaced distally compared to the contralateral ear. Patient grew hair longer to hide the defect. (**b**) An impression was made of the ear tag, being careful not to distort the remnants with the weight of the impression material. A small amount of light body polyvinyl siloxane (PVS) material was dispensed at a time and allowed to set in order to hold the tag in the proper position. (**c**) The impression was carefully removed, and a stone mold master cast was poured from the impression. (**d**) A stone mold master cast was poured from the cast with the addition of polyvinyl siloxane used to capture the ear tag portion of the mold. The ear tag was flexible so that it would not break during the mold-making process. The wax sculpture of the partial ear was checked for adaptation and sculpting match accuracy directly on the patient. Once acceptable, molds were made of the wax sculpture, and a color-matched silicone ear was processed. (**e**) Extrinsic coloration was added to the silicone prosthesis to match his contralateral ear. (**f**) Secure adaptation was achieved by sliding the prosthesis onto the ear remnant and using double-sided surgical tape on the posterior side of the prosthesis. (**g**) Right ear projection was slightly more prominent due to the postsurgical projection of the remnant. Patient was satisfied with esthetics

of the impression for adaptation onto the defect. The patient will be asked to open and close their mouth, move the jaw from side to side, look down, and any other normal movements of the head and mouth. It may be necessary to adjust the stone cast due to movement of soft tissue to achieve an intimate adaptation. Once adaptation is achieved, the wax sculpting of the ear can begin. During the sculpting phase, several patient try-ons will be needed to determine correct scale, shape, vertical angulation, and projection based on the contralateral ear dimensions.

Once the wax sculpting is satisfactory, the margins of the sculpting must be adapted to ensure good integrity with underlying skin tissue. With the patient present, the intrinsic silicone colors are mixed to match the patient's contralateral ear, and a color-packing guide is created. The completed sculpting is sealed to the stone model ready for construction of a mold. A maxillofacial flask or three-part mold is used to complete the transformation process of the wax sculpting. The laboratory procedure required to transform the sculpting to a silicone prosthesis is technique-sensitive and requires multiple steps. There are several commercially available medical grade silicone elastomers for the technician to choose from to produce the final-colored silicone prosthesis. After the curing of the chosen silicone material, the prosthesis is removed from mold, trimmed, and adapted to the patient's defect. Additional extrinsic coloration is added, as needed, for the final skin match. The average life expectancy of the silicone prosthesis is 12 months due to daily wear and removal, removing adhesive, tearing of material, and ultraviolet light degradation.

Summary

A full or partial auricular prosthesis is beneficial to those patients who are unable to undergo autologous reconstruction. Such benefit is achieved if acceptable esthetics and retention occur. Greater success is usually achieved with a full prosthesis due to the complications arising from soft tissue movement and patient dexterity in positioning the partial prosthesis. Hence, patient assessment is critical to ensure eventual success particularly in regard to movement and displacement of remnant tissue. Patient education and follow-up assessments are very important to the proper use of a full or partial auricular prosthesis. Implants provide patients with a safe and reliable method of anchoring auricular prostheses that enables restoration of normal appearance and higher quality of retention. Through multidisciplinary care, esthetic outcomes can be achieved for facial disfigured individuals.

References

1. Giot JP, Labbé D, Soubeyrand E, et al. Prosthetic reconstruction of the auricle: indications, techniques, and results. Semin Plast Surg. 2011;25:265–72.
2. Allen R. Auricular prostheses. In: McKinstry RE, editor. Fundamentals of facial prosthetics, vol. 11. Arlington, VA: ABI professional Publications; 1995. p. 152.
3. Gonzales JB. Evaluation and treatment planning for the facially disfigured. In: Lefkowitz W, editor. Proceedings of the Second International Prosthodontic Congress. St. Louis: The C.V. Mosby Co.; 1979. p. 240–1.
4. Thomas KF. Chapter 5. Auricular prosthesis. In: The art of clinical anaplastology. Great Britain: 4Edge Ltd; 2006. p. 78–96.
5. Kubon TM, Kurtz KS, Piro JD. Impression procedure for creating a partial auricular prosthesis. J Prosthet Dent. 2000;83:648–51.
6. Lemon JC, Chambers MS. Conventional methods of retention of facial prostheses. In: Beumer J, Zlotolow I, Esposito S, editors. Proceedings of the 1st International Congress on Maxillofacial Prosthetics. Memorial Sloan-Kettering Cancer Center 1; 1995. p. 116–9.
7. Parel SM, Holt GR, Brånemark PI, et al. Osseointegration and facial prosthetics. Int J Oral Maxillofac Implants. 1986;1:27–9.
8. Kiat-amnuay S, Gettleman L, Khan Z, Goldsmith LJ. Effect of adhesive retention on maxillofacial prostheses, Part 1: Skin dressings and solvent removers. J Prosth Dent. 2000;84:335–40.
9. Beumer J III, Reisberg DJ, Marunick MT, et al. Maxillofacial rehabilitation: Prosthodontic and surgical management of cancer-related, acquired, and congenital defects of the head and neck. In: Beumer III J, Marunick MT, Esposito SJ, editors. Rehabilitation of facial defects. 3rd ed. Chicago: Quintessence Publishing Co, Inc.; 2011. p. 255–314.
10. Reisberg DJ, Habakuk SW. Use of a surgical positioner for bone-anchored facial prostheses. Int J Oral Maxillofac Implants. 1997;12:376–9.
11. Wolfaardt JF, Troppmann R, Wilkes GH, Coss P. Surgical templates for auricular reconstruction. J Facial Somato Prosthet. 1996;2:131–6.
12. Edge MJ. Surgical placement guide for use with osseointegrated implants. J Prosthet Dent. 1987;57:719–22.
13. Tan KB, Loh FC, Loh KK. Use of a modified ear-bow for surgical stent location during ear implant placement: a clinical report. J Prosthet Dent. 1996;75:117–21.
14. Weissler JM, Sosin M, Dorafshar AH, Garcia JR. Combining virtual surgical planning, intraoperative navigation, and 3 dimensional printing in prosthetic-based bilateral microtia reconstruction. J Oral Maxillofac Surg. 2017;75:1491–7. https://doi.org/10.1016/j.joms.2016.12.037. Epub ahead of print
15. Huang YH, Seelaus R, Zhao L, Patel PK, Cohen M. Virtual surgical planning and 3D printing in prosthetic orbital reconstruction with percutaneous implants: a technical report. Int Med Case Rep J. 2016;P9:341–5.
16. Nickenig HJ, Eitner S. Reliability of implant placement after virtual planning of implant positions using cone beam CT data and surgical (guide) templates. J Craniomaxillofac Surg. 2007;35(4-5):201–11.
17. Al Mardini M, Ercoli C, Graser GN. A technique to produce a mirror-image wax pattern of an ear using rapid prototyping technology. J Prosth Dent. 2005;94:195–7.
18. Coward TJ, Watson RM, Wilkinson IC. Fabrication of a wax ear by rapid-process modeling using stereolithography. INT J Prosthodont. 1999;12:20–7.

Radiotherapy for Temporal Bone Cancers

29

Sweet Ping Ng and G. Brandon Gunn

Abbreviations

CRT	Chemoradiotherapy
CT	Computed tomography
FDG	Fluorodeoxyglucose
Gy	Gray
IMPT	Intensity-modulated proton therapy
IMRT	Intensity-modulated radiation (photon) therapy
IORT	Intraoperative radiation therapy
MRI	Magnetic resonance imaging
PET	Positron emission tomography
PORT	Postoperative radiotherapy
SCC	Squamous cell carcinoma
VMAT	Volumetric modulated arc therapy

Introduction

Temporal bone cancer is an extremely rare head and neck cancer with relatively poor prognosis in advanced cases. Although squamous cell carcinoma (SCC) is the most common pathology in temporal bone cancer, temporal bone SCC only accounts for 0.2% of all head and neck SCCs [1]. Given its rarity, meaningful comparison of different staging systems and treatment outcomes has proven to be challenging. To date, there has been no universally accepted staging system or consensus of optimal treatment strategies.

Radiotherapy plays a major role in the multimodality management of head and neck cancer patients. There has been retrospective case series in temporal bone cancers suggesting that the addition of postoperative radiotherapy (PORT) to definitive surgery improves outcomes [2–7]. In the postoperative setting, the general indications for adjuvant radiotherapy include positive or close (<5 mm) margins [8], nodal involvement, nodal extracapsular extension, T3 or T4 disease [9, 7], and perineural and lymphovascular invasion [8].

The use of radiotherapy, with or without concurrent chemotherapy, in the definitive setting has been examined recently in patients with locally advanced disease. A recent study by Morita et al. [10] showed a similar 5-year overall survival for patients with T3 and T4 disease treated with definitive chemoradiotherapy (CRT) (52.1%) and those who had surgery followed by adjuvant radiotherapy with/without chemotherapy (55.6%). Shinomiya et al. [11] observed similar clinical outcomes (5-year overall survival 60%; 5-year disease-free survival 60%) in their cohort of 10 patients who had modern staging with CT, MRI, and PET and treated with modern radiotherapy techniques. Takenaka et al. [12] evaluated the use of CRT in a meta-analysis on 752 locally advanced SCCs of the external auditory canal cases in 28 papers published between 2006 and 2013. They reported better 5-year overall survival in the preoperative CRT (85.7%) group compared to surgery ± radiotherapy (53.3%), definitive CRT (43.6%), and adjuvant CRT (0%). Although this meta-analysis showed no patients who had adjuvant CRT alive at 5 years, there were only eight patients included in the analysis. Therefore, the number of adjuvant CRT patients was too small to come to any significant or definitive conclusions with regard to the efficacy of adjuvant CRT in this meta-analysis.

Apart from external beam radiotherapy, brachytherapy has been used as boost treatment in cases where tumors were excised with positive margins or in cases of recurrences after external beam radiotherapy [6]. However, caution will need to be taken with brachytherapy to this area, as there is a moderate to high risk of soft tissue necrosis and osteonecrosis of the temporal bone.

Intraoperative radiotherapy (IORT) was explored by Cristalli et al. [5] as an approach to improve local control in middle ear tumors. In this retrospective study, the team delivered IORT (12 Gy) followed by postoperative radiotherapy

S. P. Ng, M.B.B.S., BMedSci (✉) · G. Brandon Gunn, M.D.
Department of Radiation Oncology, The University of Texas M.D. Anderson Cancer Center, Houston, TX, USA
e-mail: SPNg@mdanderson.org; GBGunn@mdanderson.org

P. W. Gidley, F. DeMonte (eds.), *Temporal Bone Cancer*, https://doi.org/10.1007/978-3-319-74539-8_29

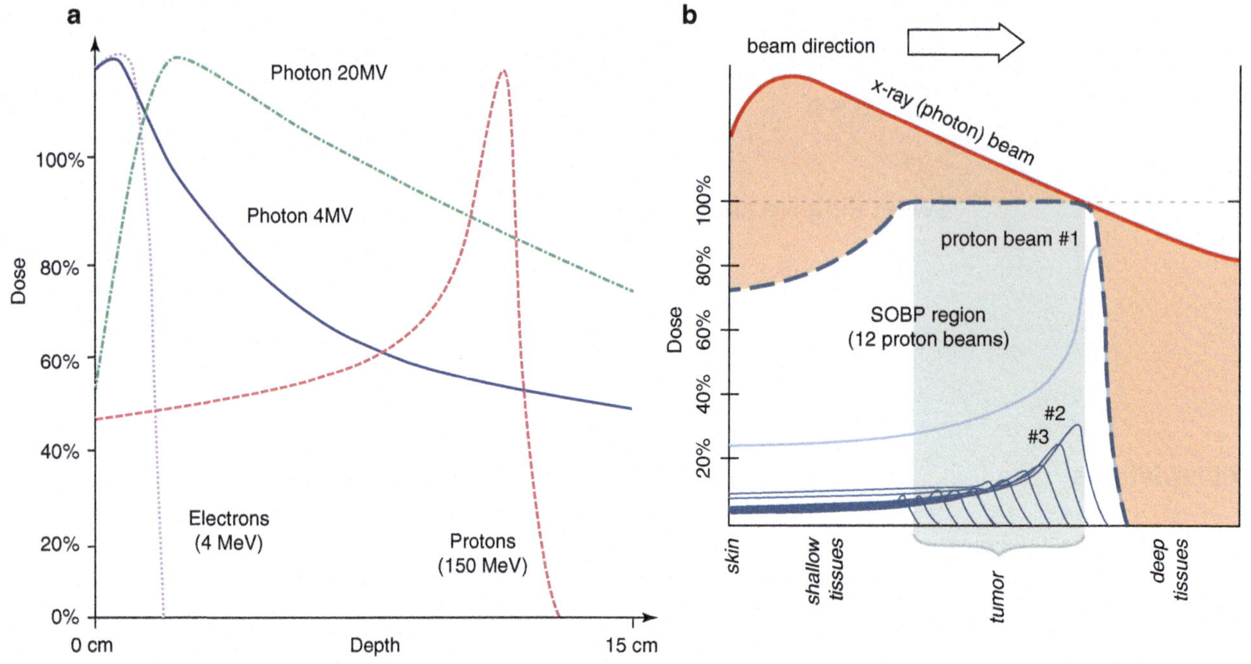

Fig. 29.1 (**a**) Depth-dose curves for photons (X-rays), electron, and proton beams, highlighting the dose distribution differences between each modality. (**b**) Depth-dose curves for photon and proton beams showing the steep dose drop-off for proton beam after the target area. Image **a** taken from https://en.wikipedia.org/wiki/Proton_therapy#/media/File:Comparison_of_dose_profiles_for_proton_v._x-ray_radiotherapy.png. Image **b** taken from https://commons.wikimedia.org/wiki/File%3ADose_Depth_Curves.svg

to 50 Gy to 13 patients. The 5-year local control, disease-free survival, and overall survival rates were 68%, 61%, and 69%, respectively. Partial necrosis of the flap was observed in three patients, although complete healing was eventually achieved with dressings.

As a general principle, the role of radiotherapy in a postoperative setting is to eliminate microscopic disease and improve locoregional control. Radiation therapy is estimated to decrease the risk of locoregional relapse by 50–60%.

The total radiation doses for a standard postoperative case with clear surgical margins are 60 Gy to postoperative tumor and involved nodal bed, 56–58 Gy to surgical bed and clinical high-risk areas, and ~54 Gy to undissected elective regions (standard clinical risk). At least 56–58 Gy will be delivered to the surgical scar with a safe margin to ensure adequate coverage of the scar. The surgical scar is typically marked with CT radiopaque wire, to improve visibility of the scar location on CT images, and a surface bolus is fabricated at simulation and used during treatment to ensure adequate surface dose when photon-based therapy is used.

There are several different radiation modalities including photons, electrons, and protons and various radiation techniques that can be utilized. The decision of which modality to use for each patient is considered on a case-by-case basis, depending on site of treatment, depth of target, field size, and surrounding normal tissues that require sparing. Generally, electrons are used for superficial targets, while photons and protons are utilized when the target also includes deeper tissues. Figure 29.1 summarizes the physical properties of each modality.

Case Studies

Here, we present several cases to highlight the different radiation modalities and techniques that can be utilized in patients with temporal bone tumors to increase the efficacy to radiation treatment delivery and reduce toxicities of treatment.

Case 1

This case showcases the use of intensity-modulated proton therapy (IMPT) treatment technique to deliver postoperative radiation to the skull base area while sparing nearby critical neural structures such as the brain stem, spinal cord, and contralateral hearing apparatus. IMPT is a highly precise technique utilizing pencil beam scanning to deliver proton treatment in a highly conformal fashion.

A 58-year-old female of good performance status presented with a history of chronic bilateral hearing loss, left ear pain, intermittent vertigo, and otorrhea, on a background of multiple tympanostomy tubes in her left ear over several years, and more recently a tympanomastoidectomy and multiple revision surgeries for an adenoma in her left middle ear. Biopsy of tumor within the left Eustachian tube from her most recent revision surgery revealed moderately differentiated intestinal-type adenocarcinoma.

Clinical examination revealed a normal left outer ear with a well-healed postauricular scar consistent with previous surgery. The left ear canal was filled with tenacious secretion, and there was a polypoid tumor within the posterior mesotympanum. There was left hypoacusis. Other cranial nerve examination was unremarkable. Nasopharyngoscopy examination revealed a tumor nodule within the left Eustachian tube.

Staging imaging including CT, MRI, and PET showed an extensive intratympanic and intramastoid tumor within the left temporal bone (Figs. 29.2, 29.3, and 29.4). The tumor was heterogeneously hypointense on T1 and hyperintense on T2 reminiscent of fluid or soft components. The left occipital bone was involved, extending posteriorly from the mastoid. There was no evidence of distant metastatic disease on PET.

Given the extent and recurrent nature of disease, she was recommended for definitive surgery followed by postoperative radiation therapy at the multidisciplinary tumor board conference.

At surgery, a lateral temporal bone resection with removal of the ear canal, excision of extratemporal soft tissue mass, resection of extradural middle and posterior fossa skull base tumor, superficial parotidectomy, and selective left neck dissection and reconstruction were performed. Operative findings described an extensive tumor with involvement into the extratemporal soft tissues of the skull base and extension along the retrosigmoid dura extratemporally. Disease involved all aspects of the temporal bone, including the middle ear, mastoid, retrofacial air cells, and along the jugular bulb into the petrous apex and Eustachian tube. Tumor was seen to extend from the mastoid into the upper sternocleidomastoid muscle.

Final histopathology confirmed intestinal-type adenocarcinoma involving skeletal muscle, soft tissue, and bone, with no evidence of lymphovascular or perineural invasion. The tumor involved the muscle and cartilage from the Eustachian tube, the retrosigmoid tissue, the stylomastoid foramen, tissue medial to the carotid, tissue from middle ear, retrofacial air cells, and the mastoid cavity. One node within the left parotid was positive for tumor. There was no tumor identified in left neck dissection levels 2A to 3. The condyle of the mandible was not involved, and resection margins were clear. Figure 29.5 showed the postoperative changes evident on CT obtained after surgery.

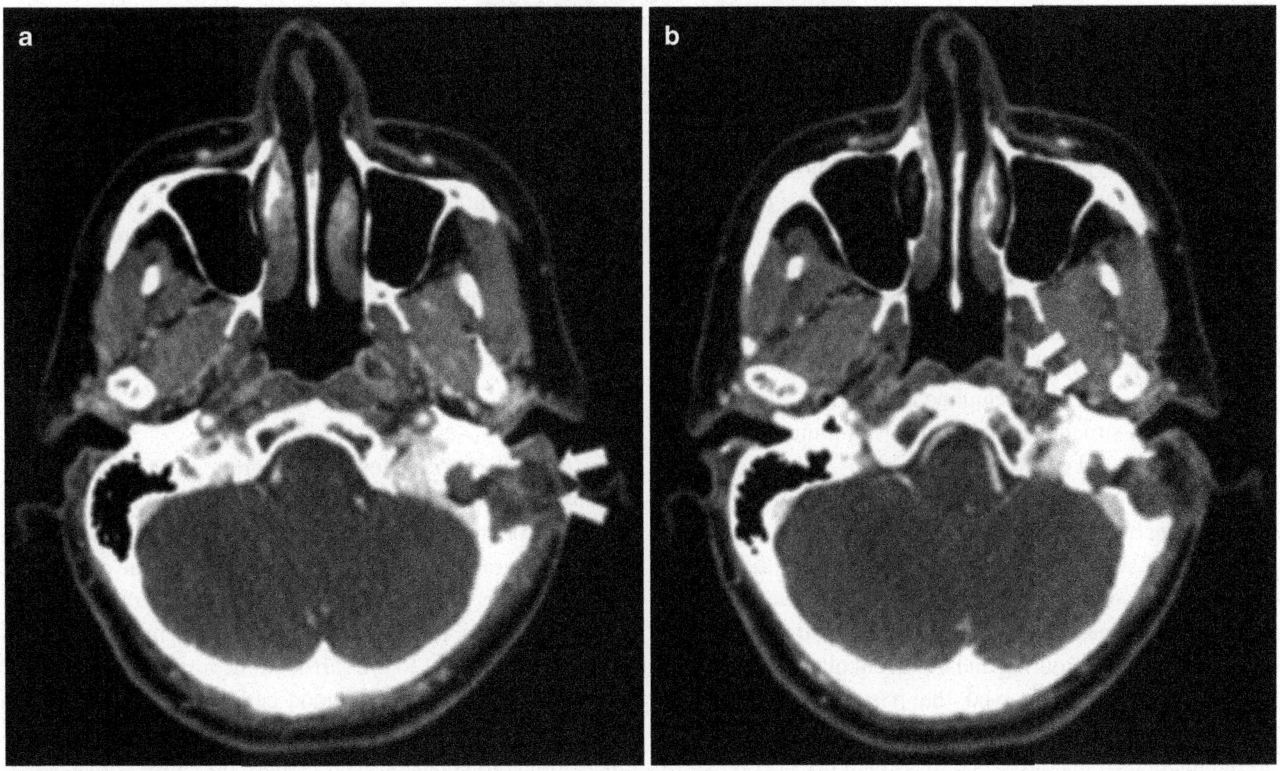

Fig. 29.2 CT of patient 1 depicting (**a**). The large mastoidectomy defect filled with tumor that enhances mildly with tumor behind the left stylomastoid foramen (arrows) and (**b**) subtly enhancing tumor in the left Eustachian tube

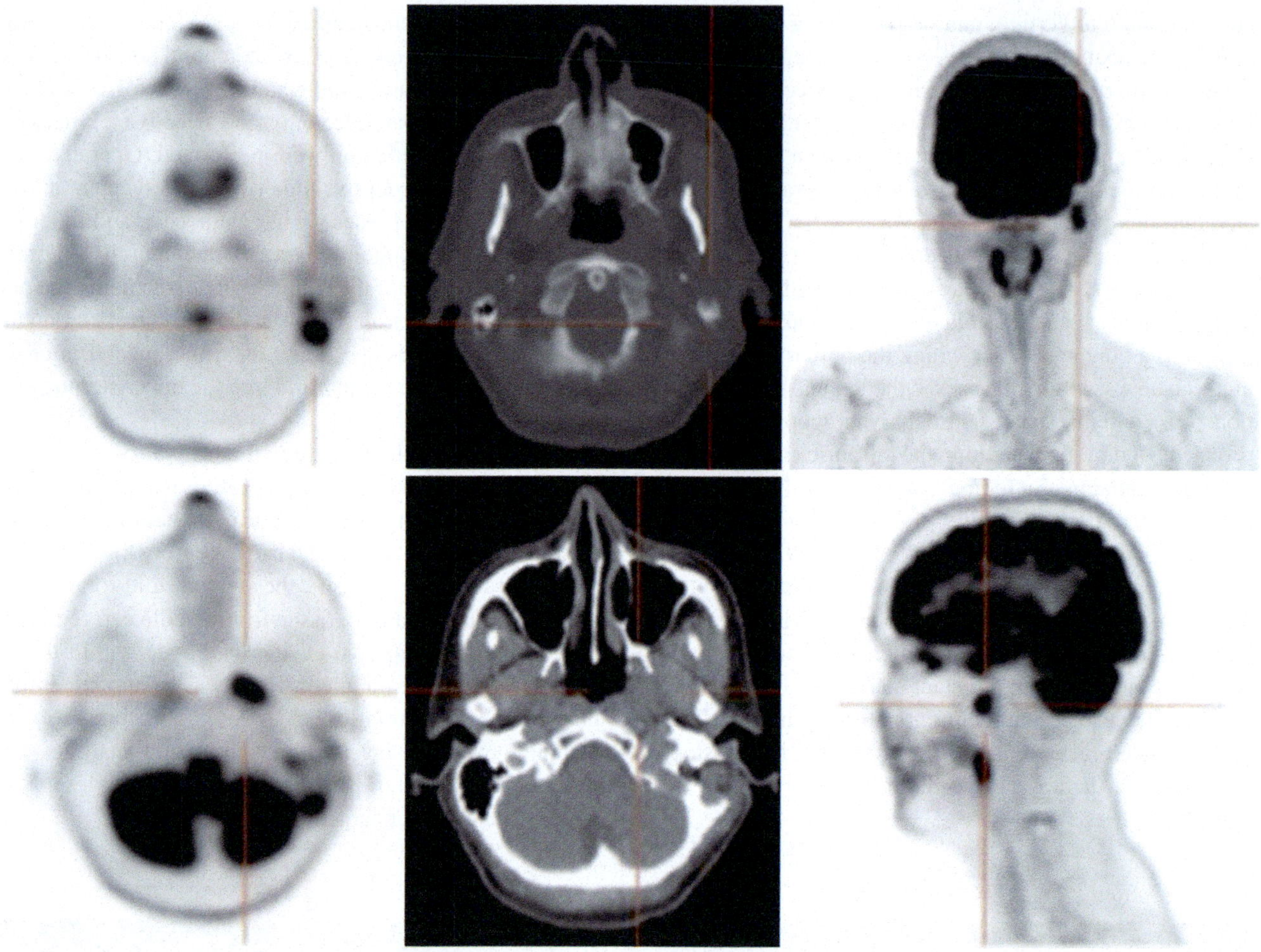

Fig. 29.3 PET showing the FDG-avid lesion correlating with the abnormality on CT within the left temporal region and left Eustachian tube

Approximately a fortnight following surgery, she was simulated for radiation therapy delivered using IMPT technique to facilitate maximal sparing of her critical structures, in particular the temporal lobe, brain stem, spinal cord, and contralateral cochlea especially when she had complete hearing loss on the affected side. The advantage of proton therapy is the rapid dose falloff after target volume; and hence, in this case, this technique maximizes sparing of her critical neural structures while delivering minute to no dose to her contralateral cochlea.

The patient was brought to the proton therapy simulation suite. A bite block was integrated, and a customized thermoplastic mask was fabricated and secured over the patient. Provisional isocenter was placed and CT images were obtained. The images were transferred to the treatment planning system for contouring and treatment planning purposes. Target volume encompassed the postoperative bed with planned 66 Gy to the high-risk areas (tumor bed) and 58 Gy to the unaffected operative bed (dissected neck) (Fig. 29.6). She was treated to a total dose of 66 Gy in 33 daily fractions over 6.5 weeks.

The patient tolerated the treatment well with grade 2 skin reaction and grade 1 oral mucositis at the end of treatment. Follow-up clinical examination and MRI at 3 years did not reveal any signs of locoregional recurrence or significant late toxicity of treatment.

Case 2

This case poses a diagnostic conundrum given the initial difficulty in detecting perineural invasion radiologically to account for the patient's symptoms. In this case, intensity-modulated radiation therapy (IMRT) technique was used. IMRT utilizes photon beams and delivers highly conformal radiation doses to the target volume via multiple beams while limiting dose to the surrounding normal tissues.

A 67-year-old male, of good performance status, with a long history of sun exposure and multiple treated non-melanomatous cutaneous carcinomas, presented with a 5-year history of gradual worsening left facial paresthesia and subsequently left facial paralysis. His past medical history revealed

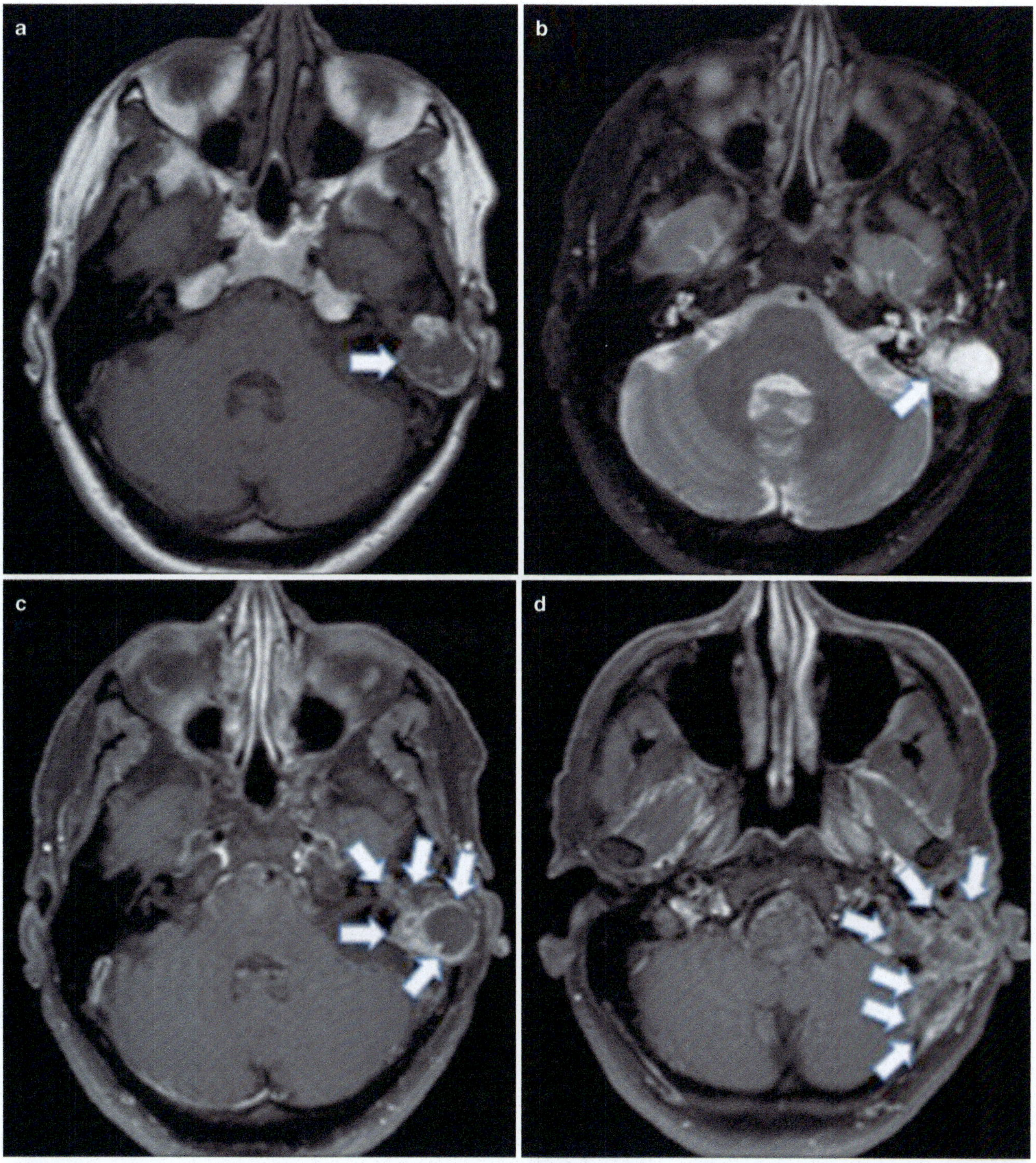

Fig. 29.4 MRI showing the extent of tumor recurrence. The tumor was heterogeneously hypointense on T1 (**a**) and hyperintense on T2 (**b**), with peripheral ring-type enhancement (**c**). Image **d** and **e** showed involvement of the left occipital bone extending posteriorly from the mastoid. The extent of disease is shown in a representative coronal section (**f**)

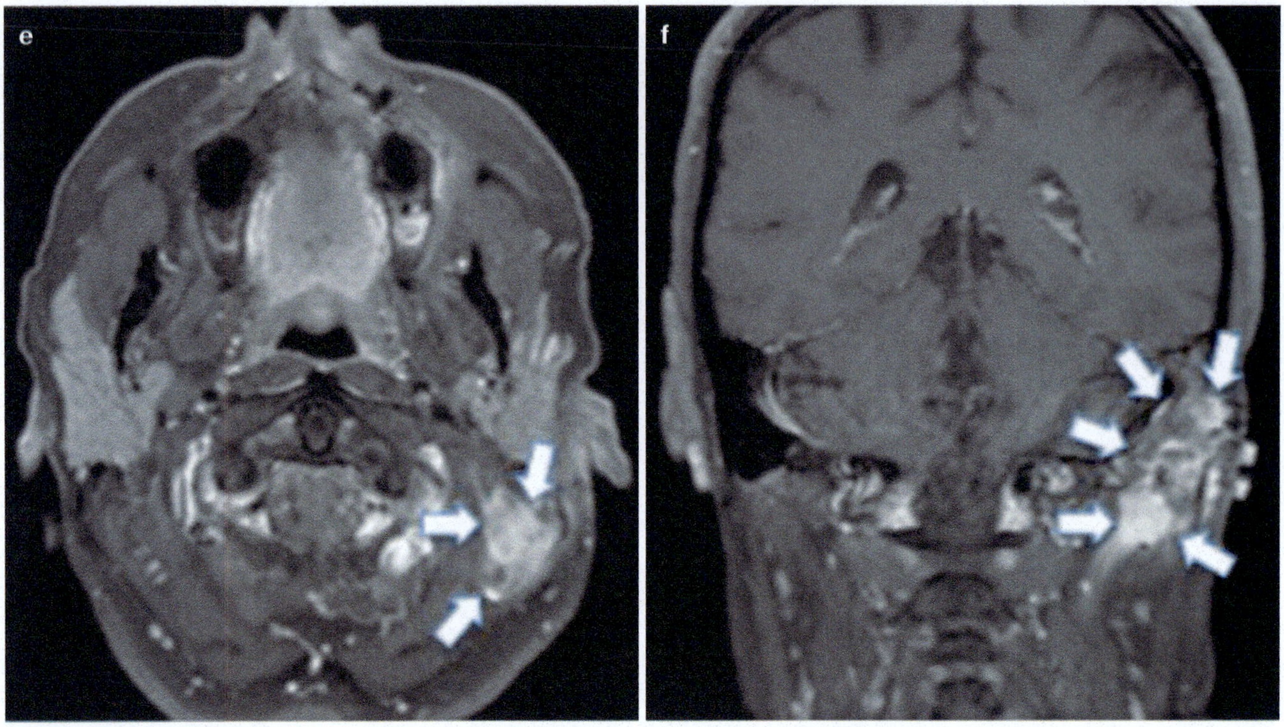

Fig. 29.4 (continued)

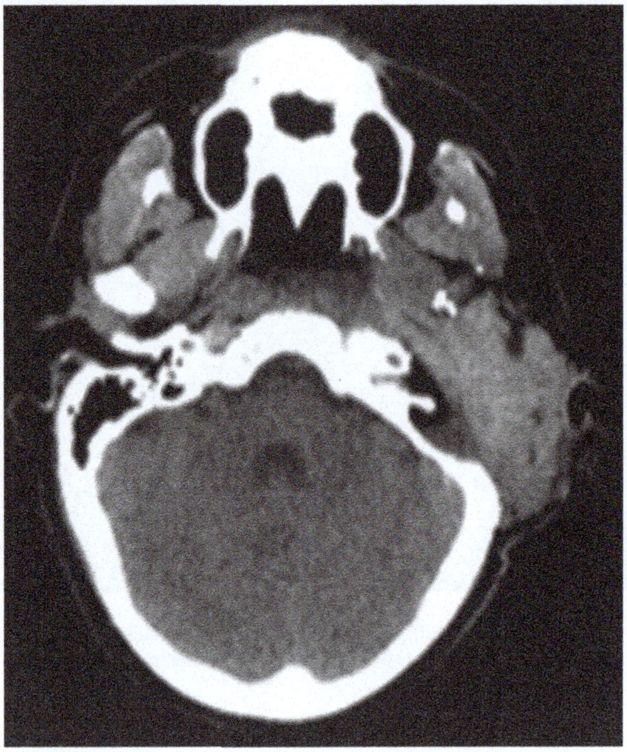

Fig. 29.5 CT after surgical resection and flap reconstruction

a previous left cheek basal cell carcinoma that was excised via Mohs surgery 10 years prior. Numerous imaging evaluations including MRIs over several years were unrevealing of a specific cause for his facial paralysis and facial paresthesia.

Physical examination revealed a complete left facial paralysis and a palpable subcutaneous nodule near the surgical scar in his left cheek. Facial sensation was intact. There was no palpable cervical lymphadenopathy.

Repeat MRI subsequently showed abnormal enhancement of the left facial nerve, posterior genu and the descending segment into the stylomastoid foramen, and the proximal extracranial main facial trunk (Fig. 29.7). There was a speculated subcutaneous mass measuring 1.6 cm within the area of previous Mohs surgery, concerning of subcutaneous skin cancer.

A fine needle aspiration and a core biopsy of the left cheek nodule yielded no malignant cells. Following discussion at the multidisciplinary tumor board conference, the patient was dispositioned to surgery followed by postoperative radiotherapy given the extent of facial nerve involvement.

The patient underwent excision of left subcutaneous nodule, total parotidectomy, selective neck dissection levels II–III, complete mastoidectomy, and resection of the left facial nerve. This was followed by reconstruction of the left cheek defect with free anterolateral thigh flap, an 11 cm nerve graft anastomosed from proximal stump of facial nerve to the marginal branch. A static sling of the left face was performed to correct the left facial palsy defect.

Histopathology confirmed poorly differentiated squamous cell carcinoma with perineural carcinomatous nests within the parotid and perineural involvement of the facial nerve including at the mastoid segment. No lymph nodes were involved.

A month following surgery, the patient was brought to the CT simulation suite. He was positioned on the simulator

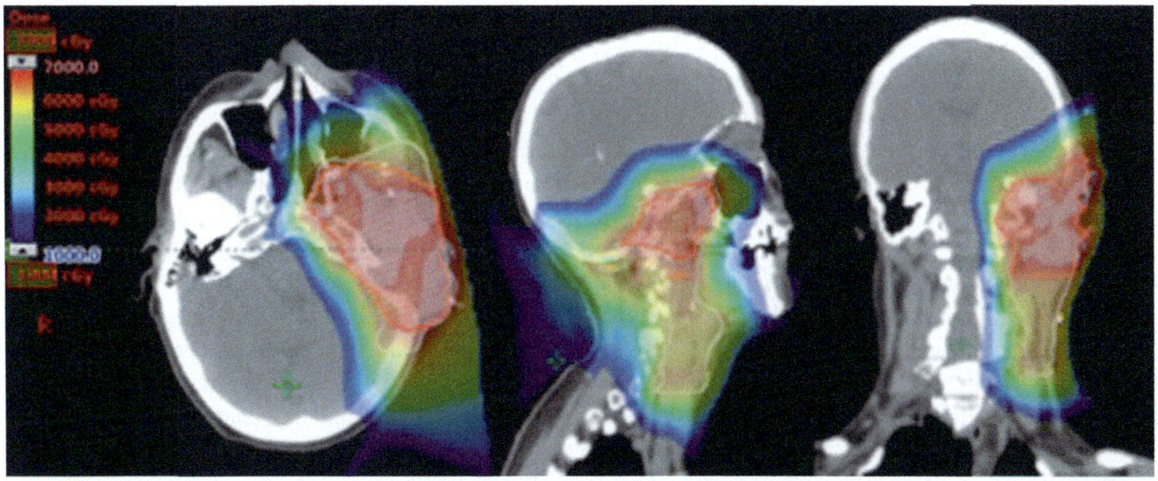

Fig. 29.6 Representative axial, sagittal, and coronal images of radiation dose distribution plan using IMPT planning, highlighting the rapid dose falloff after target volume contoured (red line,66 Gy; yellow line, 58 Gy)

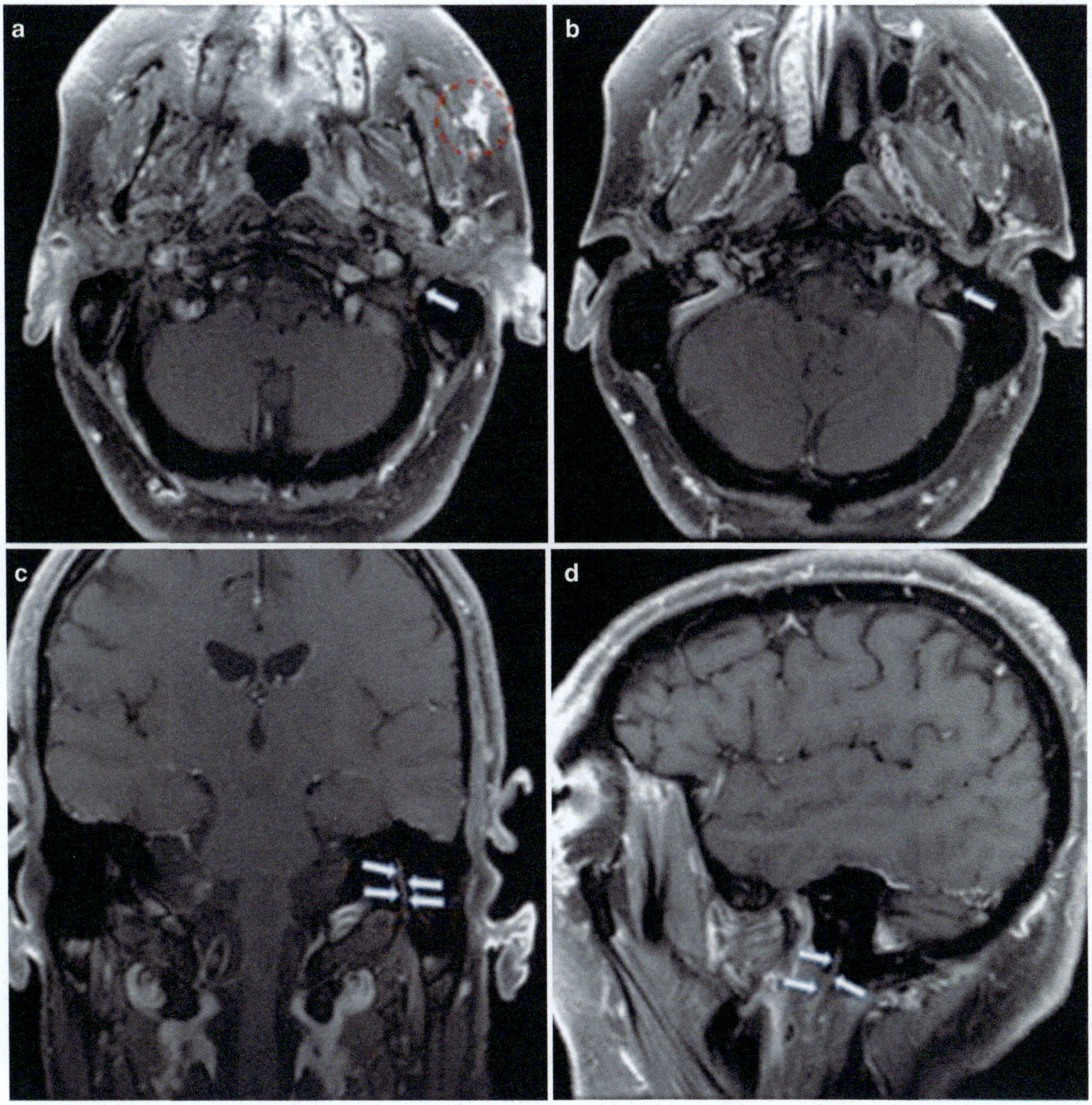

Fig. 29.7 T1 with contrast MRI images illustrating the subcutaneous mass (dotted red line in image **a**) and the enhancement of the left facial nerve (arrows)

table in the supine position on a headrest. As for most postoperative cases, the surgical scar and flap reconstruction was wired with CT radiopaque marker to assist with target volume delineation. A custom tongue-deviating stent was placed into the oral cavity. A 5 mm custom bolus was fabricated with a 1–1.5 cm margin to the surgical scar. The bolus is made of soft tissue-equivalent material and is used to ensure sufficient surface dose. A tissue-equivalent material was placed into the left ear and taped the ear flat to the neck to reduce contour irregularities and tissue inhomogeneity during radiation treatment planning and delivery. A 2 mm custom bolus was placed over the neck dissection scar. A customized thermoplastic mask was used for immobilization (Fig. 29.8). Non-contrast CT images were taken from the top of the head to the carina. These images were transferred to the treatment planning software system for contouring and CT-based treatment planning.

The patient was treated using IMRT technique. A total dose of 60 Gy was delivered to the tumor bed with a boost to facial canal and to the soft tissue under the flap to 66 Gy. Areas at intermediate risk (dissected uninvolved areas) received 57 Gy, and low-risk (uninvolved undissected unilateral neck) regions received a dose of 54 Gy. The target volume encompassed the postoperative tumor bed and the facial nerve tracking all the way to its site of origin at the brain stem (Fig. 29.9). Radiation therapy was delivered under daily kV imaging guidance and with concurrent cisplatin (40 mg/m^2 weekly).

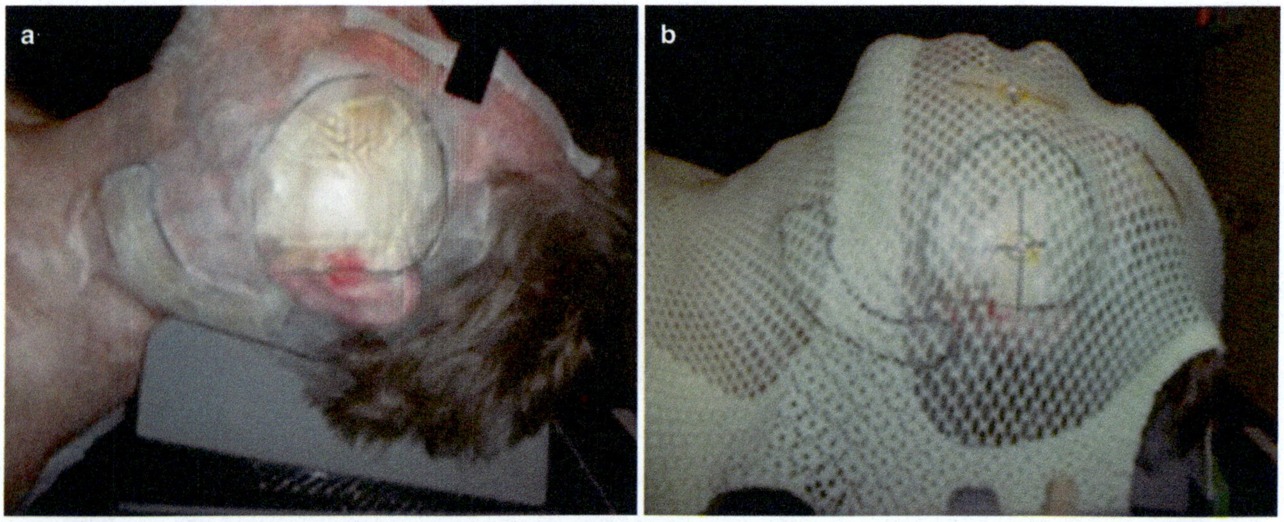

Fig. 29.8 Simulation. Surgical scars were wired and a custom bolus placed over the scar with a margin to improve dose delivery to skin surface. Tissue-equivalent material (pink) was placed into left ear to reduce tissue inhomogeneity. Finally a thermoplastic mask was placed over patient for immobilization

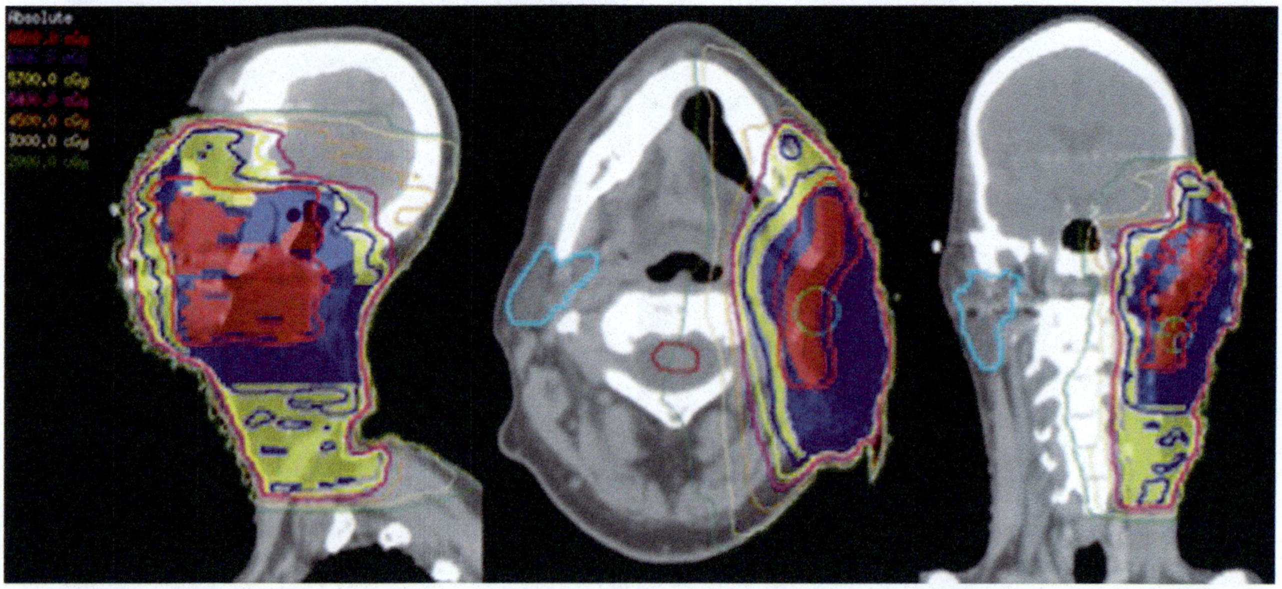

Fig. 29.9 Final dose distribution plan utilizing IMRT. Note sparing of contralateral parotid gland. Shaded areas indicate contoured target volumes, and lines indicate isodose lines (red, 66 Gy; blue, 60 Gy; yellow, 57 Gy)

He tolerated the treatment well with grade 3 skin reaction and grade 1 oral mucositis at the end of treatment. At 5-year follow-up, he remained disease-free, with no significant late toxicities of treatment.

Case 3

This case demonstrates the use of IMRT in the definitive setting for a locally advanced non-operable case. Unfortunately, the patient in case 3 subsequently relapsed within the low to no dose region after completion of radiotherapy.

An 81-year-old male, of average performance status (ECOG 2), with a long history of treated non-melanomatous cutaneous carcinomas of the head and neck region, presented with a 1-year history of left-sided facial paralysis. He had a history of biopsy-proven and recurrent left temple squamous cell carcinoma, for which he had superficial therapies and local excision to that region.

Physical examination revealed a complete left facial paralysis with left upper, mid, and lower face asthenia. There was no palpable parotid or cervical lymphadenopathy. There was a surgical scar and lesion within the left temporal scalp.

Biopsy of a left temporal scalp lesion showed moderately differentiated squamous carcinoma invading deep dermis, with no perineural invasion. CT imaging showed postsurgical changes within the left temporal scalp with nodular enhancement along the posterior margin of the left preauricular region (Fig. 29.10).

MRI (Fig. 29.11) showed an extensive lesion extending from the left temporal skin surface to the periosteum of the skull with extensive perineural enhancement and to the vertical portion of the facial nerve within the stylomastoid foramen as well as bright enhancement along the anterior genu of the facial nerve and of the greater superficial petrosal nerve. Additionally, there was abnormal enhancement in left Meckel's cave and along the branches of left cranial nerve V with involvement of V3 and the vidian canal. The left pterygoid muscles and the soft tissues surrounding the glenoid fossa and the temporomandibular joint had abnormal soft tissue involvement or inflammation. Diffuse edema and inflammation around the coronoid process and the fibers of the temporalis muscle were also seen. There was no radiological or clinical evidence of regional nodal or distant metastatic disease.

Given the extensive skull base perineural involvement, the patient was deemed not a surgical candidate and was dispositioned to radiotherapy following discussion at the multidisciplinary tumor board conference with the aim of achieving local control, as progression of perineural disease will undoubtedly be a detriment to his quality of life.

The patient was brought to the CT simulation suite. The nodule along the left temple was palpated, and a CT radiopaque marker was used to wire-out this area with a generous margin of 2–3 cm. The area along this region was covered with a custom 5 mm bolus to ensure adequate surface dose to this region. Similarly, a 3 mm bolus was used in the preauricular region to ensure adequate dose in that region given

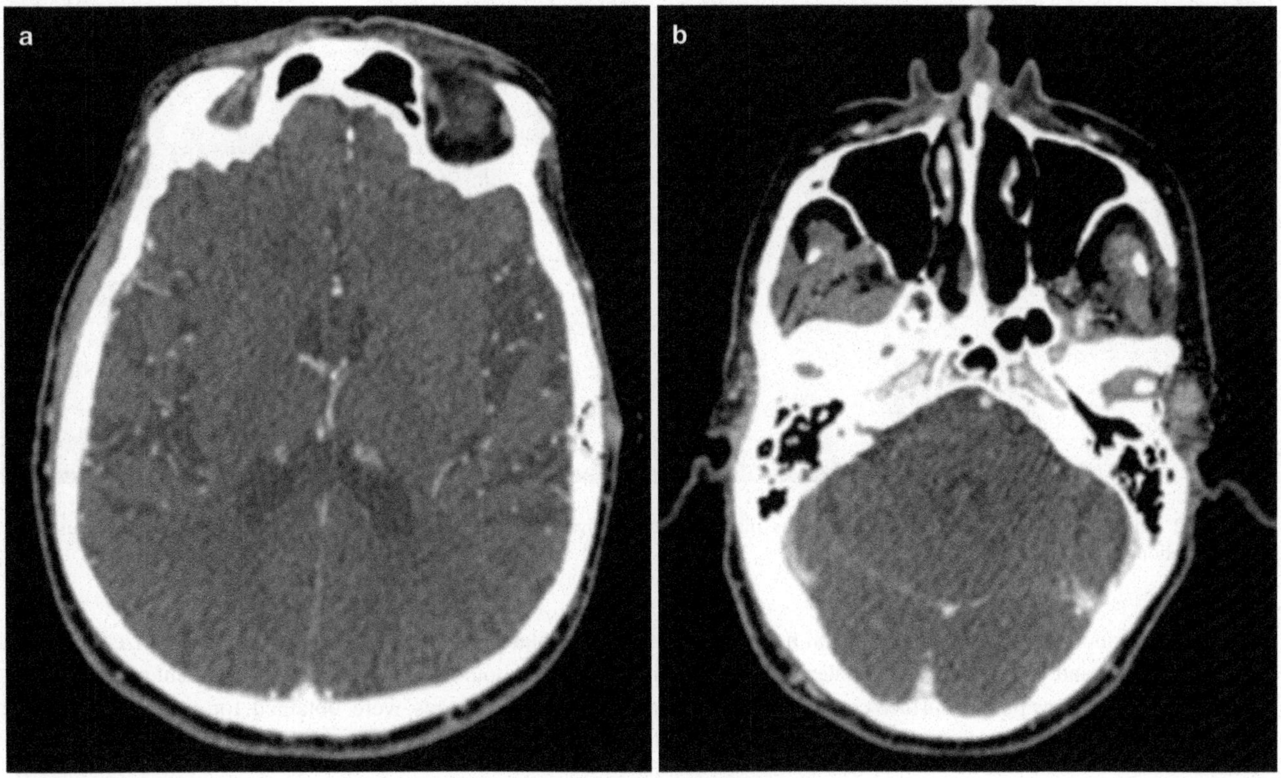

Fig. 29.10 CT images showing left temporal scalp and preauricular lesion (red dashed circle)

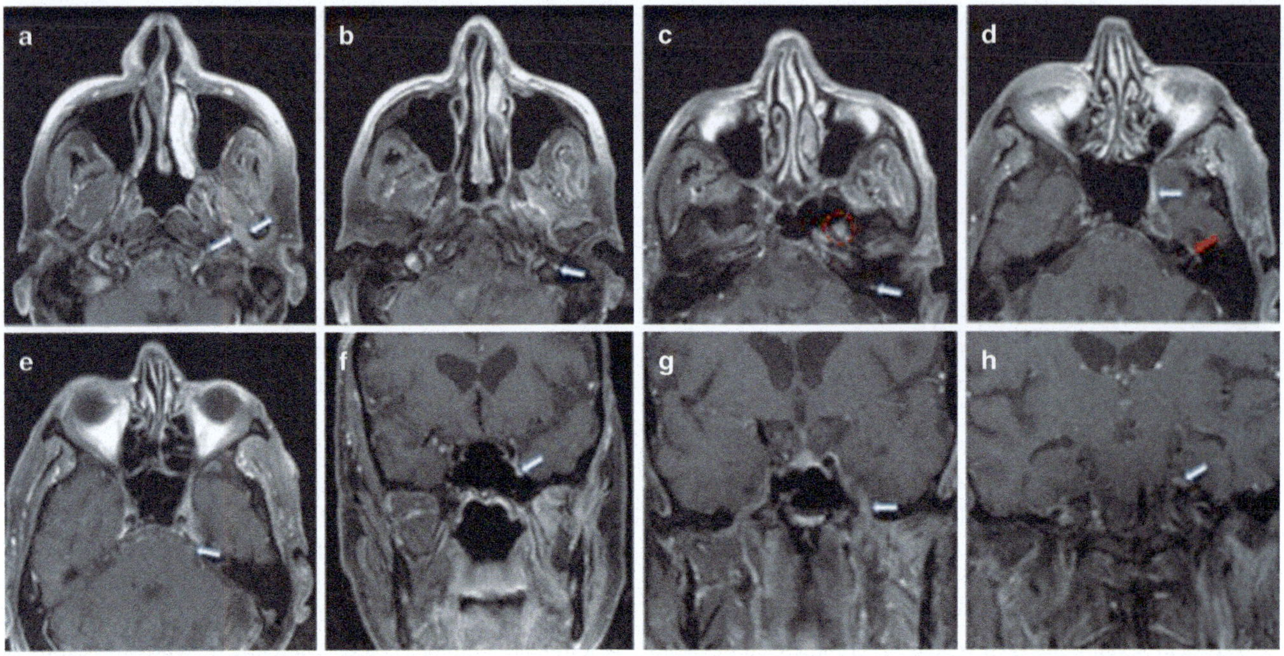

Fig. 29.11 Pertinent findings on MRI: (**a**) soft tissue involvement surrounding temporomandibular joint. (**b**) Enhancement of facial nerve within the stylomastoid foramen. (**c**) Facial nerve enhancement (arrow) and involvement of temporalis tendon on the coronoid process (red dashed line). (**d**) Enhancement along anterior genu of the facial nerve (white arrow) and the greater petrosal nerve (red arrow). (**f**) Vidian canal involvement. (**g**) Involvement of the V3 nerve through foramen ovale. (**h**) Thickening of the dural folds of Meckel's cave

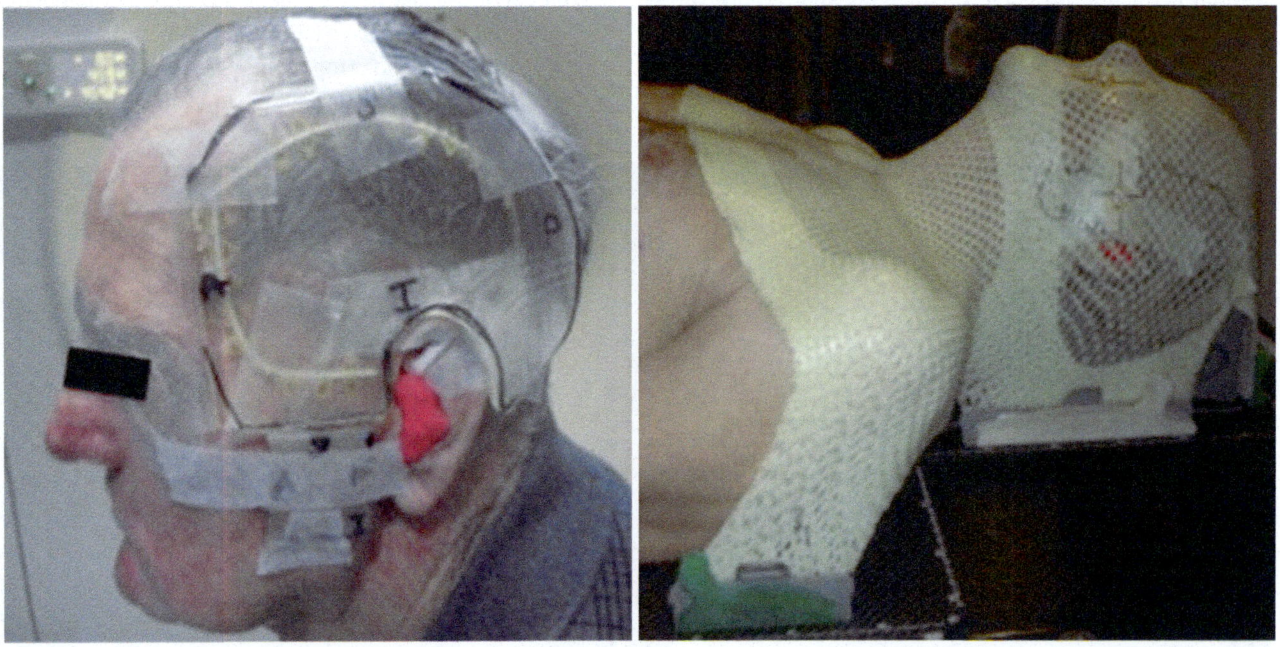

Fig. 29.12 Simulation. Surgical scar wired and bolus placed. Tissue-equivalent material placed in his ear. Thermoplastic mask used for immobilization

concern for perineural spread along the facial nerve. His ear was taped back, and tissue-equivalent material was placed within the ear to reduce patient surface contour irregularities (Fig. 29.12). An intraoral stent was placed, and a customized thermoplastic mask was created to immobilize his head, neck, and shoulders in the intended treatment position. Noncontrast CT images were obtained for treatment planning purposes.

The patient was treated using intensity modulation therapy to a total dose of 69.96 Gy in 33 fractions with concurrent erlotinib on a clinical trial. Intermediate- and lower-risk sites were also treated simultaneously to lower doses. The target volume encompassed the left temple region as well as the sites of involvement along cranial nerves V and VII tracking all the way to their origin at the brain stem (Fig. 29.13). Treatment was delivered under daily kV imaging guidance allowing daily bony alignment to reproduce position at simulation and ensure treatment delivery accuracy.

The patient tolerated the treatment well with grade 3 skin reaction and grade 1 oral mucositis at the end of treatment. The patient remained disease-free for 18 months posttreatment. He subsequently developed symptomatic left-sided neck swelling and neuropathic pain. Imaging was concerning for perineural tumor spread along the left greater auricular nerve to C2 (Fig. 29.14). The patient passed away 3 months after.

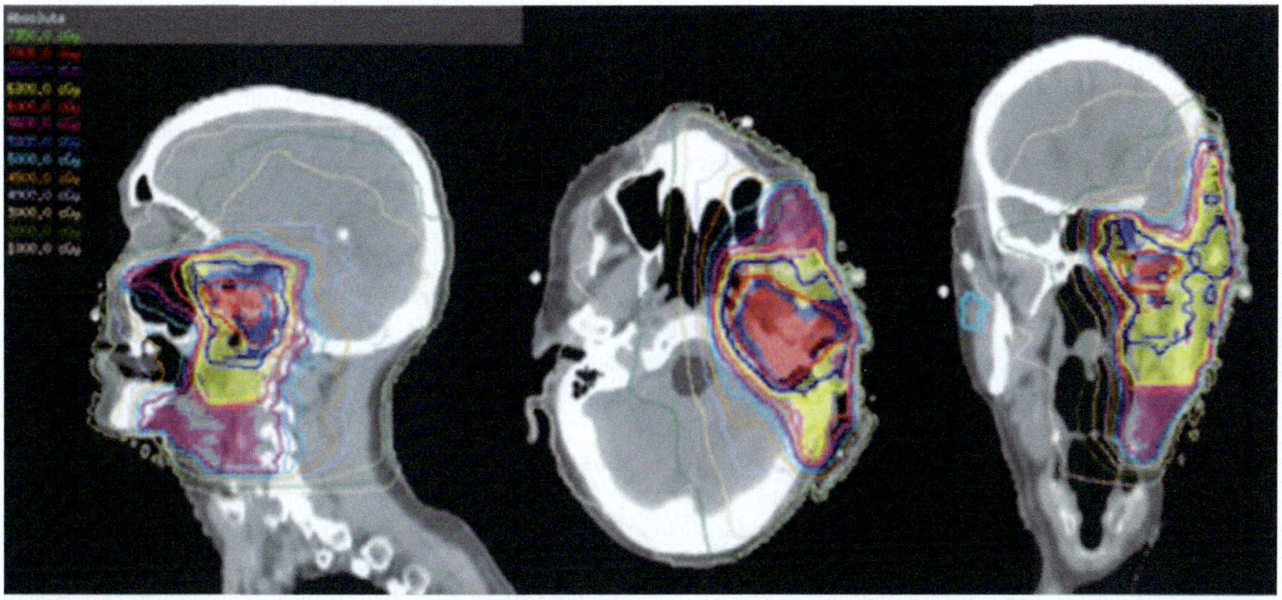

Fig. 29.13 Representative images of dose distribution. Shaded area: red, 69.96 Gy; blue, 66 Gy; yellow 63 Gy; pink, 55 Gy

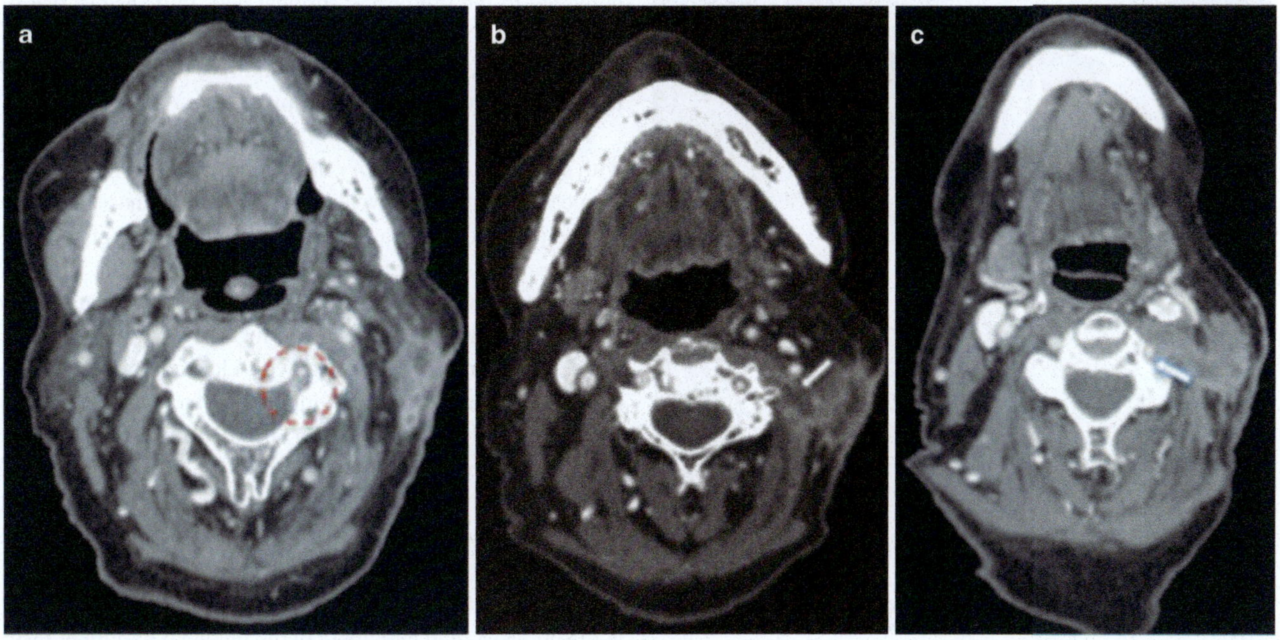

Fig. 29.14 Recurrence seen on CT imaging. (**a**) Epidural extension via neural foramen at C2. (**b**) Involvement of C2 spinal nerve and mass behind sternocleidomastoid muscle. (**c**) Tumor surrounding left vertebral artery at level of vertebral foramen

Case 4

This case demonstrates the use of IMRT in the definitive setting for a locally advanced non-operable case. This patient had no evidence of disease at 5-year follow-up after treatment. Cases 3 and 4 highlight that a high dose of radiation is effective in providing local control and the extent of treatment fields/volumes needs considerable thought during treatment planning to achieve a balance between larger treatment fields (i.e., probable better local control) and increased treatment toxicity.

An 88-year-old male, of good performance status (ECOG 1), with significant cardiovascular disease history, presented with recurrent basal cell carcinoma of his right ear for which he had at least seven surgeries over the past 30 years. He was found to have a right preauricular lesion which was excised with positive radial and deep margins. Histology once again confirmed infiltrating basal cell carcinoma.

Physical examination revealed a shortened and narrowed right external auditory meatus consistent with surgical changes. The bony ear canal and tympanic membrane appeared normal. The left external ear, meatus, and tympanic membrane were normal. There was no gross cranial neuropathy or palpable cervical lymphadenopathy. CT imaging showed the soft tissue recurrence abutting the mandibular condyle and temporomandibular joints without obvious bony involvement (Fig. 29.15). Formal audiology assessment revealed moderate to severe bone conduction hearing loss in the right ear.

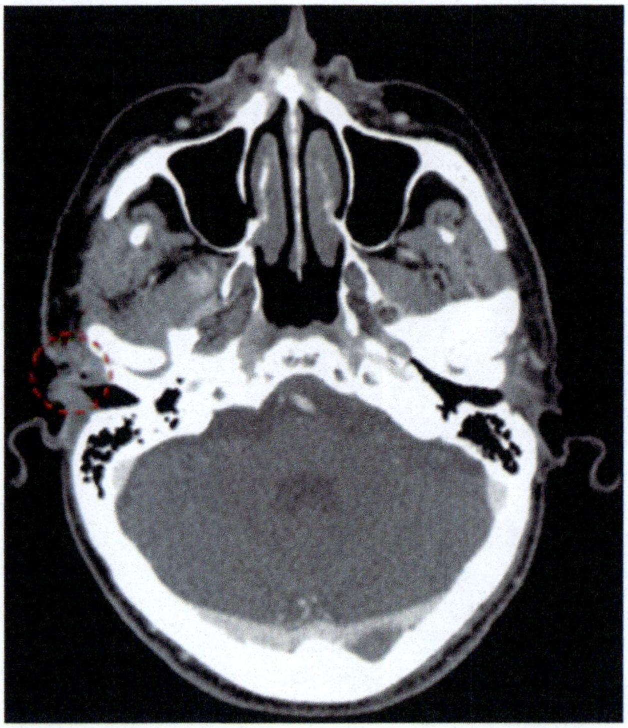

Fig. 29.15 Representative CT image showing right preauricular lesion (red dashed circle)

He was deemed not a suitable surgical candidate due to his extensive cardiovascular history and was dispositioned to definitive radiotherapy following discussion at the multidisciplinary tumor board conference.

The patient was brought to the CT simulation suite. His ear was taped back, and tissue-equivalent material was placed within the ear to reduce any contour irregularities (Fig. 29.16). A customized thermoplastic mask was created to immobilize his head in the intended treatment position. Non-contrast CT images were obtained for treatment planning purposes.

He was treated using IMRT technique to a total dose of 66 Gy in 30 fractions to the gross tumor, with 60 Gy to surgical bed and 57 Gy to adjacent at-risk soft tissues (Fig. 29.17).

He tolerated radiotherapy very well with grade 3 skin reaction within the posterior aspect of the auricle. His 3-year follow-up imaging (Fig. 29.18) and his 5-year clinical follow-up showed no evidence of tumor recurrence. Audiology assessment at 3 years after radiotherapy revealed no significant change in his hearing function compared to pre-radiotherapy levels.

Case 5

This case highlights the fact that each radiotherapy plan is considered on a case-by-case basis, tailoring treatment target volumes to an educated estimate of each patient's risk of locoregional relapse. This patient had a localized low-grade ear canal tumor whereby postoperative radiotherapy was delivered to the tumor and surgical beds only, as her risk of regional nodal relapse is estimated to be low, thereby reducing the volume of tissue treated and risk of acute and long-term complication of radiotherapy.

A 62-year-old lady of good performance status presented with several months history of left ear fullness and drainage. Clinical examination revealed a left ear canal mass.

She proceeded to have a left temporal bone excision, left parotidectomy, and left facial nerve biopsy. Final histopathology confirmed low-grade squamous cell carcinoma within the temporal bone involving the external auditory canal. The tumor was excised with clear margins, with no evidence of perineural or lymphovascular invasion. Given the bony involvement of tumor, postoperative radiotherapy was recommended.

She was brought to the CT simulation suite. The surgical scar was wired-out with a CT radiopaque marker, and a tissue-equivalent material was placed in the left ear canal. A customized thermoplastic mask was created to immobilize her head, neck, and shoulders in the intended treatment position (Fig. 29.19). Non-contrast CT images were obtained for treatment planning purposes.

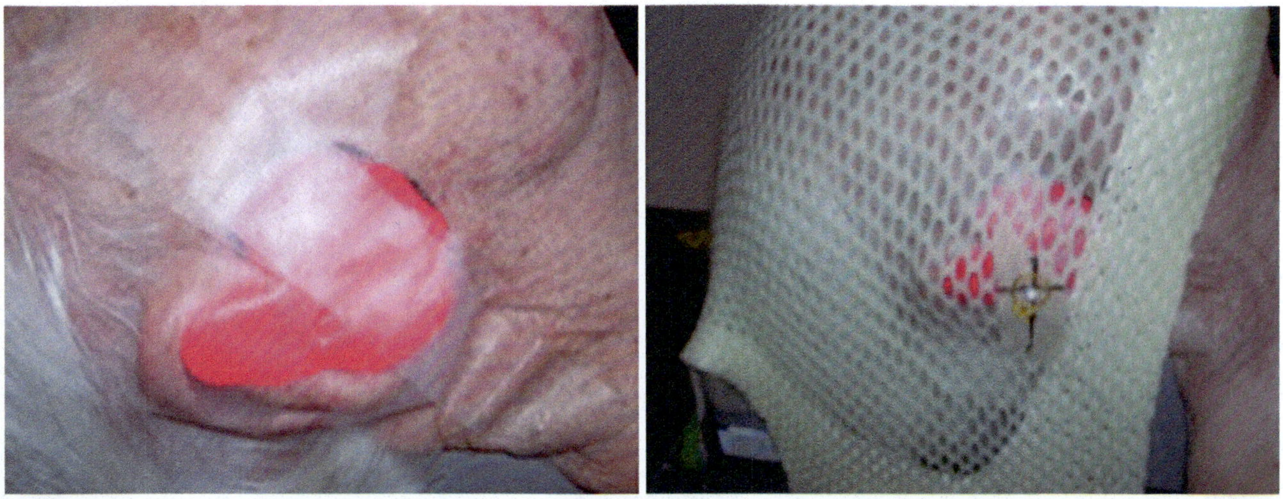

Fig. 29.16 Simulation. Tissue-equivalent material placed in his ear. Thermoplastic mask used for immobilization

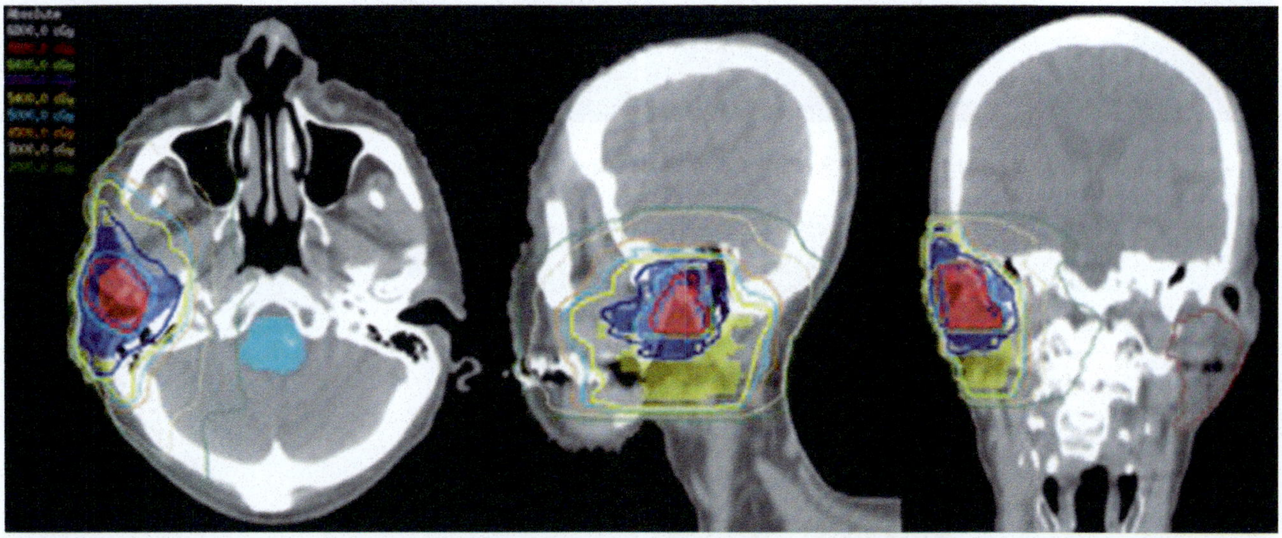

Fig. 29.17 Representative images of dose distribution. Shaded area: red, 66 Gy; blue, 60 Gy; yellow, 56 Gy

The patient was treated using volumetric arc therapy (VMAT) to a total dose of 60 Gy in 30 fractions. VMAT technique, a way of delivering photon radiation in an arc fashion, was chosen in this case to improve dose homogeneity delivered to the target volume while limiting dose to the contralateral normal tissues. The non-involved surgical bed was treated to a lower dose of 56 Gy. The target volume encompassed the tumor bed and non-involved surgical bed (Fig. 29.20). The draining nodal groups were not electively covered since her risk of nodal metastases was estimated as low (<15%), her tumor was low grade with no adverse features, and her tumor was excised with clear margins. Treatment was delivered under daily kV imaging guidance.

The patient tolerated the treatment very well with skin erythema and mild desquamation at the end of treatment. She recovered well from the acute effects of radiotherapy. She has ongoing follow-up with her surgical team.

Acute Effects of Radiotherapy During Treatment

In general, apart from fatigue, the acute effects of radiotherapy are local and limited to the radiotherapy treatment fields. Therefore, the side effect profile of radiotherapy can vary from patient to patient, depending on the patient's general status (comorbidities, performance status, medications, nutritional status), surgical site and healing, radiological and pathological findings, and radiotherapy treatment factors (total dose, dose/fraction, fields, treatment modality).

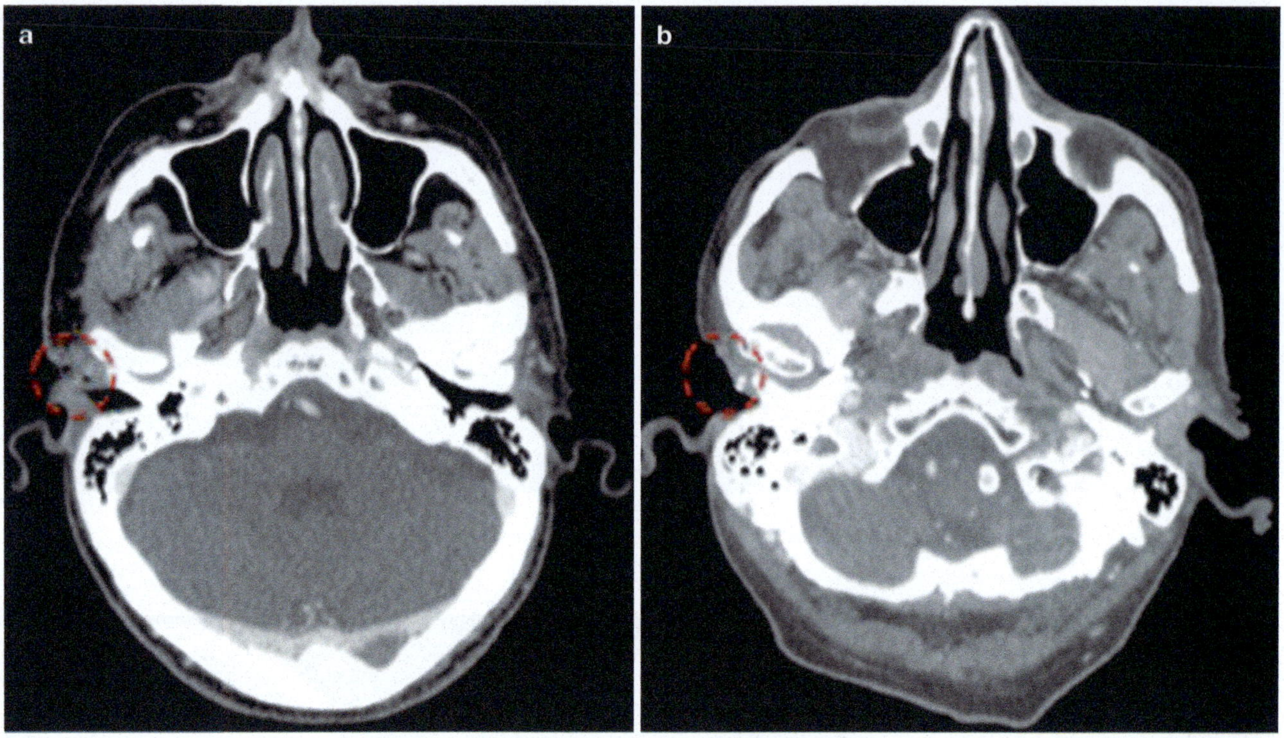

Fig. 29.18 Comparison of images before (**a**) and 3 years after (**b**) radiotherapy, highlighting the absence of tumor

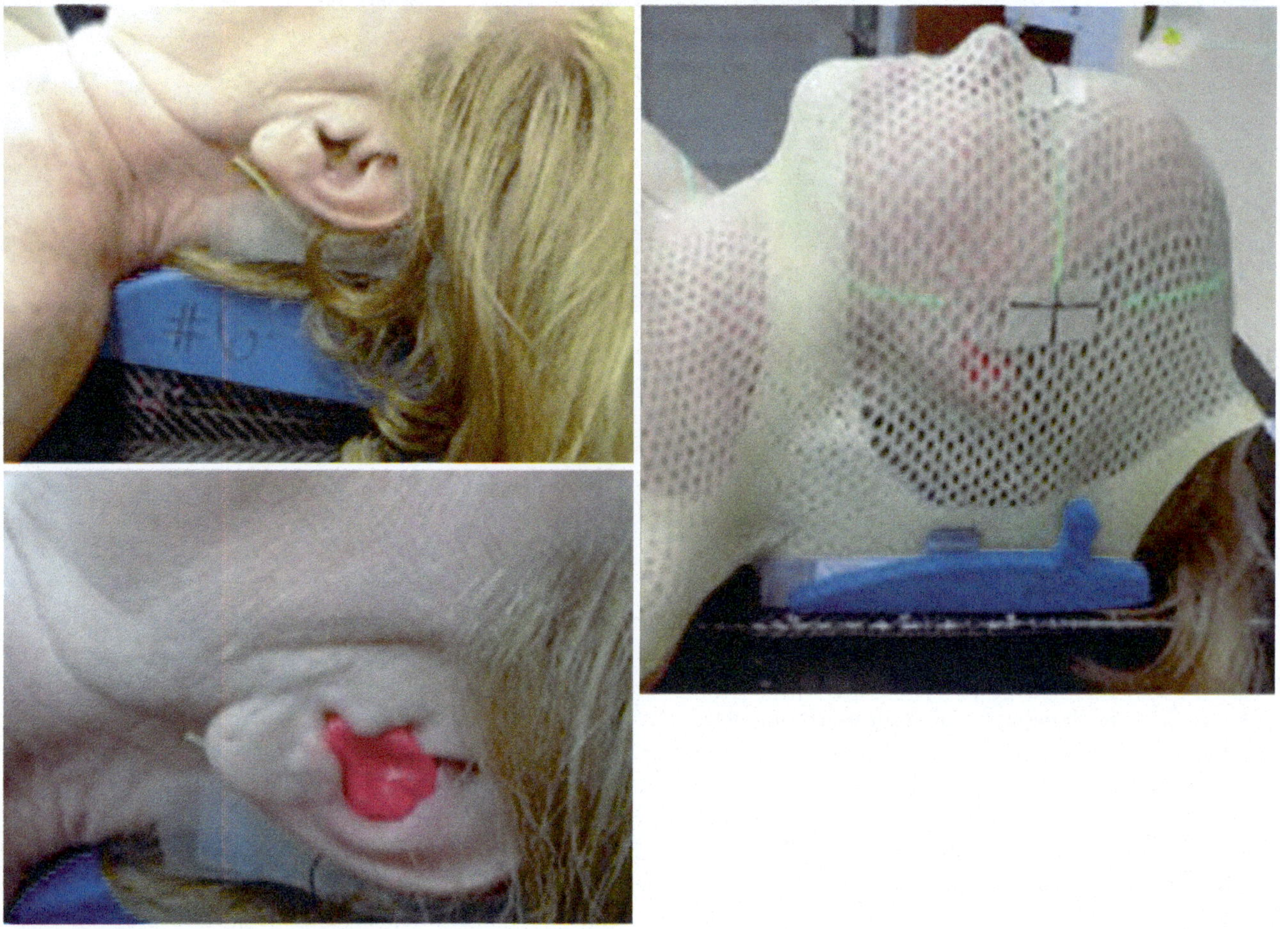

Fig. 29.19 Simulation. Postauricular surgical scar wired and tissue-equivalent material place within the left ear canal to reduce tissue inhomogeneity. Thermoplastic mask used for immobilization

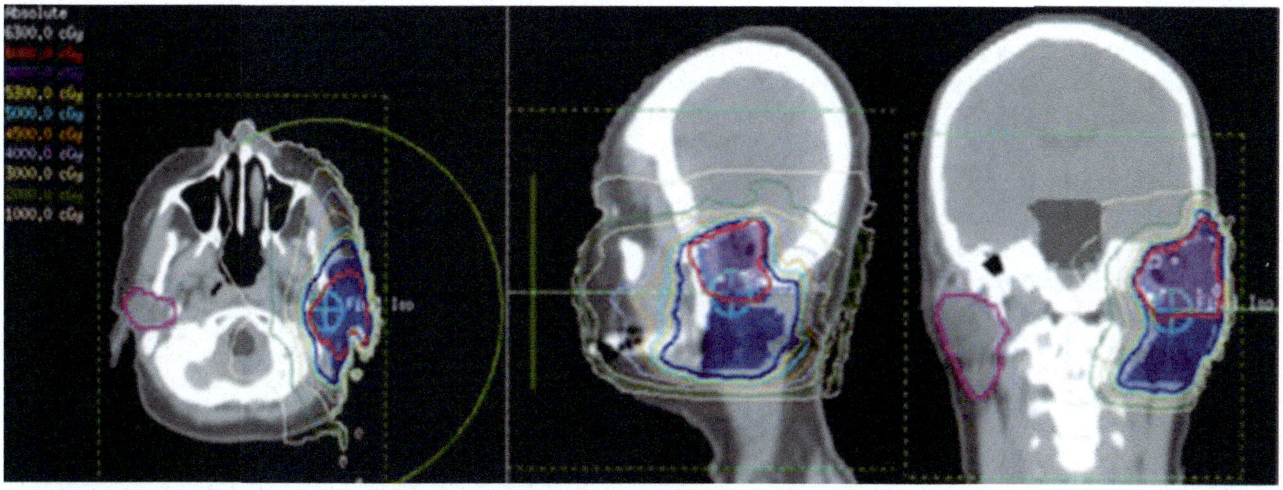

Fig. 29.20 Final dose distribution plan. Red, tumor bed, 60 Gy; blue, non-involved surgical bed, 56 Gy. Note excellent dose sparing of contralateral parotid gland and minimal dose to the left temporal lobe

Common local side effects for radiotherapy to the temporal bone region include radiation dermatitis, reduced hearing due to swelling of the ear canal, and thickened saliva and/or xerostomia. Oral mucositis and altered sense of taste can be common if the oral cavity, particularly the oral tongue, receives more than 30 Gy. Esophagitis is less common in this group of patients as they tend to receive unilateral neck treatment, reducing the dose to the esophagus compared to other head and neck cancer patients with bilateral neck irradiation.

These side effects typically increase in severity over the treatment course and resolve in approximately 4–6 weeks after completion of treatment. Fatigue and dysgeusia may take several months to resolve.

Radiation-Associated Long-Term Effects on the Temporal Bone

For long-term head and neck cancer survivors who received radiotherapy to the temporal bone, vigilant surveillance of late complications to the temporal bone is of upmost importance to allow optimal management.

Radiation therapy can cause tissue fibrosis, in particular vascular fibrosis and intimal hyperplasia leading to decreased vascular supply to the irradiated normal tissue. Within the temporal bone region, this contributes to the risk of long-term injury to bone (osteonecrosis), cartilage (chondronecrosis), cochlea (sensorineural hearing loss), and Eustachian tube/middle ear (serous otitis media and/or conductive hearing loss). Although the risk of developing these long-term effects is dependent on the total radiation dose and dose/fraction received, the patient's age, smoking status, comorbidities, and previous surgery to the area are also contributing factors.

Typically, sensorineural hearing loss and otitis media tend to develop within months after radiation treatment due to the fibrosis of the cochlea and Eustachian tube. A total cochlear dose of 30–50 Gy is an independent risk factor for sensorineural hearing loss, while the dose-effect relationship for the Eustachian tube is less well-established and is estimated at approximately 43–50 Gy [13].

Osteonecrosis of the temporal bone can develop 5–10 years after radiotherapy. Patients usually have non-specific symptoms such as crusting of external auditory canal, otorrhea, otalgia, and/or hearing loss. Physicians need to have high index of suspicion to identify and diagnose these patients as early osteonecrosis can be managed conservatively or with hyperbaric oxygen, whereas advanced or symptomatic osteonecrosis, in most cases, will require surgical intervention. It is estimated that a dose of 50Gy and above is a risk factor [13].

Radiation therapy can cause vascular changes including microangiopathy in the brain [14]. The temporal lobe is at risk, although low, of developing radiation necrosis given its location adjacent to the temporal bone. Encephalomalacia of the temporal lobe is usually asymptomatic but can manifest with non-specific symptoms such as headaches, mood changes, gradual memory impairment, fatigue, and poor concentration. Given the rarity of radiation necrosis of the brain, the majority of cases of temporal lobe necrosis tend to be reported in patients who received definitive radiotherapy for nasopharyngeal carcinoma. The median time to develop temporal lobe necrosis is typically 5 years [15]. A large imaging study on 1916 patients who received definitive radiotherapy for nasopharyngeal carcinoma over a 5-year period showed only 47 (2.5%) patients demonstrated temporal lobe changes on imaging [15].

Conclusion

Overall, radiation therapy improves locoregional control in patients with temporal bone tumors. For unresectable locally advanced tumors, radiotherapy can be utilized upfront as a definitive treatment. Regardless, in all cases, careful radiation treatment planning is necessary due to the presence of critical radiosensitive normal structures within the region. Various methods of treatment delivery and radiation modalities can be used to achieve the optimal radiotherapy plan for the patient.

References

1. Zanoletti E, Lovato A, Stritoni P, Martini A, Mazzoni A, Marioni G. A critical look at persistent problems in the diagnosis, staging and treatment of temporal bone carcinoma. Cancer Treat Rev. 2015;41(10):821–6. https://doi.org/10.1016/j.ctrv.2015.10.007.
2. Masterson L, Rouhani M, Donnelly NP, Tysome JR, Patel P, Jefferies SJ, et al. Squamous cell carcinoma of the temporal bone: clinical outcomes from radical surgery and postoperative radiotherapy. Otol Neurotol. 2014;35(3):501–8. https://doi.org/10.1097/MAO.0000000000000265.
3. Moffat DA, Wagstaff SA, Hardy DG. The outcome of radical surgery and postoperative radiotherapy for squamous carcinoma of the temporal bone. Laryngoscope. 2005;115(2):341–7. https://doi.org/10.1097/01.mlg.0000154744.71184.c7.
4. Zhang T, Li W, Dai C, Chi F, Wang S, Wang Z. Evidence-based surgical management of T1 or T2 temporal bone malignancies. Laryngoscope. 2013;123(1):244–8. https://doi.org/10.1002/lary.23637.
5. Cristalli G, Mercante G, Marucci L, Soriani A, Telera S, Spriano G. Intraoperative radiation therapy as adjuvant treatment in locally advanced stage tumours involving the middle ear: a hypothesis-generating retrospective study. Acta Otorhinolaryngol Ital. 2016;36(2):85–90. https://doi.org/10.14639/0392-100X-486.
6. Pfreundner L, Schwager K, Willner J, Baier K, Bratengeier K, Brunner FX, et al. Carcinoma of the external auditory canal and middle ear. Int J Radiat Oncol Biol Phys. 1999;44(4):777–88.
7. Bibas AG, Ward V, Gleeson MJ. Squamous cell carcinoma of the temporal bone. J Laryngol Otol. 2008;122(11):1156–61. https://doi.org/10.1017/S0022215107001338.
8. Prasad SC, D'Orazio F, Medina M, Bacciu A, Sanna M. State of the art in temporal bone malignancies. Curr Opin Otolaryngol Head Neck Surg. 2014;22(2):154–65. https://doi.org/10.1097/MOO.0000000000000035.
9. Ogawa K, Nakamura K, Hatano K, Uno T, Fuwa N, Itami J, et al. Treatment and prognosis of squamous cell carcinoma of the external auditory canal and middle ear: a multi-institutional retrospective review of 87 patients. Int J Radiat Oncol Biol Phys. 2007;68(5):1326–34. https://doi.org/10.1016/j.ijrobp.2007.01.052.
10. Morita S, Homma A, Nakamaru Y, Sakashita T, Hatakeyama H, Kano S, et al. The outcomes of surgery and chemoradiotherapy for temporal bone cancer. Otol Neurotol. 2016;37(8):1174–82. https://doi.org/10.1097/MAO.0000000000001152.
11. Shinomiya H, Hasegawa S, Yamashita D, Ejima Y, Kenji Y, Otsuki N, et al. Concomitant chemoradiotherapy for advanced squamous cell carcinoma of the temporal bone. Head Neck. 2016;38(Suppl 1):E949–53. https://doi.org/10.1002/hed.24133.
12. Takenaka Y, Cho H, Nakahara S, Yamamoto Y, Yasui T, Inohara H. Chemoradiation therapy for squamous cell carcinoma of the external auditory canal: a meta-analysis. Head Neck. 2015;37(7):1073–80. https://doi.org/10.1002/hed.23698.
13. Lambert EM, Gunn GB, Gidley PW. Effects of radiation on the temporal bone in patients with head and neck cancer. Head Neck. 2016;38(9):1428–35. https://doi.org/10.1002/hed.24267.
14. Valk PE, Dillon WP. Radiation injury of the brain. AJNR Am J Neuroradiol. 1991;12(1):45–62.
15. Chong VF, Fan YF, Mukherji SK. Radiation-induced temporal lobe changes: CT and MR imaging characteristics. AJR Am J Roentgenol. 2000;175(2):431–6. https://doi.org/10.2214/ajr.175.2.1750431.

Radiation Effects on the Temporal Bone

30

Christopher D. Frisch, Beth M. Beadle, and Paul W. Gidley

Introduction

History

Radiation has been used as a treatment method in many head and neck cancers for decades [1]. Due to the proximity of the temporal bone to many primary head and neck tumors, including nasopharynx, oral cavity, and oropharynx cancers, radiation dose is often delivered to the temporal bone, and it is at risk for radiation toxicity. In the past several decades, radiation therapy treatment planning and delivery has evolved, with a goal of minimizing doses to nontarget structures. This evolution has included transition from two-dimensional (2D) radiation planning using simple radiographs to three-dimensional planning using cross-sectional imaging (typically CT scans). As well, treatment delivery has evolved from simple conventional external beam therapy, which had a large target volume, to more conformal radiation techniques, including intensity-modulated radiotherapy (IMRT) and, most recently, proton beam therapy. The latter techniques specifically attempt to deliver dose to the targets while protecting normal tissues, including the adjacent bone, salivary glands, brain, inner ear, and spinal cord (among others).

Early complications to the temporal bone, such as soft tissue injury, chronic otitis media, and hearing loss, have been recognized as far back as the initiation of radiation delivery to the temporal bone, but the delayed complications of osteoradionecrosis and radiation-induced malignancy were not documented until much later [2, 3]. As therapy becomes further refined, with lesser radiation dose delivered to adjacent normal tissues, the hope is that these complications will decrease.

Sites Receiving Radiation

Radiation injury to the temporal bone and its contained structures can occur as a result of therapy directed precisely to the temporal bone (for treatment of squamous cell and other carcinomas) or as a consequence of radiation treatment to nearby head and neck subsites, such as the nasopharynx, oropharynx, parotid gland, upper neck, and brain [4–6]. The site, total dose, and type of radiation have an impact on the development and severity of temporal bone-related complications [7].

For example, primary radiotherapy as treatment for temporal bone squamous cell carcinoma, delivered daily over the course of 6 weeks, will cause more severe problems in the ear than de-escalated adjuvant radiation given for an oropharyngeal carcinoma, in which the temporal bone is an adjacent site but not a target. Malignancies treated primarily by radiation or chemoradiation are likely to be more associated with temporal bone complications than those receiving surgery and postoperative radiation, in which the dose is typically lower than in cases in which radiation itself is curative.

Types of Radiation

The key factor in the development of radiation-associated complications is the total dose and dose per fraction delivered to the area of interest [8]. The most common way for radiation to be delivered is using conventional external beam radiation (3DRT) or intensity-modulated radiotherapy (IMRT) [1]. IMRT has widely been adopted since 2000 as a method of treatment with the goal of minimizing dose to adjacent normal tissues for cancers of the head and neck [9]. There is randomized data in head and neck cancers showing

C. D. Frisch, M.D.
Department of Otolaryngology, Olmsted Medical Center, Rochester, MN, USA

B. M. Beadle, M.D., Ph.D.
Department of Radiation Oncology, Stanford University, Palo Alto, CA, USA
e-mail: bbeadle@stanford.edu

P. W. Gidley, M.D., F.A.C.S. (✉)
Department of Head and Neck Surgery, The University of Texas M.D. Anderson Cancer Center, Houston, TX, USA
e-mail: pwgidley@mdanderson.org

P. W. Gidley, F. DeMonte (eds.), *Temporal Bone Cancer*, https://doi.org/10.1007/978-3-319-74539-8_30

its benefit in reduction of xerostomia with a suggestion of improved survival [10, 11].

In the modern era, patients with head and neck cancer are planned for radiation therapy using a computed tomographic (CT) scan. This allows delineation of the targets (gross tumor and adjacent areas at risk for microscopic spread) as well as delineation of the normal tissues that are to be avoided, including the spinal cord, mandible, brainstem, and salivary glands [1]. After the target volumes and normal tissues are delineated, a team of dosimetrists and medical physicists use inverse planning and elegant radiation treatment planning software to design an array of beams that maximize the target coverage while minimizing dose to the adjacent normal tissues (Fig. 30.1). The doses for curative treatment in the head and neck, without surgery, are typically 66–70 Gy in 33–35 fractions. The doses for postoperative treatment in the head and neck are typically 60 Gy in 30 fractions. There are well-known limits for normal tissues, based on prior data and scientific experiments, which determine the acceptable doses with minimal complications for normal tissues [12]. The treating radiation oncology physician must then assess the plan and make judgments about optimizing target coverage versus protecting normal tissues, based on careful risk/benefit analysis. Once a plan is approved by the physician, the plan typically undergoes careful quality assurance to ensure that the computer model represents the delivered dose coming out of the radiation treatment machine. In the modern era, radiation treatment is typically delivered using a linear accelerator; the patient is aligned every day in the same position as when the plan was created. Treatment is then delivered daily (Monday to Friday) until the completion of therapy. Every effort is made to minimize treatment breaks or interruptions, which reduce the chances of cancer control.

Proton beam therapy has emerged as another radiation therapy technique, with the goals of maximizing coverage of the tumor target while minimizing treatment of adjacent normal tissues. Proton therapy must be delivered using a specialized machine; the availability of these machines has increased considerably over the last decade in the United States [13]. As opposed to conventional radiation or IMRT, proton therapy uses protons (which are particles) rather than electromagnetic radiation, to deliver treatment. Protons have different physical properties, with the majority of the energy being delivered at the end of range. The potential advantage of proton therapy is that these physical properties may deliver less low-dose radiation to normal tissues in the treated area. However, the impact of this is unknown. Ongoing clinical trials in the head and neck seek to answer the questions regarding the long-term effects of proton therapy in both cancer control and toxicity.

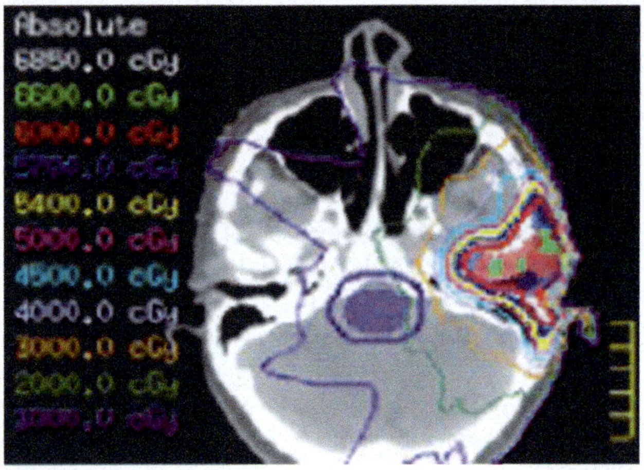

Fig. 30.1 Radiotherapy plan. Colored lines indicate isodose levels

Mechanism of Radiation-Induced Injury

The basic principle behind the efficacy of radiation as a treatment modality in head and neck cancer is its ability to induce damage to cancer cells. This damage occurs either directly, as occurs when radiation induces breaks within the DNA of cancer cells, or indirectly, as a result of the production of free radicals, which damage cancer DNA. Because cancer cells are dividing at a rate faster than adjacent normal tissue, they are more likely to be affected.

Cancer cells' susceptibility to the effects of ionizing radiation is determined by other principles, often referred to as the four "Rs" of radiation: Repair of sublethal DNA damage, cell Repopulation, Redistribution of cells in the cell cycle, and Reoxygenation of previously hypoxic tumor areas [14]. Some radiation scientists have referred to a fifth "R" known as the relative Radiosensitivity of a particular tumor. Other factors play a role, such as the overall tumor size (tumor burden), vascularity, tumor properties (solid versus cystic or necrotic), as well as the individuals' particular inflammatory response. Some cancerous cells are also more affected by radiation if they have been "radiosensitized" by the use of chemotherapy [1]. Treatment effect and the incidence of complications observed are determined by the damage induced by radiotherapy and the individuals' repair response.

Dose-Response Relationship and Radiation Repair

The ratio between radiation-induced damage and radiation-repair response determines clinical efficacy and associated side effects. Some evidence suggests that higher doses of radiation result in increased death of cancer cells and hence treatment response; however, concomitant increases in toxicity result from higher doses being delivered to adjacent normal tissues. Nevertheless, normal tissues do have the ability

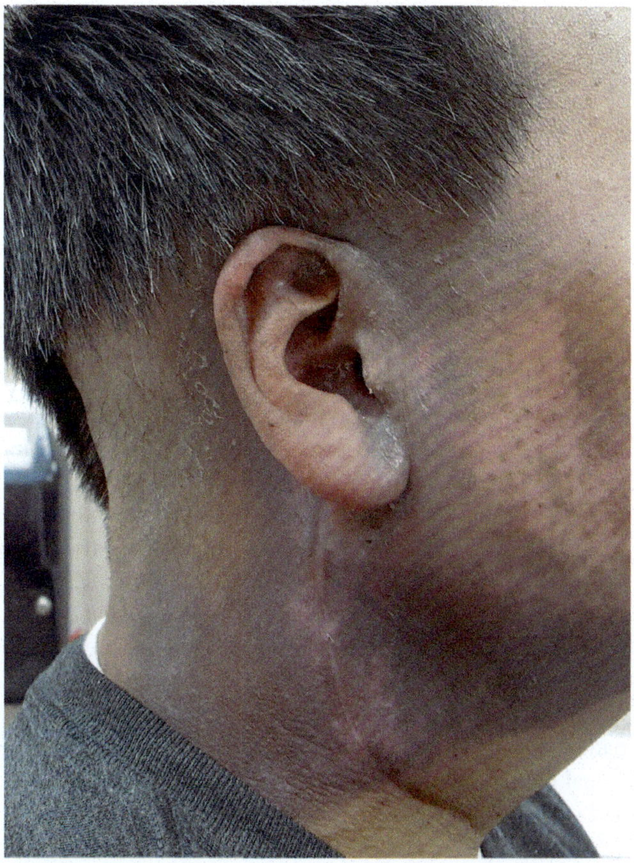

Fig. 30.2 Acute radiation effects on the skin of the ear, face, and neck. This patient is 2 weeks after completing 60 Gy of radiation

to repair DNA damage caused by radiation therapy, resulting in the ratio observed. The ability of normal tissues to repair damage inflicted by radiation therapy is dependent on several factors, most notably the tissue type. Tissues with quick cellular turnover, including mucosa (in which damage causes mucositis with associated pain, sloughing of tissue, and ulceration) and skin (in which damage causes dermatitis and/or radiation burns) (Fig. 30.2), demonstrate more obvious toxicity than those with more stable cell populations and less turnover such as muscles, nerves, and bone [15].

Variability in Patient Response

Despite data on normal tissue tolerance and tumor response to radiation therapy in multiple cell lines and in vitro experiments, variability exists between individual patient responses, even when comparing tumors of identical histology and subsite location. This variability is likely explained by underlying genetic factors, as well as environmental risk factors. Genetic factors that play a role include those involved in repair of DNA damage and determining an individual's inflammatory response. Genetic mutations that result in compromised DNA repair result in readily observed and sometimes severe syndromes such as xeroderma pigmentosum [16]. Any mutation resulting in a more robust inflammatory response in normal tissue exposed to radiation will similarly result in less tolerance of standard radiation doses.

External environmental factors that predispose certain individuals to increased side effects include those involved in wound healing [17]. Compromised wound healing may occur as a result of poor local circulation (atherosclerosis, diabetes, tobacco use), malnutrition (vitamin deficiencies, cancer treatment-associated anorexia), and states resulting in poor metabolism (i.e., hypothyroidism).

Duration of Effect

There are two phases of toxicity to radiation therapy. The acute phase develops during radiation therapy (approximately week 2–3) and lasts for approximately 2 weeks after the end of treatment and then resolves. The chronic phase develops months to years after radiation therapy, and these side effects may not be seen in any severity until that time. Radiation techniques must attempt to reduce both of these; however, the major goal is to minimize long-term or chronic toxicity, which can be much more devastating.

The acute effects of radiation are most quickly seen in certain types of tissues, such as skin and mucosa, which have rapidly dividing cells [15]. A larger proportion of cells in these tissues are in the synthesis phase of the cell cycle (the point in which cell DNA is most susceptible to the toxic effects of radiation) [1]. For tumors involving or adjacent to the otic structures, side effects are often seen early in these tissues, including radiation dermatitis, with drying, reddening, and often burning of skin in and around the ear on the surface of the temporal bone (Fig. 30.2) [18]. Damage to the mucosa can quickly induce an inflammatory response in the middle ear, with a resultant increase in mucous production. This may lead to development of serous otitis media and conductive hearing loss, which may become secondarily infected, leading to acute otitis media and possibly chronic serous otitis media (Fig. 30.3) [19].

The chronic effects are typically more related to damage to other tissues, such as the salivary glands and bone. In fact, radiation-induced damage to the inner ear, bone, and vasculature may not present acutely or be obvious clinically. Damage to these tissue types is particularly problematic since these changes occur over the course of years rather than days or weeks and require diligent follow-up.

Damage to the inner hair cells of the cochlea has been well documented, and clinically significant sensorineural hearing loss may develop years after treatment [20]. Damage to bone results in a derangement of the complex interplay between osteoblast and osteoclast activity and an imbalance of the

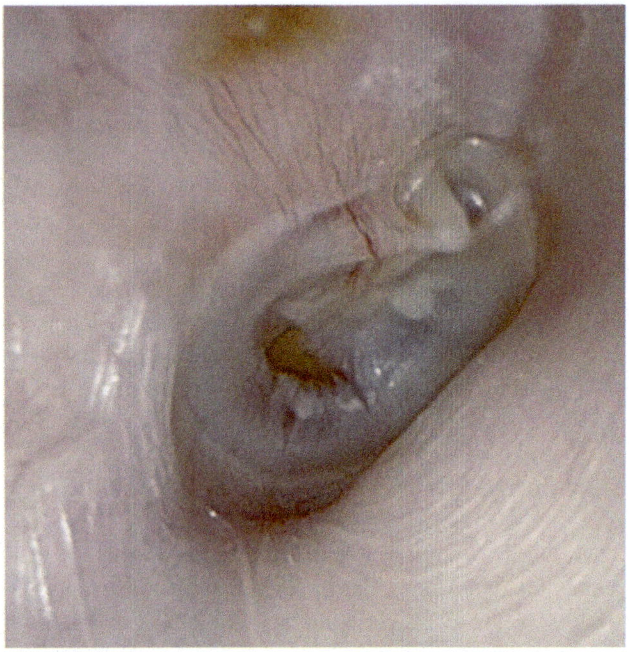

Fig. 30.3 Radiation-induced chronic serous otitis media

relative proportions of these cells due to altered differentiation from progenitor stem cells [6, 21, 22]. This ultimately leads to changes in the overall composition of bone after radiation-induced repair, resulting in unstable, fibrotic bone [23]. Damage to vascular tissue in the temporal bone may occur as a result of both periarteritis and obliterative endarteritis [7]. This vascular pathology may contribute to other secondary issues, such as inflammation and infection, due to poor delivery of wound-healing factors. Impaired vascularity may accelerate hearing loss due to the resulting bone erosion [24]. By a similar mechanism, accelerated bone erosion may contribute to developing osteoradionecrosis at a later stage.

Lastly, direct damage to DNA induced by radiation may eventually lead to the development of a secondary, radiation-associated malignancy (RAM). This is exceedingly rare; however, radiation to the head and neck may predispose to the development of squamous cell carcinoma or sarcomas in the temporal bone. In the rare occasions of this development, it typically is many years after the initial treatment [3, 7].

Clinical Manifestations and Treatment

The use of radiotherapy delivered directly to the temporal bone, or to adjacent subsites, can result in damage of any of the structures housed within the temporal bone. The range of possible sequelae can be classified into those that may occur to the external soft tissue, the middle ear mucosa and ossicles, the cochlea and vestibular apparatus, and the temporal bone itself. Radiation effects can also be classified based on the time of occurrence (Fig. 30.4). Acute effects, like dermatitis, happen either during or shortly after radiation treatment (during treatment or the following 6 weeks following treatment). Subacute effects like sensorineural hearing loss occur 6 weeks to 1 year posttreatment. Chronic effects, like osteoradionecrosis or radiation-associated malignancy, occur years after radiotherapy has ceased. Prior to discussing the different pathologies, it would be beneficial to review the relevant anatomy.

Acute Effects of Radiotherapy

Soft Tissue Injury

Injury to the soft tissue overlying the temporal bone is common following radiotherapy to the temporal bone and cancers of adjacent subsites [15]. As discussed previously, the skin is a rapidly dividing organ and hence demonstrates the acute effects of radiation therapy more quickly. Skin atrophy, loss of hair follicles, and cerumen glands may all occur (Fig. 30.5). Alterations in the normal physiology and flora of the ear canal skin may lead to the development of otitis externa (OE). This presents like OE in the nonirradiated patient, with purulent drainage, itching, fullness, and occasional pain. This is treated by frequent, careful debridement and steroid/antibiotic combination ototopical drops.

Radiation-associated dermatitis is seen acutely with radiation doses delivered to the periauricular skin, the outer ear, and ear canal [7]. This is considered a normal and expected side effect of radiation treatment, but supportive care must be given to ensure that it heals well. Clinical manifestations include red, scaly, and sloughing skin with associated pain, ulceration, bleeding, and increased risk of infection. On exam, reddened, scaly skin that readily shears and is painful to the touch is often found. Sloughing of ear canal skin can lead to blockage and otitis externa (Fig. 30.6). The skin may have an increased temperature, and there may be an associated purulent, malodorous drainage. Prompt recognition and treatment of this pathology is needed to prevent further complications associated with excessive ulceration, breakdown, and bone exposure.

Aggressive wound care management with frequent wet-dry dressing changes, as well as application of topical steroid-containing or antibiotic-impregnated creams, will assist in preventing the aforementioned worsening complications of advanced soft tissue breakdown [25]. Certain silver-containing creams also have been used with varying success for associated burns [26]; however, these should not be used during radiation treatment and should only be considered after the conclusion of the entire course. Active purulent drainage, redness, and odor with or without fever might be indications of a more serious infection requiring the administration of topical antibiotic therapy. Careful administration of drops without the use of earwicks is recommended, as the wicks can result in further damage and sloughing of fragile postirradiated skin, leaving exposed bone.

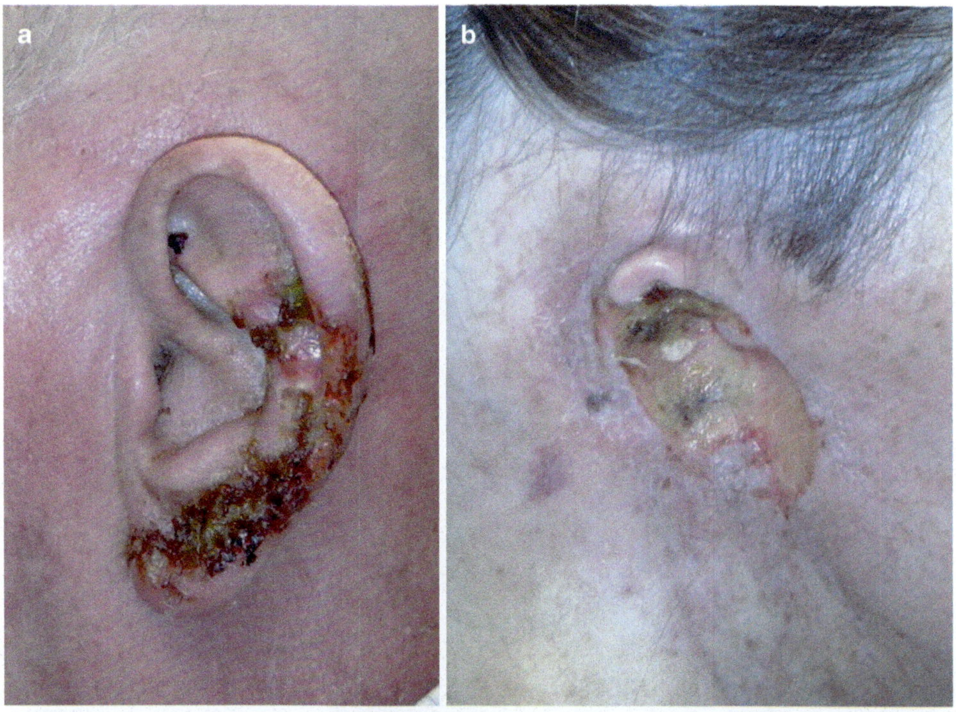

Fig. 30.4 (**a**) Acute effects of radiation to the external ear including ulceration and skin breakdown. (**b**) Late effect of radiation resulting in loss of external ear

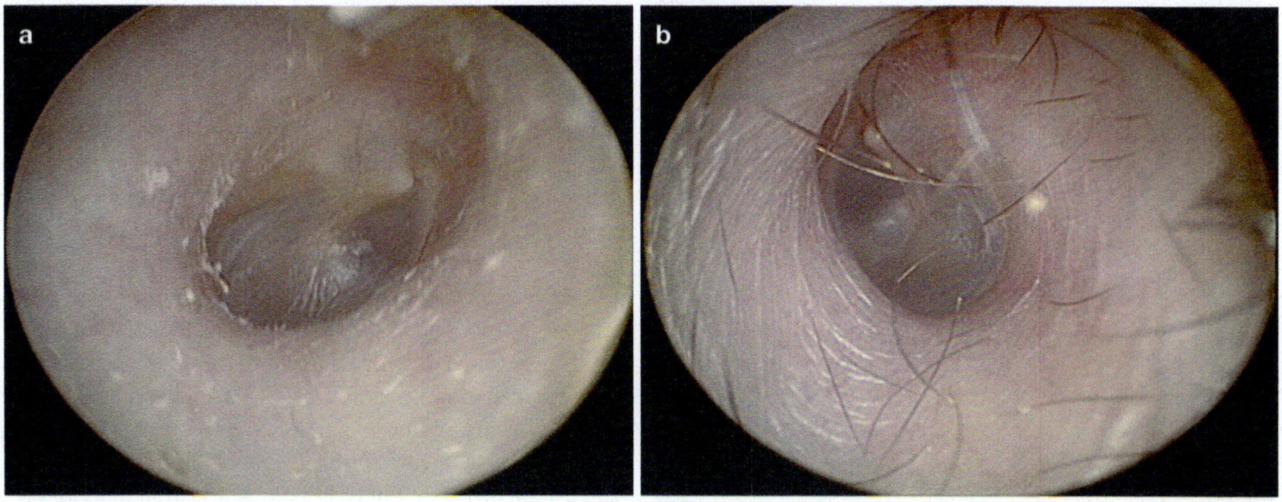

Fig. 30.5 Loss of hair follicles observed in the right ear (**a**) following radiation to the right parotid, compared to the normal left (**b**) side

Radiation-associated soft tissue injury may occur early in treatment and persist through treatment, but these toxicities will typically heal without long-term issues if managed early and aggressively.

Subacute Effects of Radiotherapy

Serous Otitis Media and Eustachian Tube Dysfunction

Otitis media can occur during radiotherapy in the form of acute serous otitis media—also called radiation-associated otitis media. This often resolves within a month or two of finishing XRT, though it can persist, resulting in chronic serous otitis media with effusion.

Radiation affects both the Eustachian tube and the middle ear mucosa. Jung et al. have outlined the changes that occur at the cellular level within the middle ear and Eustachian tube after radiation [27]. The Eustachian tube is critical to the equilibrium within the middle ear, and malfunction of this conduit leads to chronic problems within the middle ear that are often difficult to fix.

Following radiation therapy, the middle ear mucosa loses much of its cytoplasmic volume, which results in wider spaces in between individual cells [19]. Additionally, cells

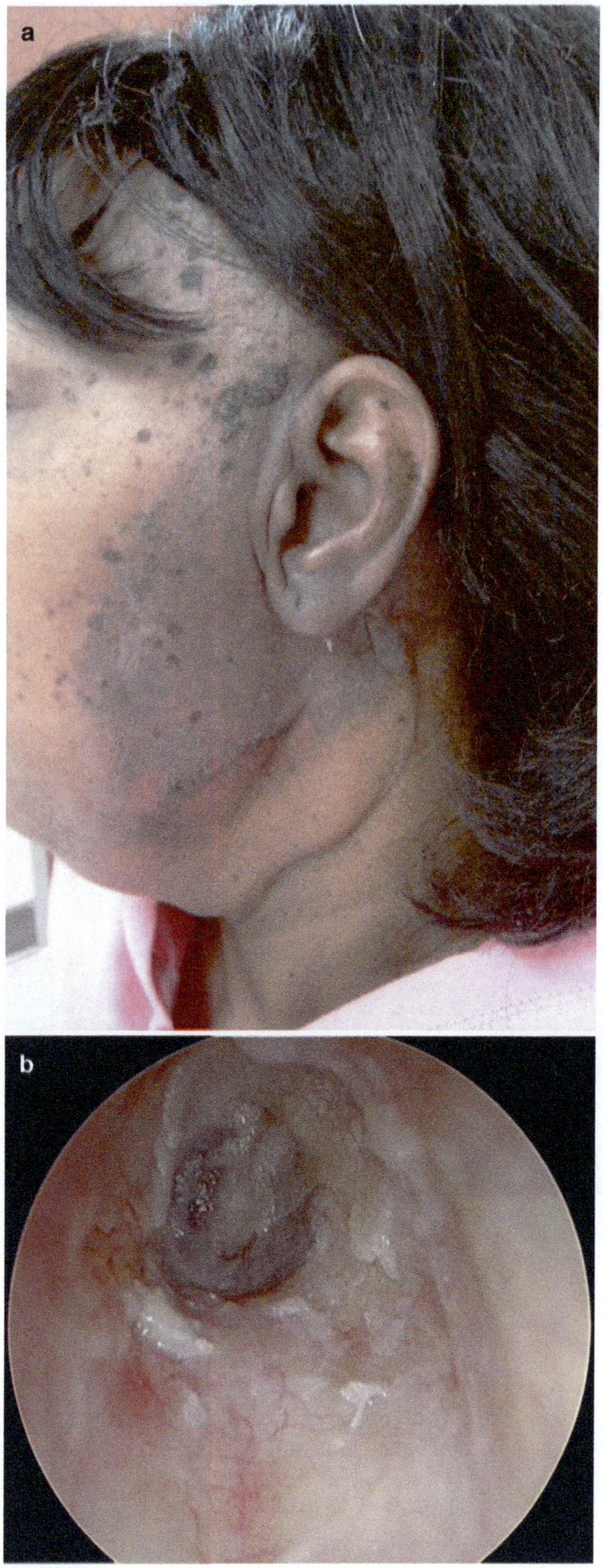

Fig. 30.6 Acute effect of radiation 2 weeks after radiotherapy for parotid cancer. (**a**) Desquamation of periauricular skin, (**b**) radiation otitis externa

lose cilia and have abnormal ciliary motion, resulting in loss of the "mucous-sweeping" function of the middle ear mucosa toward the Eustachian tube [27]. Eventually, this may lead to trapping of dry, inspissated mucous within the middle ear. Studies have shown that doses as low as 30 Gy will cause an increase rate of opacification of the mastoid and middle ear, as noted on magnetic resonance imaging [28].

Damage to the Eustachian tube may further compound damage to the middle ear mucosa. The Eustachian tube is nearly 4 cm in length and runs from the anterior mesotympanum to the nasopharynx at an angle of approximately 30° in the adult [29]. The lateral one third of the tube is a bony canal, whereas the more medial two thirds is cartilaginous. The narrowest point is the junction of these two areas, known as the isthmus. Further narrowing of this area, or a decrease in function of the adjacent tensor veli palatini muscle, which acts to open the tube, leads to Eustachian tube obstruction. Similar to the middle ear, the Eustachian tube may lose normal ciliary function and cellular composition following radiotherapy [27]. In addition, the surrounding muscles and tube itself undergo a transformation with increased deposition of fibrotic tissue [30].

Radiation to the middle ear and Eustachian tube may cause damage at the cellular level, which can become clinically significant and challenging to manage. Abnormal middle ear mucosal composition, ciliary function, and Eustachian tube problems can result in the formation of thickened, stagnant middle ear effusion. Treatment of radiation-associated otitis media and its associated hearing loss can risk further complications; therefore, pretreatment counseling with patients should be directed at individual goals and expectations in relation to expected risk versus benefit.

The improved focal delivery of radiation via the use of IMRT may prove to mitigate much of this damage. The rates of otitis media and hearing loss in nasopharyngeal cancer (NPC) patients is lower in those treated with IMRT than those treated with conventional external beam therapy [31]. The use of IMRT, not only in NPC but also in parotid, oropharyngeal, and temporal bone carcinoma, may reduce the rates of radiation-induced complications of the middle ear and Eustachian tube.

Treatment of radiation-induced Eustachian tube dysfunction and chronic otitis media with effusion is a challenge, and controversy exists over standard management. Tympanostomy tube placement is a time-honored means of treating chronic serous otitis media in the nonirradiated population. However, in the irradiated population, the use of tympanostomy tubes is controversial, because tubes have been associated with higher rates of persistent tympanic membrane perforation, chronic otorrhea, and conductive hearing loss (Fig. 30.7). Chronic otorrhea, while not dangerous, is cumbersome for patients to deal with. Chronic TM perforation requires practicing water precautions to reduce the incidence of middle ear infection.

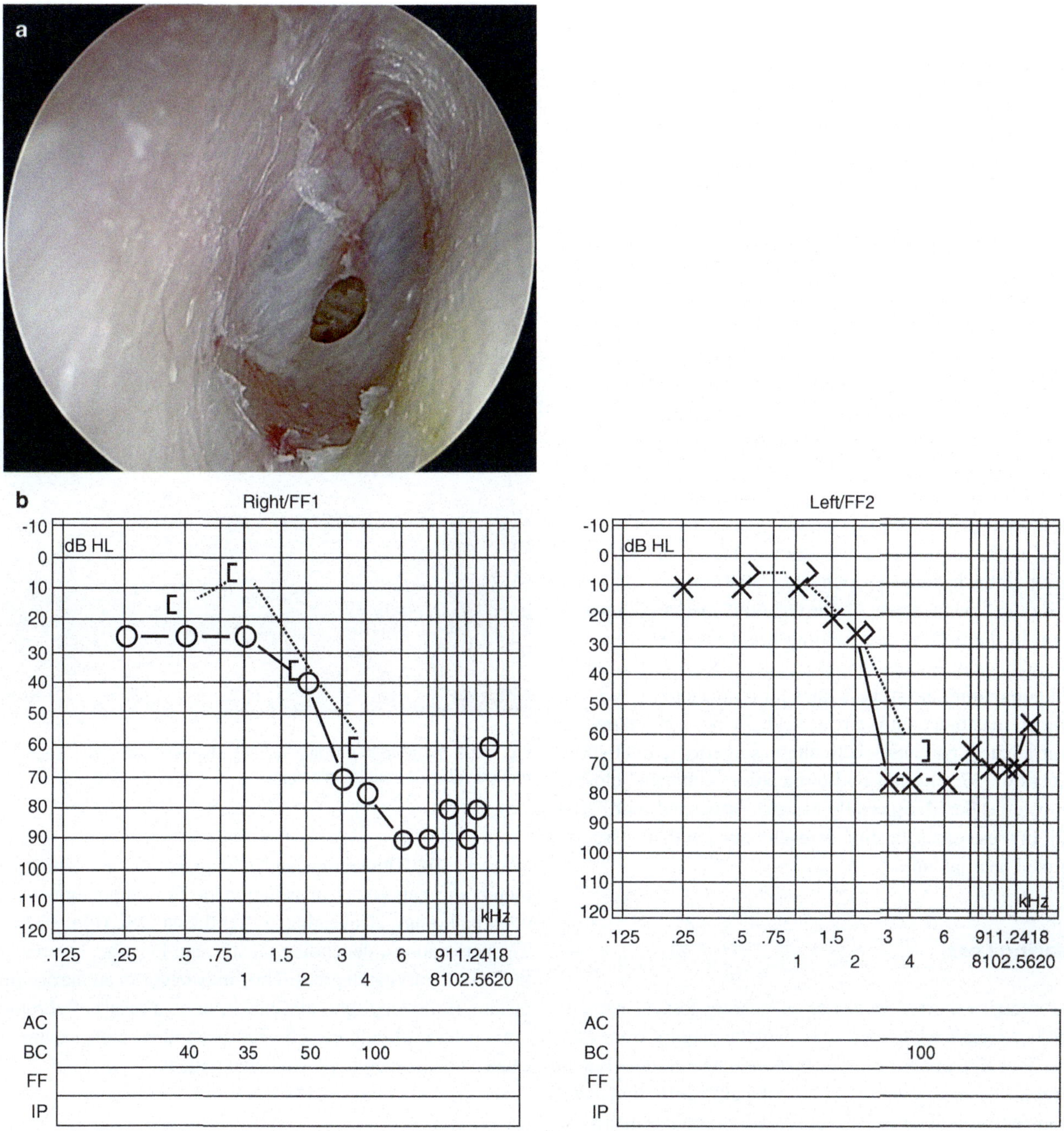

SRT PTA Right:- PTA Left:-					
Transducer	Test type	Intensity	Masking	Aided	ISF440 list
Right	HL	30			Spondee A
Left	HL	10			Spondee A

WR PTA Right:- PTA Left:-						
Transducer	WR	Intensity	Masking	Score	Aided	ISF440 List
Left	WR1	50		92		NU-6 LIST 1A
Right	WR1	70	40	92		NU-6 LIST 2A

Fig. 30.7 TM perforation. This 57-year-old man had a tube placed prior to treatment for nasopharyngeal cancer. He completed concurrent chemoradiotherapy. (**a**) Persistent dry perforation 2 years after completing cancer therapy. (**b**) Audiogram, showing minimal conductive loss from perforation

Additionally, while not commonly observed, cholesteatoma development can be associated with chronic tympanic membrane perforation [32].

Despite these risks, certain studies have shown that the insertion of ventilation tubes results in a higher rate of resolution of otitis media with effusion [33]. To contrast, Morton et al. found no difference in rates of persistent OME in irradiated patients who were observed versus who underwent tube insertion [34]. Therefore, a thorough discussion of risk versus benefit in relation to expected goals of therapy should be shared with each patient.

If correcting hearing loss is the main objective, then alternatives to tube insertion should be explored. An example is the use of a conventional hearing aid or an osseointegrated hearing aid [35]. Conventional in-the-ear hearing aid use in the irradiated patient may lead to canal irritation, breakdown, and increased incidence of otitis externa which can itself also become chronic resulting in chronic otorrhea [7]. Additionally, osseointegrated device placement may be associated with wound-healing issues and failure of osseointegration in the irradiated patient (Fig. 30.8) [36].

Surgical management of chronic otitis media with perforation in the postradiation setting has a lower success rate than in the nonirradiated population (Fig. 30.9). In the irradiated population, the success rates for tympanoplasty with or without mastoidectomy are around 50–60% compared to nonirradiated patients where these surgeries are 80–90% successful [37, 38]. Mastoid obliteration with canal closure can be considered, especially in cases associated with ORN [39]. In these cases, hearing is rehabilitated with an osseointegrated hearing aid.

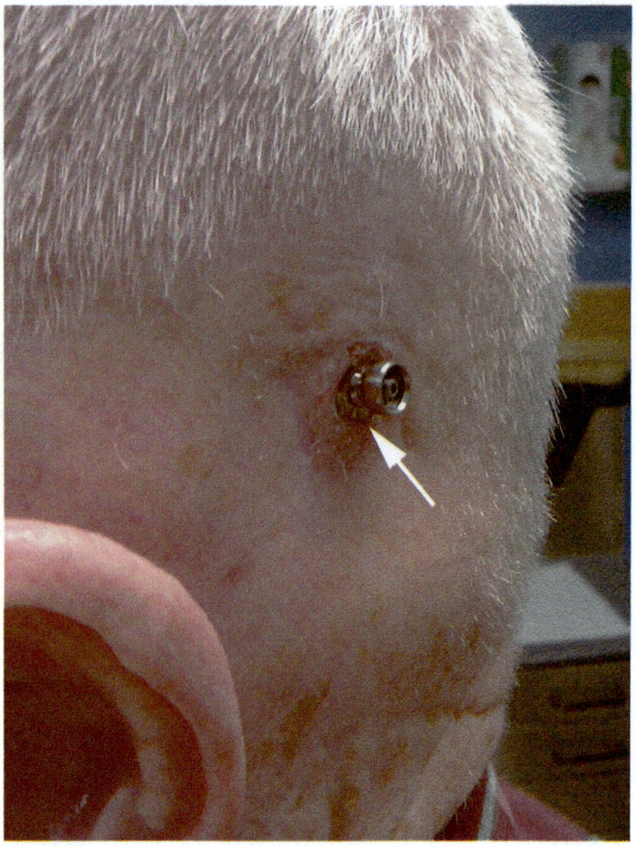

Fig. 30.8 Skin loss (arrow) around abutment of osseointegrated implant following radiation therapy

Hearing Loss

The overall reported incidence of hearing loss in patients with head and neck cancer varies widely, ranging from 24% to 67% of all patients [40]. The pattern of hearing loss is also variable. Acute hearing loss, like conductive loss from acute serous otitis media, typically improves. Chronic sensorineural hearing loss related to radiation therapy is typically a chronic complication, which may develop and progress months to years following treatment [20]. Hearing loss can be conductive or progressive sensorineural [41].

Conductive Hearing Loss (CHL)

Conductive hearing loss may occur as a result of damage to any component of the sound transmission pathway. Stenosis of the external auditory canal due to either soft tissue thickening or buildup of keratinous debris can cause a CHL, as can blunting of the anterior sulcus of the tympanic ring (Fig. 30.10). Thickening and effacement of the tympanic membrane can occur in isolation or in combination with other pathology, also leading to significant CHL (Fig. 30.11). TM perforations, depending on size and location, can result in CHL of varying degrees. They may occur in an iatrogenic fashion, following tube placement, or as a result of chronic otitis media. Middle ear effusion is another, more common cause of CHL seen in postradiated patients.

Sensorineural Hearing Loss (SNHL)

Damage to the cochlea leading to hearing loss has been well described. Radiation causes changes to the neuroepithelium of the cochlea, the supporting cells, and the stria vascularis, leading to direct damage to the structures involved in neural transmission of sound or to the structures contributing to the tenuous local homeostatic environment [42, 43]. Additionally, the inner and outer hair cells along with spiral ganglion cells have been shown to degenerate. These cellular changes are accompanied by progressive fibrosis within the organ of Corti and perilymph spaces, ultimately leading to partial obliteration within the inner ear [43].

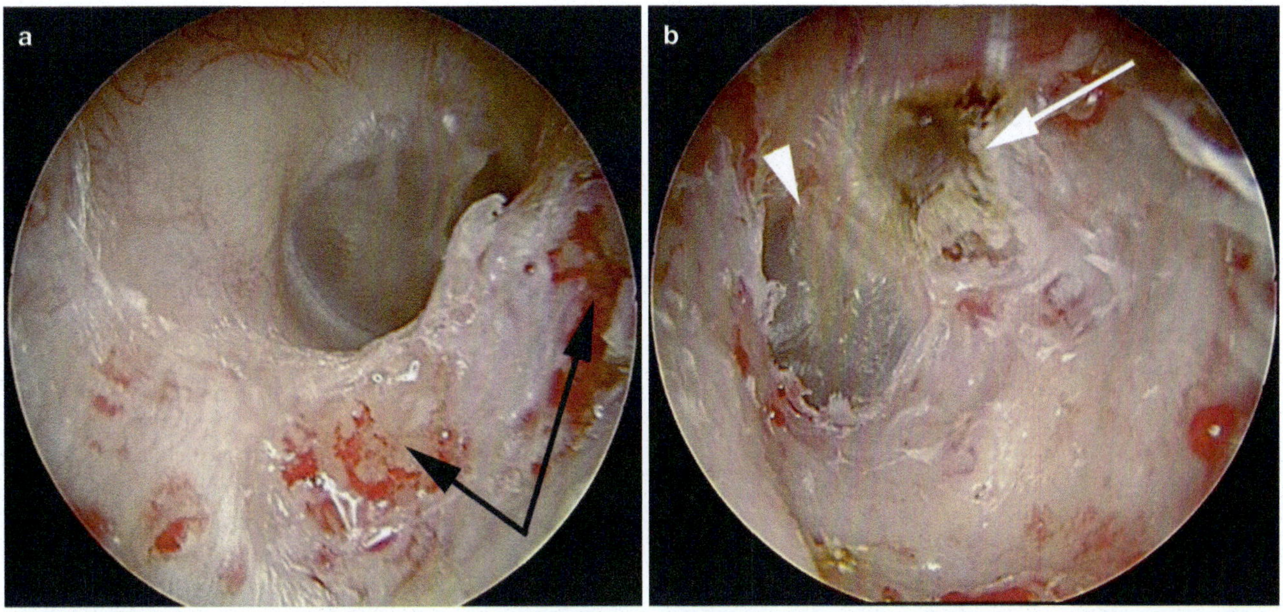

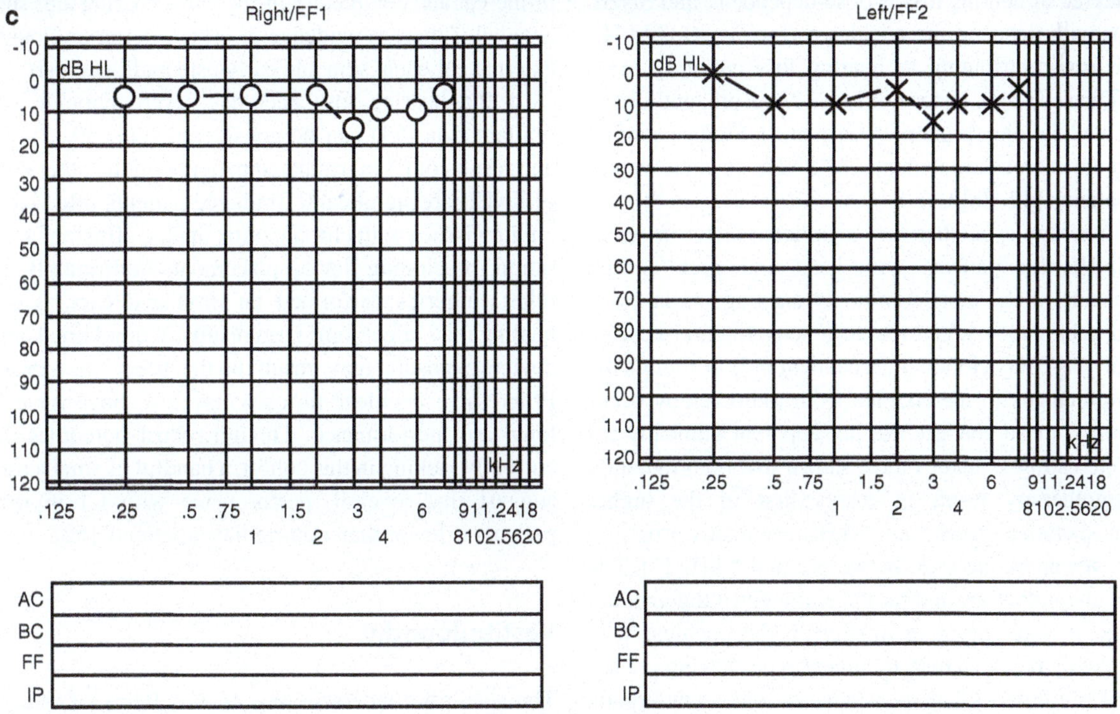

SRT PTA Right:- PTA Left:-					
Transducer	Test type	Intensity	Masking	Aided	ISF440 list
Left	HL	15			Spondee A
Right	HL	5			Spondee A

WR PTA Right:- PTA Left:-						
Transducer	WR	Intensity	Masking	Score	Aided	ISF440 List
Left	WR1	55		100		NU-6 LIST 1A
Right	WR1	55		100		NU-6 LIST 2A

Fig. 30.9 Cholesteatoma. A 38-year-old man who was treated for medulloblastoma 8 years earlier with surgery and radiation therapy. (**a**) Exposed bone in the right ear canal (black arrows). (**b**) Pars flaccida cholesteatoma (white arrow) in the left ear. Malleus is indicated by white arrowhead. (**c**) Audiogram shows normal hearing bilaterally. (**d**) Coronal CT showing disease in surrounding malleus (arrow)

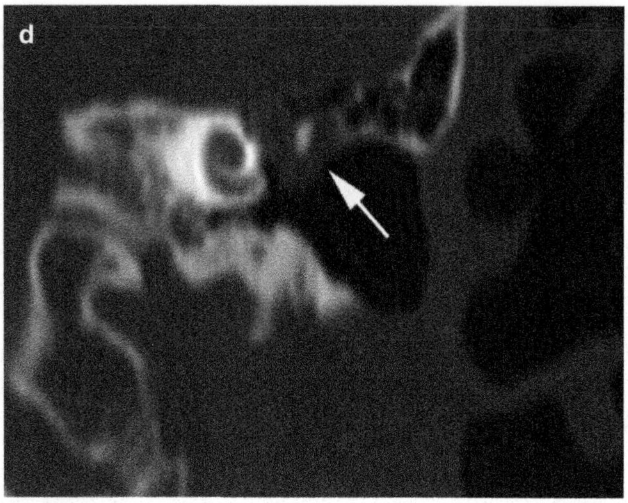

Fig. 30.9 (continued)

The degree of hearing loss is dose-dependent, and SNHL can occur with doses to the cochlea as low as 30 Gy [44]. Other factors contributing to hearing loss certainly exist, such as advanced age, history of noise exposure, and use of ototoxic medications (principally cisplatin). Studies conflict regarding an increased incidence of SNHL in male versus female patients [45, 46].

Chemotherapy is another very significant factor in developing SNHL for patients with head and neck cancer. Cisplatin, one of the most commonly used agents in many head and neck cancers, can result in sensorineural hearing loss as early as 3 days following treatment [47]. Although the histologic changes to the cochlea from radiotherapy occur within hours, these changes are not apparent clinically for weeks. Interestingly, studies have shown that both radiation and chemotherapy result in losses first in the higher frequencies, often between 6 and 8 kHz, eventually progressing to the lower frequencies, between 2 and 4 kHz [7]. The effects of chemotherapy and radiotherapy given together are synergistic in their negative impact on the cochlea, with patients having received both treatment types having greater degrees of hearing loss than their radiation-only counterparts [48]. In fact, the radiation dose required to produce a clinically significant SNHL when combined with chemotherapy may be as little as 10 Gy [47].

Limiting cochlear radiation dose by IMRT has been studied as a way to prevent radiation-induced SNHL. Since the total dose delivered to the cochlea is the most important factor in developing SNHL, limiting radiation dose to the cochlea is the primary way of preventing SNHL. For example, in nasopharyngeal carcinoma patients, a lower dose is delivered to the cochlea by IMRT, and the incidence of SNHL appears to be lower as compared to patients receiving conventional external beam therapy. These studies have shown that the total dose delivered to the cochlea is as low as 19–37 Gy in the IMRT-treated groups [49, 50]. In comparing the incidence of SNHL in the IMRT group versus conventional group, lower rates of SNHL were observed among the IMRT groups, though the differences did not reach statistical significance.

Steroid therapy has been studied as another measure to prevent the occurrence of SNHL following radiation therapy. Animal studies have shown the success of pre-chemotherapy steroid administration in preventing SNHL [51]. However, data on this topic is lacking in human studies, and prospective trials must be conducted to document clinical efficacy.

Management of radiation-associated SNHL is similar to the treatment of other etiologies of SNHL, with a couple of exceptions. First, patients should be followed with yearly audiograms for an extended duration, as the hearing loss can be progressive for many years. Secondly, patients may be treated with conventional hearing aids, though the use of these devices can be problematic in irradiated ears as irritation to fragile EACs may result in chronic otitis externa. Thus, in-the-ear and completely-in-the-canal hearing aids should be avoided if there is evidence of otitis externa or sloughing of external ear canal skin and early osteoradionecrosis.

If the hearing loss becomes severe enough, cochlear implantation (CI) can be considered (Fig. 30.12). The use and results of CI in irradiated patients versus other etiologies of SNHL are significant. Irradiated patients often have challenging issues with chronic otitis media, effusion, and perforation, precluding device placement. Additionally, as with other surgeries performed on irradiated ears, issues with healing may affect long-term results. Wound breakdown and device exposure may result in the need for explantation. Progressive cochlear fibrosis may also have an effect on long-term performance. Though robust outcomes data are currently lacking in this cohort, a handful of small case series suggest that, overall, performance with CI in irradiated patients is lower than nonirradiated patients [52].

Vestibulopathy

The scientific understanding of the effects of radiation on the vestibular apparatus is lacking compared to our understanding of its association with sensorineural hearing loss [7]. While radiation can presumably cause damage to the hair cells of the vestibule and semicircular canals, an understanding of dose effects and long-term sequelae does not exist. Postradiation vestibular effects are typically seen about 6 months following radiotherapy, with caloric weakness seen in up to 10% of patients [6]. Patients who have received unilateral vestibular radiation exposure will have symptoms of unilateral vestibular weakness: brief off-balance sensation for 1–2 s with quick turning or veering off a straight line while walking (Fig. 30.13). Patients with bilateral radiation exposure to the vestibule can develop symptoms of bilateral vestibular weakness such as oscillopsia.

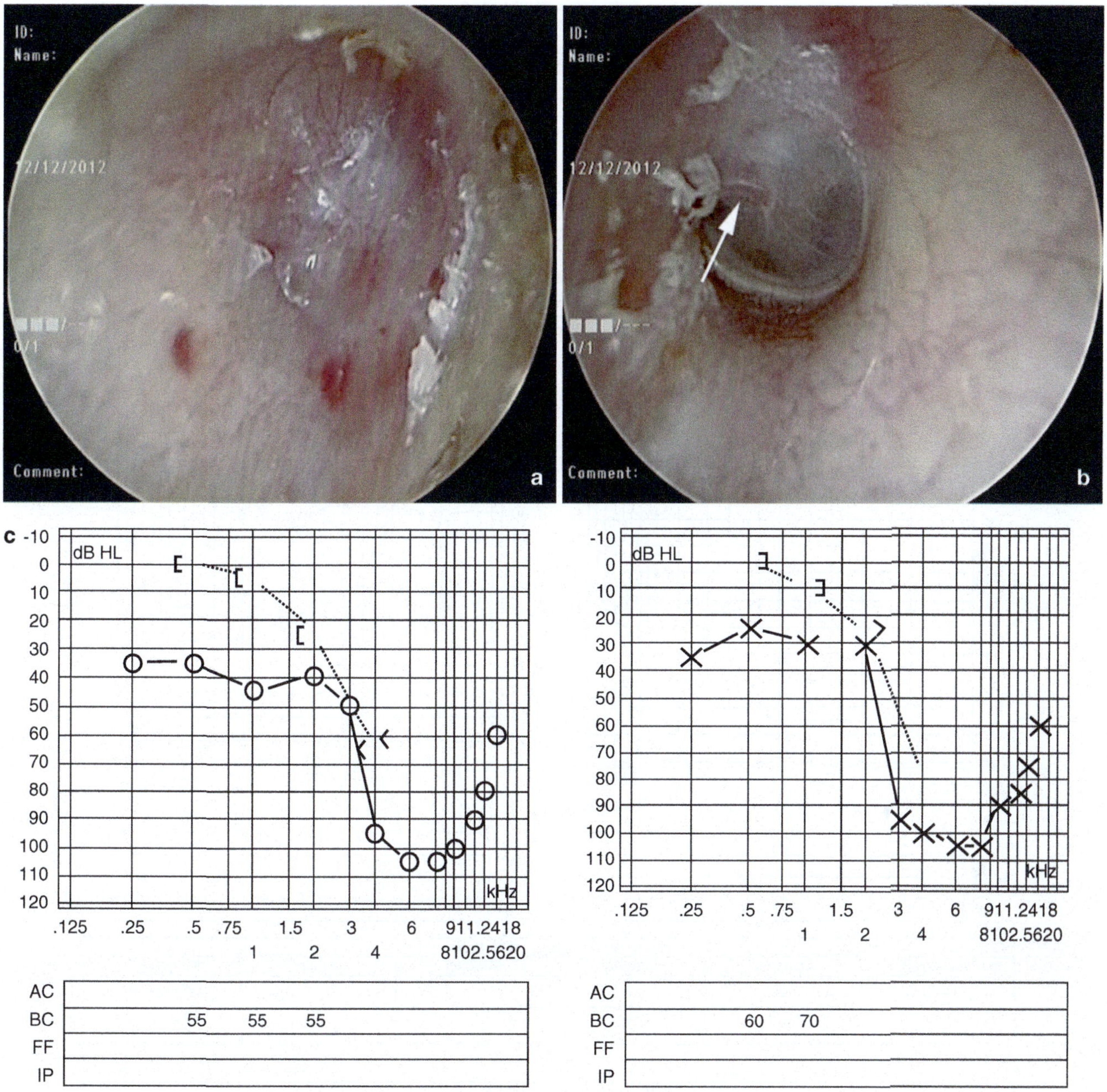

SRT PTA Right:- PTA Left:-					
Transducer	Test type	Intensity	Masking	Aided	ISF440 list
Right	HL	40			Spondee A
Left	HL	20			Spondee A

WR PTA Right:- PTA Left:-						
Transducer	WR	Intensity	Masking	Score	Aided	ISF440 List
Left	WR1	60		96		NU-6 LIST 1A
Right	WR1	80	50	100		NU-6 LIST 2A

Fig. 30.10 Ear canal blunting. A 57-year-old man with T4 oral cavity cancer, treated with surgery and postoperative radiotherapy (total dose 60 Gy). He developed progressive hearing loss due to canal blunting. (**a**) Right ear canal and TM showing complete effacement of the normal landmarks. (**b**) Left ear canal and TM showing scar band from anterior canal wall to TM (arrow). (**c**) Audiogram showing bilateral low-frequency conductive hearing loss

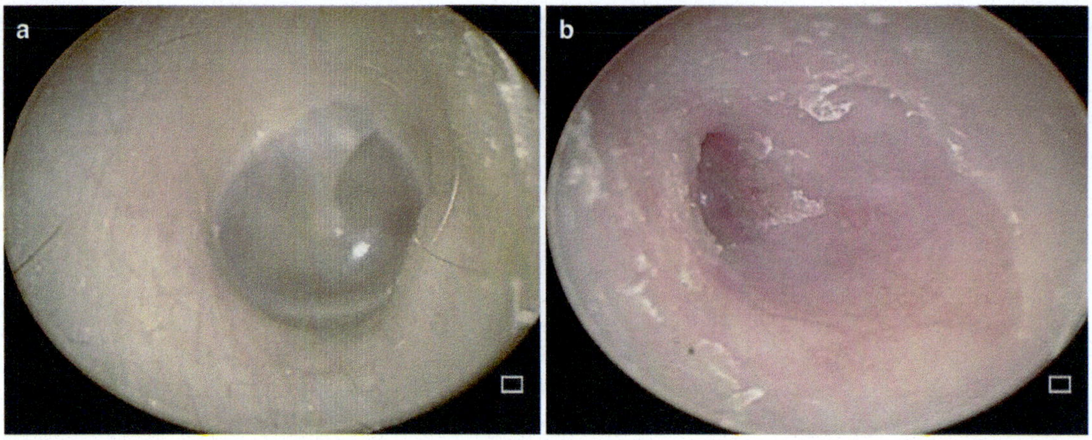

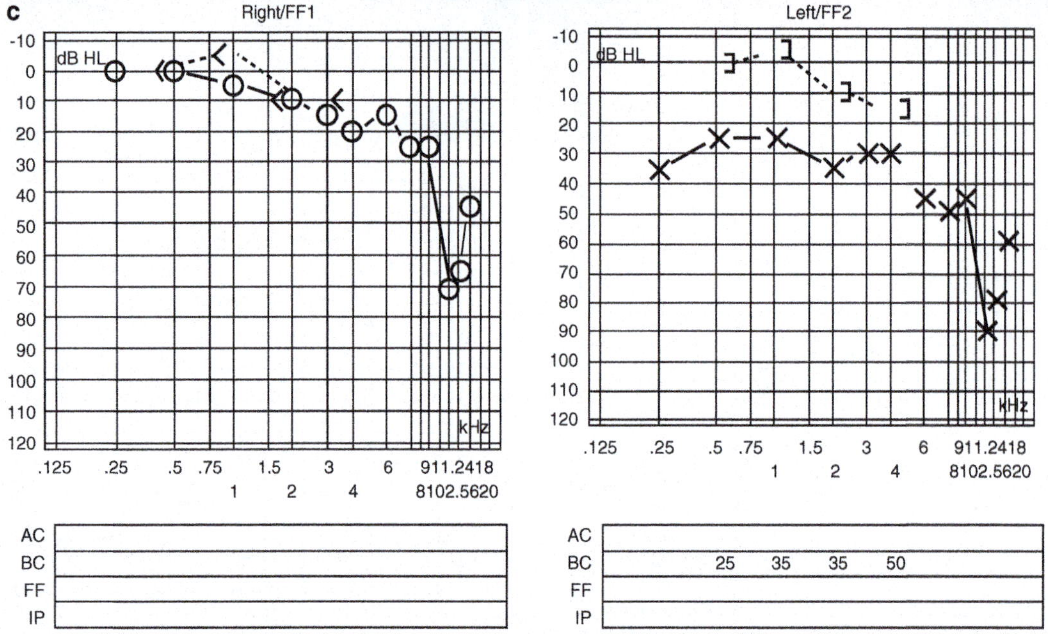

SRT PTA Right:- PTA Left:-					
Transducer	Test type	Intensity	Masking	Aided	ISF440 list
Right	HL	5			Spondee A
Left	HL	25			Spondee A

WR PTA Right:- PTA Left:-						
Transducer	WR	Intensity	Masking	Score	Aided	ISF440 List
Right	WR1	45		100		NU-6 LIST 1A
Left	WR1	65	35	100		NU-6 LIST 2A

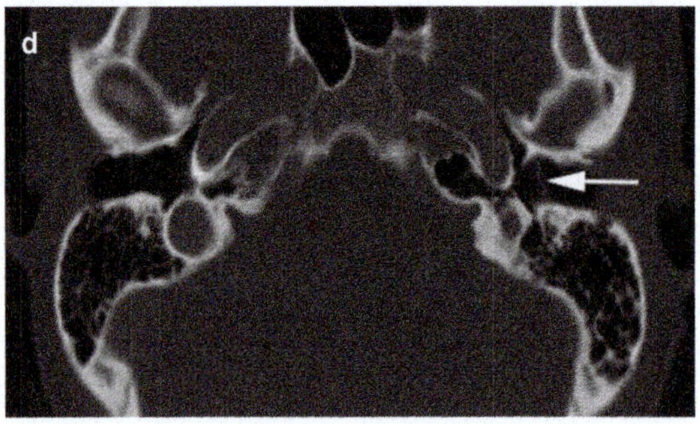

Fig. 30.11 Conductive hearing loss. This 44-year-old woman was treated with surgery and postoperative radiotherapy for left parotid cancer 3.5 years earlier. (**a**) Normal right TM. (**b**) Left ear canal and TM showing complete effacement. (**c**) Audiogram showing left-sided mild conductive hearing loss. (**d**) CT showing thickened TM (arrow) and aerated middle ear and mastoid

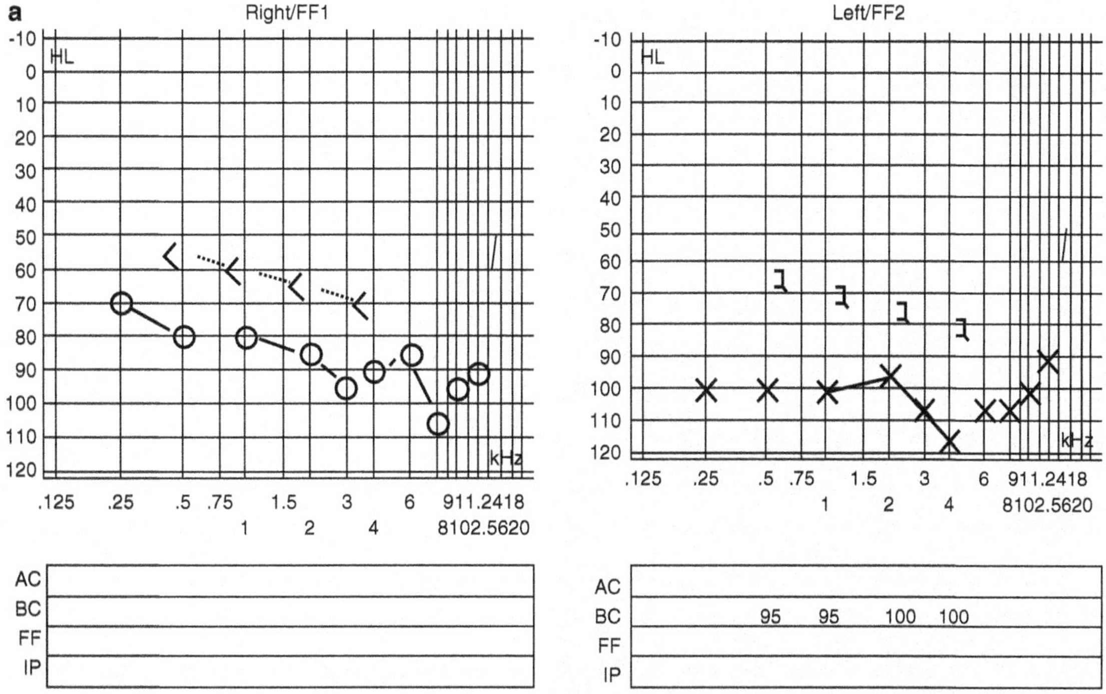

SRT				
Transducer	Test type	Intensity	Masking	Aided
Right	HL	75		
Left	HL	90		

Transducer	WR	Intensity	Masking	Score	Aided
	WR1	90		56	

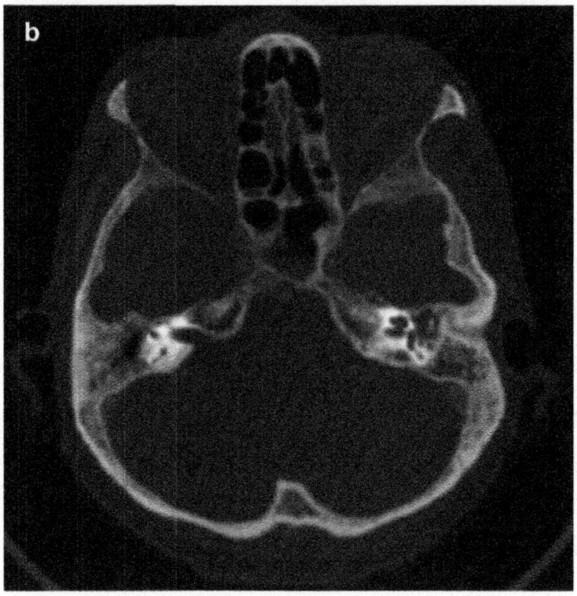

Fig. 30.12 Cochlear implantation. A 67-year-old woman with a history of nasopharyngeal carcinoma treated with concurrent chemoradiotherapy 8 years earlier. She developed chronic otitis media bilaterally. The right ear was chronically draining. The left ear was implanted. (**a**) Preimplantation audiogram. (**b**) Preimplantation CT scan. Intraoperative findings included serous fluid, thick fibrous tissue and granulation tissue filling air spaces and middle ear, and a dehiscent facial nerve. Complete electrode insertion. Postoperative HINT sentences were 68% and CUNY sentences 52% 4 months following her implantation

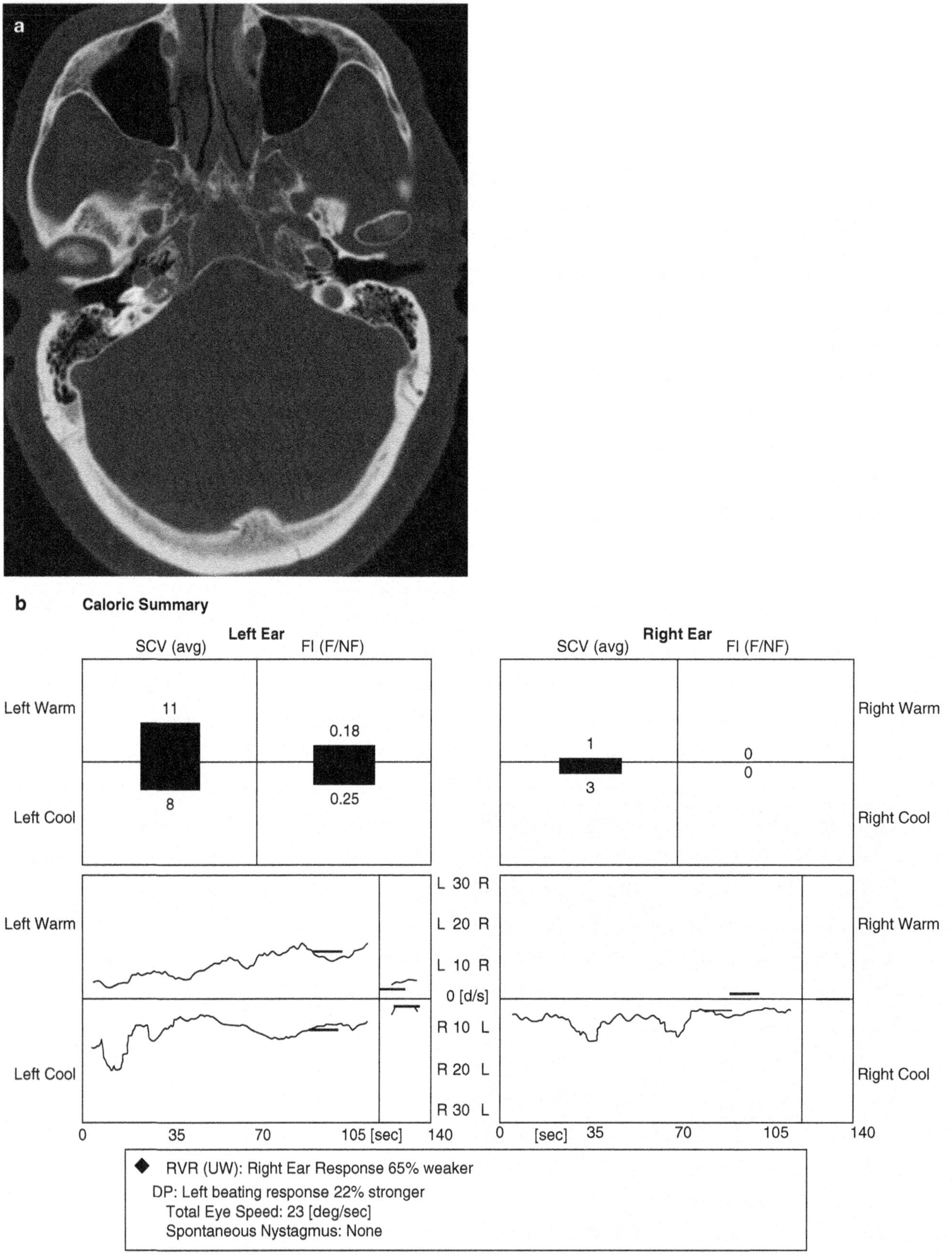

Fig. 30.13 Vestibular weakness. A 77-year-old man with a history of metastatic squamous cell cancer of the skin status post a right parotidectomy and neck dissection followed by postoperative radiotherapy (60 Gy). He began to have balance problems about 6 months after completing his radiotherapy. It has been a slow and gradual in onset. He denies any dizziness or vertigo. (**a**) CT shows aerated mastoids and middle ears. (**b**) Videonystagmography shows 65% caloric weakness; central and positional tests were normal

Some of these patients will eventually need a cane or walker for ambulation.

Late Complications of Radiotherapy

Osteoradionecrosis

Radiation-induced necrosis of the temporal bone is an important topic as the disease presentation may occur many years after treatment, degree of involvement is highly variable, and the range of possible morbidity is great. As mentioned previously, the thin overlying skin of the temporal bone may present a risk to the underlying bone following delivery of radiotherapy. If skin breakdown occurs, bone necrosis is more likely to occur [53]. The clinical manifestations of this problem are highly variable, depending on the location and amount of bone exposed. If directly visible and of small area, localized debridement is possible [54]. However, if widespread temporal bone involvement occurs, particularly in deeper areas, extensive resection may be required to prevent widespread osteomyelitis and the possible associated complications of meningitis, neck or brain abscess, carotid artery erosion, or fistula formation [55].

Localized temporal bone osteoradionecrosis occurs when small areas of bone are exposed, often resulting in pain localized to the area of exposed bone, as well as otorrhea [54]. This localized disease is often effectively managed with aggressive and frequent debridement performed in the office in conjunction with topical and/or systemic antibiotic administration (Fig. 30.14).

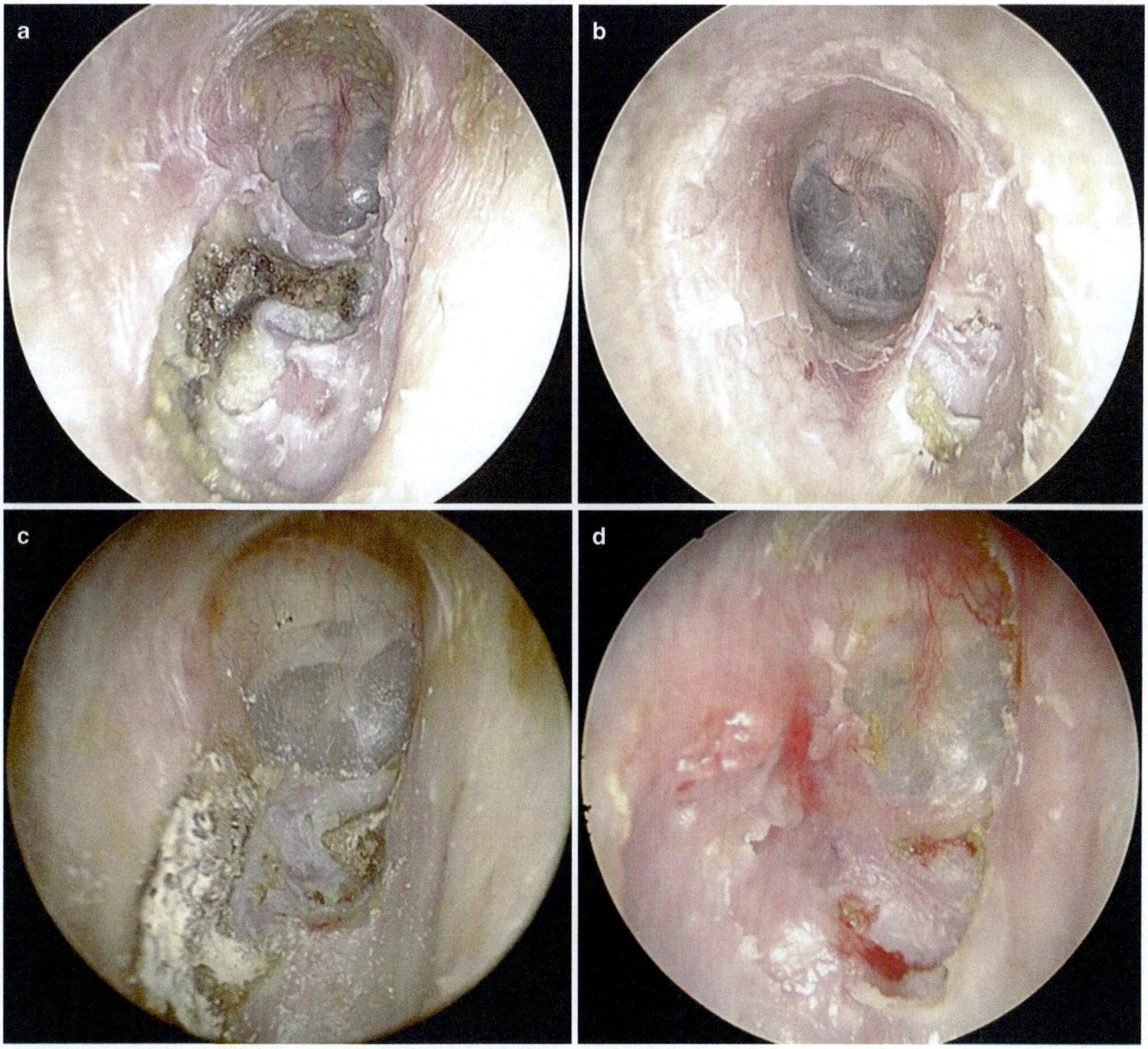

Fig. 30.14 Localized osteoradionecrosis (ORN) . A 50-year-old woman with a history of metastatic breast cancer first diagnosed in April 1988. She developed a metastatic lesion in the cerebellum in August 1998, which was resected and treated with postoperative radiotherapy. (**a**) Right ear canal (February 2013). (**b**) Left ear canal (February 2013). (**c**) Right ear canal 1 week later, following debridement of dead bone (sequestrectomy). (**d**) Right ear canal 6 months later, showing healing and epithelium covering bone

More diffuse temporal bone osteoradionecrosis is a much more serious and challenging problem for the clinician to manage (Fig. 30.15). As opposed to localized bone exposure, the hallmark of diffuse disease is involvement of the mastoid, with coalescence and breakdown of bony septae [56]. Diffuse disease results in widespread exposed bone within the middle ear and mastoid bone. This can result in increased inflammatory reaction, mucous production, and often secondary infection. The local flora of the middle ear, or the adjacent Eustachian tube, may uncontrollably proliferate resulting in more serious conditions such as widespread osteomyelitis, abscess formation, fistula formation (Fig. 30.16), meningitis, subdural abscess, and encephalitis [54]. The likelihood of developing this problem is increased in the head and neck cancer patient population who may be immunocompromised from a long-term malnourished state [57].

Once widespread disease occurs, management becomes more difficult and requires a more aggressive approach. Long-term IV antibiotic treatment is an option for moderate degrees of infection. However, more severe, diffuse disease involving most or all of the temporal bone will require surgical debridement. Surgery entails radical mastoidectomy or lateral temporal bone resection with obliteration of the mastoid with either a temporalis flap or microvascular free flap (Fig. 30.17) [58].

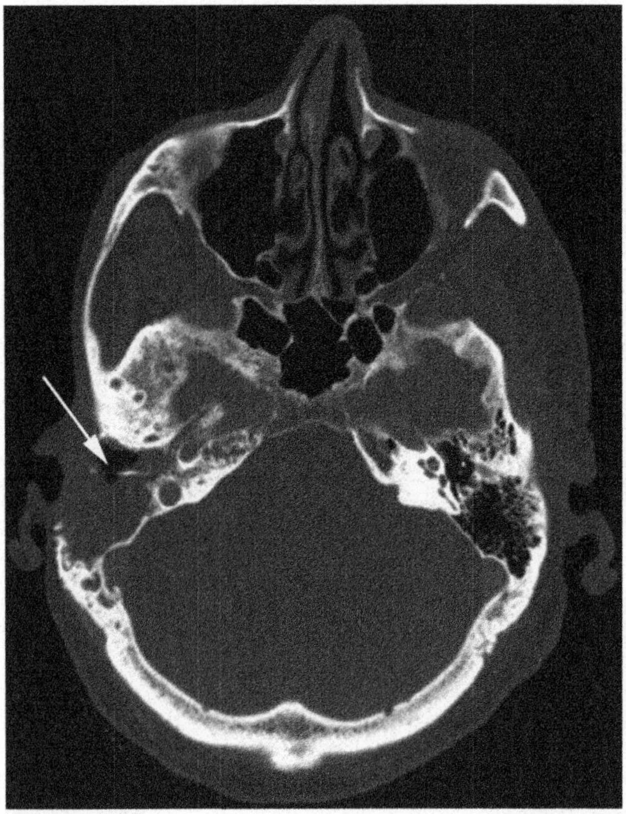

Fig. 30.15 Diffuse ORN. Axial CT showing canal-mastoid fistula (arrow) and opacification of mastoid and middle ear, 10 years after radiation for parotid malignancy

Temporal Lobe Radionecrosis

On rare occasion, necrosis of the temporal lobe of the brain can develop [59]. This is most common for diseases which require treatment of that area or adjacent to it, such as primary tumors of the deep lobe of the parotid or nasopharynx. This complication may range in severity, from asymptomatic to frankly devastating. In the most severe (and rare) cases, it may require temporal lobectomy (Fig. 30.17).

Abscess Formation

Another highly unusual but potential complication of radiation is abscess formation. This can occur in the infratemporal fossa (Fig. 30.18) or in the neck (Bezold's abscess) (Fig. 30.19). Their presentation is variable, depending on the location and involvement of adjacent structures. In our experience, surgical management and concurrent long-term IV antibiotic therapy are the mainstays of treatment for this rare complication.

Carotid Artery Rupture

One of the most severe, and dreaded, potential complications of radiation therapy to the head and neck is carotid artery rupture (or "carotid blowout"). This is extremely rare for patients that receive a single definitive course of radiation therapy to the head and neck, since the doses received are within tolerance of the carotid artery. However, this is more common in patients who receive a second course of radiation (re-irradiation) of the same area for recurrence or a second primary cancer. In these cases, patients should be counseled that repeat radiation has a heightened level of side effects, some of which may be fatal; only when the benefits outweigh the risks (and the patient understands the risks) should this be performed. Carotid artery rupture, even in this setting, is relatively rare [60]. Patients may present with sentinel bloody otorrhea followed by hemorrhage from the ear canal (Fig. 30.20). Surgery is generally not employed in these cases, with management deferred to interventional vascular specialists. If not recognized and managed appropriately, this event can be fatal.

Radiation-Associated Malignancy

The development of a secondary malignancy following radiation to the temporal bone is a rare but devastating complication [61]. Radiation-induced malignancies have been well described, and classification schemes have been

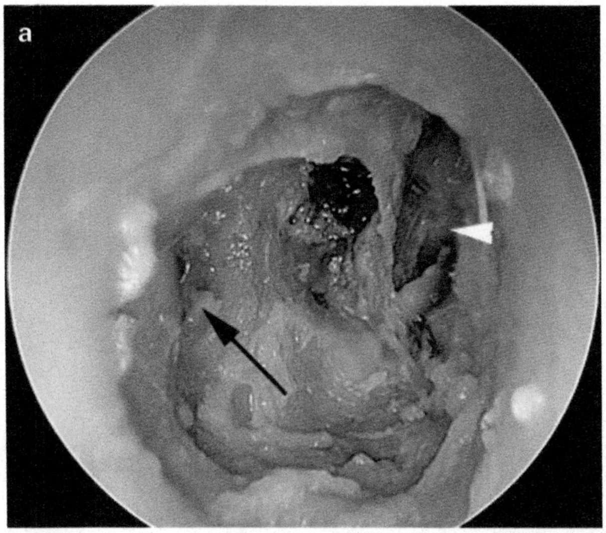

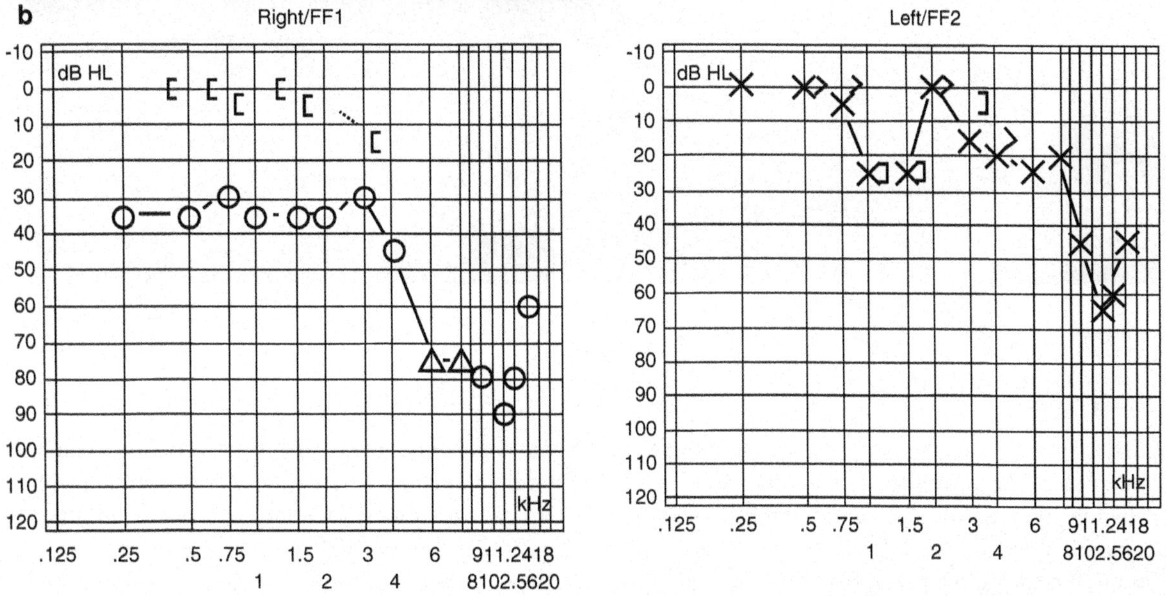

Right	
AC	40 40
BC	30 35 75 55 30 50
FF	
IP	

Left	
AC	
BC	75 75 65
FF	
IP	

SRT PTA Right:- PTA Left:-

Transducer	Test type	Intensity	Masking	Aided	ISF440 list
Left	HL	10			N/A
Right	HL	30			N/A

WR PTA Right:- PTA Left:-

Transducer	WR	Intensity	Masking	Score	Aided	ISF440 List
Right	WR1	70	70	100		N/A
Left	WR1	50	50	100		N/A

Fig. 30.16 Localized ORN progressing to diffuse ORN. (**a**) Oto-endoscopic photo showing canal-mastoid fistula (arrow) and TM (white arrowhead). (**b**) Audiogram, showing right-sided mixed hearing loss. (**c**) CT scan showing localized disease (arrow) two years earlier. (**d**) CT scan at the time of otoendoscopic photos later showing diffuse ORN (arrowheads). This patient was treated with mastoid obliteration using a temporalis muscle flap and an osseointegrated implant for cochlear stimulation

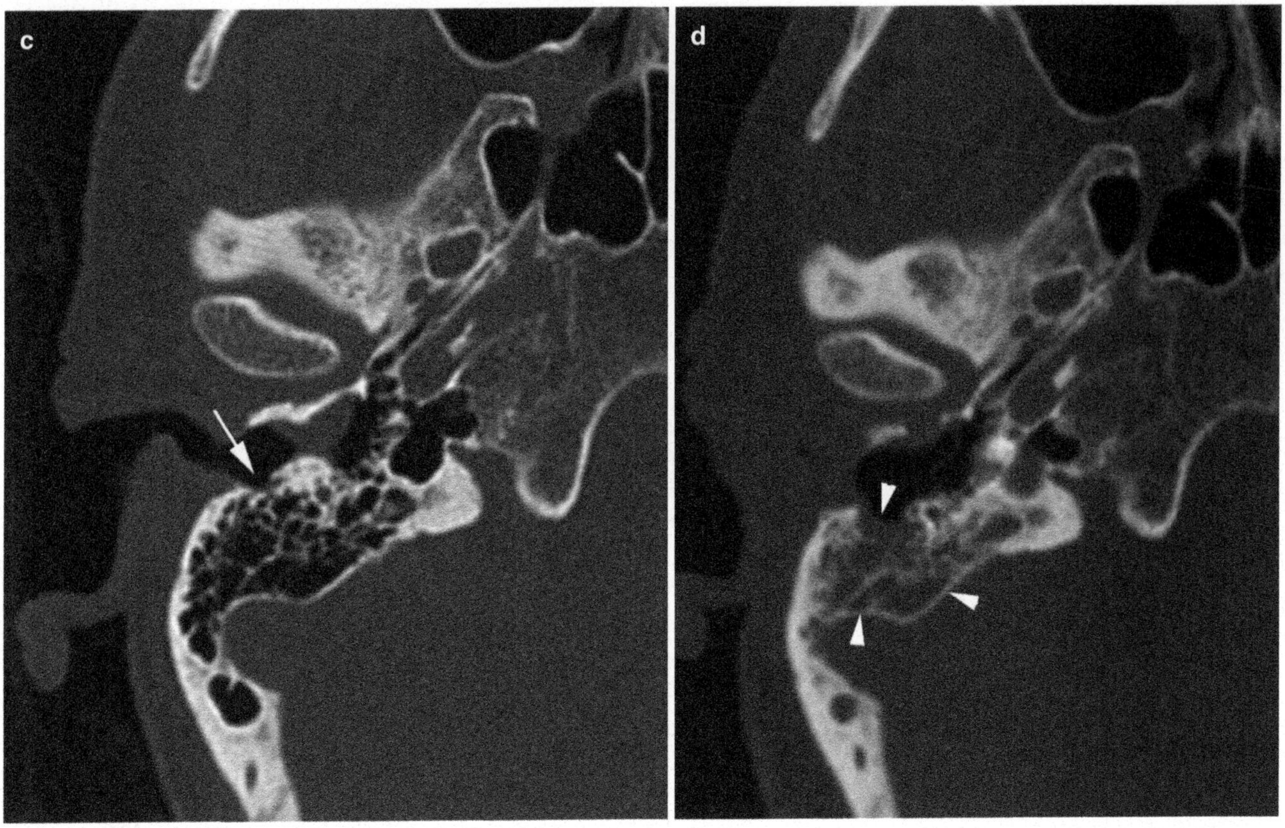

established to differentiate them from other pathologies or tumor recurrence. An example is the modified Cahan's criteria, which state that the following conditions be met before a tumor may be considered "radiation induced": (1) the tumor must have not been present before radiation, (2) the tumor must arise within the previously irradiated field, (3) there must be a reasonable interval between radiotherapy and the detection of the second tumor (usually more than 5 years), and (4) a histologic difference must exist between the primary and secondary lesions [62]. Though not fully elucidated, radiation-induced tumors likely develop due to damage to tumor suppressor genes [63]. Statistics regarding distribution of radiation-induced tumor histology in this cohort are lacking, but a survey of existing literature would suggest that squamous cell carcinoma in the temporal bone is more common than sarcoma [61, 64].

Radiation-induced malignancy of the temporal bone presents in a way similar to primary malignancy of the temporal bone, depending on the site of the temporal bone involved. Cancer within the external ear canal may present with bloody otorrhea, ear fullness, hearing loss, pain, and mass growth (Fig. 30.21). Tumors within the middle ear may present similarly but may also present with chronic otitis media, hearing loss, or even facial weakness (Fig. 30.22). If advanced, these tumors may erode into the inner ear, resulting in a more significant hearing loss and vestibulopathy. Tumors in the petrous apex or internal auditory canal may present with multiple cranial neuropathies.

As discussed previously, the other more commonly seen complications of radiation to the temporal bone present with symptoms overlapping those of radiation-induced malignancy. The clinician must remain aware of the possibility of malignancy and proceed with biopsy for suspicious lesions, if accessible. Other diagnostic considerations in this situation are benign growths, chronic otitis media, osteoradionecrosis, osteomyelitis, primary tumor recurrence (if the primary was in fact in the temporal bone), and possibly metastasis [7].

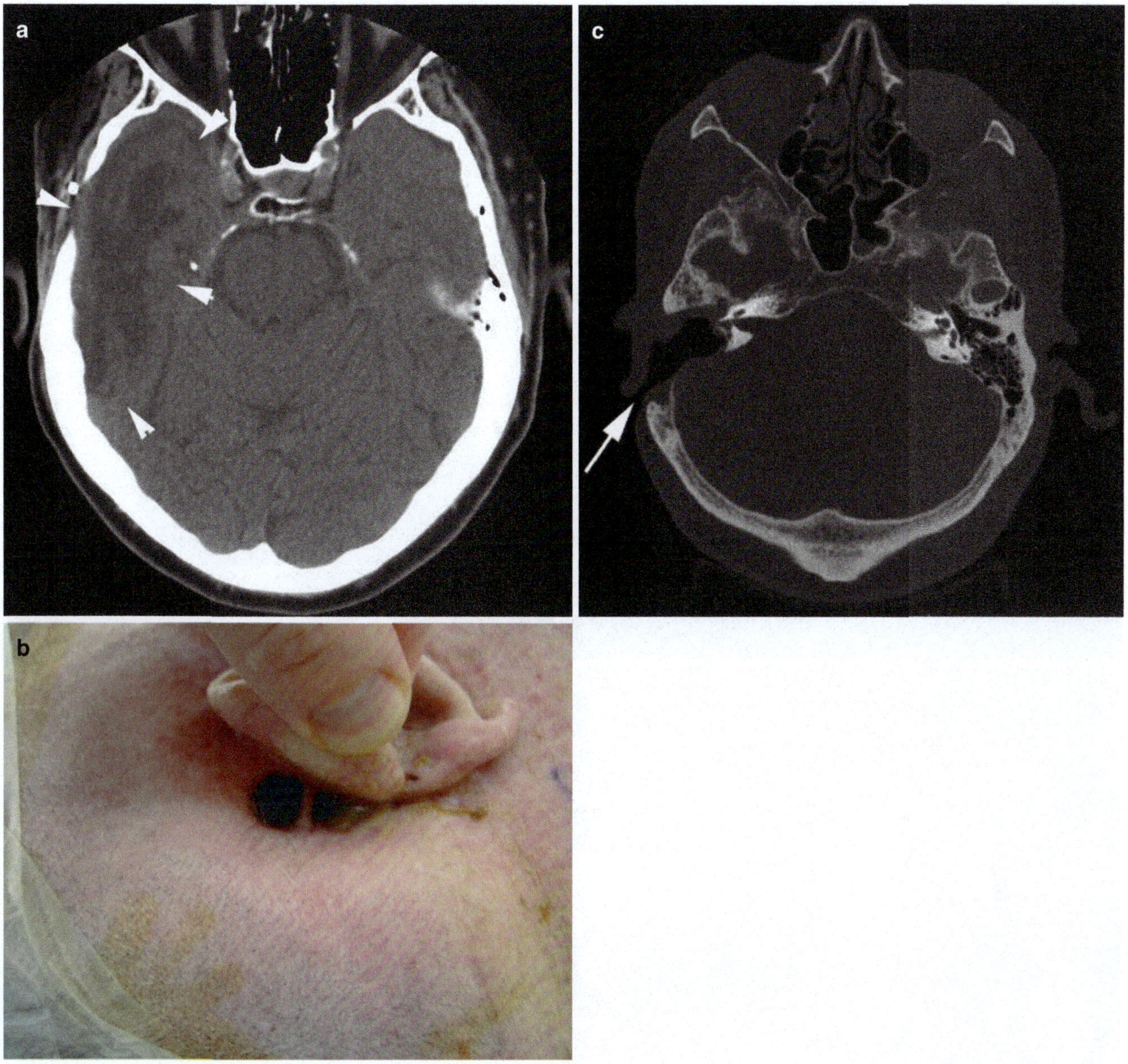

Fig. 30.17 Temporal lobe necrosis. A 72-year-old man with salivary duct carcinoma of right parotid, diagnosed in October 24, 2001 and treated with parotidectomy and postoperative radiotherapy. In February 2005, he had craniotomy for brain radionecrosis of the right temporal, parietal, and frontal regions. (**a**) CT showing temporal lobe necrosis (arrowheads). Shortly after this, he developed drainage from his right ear. He was treated with long-term IV Abx followed by HBO. In August 2005, he underwent a right tympanomastoidectomy for persistent drainage. In 2009, he underwent a lateral temporal bone resection, but his postauricular wound broke down. (**b**) In 2010, he presented to us with cutaneous mastoid fistula. (**c**) CT showing cutaneous mastoid fistula (arrow)

The time range for developing a radiation-induced tumor is wide, with latencies as long as 30 years having been described [7]. Physicians must bear in mind that a past history of radiation exposure to the temporal bone raises the risk of radiation-associated malignancy. Treatment of radiation-induced tumors of the temporal bone follows the principles used to treat those tumors as a primary entity. Resection remains the mainstay of treatment in the vast majority of cases, with some requiring adjuvant therapy afterward.

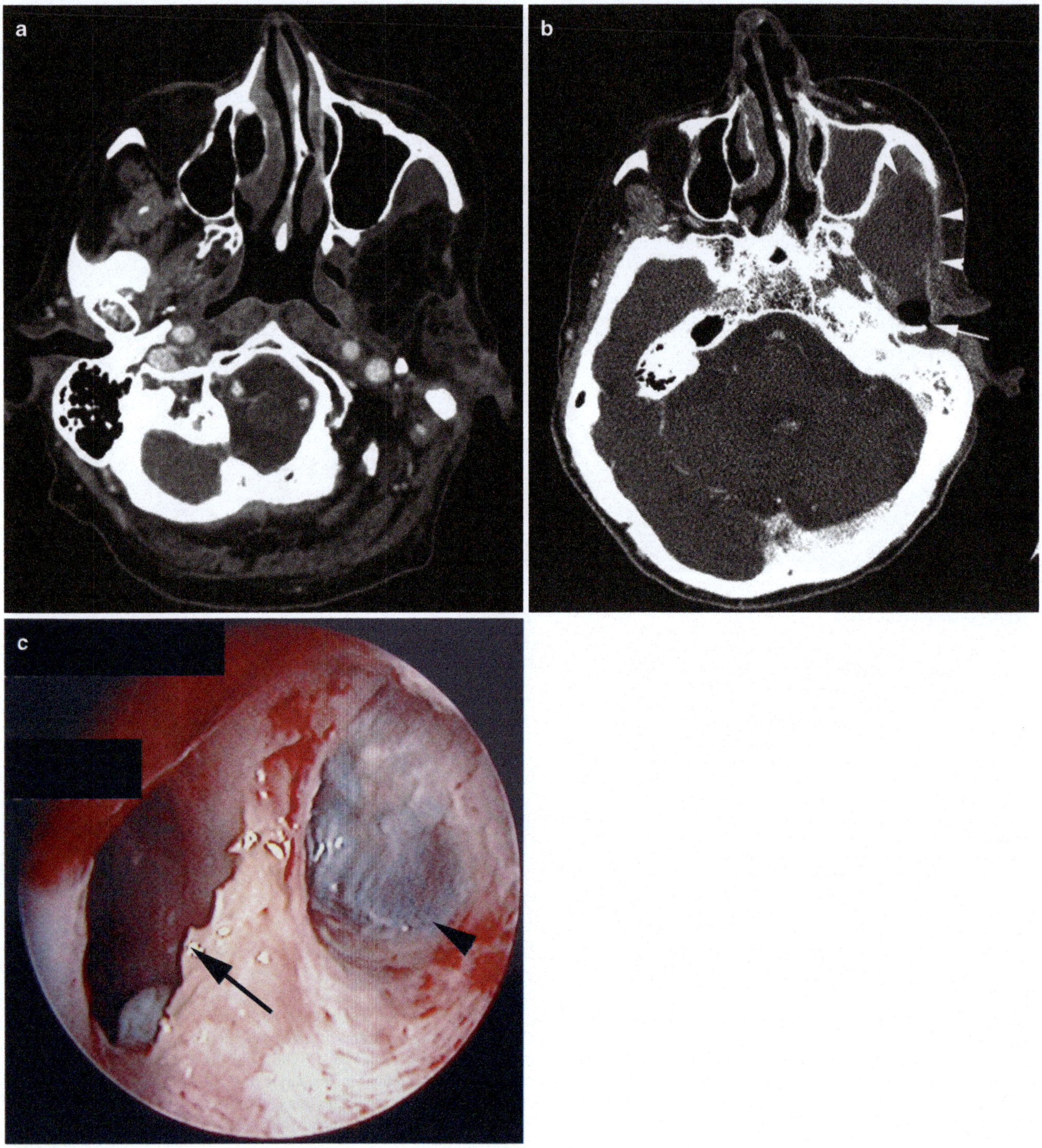

Fig. 30.18 Infratemporal fossa abscess. A 92-year-old woman with a history of left retromolar trigone cancer T4 N2b, treated with induction chemotherapy followed by hemimandibulectomy, infratemporal fossa dissection, neck dissection, and free flap reconstruction in March 2008. PORT completed in June 2008. (**a**) Posttreatment CT. Three years later she developed chronic ear drainage. (**b**) CT showing left infratemporal fossa abscess (arrowheads). A canal fistula is marked with an arrow. (**c**) Otoendoscopic view of the ear canal, showing breakdown of the anterior ear canal (arrow). Arrowhead marks the TM. She was treated with oral antibiotics for 2 weeks and then managed with vinegar and water irrigations

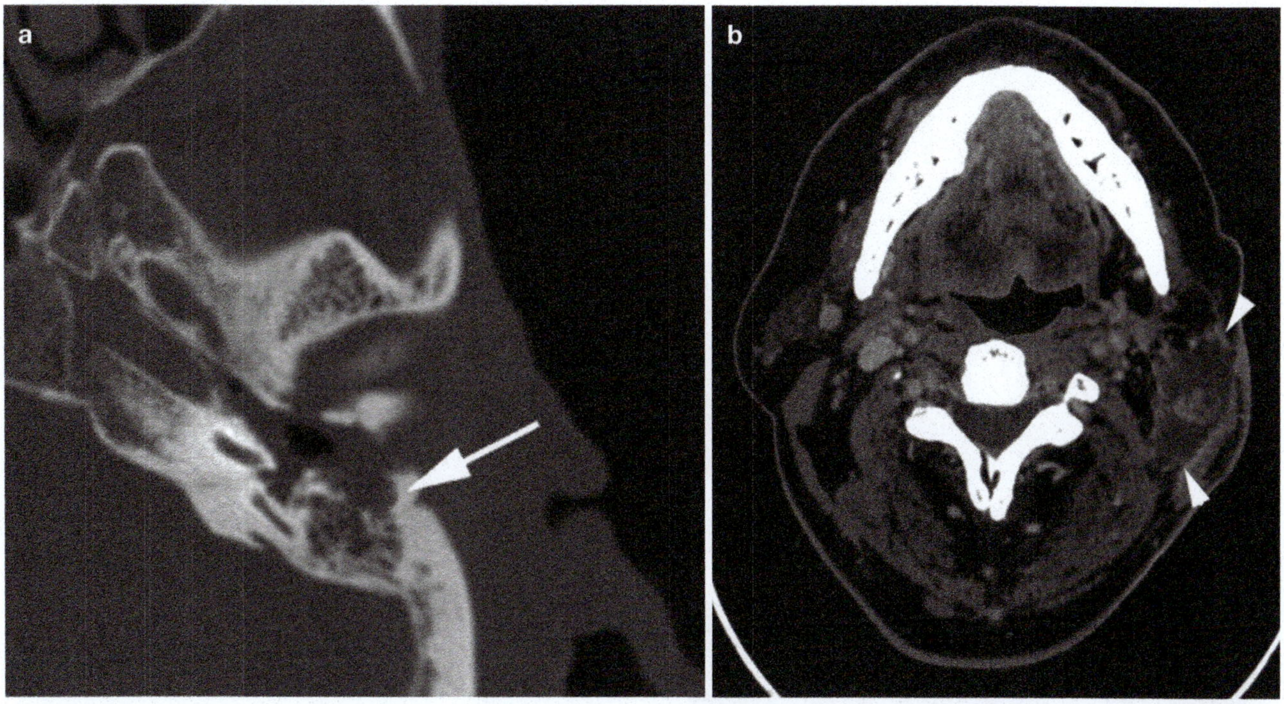

Fig. 30.19 Bezold's abscess complicating osteoradionecrosis of the left temporal bone. (**a**) CT temporal bone showing breakdown of the ear canal (arrow) and mastoid opacification. (**b**) CT neck showing abscess (arrowheads). This patient was treated with drainage of the abscess, lateral temporal bone resection, free flap reconstruction, and IV antibiotics. His wound cultures showed a polymicrobial infection

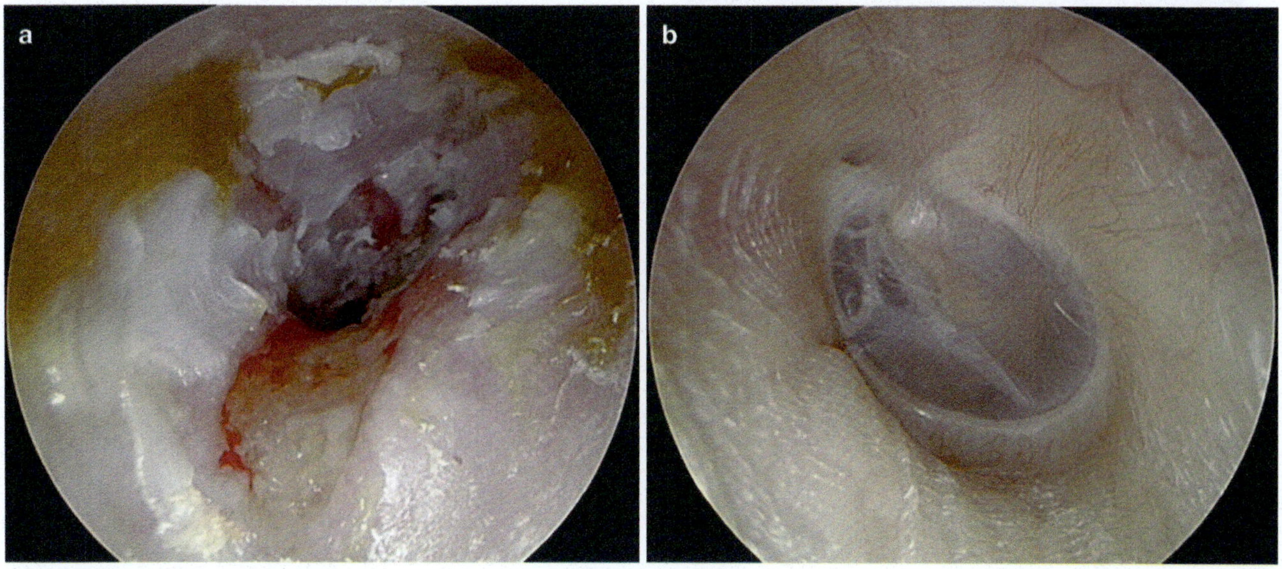

Fig. 30.20 Carotid artery rupture. A 57-year-old man with a history of nasopharyngeal cancer, treated with concurrent chemoradiotherapy (cisplatin 100 mg/M2, IMRT 70 Gy). Four years later, he presented with intermittent bleeding from his right ear. Oto-endoscopic photos of the (**a**) right ear and (**b**) left ear. One week later he presented with significant bleeding from the right ear and was referred for angiography where an impending carotid artery rupture was found. The artery was coiled, and the patient experienced no neurologic complication

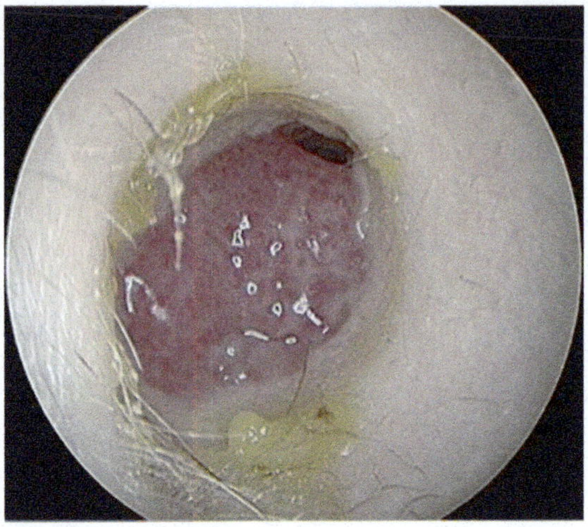

Fig. 30.21 Radiation-induced squamous cell carcinoma of the right ear canal

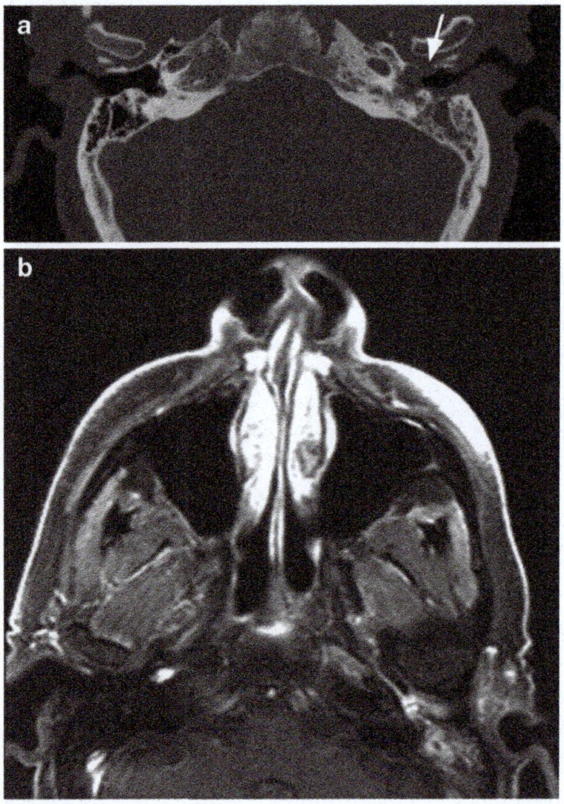

Fig. 30.22 Radiation-associated SCC of the left middle ear and mastoid presenting with left facial weakness. A 60-year-old man with history of T4 N2c left nasopharyngeal cancer treated 13 years prior with chemoradiation therapy. For about 6 months, he has had intense, deep pain in his left ear (8/10 severity); and recently he developed some very mild weakness of the left face. (**a**) CT showing opacified middle ear and mastoid, arrow points to erosion in the anterior ear canal. (**b**) Contrast-enhanced MRI showing enhancement in the middle ear and mastoid. He was treated with preoperative chemotherapy (carboplatin and paclitaxel), subtotal temporal bone resection and free flap reconstruction, and postoperative re-irradiation with weekly cisplatin. He remains free of disease 10 years later

Surveillance

As discussed throughout this chapter, the effects of radiation are lifelong, and radiation-associated complications can occur years following the completion of treatment. It is incumbent on treating physicians to be aware of these complications, to treat them appropriately, and to make prompt referral when these complications do not respond to treatment.

Conclusions

Radiotherapy is a commonly used and highly effective treatment in patients with head and neck cancer. Advances in the delivery of radiation, including use of IMRT, decrease the incidence of radiation-induced complications of the temporal bone. The most important factor in the development of these complications appears to be the dose of radiation delivered. Though management of these complications can be challenging, treatment options exist in all categories, with prognosis generally being favorable.

References

1. Popovtzer A, Eisbruch A. Radiotherapy for head and neck cancer. In: Flint PW, Haughey BH, Lund VJ, Niparko JK, Robbins KT, Thomas JR, et al., editors. Cummings otolaryngology, head and neck surgery. 2. 6th ed. Philadelphia: Elsevier; 2015. p. 1088–109.
2. Schuknecht HF, Karmody CS. Radionecrosis of the temporal bone. Laryngoscope. 1966;76(8):1416–28.
3. Lustig LR, Jackler RK, Lanser MJ. Radiation-induced tumors of the temporal bone. Am J Otol. 1997;18(2):230–5.
4. Ondrey FG, Greig JR, Herscher L. Radiation dose to otologic structures during head and neck cancer radiation therapy. Laryngoscope. 2000;110(2 Pt 1):217–21.
5. Leonetti JP, Marzo SJ, Zender CA, Porter RG, Melian E. Temporal bone osteoradionecrosis after surgery and radiotherapy for malignant parotid tumors. Otol Neurotol. 2010;31(4):656–9.
6. Johannesen TB, Rasmussen K, Winther FØ, Halvorsen U, Lote K. Late radiation effects on hearing, vestibular function, and taste in brain tumor patients. Int J Radiat Oncol Biol Phys. 2002;53(1):86–90.
7. Lambert EM, Gunn GB, Gidley PW. Effects of radiation on the temporal bone in patients with head and neck cancer. Head Neck. 2016;38(9):1428–35.
8. Jereczek-Fossa BA, Rondi E, Zarowski A, D'Onofrio A, Alterio D, Ciocca M, et al. Prospective study on the dose distribution to the acoustic structures during postoperative 3D conformal radiotherapy for parotid tumors: dosimetric and audiometric aspects. Strahlenther Onkol. 2011;187(6):350–6.
9. Guadagnolo BA, Liu CC, Cormier JN, Du XL. Evaluation of trends in the use of intensity-modulated radiotherapy for head and neck cancer from 2000 through 2005. Cancer. 2010;116(14):3505–12.
10. Miah AB, Gulliford SL, Clark CH, Bhide SA, Zaidi SH, Newbold KL, et al. Dose–response analysis of parotid gland function: what is the best measure of xerostomia? Radiother Oncol. 2013;106(3):341–5.
11. Beadle BM, Liao KP, Elting LS, Buchholz TA, Ang KK, Garden AS, et al. Improved survival using intensity-modulated radiation

therapy in head and neck cancers: a SEER-Medicare analysis. Cancer. 2014;120(5):702–10.

12. Beetz I, Steenbakkers RJ, Chouvalova O, Leemans CR, Doornaert P, van der Laan BF, et al. The QUANTEC criteria for parotid gland dose and their efficacy to prevent moderate to severe patient-rated xerostomia. Acta Oncol. 2014;53(5):597–604.
13. The National Association for Proton Therapy. Patient resources [cited 2016, 12/1/2016]. Available from: http://www.proton-therapy.org/patient_resources.htm.
14. Pasha R, Golub JS. Otolaryngology-head and neck surgery: clinical reference guide. San Diego, CA: Plural Publishing; 2013.
15. Trotti A. Toxicity in head and neck cancer: a review of trends and issues. Int J Radiat Oncol Biol Phys. 2000;47(1):1–12.
16. Black JO. Xeroderma pigmentosum. Head Neck Pathol. 2016;10(2):139–44.
17. Porock D, Nikoletti S, Cameron F. The relationship between factors that impair wound healing and the severity of acute radiation skin and mucosal toxicities in head and neck cancer. Cancer Nurs. 2004;27(1):71–8.
18. Zenda S, Ota Y, Tachibana H, Ogawa H, Ishii S, Hashiguchi C, et al. A prospective picture collection study for a grading atlas of radiation dermatitis for clinical trials in head-and-neck cancer patients. J Radiat Res. 2016;57(3):301–6.
19. Elwany S. Delayed ultrastructural radiation induced changes in the human mesotympanic middle ear mucosa. J Laryngol Otol. 1985;99(4):343–53.
20. Carlson ML, Jacob JT, Pollock BE, Neff BA, Tombers NM, Driscoll CL, et al. Long-term hearing outcomes following stereotactic radiosurgery for vestibular schwannoma: patterns of hearing loss and variables influencing audiometric decline. J Neurosurg. 2013;118(3):579–87.
21. Williams H, Davies A. The effect of X-rays on bone: a pictorial review. Eur Radiol. 2006;16(3):619–33.
22. Cao X, Wu X, Frassica D, Yu B, Pang L, Xian L, et al. Irradiation induces bone injury by damaging bone marrow microenvironment for stem cells. Proc Natl Acad Sci U S A. 2011;108(4):1609–14.
23. Xie X, Qiu W, Yuan W, Wang Z. Experimental study of radiation effect on the mandibular microvasculature of the guinea pig. Chin J Dent Res. 1998;1(2):46–51.
24. Milliat F, François A, Isoir M, Deutsch E, Tamarat R, Tarlet G, et al. Influence of endothelial cells on vascular smooth muscle cells phenotype after irradiation: implication in radiation-induced vascular damages. Am J Pathol. 2006;169(4):1484–95.
25. Bray FN, Simmons BJ, Wolfson AH, Nouri K. Acute and chronic cutaneous reactions to ionizing radiation therapy. Dermatol Ther. 2016;6(2):185–206.
26. Hemati S, Asnaashari O, Sarvizadeh M, Motlagh BN, Akbari M, Tajvidi M, et al. Topical silver sulfadiazine for the prevention of acute dermatitis during irradiation for breast cancer. Support Care Cancer. 2012;20(8):1613–8.
27. Jung TT, Park YM, Panossian D, Weeks D, Miller SK, Sandefur J, et al. Effect of the radioprotector WR2721 on irradiation-induced injury to ciliated cells of eustachian tube. Ann Otol Rhinol Laryngol. 1992;101(5):395–402.
28. Walker GV, Ahmed S, Allen P, Gidley PW, Woo SY, DeMonte F, et al. Radiation-induced middle ear and mastoid opacification in skull base tumors treated with radiotherapy. Int J Radiat Oncol Biol Phys. 2011;81(5):e819–23.
29. Takasaki K, Takahashi H, Miyamoto I, Yoshida H, Yamamoto-Fukuda T, Enatsu K, et al. Measurement of angle and length of the eustachian tube on computed tomography using the multiplanar reconstruction technique. Laryngoscope. 2007;117(7):1251–4.
30. Pulec JL, Simonton KM. Abnormal patency of the eustachian tube: report on 41 cases. Laryngoscope. 1964;74(2):267–71.
31. Wang SZ, Li J, Miyamoto CT, Chen F, Zhou LF, Zhang HY, et al. A study of middle ear function in the treatment of nasopharyngeal carcinoma with IMRT technique. Radiother Oncol. 2009;93(3):530–3.
32. Yamamoto K, Yaguchi Y, Kojima H. Clinical analysis of secondary acquired cholesteatoma. Am J Otolaryngol. 2014;35(5):589–93.
33. Xu YD, Ou YK, Zheng YQ, Chen Y, Ji SF. The treatment for post-irradiation otitis media with effusion: a study of three methods. Laryngoscope. 2008;118(11):2040–3.
34. Morton RP, Woollons AC, McIvor NP. Nasopharyngeal carcinoma and middle ear effusion: natural history and the effect of ventilation tubes. Clin Otolaryngol Allied Sci. 1994;19(6):529–31.
35. Soo G, Tong MC, Tsang WS, Wong TK, To KF, Lueng SF, et al. The BAHA hearing system for hearing-impaired postirradiated nasopharyngeal cancer patients: a new indication. Otol Neurotol. 2009;30(4):496–501.
36. Nader ME, Beadle BM, Roberts DB, Gidley PW. Outcomes and complications of osseointegrated hearing aids in irradiated temporal bones. Laryngoscope. 2015;126(5):1187–92.
37. Hsu YC, Su CY. Tympanoplasty for chronic otitis media in post-irradiated nasopharyngeal carcinoma patients. Ann Otol Rhinol Laryngol. 2006;115(5):330–3.
38. Bennett M, Kaylie D, Warren F, Jackson CG. Chronic ear surgery in irradiated temporal bones. Laryngoscope. 2007;117(7):1240–4.
39. Oghalai JS, Driscoll CL. Temporal bone surgery for infectious disease. Atlas of neurotologic and lateral skull base surgery. Berlin: Springer; 2016. p. 193–220.
40. Yilmaz YF, Aytas FI, Akdogan O, Sari K, Savas ZG, Titiz A, et al. Sensorineural hearing loss after radiotherapy for head and neck tumors: a prospective study of the effect of radiation. Otol Neurotol. 2008;29(4):461–3.
41. Chen WC, Jackson A, Budnick AS, Pfister DG, Kraus DH, Hunt MA, et al. Sensorineural hearing loss in combined modality treatment of nasopharyngeal carcinoma. Cancer. 2006;106(4):820–9.
42. Nitta Y, Araki N, Nitta K, Harada T, Ishizaki F, Ando J. Effects of high linear energy transfer radiation on the cochlea of C3H/He mouse during postnatal developmental course. J Radiat Res. 2005;46(1):75–81.
43. Hoistad DL, Ondrey FG, Mutlu C, Schachern PA, Paparella MM, Adams GL. Histopathology of human temporal bone after cis-platinum, radiation, or both. Otolaryngol Head Neck Surg. 1998;118(6):825–32.
44. Honoré HB, Bentzen SM, Møller K, Grau C. Sensori-neural hearing loss after radiotherapy for nasopharyngeal carcinoma: individualized risk estimation. Radiother Oncol. 2002;65(1):9–16.
45. Ho WK, Wei WI, Kwong DL, Sham JS, Tai PT, Yuen AP, et al. Long-term sensorineural hearing deficit following radiotherapy in patients suffering from nasopharyngeal carcinoma: a prospective study. Head Neck. 1999;21(6):547–53.
46. Kwong DL, Wei WI, Sham JS, Ho WK, Yuen PW, Chua DT, et al. Sensorineural hearing loss in patients treated for nasopharyngeal carcinoma: a prospective study of the effect of radiation and cisplatin treatment. Int J Radiat Oncol Biol Phys. 1996;36(2):281–9.
47. Hitchcock YJ, Tward JD, Szabo A, Bentz BG, Shrieve DC. Relative contributions of radiation and cisplatin-based chemotherapy to sensorineural hearing loss in head-and-neck cancer patients. Int J Radiat Oncol Biol Phys. 2009;73(3):779–88.
48. Wang SZ, Wang WF, Zhang HY, Guo M, Hoffman MR, Jiang JJ. Analysis of anatomical factors controlling the morbidity of radiation-induced otitis media with effusion. Radiother Oncol. 2007;85(3):463–8.
49. Jereczek-Fossa BA, Zarowski A, Milani F, Orecchia R. Radiotherapy-induced ear toxicity. Cancer Treat Rev. 2003;29(5):417–30.
50. Hsin CH, Chen TH, Young YH, Liu WS. Comparison of otologic complications between intensity-modulated and two-dimensional

radiotherapies in nasopharyngeal carcinoma patients. Otolaryngol Head Neck Surg. 2010;143(5):662–8.

51. Murphy D, Daniel SJ. Intratympanic dexamethasone to prevent cisplatin ototoxicity: a guinea pig model. Otolaryngol Head Neck Surg. 2011;145(3):452–7.
52. Adunka OF, Buchman CA. Cochlear implantation in the irradiated temporal bone. J Laryngol Otol. 2007;121(1):83–6.
53. Pathak I, Bryce G. Temporal bone necrosis: diagnosis, classification, and management. Otolaryngol Head Neck Surg. 2000;123(3):252–7.
54. Ramsden RT, Bulman CH, Lorigan BP. Osteoradionecrosis of the temporal bone. J Laryngol Otol. 1975;89(9):941–55.
55. Lau WY, Chow CK. Radiation-induced petrous internal carotid artery aneurysm. Ann Otol Rhinol Laryngol. 2005;114(12):939–40.
56. Ahmed S, Gupta N, Hamilton JD, Garden AS, Gidley PW, Ginsberg LE. CT findings in temporal bone osteoradionecrosis. J Comput Assist Tomogr. 2014;38(5):662–6.
57. Birzgalis AR, Ramsden RT, Farrington WT, Small M. Severe radionecrosis of the temporal bone. J Laryngol Otol. 1993;107(3):183–7.
58. Xu YD, Ou YK, Zheng YQ, Zhang SY. Surgical treatment of osteoradionecrosis of the temporal bone in patients with nasopharyngeal carcinoma. J Laryngol Otol. 2008;122(11):1175–9.
59. Zhou X, Ou X, Xu T, Wang X, Shen C, Ding J, et al. Effect of dosimetric factors on occurrence and volume of temporal lobe necrosis following intensity modulated radiation therapy for nasopharyngeal carcinoma: a case-control study. Int J Radiat Oncol Biol Phys. 2014;90(2):261–9.
60. McDonald MW, Moore MG, Johnstone PA. Risk of carotid blowout after reirradiation of the head and neck: a systematic review. Int J Radiat Oncol Biol Phys. 2012;82(3):1083–9.
61. Lambert EM, Garden AS, DeMonte F, Roberts DB, Gidley PW. Radiation-associated malignancies of the ear canal and temporal bone. Laryngoscope. 2015;125(5):1198–204.
62. Frisch CD, Carlson ML, Link MJ. Synchronous head and neck tumors after low-dose radiation to the temporal bone. Otol Neurotol. 2012;33(1):e3–4.
63. Patel SG, See AC, Williamson PA, Archer DJ, Rhys Evans PH. Radiation induced sarcoma of the head and neck. Head Neck. 1999;21(4):346–54.
64. Shu M-T, Lin H-C, Lee J-C, Chen B-F. Radiation-induced squamous cell carcinoma of the external auditory canal. Otol Neurotol. 2011;32(3):e24–e5.

Chemotherapy for Temporal Bone Cancer

31

Renata Ferrarotto and Merrill S. Kies

Introduction

Temporal bone cancer (TBC) encompasses a group of rare malignancies, with a reported incidence of 1 in 1,000,000 individuals per year [1]. It includes cancers arising from the skin of the pinna that invades the temporal bone; primary tumors of the external auditory canal (EAC), middle ear, mastoid, or petrous apex; and metastatic lesions.

The most frequent TBC are basal cell and squamous cell carcinoma (SCC) arising from the pinna and lateral concha or parotid gland carcinoma invading the temporal bone; however, the most common primary neoplasm of the EAC is SCC [2]. Other rarer TBC histologies include adenoid cystic carcinoma, Merkel cell carcinoma, adenocarcinoma, and rhabdomyosarcoma.

While surgical resection often followed by adjuvant radiotherapy is the most accepted therapeutic option for patients with early stage TBC, surgery can be challenging for patients with more advanced tumors due to the anatomical site [3]. Surgery can significantly impair a patient's quality of life through disfiguration, deafness, facial palsy, or more serious complications such as meningitis [4]. Furthermore, patients with stage III or IV disease as proposed by the Pittsburgh staging system [5] (Table 31.1) have a poor prognosis.

In this chapter, we will discuss the available evidence regarding systemic therapy options for curative intent and for palliation in patients with TBC, with a special focus on SCC of the temporal bone.

Table 31.1 Modified Pittsburgh staging system for SCC of the temporal bone [5]

T classification	
T1	Limited to the EAC without bony erosion or evidence of soft tissue involvement
T2	Limited to the EAC with bone erosion (not full thickness) or limited soft tissue involvement (<0.5 cm)
T3	Erosion through the osseous EAC (full thickness), with limited soft tissue involvement (<0.5 cm) or tumor involvement in the middle ear or mastoid
T4	Erosion of the cochlea, petrous apex, medial wall of the middle ear, carotid canal, jugular foramen, or dura, with extensive soft tissue involvement (>0.5 cm, such as involvement of the TMJ or styloid process), or evidence of facial paresis
N classification	
N0	No regional nodes involved
N1	Single metastatic regional node <3 cm
N2a	Single ipsilateral metastatic node 3–6 cm
N2b	Multiple ipsilateral metastatic lymph nodes
N2c	Contralateral metastatic lymph node
N3	Metastatic lymph node >6 cm
Overall stage	
I	T1N0
II	T2N0
III	T3N0
IV	T4N0 or T1-4N+

Squamous Cell Carcinoma of the Temporal Bone

SCC accounts for 60–80% of the tumors arising in the ear canal, middle ear, or mastoid cavity. The 5-year overall survival for patients with temporal bone SCC is approximately 57–73% [5, 6]; however, only approximately 30% of patients with stage IV disease are alive after 5 years [5–7].

R. Ferrarotto, M.D. (✉) · M. S. Kies, M.D.
Thoracic-Head and Neck Medical Oncology, Houston, TX, USA
e-mail: rferrarotto@mdanderson.org; mkies@mdanderson.org

P. W. Gidley, F. DeMonte (eds.), *Temporal Bone Cancer*, https://doi.org/10.1007/978-3-319-74539-8_31

Chemotherapy in the Curative Intent Setting

Neoadjuvant Chemotherapy

The use of effective systemic therapy in the neoadjuvant setting has the potential to allow for a more conservative surgery or provide a chance of curative intent surgery for patients initially deemed unresectable, if significant response is achieved.

Joshi et al. [8] reported a series of four patients, not eligible for surgery at presentation due to extensive disease, who were treated with neoadjuvant chemotherapy. Three patients received a combination of docetaxel, cisplatin, and 5-fluorouracil (TPF), and one patient received cisplatin and paclitaxel. All three patients treated with TPF achieve a partial response (PR) by Response Evaluation Criteria in Solid Tumors (RECIST 1.1) [9], and one was able to undergo surgery. The single patient that received the two-drug combination achieved stable disease with minor tumor shrinkage but was able to undergo resection. In the short term, the two patients who underwent surgery recurred in 3 and 6 months, and one eventually died of disease progression, raising the question if neoadjuvant chemotherapy can improve patient's outcomes. The other two patients who underwent concurrent chemoradiation after achieving a partial response to induction chemotherapy were alive with controlled disease in the short-term follow-up.

Concurrent Chemoradiation

Concurrent chemoradiation has been studied in patients with locally advanced TBC, in the neoadjuvant, definitive, and adjuvant settings.

A meta-analysis including 752 patients with temporal bone SCC reported on 174 of them with locally advanced disease, 42 with stage III (T3N0), and 132 with stage IV (T3N1, T4N0, or T4N1) [6]. Surgery was performed in 124 patients: seven received neoadjuvant concurrent chemoradiation (CRT) and eight received adjuvant CRT. Definitive CRT was performed in 37 patients. Various chemotherapy regimens were used, the majority of them platinum based. Interestingly, the 5-year overall survival of patients who underwent definitive CRT was comparable to that of patients treated with standard of care surgery with or without adjuvant radiotherapy (43.6% vs. 53.3%, respectively, $P = 0.2$) despite the majority of them having unresectable disease and poor prognosis.

When CRT was used in combination with surgery, the 5-year OS was better for patients who received it in the neoadjuvant setting compared to the adjuvant setting (85.7% vs. 0%, respectively), although the difference was not statistically significant. Given that positive margins are associated with poor prognosis, it is reasonable to consider adjuvant CRT for patients with R1 resection (microscopic residual tumor) [10].

A recent series published by Morita et al. including 28 patients with T3/T4 TBC demonstrated similar findings to the meta-analysis [10]. The 5-year overall survival was 52.1% for those receiving CRT and 55.6% for patients treated with surgery followed by radiotherapy with or without chemotherapy. There were no statistically significant differences in the rate of grade 3–4 adverse events between the two treatment groups.

Super-selective Intra-arterial Chemotherapy

Super-selective intra-arterial chemotherapy administered via the posterior auricular and/or superficial temporal artery combined with radiotherapy has been used in selected cases of temporal bone SCC with the intent of organ preservation. The theoretical advantage of intra-arterial chemotherapy over the standard intravenous administration is the higher concentration of the cytotoxic agent administered directly to the tumor with consequent lower systemic exposure.

The two published series included nine patients with temporal bone SCC [11, 12]. All patients were treated with 2–4 doses of intra-arterial cisplatin concurrently with external beam radiotherapy. With a median follow-up of 28–30 months, seven out of the nine patients achieved a complete response with no recurrence, one patient recurred distantly, and one patient recurred locally, with an overall local control rate of 89%.

While these results seem promising, in a phase III randomized trial including functionally unresectable head and neck SCC, cisplatin administered intra-arterially (four doses of 150 mg/m^2) was not found to be superior to intravenous systemic cisplatin (three cycles of 100 mg/m^2) administered concurrently with radiotherapy. Subset analysis suggested that the local control rate with high-dose intra-arterial cisplatin was better against tumors that did not cross the midline. The subset analysis was unplanned and should be interpreted with caution [13].

Chemotherapy Agents Commonly Used in Temporal Bone SCC

Given the disease's rarity, there are no randomized, prospective trials testing chemotherapy agents in temporal bone SCC. Based on case reports and extrapolating from the head and neck SCC literature, the most frequently used cytotoxic agents are platinum, taxanes, 5-fluorouracil, and cetuximab given in the neoadjuvant setting, in patients with recurrent disease not amenable to a curative intent salvage approach, or in patients with distant metastasis (Table 31.2) [14, 15]. While the combination of three agents, such as docetaxel, cisplatin, and 5-fluorouracil (so-called TPF), can be justified in a curative intent approach, platinum doublets and single agent are preferred to avoid significant toxicity in the palliative setting. In the concurrent setting, cisplatin single agent is the most commonly used chemotherapy agent.

Table 31.2 Chemotherapy agents frequently used for temporal bone cancers

Agent	Mechanism of action	Typical dose/route/schedule	Main toxicities[a]
Chemotherapy			
Cisplatin	Alkylating	75 mg/m² IV Q3W 100 mg/m² IV Q3W (with RT) 40 mg/m² IV Q1W (with RT)	Nausea, vomiting, nephrotoxicity, myelosuppression, peripheral neuropathy, ototoxicity
Carboplatin	Alkylating	AUC 6 IV Q3W AUC 2 IV Q1W (with RT)	Myelosuppression, nausea, hyponatremia, increase transaminases, nephrotoxicity
Cyclophosphamide	Alkylating	1200 mg/m² IV Q3W (for RMS)	Nausea, myelosuppression, fatigue, mucositis, diarrhea
Dactinomycin	Antibiotic	0.045 mg/kg IV Q3W (for RMS)	Fatigue, myelosuppression, abdominal pain, diarrhea, muscle ache
5-Fluorouracil	Antimetabolite	1000 mg/m² CI IV D1–4 Q3W	Stomatitis, diarrhea, myelosuppression, anorexia, alopecia
Docetaxel	Antimicrotubular	75 mg/m² IV Q3W	Myelosuppression, fatigue, fluid retention, stomatitis, peripheral neuropathy
Paclitaxel	Antimicrotubular	175 mg/m² IV Q3W	Peripheral neuropathy, myelosuppression, alopecia, nausea, hypersensitivity reaction
Vinorelbine	Antimicrotubular	25 mg/m² IV D1/D8 Q3W	Constipation, myelosuppression, nausea, fatigue, increase transaminases
Vincristine	Antimicrotubular	1.5 mg/m² IV Q1W (for RMS)	Nausea, abdominal pain, myelosuppression, peripheral neuropathy, weight loss
Adriamycin	Topoisomerase II inhibitor	60 mg/m² IV Q3W	Cardiovascular, myelosuppression, fatigue, alopecia, nausea
Etoposide	Topoisomerase II inhibitor	100 mg/m² IV D1–3 Q3W	Myelosuppression, nausea, vomiting, alopecia, diarrhea
Topotecan	Topoisomerase I inhibitor	1.5 mg/m² IV D1–5 Q3W 2.3 mg/m² PO D1–5 Q3W	Myelosuppression, nausea, anorexia, diarrhea, fatigue
Targeted therapy			
Vismodegib	Hedgehog inhibitor	150 mg PO QD	Muscle spasm, dysgeusia, alopecia, fatigue, weight loss
Sonidegib	Hedgehog inhibitor	200 mg PO QD	Increase BUN, increase in CPK, muscle spasm, dysgeusia, hyperglycemia
Cetuximab	EGFR inhibitor	400 mg/m² IV loading dose, 250 mg/m² IV maintenance Q1W	Desquamation, acneiform rash, fatigue, diarrhea, weight loss
Panitumumab	EGFR inhibitor	6 mg/kg Q2W	Acneiform rash, fatigue, paronychia, pruritus, nausea
Gefitinib	EGFR inhibitor	250 mg PO QD	Dermatologic reaction, diarrhea, proteinuria, increase in transaminases, anorexia
Sorafenib	VEGF inhibitor	400 mg PO BID	Fatigue, palmar-plantar erythrodysesthesia, fatigue, diarrhea, increase transaminases
Sunitinib	VEGF inhibitor	50 mg PO QD (4 W on—2 W off)	Fatigue, diarrhea, hypertension, anemia, skin discoloration
Axitinib	VEGF inhibitor	5 mg PO BID	Diarrhea, hypertension, fatigue, increase creatinine, hypocalcemia
Immunotherapy			
Avelumab	Anti-PD-L1	10 mg/kg IV Q2W	Fatigue, lymphocytopenia, diarrhea, skin rash, peripheral edema
Pembrolizumab	Anti-PD-1	200 mg IV Q3W	Fatigue, hyperglycemia, anemia, hypoalbuminemia, pruritus
Nivolumab	Anti-PD-1	240 mg IV Q2W	Fatigue, hyperglycemia, lymphocytopenia, anemia, diarrhea
Ipilimumab	Anti-CTLA-4	10 mg/kg IV Q3W × 4 (adjuvant) 3 mg/kg IV Q3W (palliative)	Diarrhea, fatigue, nausea, pyrexia, vomiting
Interferon alpha	Immunomodulator	20 million U/m² IV D1–5 Q1W × 4 (induction), 10 million U/m² SQ 3×/W × 48W (maintenance)	Flu-like symptoms, fever, myalgia, myelosuppression, depression

IV intravenously, *W* weeks, *RT* radiotherapy, *AUC* area under the curve, *D* day, *CI* continuous infusion, *RMS* rhabdomyosarcoma, *PO* per oral, *QD* once a day, *BID* twice a day

[a]Five among the most common toxicities reported with the drug when administered as a single agent

Other TBC Histologies

Basal Cell Carcinoma

Basel cell carcinoma (BCC) is the most common skin cancer. Seventy to eighty percent of the cases occur in the face, with ear being the fifth most common site, particularly in the helix [16].

The vast majority of BCC have mutations in genes involved in the hedgehog signaling pathway, particularly in the cell surface receptor patched homolog 1 (PTCH1) and in the smoothened homolog (SMO) receptor, which leads to constitutive hedgehog pathway activation [17, 18].

Vismodegib, the first-in-class SMO inhibitor, has significant clinical activity in patients with BCC rendering objective responses in approximately 48–60% of patients with locally advanced disease and 34–45% of patients with metastatic disease, with a median response duration of approximately 8 months [19, 20]. Adverse events particularly muscle spasms, dysgeusia, and weight loss lead to treatment discontinuation in 10–20% of the cases.

Interim results of a phase II trial with sonidegib, another SMO inhibitor, have shown similar activity and toxicity profile to vismodegib and represent another therapeutic option in inoperable basal cell carcinoma [21].

Cutaneous SCC

Cutaneous SCC (cSCC) is the second most common malignancy in the USA after BCC. Advanced disease usually affects the elderly and immunosuppressed patients, posing an additional challenge to treatment. There is limited data on the role of chemotherapy in the treatment of locally advanced, recurrent, or metastatic cSCC. In terms of cytotoxic chemotherapy, platinum-based combinations usually with 5-fluorouracil or taxanes are the most commonly used agents (Fig. 31.1). The evidence comes mostly from small retrospective studies and case reports [22, 23]. Aside from chemotherapy, monoclonal antibodies targeting the epidermal growth factor receptor (EGFR) such as cetuximab and panitumumab have shown activity in cSCC.

A retrospective study evaluating cetuximab-based systemic therapy in the neoadjuvant setting for patients with locally advanced unresectable disease reported that cetuximab single agent led to objective response in five out of nine patients (three complete and two partial responses), allowing these patients to undergo surgery. When cetuximab was combined with platinum and 5-fluorouracil, 23 out of 25 patients were able to undergo surgery, and complete pathological response was achieved in 15 patients (60%) [24].

In a phase II study of cetuximab in 36 patients with locally advanced or metastatic cSCC, objective response rate was 28% (eight partial and two complete responses). Three patients became surgical candidates after treatment with cetuximab. Benefit correlated with the development of acneiform rash [25].

Panitumumab was studied in a phase II trial enrolling 16 cSCC patients. Response was documented in five (30%) patients (three partial and two complete), similar to the response rate seen with cetuximab [26].

Gefitinib, an EGFR tyrosine kinase inhibitor, has also been investigated in the neoadjuvant setting in a phase II study including 23 cSCC patients. Complete response was documented in 18% of the patients and partial response was seen in 27% [27].

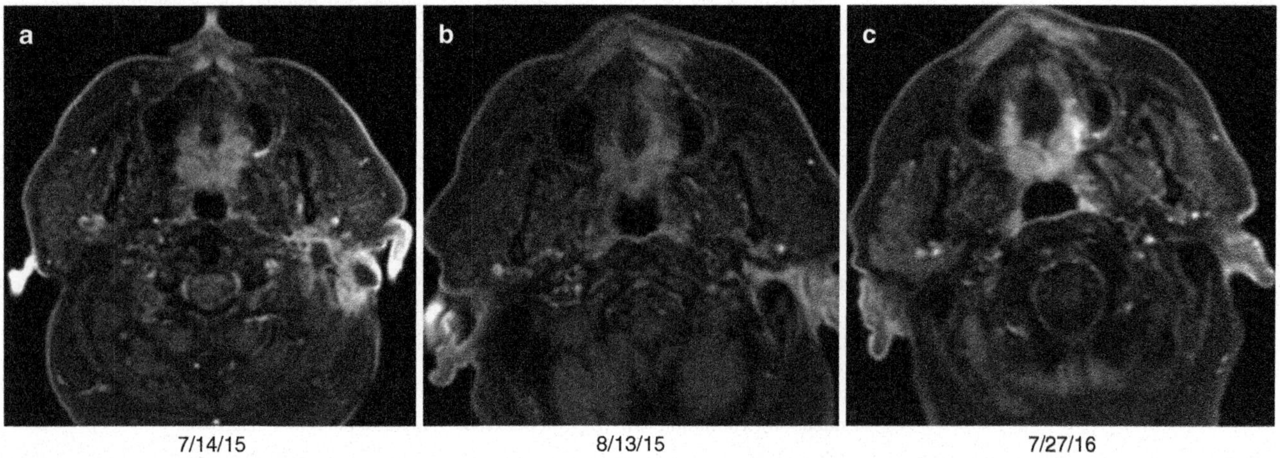

Fig. 31.1 A 66-year-old gentleman with multiple comorbidities diagnosed with a T3N2b SCC of the left auricle. He was treated with three cycles of induction chemotherapy with carboplatin and paclitaxel followed by concurrent chemoradiation with the same drug regimen. He had significant improvement in pain after one cycle of induction chemotherapy and achieved a partial response after two cycles. (**a**) baseline MRI; (**b**) MRI after two cycles of neoadjuvant chemotherapy; (**c**) MRI approximately 8 months after completion of concurrent chemoradiation

Adenoid Cystic Carcinoma

Adenoid cystic carcinoma (ACC) is the second most common malignant salivary gland tumor, but it can arise from any secretory gland. It is known to be chemoresistant, and there is no standard of care systemic therapy for patients with recurrent and/or metastatic disease [28]. Given the usually slow-growing nature of this disease, close observation is a widely accepted approach. For patients that are symptomatic, have a high disease burden, or have an aggressive phenotype, the chemotherapy regimens of cisplatin and vinorelbine or of cyclophosphamide, Adriamycin, and cisplatin (CAP) are frequently used, based on retrospective studies and small single-arm phase II trials [29, 30]. Anti-angiogenic agents such as sorafenib, sunitinib, and axitinib have shown some activity in ACC, mostly in terms of disease stability [28]. Recently, genomic profiling of ACC samples revealed novel targetable genomic alterations such as *FGFR* and *NOTCH1* activating mutations. Targeted therapy against these mutations holds promise and warrants investigation in prospective trials [28, 31].

Merkel Cell Carcinoma and Other High-Grade Neuroendocrine Tumors

Merkel cell carcinoma (MCC) is a high-grade neuroendocrine carcinoma of the skin frequently associated with Merkel cell polyomavirus (MCPyV). It affects mainly elderly, light-skinned males and 10% of patients are immunosuppressed. Disease recurrence following curative intent surgery and/or radiotherapy occurs in at least 35% of cases [32]. Patients with advanced disease stage have a dismal prognosis with a 5-year survival ranging from 0% to 18%.

Extrapolating from small cell lung cancer, locally advanced, inoperable MCC or other high-grade neuroendocrine carcinomas involving the temporal bone are treated with concurrent chemoradiation usually with cisplatin and etoposide. Distant failure is common, and patients with metastatic disease are frequently treated with cisplatin and etoposide or topotecan [33, 34]. Response rate with platinum and etoposide is approximately 60% as first-line therapy; however, the response is usually of short duration and with questionable benefit in survival [35]. Checkpoint inhibitors, particularly anti-programed death 1 (PD-1), have shown promise in MCC and will be discussed in section "Checkpoint Inhibitors."

Papillary Adenocarcinoma Tumors

Aggressive papillary tumor of the temporal bone (also called endolymphatic sac tumor) arises in the vicinity of the inner ear and may extend to the posterior fossa as well as the middle ear and the external ear canal. It can be encountered sporadically or in von Hippel-Lindau disease. They are slow-growing but locally aggressive tumors, with many patients presenting with audiovestibular or facial nerve dysfunction [36]. EGFR has been identified in specimens of aggressive papillary ear tumors. Furthermore, the EGFR inhibitor cetuximab has shown encouraging activity in a genetically engineered mouse model of aggressive papillary ear tumor [37]. In the absence of standard of care systemic therapy for this patient population, EGFR inhibitor seems like a reasonable approach for patients not amenable to curative intent local therapy.

Rhabdomyosarcoma

Rhabdomyosarcoma (RMS), particularly the embryonal subtype, is the most common malignancy of the temporal bone in children. It usually manifests as chronic otitis media refractory to treatment [38]. Prior to 1970, the prognosis of children with RMS was dismal, with a 20% cure rate from surgery, with or without adjuvant radiotherapy. Outcomes have significantly improved with the addition of chemotherapy with a 5-year survival rate around 70%. Patients with locally advanced disease undergo a combined modality approach that incorporates initial chemotherapy, surgery if feasible, and radiotherapy to control microscopic local residual disease. The treatment recommendation is based on a prognostic stratification (risk-adapted). The most commonly used cytotoxic agents in RSM are vincristine and dactinomycin plus or minus cyclophosphamide [39–41].

Melanoma

Melanoma is an aggressive cutaneous neoplasia. Wide local excision with margins of 1–2 cm is recommended, depending on the thickness, but is not always attainable in primaries of the head and neck, as it may lead to significant functional and cosmetic disability. Adjuvant radiotherapy is frequently used, particularly when satisfactory margins are not obtained [42].

Patients with high-risk disease without lymph node involvement (seventh TNM stage IIB or IIC) and a good performance status can receive adjuvant high-dose interferon alpha (INFα), with a 5-year absolute benefit in survival of 9% [43]. For patients with high-risk stage III disease, defined as macroscopic lymph node involvement, multiple positive nodes, or a single node with more than 1 mm of microscopic disease, ipilimumab, a cytotoxic T-lymphocyte-associated antigen 4 [CTLA-4] checkpoint inhibitor, (see section on "Checkpoint Inhibitors"), has demonstrated an 11% survival benefit at 5 years and should be considered the agent of choice [44].

In the metastatic setting, molecular targeted therapies with specific inhibitors for BRAF or KIT mutants or checkpoint inhibitors, specifically anti-CTLA-4 (ipilimumab) and/or anti-PD-1 (nivolumab/pembrolizumab), are the main therapeutic options. The combination of anti-CTLA-4 and anti-PD-1 in the first-line setting for non-BRAF and non-KIT mutants is preferred given increased response rate and progression-free survival than either agent alone [45]. The optimal sequencing of systemic therapy for patients with actionable driver mutations is yet to be determined. Chemotherapy has a limited role in the treatment of melanoma.

Metastatic Tumors

The temporal bone may be a site for metastasis from lymphoma or solid tumors such as breast, lung, kidney, or prostate carcinoma [46]. Systemic therapy for these lesions is the same indicated for the underlying malignant disease. Temporal bone resection can be used exceptionally in the treatment of oligometastatic disease.

Checkpoint Inhibitors

In many cancers, immune checkpoint proteins such as CTLA-4 and PD-1/PD-L1 can be dysregulated, allowing for immune evasion. CTLA-4 is expressed by activated T cells. It binds to CD80 and CD86 on antigen-presenting cells, transmitting an inhibitory signal to T cells. Blockage of CTLA-4 with antibodies such as ipilimumab has shown activity in melanoma, being approved in the adjuvant and metastatic setting in this disease [44, 45]. PD-1 is a negative regulator of T cell that can interact with two ligands: PD-L1 or PD-L2. When engaged by ligand, PD-1 inhibits signaling pathways that normally lead to T cell activation [47]. Antibodies blocking PD-1 or PD-L1 have shown activity in multiple tumor types, including head and neck SCC, leading to its approval in the recurrent/metastatic setting, after progression to first-line chemotherapy [48, 49]. In Merkel cell carcinoma, the anti-PD-L1 avelumab and the anti-PD-1 pembrolizumab led to response rates ranging between 32% and 56%, usually of prolonged duration. Avelumab has been recently approved by the Food and Drug Administration for patients with recurrent or metastatic Merkel cell carcinoma [50, 51].

Predictive markers of activity of checkpoint inhibitors are currently being investigated; however, a strong correlation exists between high mutational burden, PD-L1 overexpression in the tumor, or immune-infiltrate cells and responses to anti-PD-1 or anti-PD-L1 therapy [47]. These agents have a very attractive toxicity profile and are currently being investigated in multiple neoplasms, such as cutaneous squamous cell carcinoma, and could be active in a variety of tumor histologies affecting the temporal bone, such as SCC.

Conclusions

Irrespective of the histological subtype, surgery remains the standard of care treatment for patients with TBC amenable to a curative intent procedure. In SCC of the temporal bone, preoperative CRT may improve survival in patients with locally advanced disease, and definitive CRT is a valid alternative to surgical treatment in patients not amenable to curative intent surgery. Adjuvant CRT may not be effective to salvage worse prognosis patients but should be considered in cases with positive margins. TBC histology is important in determining systemic therapy options. Checkpoint inhibitors hold promise in multiple cancer types and might became a therapeutic option in TBC. Prospective, multicenter, international trials evaluating systemic therapy for patients with TBC are warranted.

References

1. Kuhel WI, Hume CR, Selesnick SH. Cancer of the external auditory canal and temporal bone. Otolaryngol Clin N Am. 1996;29(5):827–52.
2. Devaney KO, Boschman CR, Willard SC, Ferlito A, Rinaldo A. Tumours of the external ear and temporal bone. Lancet Oncol. 2005;6(6):411–20.
3. Pfreundner L, Schwager K, Willner J, Baier K, Bratengeier K, Brunner FX, et al. Carcinoma of the external auditory canal and middle ear. Int J Radiat Oncol Biol Phys. 1999;44(4):777–88.
4. Lobo D, Llorente JL, Suarez C. Squamous cell carcinoma of the external auditory canal. Skull Base. 2008;18(3):167–72.
5. Moody SA, Hirsch BE, Myers EN. Squamous cell carcinoma of the external auditory canal: an evaluation of a staging system. Am J Otol. 2000;21(4):582–8.
6. Takenaka Y, Cho H, Nakahara S, Yamamoto Y, Yasui T, Inohara H. Chemoradiation therapy for squamous cell carcinoma of the external auditory canal: a meta-analysis. Head Neck. 2015;37(7):1073–80.
7. Yin M, Ishikawa K, Honda K, Arakawa T, Harabuchi Y, Nagabashi T, et al. Analysis of 95 cases of squamous cell carcinoma of the external and middle ear. Auris Nasus Larynx. 2006;33(3):251–7.
8. Joshi A, Tandon N, Noronha V, Dhumal S, Patil V, Arya S, et al. Neoadjuvant chemotherapy in technically unresectable carcinoma of external auditory canal. Indian J Med Paediatr Oncol. 2015;36(3):172–5.
9. Eisenhauer EA, Therasse P, Bogaerts J, Schwartz LH, Sargent D, Ford R, et al. New response evaluation criteria in solid tumours: revised RECIST guideline (version 1.1). Eur J Cancer. 2009;45(2):228–47.
10. Morita S, Homma A, Nakamaru Y, Sakashita T, Hatakeyama H, Kano S, et al. The outcomes of surgery and chemoradiotherapy for temporal bone cancer. Otol Neurotol. 2016;37(8):1174–82.
11. Ueda Y, Kurita T, Matsuda Y, Ito S, Nakashima T. Superselective, intra-arterial, rapid infusion chemotherapy for external auditory canal carcinoma. J Laryngol Otol Suppl. 2009;(31):75–80.
12. Sugimoto H, Ito M, Yoshida S, Hatano M, Yoshizaki T. Concurrent superselective intra-arterial chemotherapy and radiotherapy for late-stage squamous cell carcinoma of the temporal bone. Ann Otol Rhinol Laryngol. 2011;120(6):372–6.
13. Rasch CR, Hauptmann M, Balm AJ. Intra-arterial chemotherapy for head and neck cancer: is there a verdict? Cancer. 2011;117(4):874. author reply; 874–5

14. Lorch JH, Goloubeva O, Haddad RI, Cullen K, Sarlis N, Tishler R, et al. Induction chemotherapy with cisplatin and fluorouracil alone or in combination with docetaxel in locally advanced squamous-cell cancer of the head and neck: long-term results of the TAX 324 randomised phase 3 trial. Lancet Oncol. 2011;12(2):153–9.
15. Vermorken JB, Mesia R, Rivera F, Remenar E, Kawecki A, Rottey S, et al. Platinum-based chemotherapy plus cetuximab in head and neck cancer. N Engl J Med. 2008;359(11):1116–27.
16. Ragi JM, Patel D, Masud A, Rao BK. Nonmelanoma skin cancer of the ear: frequency, patients' knowledge, and photoprotection practices. Dermatol Surg. 2010;36(8):1232–9.
17. Xie J, Murone M, Luoh SM, Ryan A, Gu Q, Zhang C, et al. Activating smoothened mutations in sporadic basal-cell carcinoma. Nature. 1998;391(6662):90–2.
18. Johnson RL, Rothman AL, Xie J, Goodrich LV, Bare JW, Bonifas JM, et al. Human homolog of patched, a candidate gene for the basal cell nevus syndrome. Science. 1996;272(5268):1668–71.
19. Sekulic A, Migden MR, Oro AE, Dirix L, Lewis KD, Hainsworth JD, et al. Efficacy and safety of vismodegib in advanced basal-cell carcinoma. N Engl J Med. 2012;366(23):2171–9.
20. Sekulic A, Migden MR, Lewis K, Hainsworth JD, Solomon JA, Yoo S, et al. Pivotal ERIVANCE basal cell carcinoma (BCC) study: 12-month update of efficacy and safety of vismodegib in advanced BCC. J Am Acad Dermatol. 2015;72(6):1021–6.e8.
21. Migden MR, Guminski A, Gutzmer R, Dirix L, Lewis KD, Combemale P, et al. Treatment with two different doses of sonidegib in patients with locally advanced or metastatic basal cell carcinoma (BOLT): a multicentre, randomised, double-blind phase 2 trial. Lancet Oncol. 2015;16(6):716–28.
22. Cartei G, Cartei F, Interlandi G, Meneghini G, Jop A, Zingone G, et al. Oral 5-fluorouracil in squamous cell carcinoma of the skin in the aged. Am J Clin Oncol. 2000;23(2):181–4.
23. Khansur T, Kennedy A. Cisplatin and 5-fluorouracil for advanced locoregional and metastatic squamous cell carcinoma of the skin. Cancer. 1991;67(8):2030–2.
24. Reigneau M, Robert C, Routier E, Mamelle G, Moya-Plana A, Tomasic G, et al. Efficacy of neoadjuvant cetuximab alone or with platinum salt for the treatment of unresectable advanced non-metastatic cutaneous squamous cell carcinomas. Br J Dermatol. 2015;173(2):527–34.
25. Maubec E, Petrow P, Scheer-Senyarich I, Duvillard P, Lacroix L, Gelly J, et al. Phase II study of cetuximab as first-line single-drug therapy in patients with unresectable squamous cell carcinoma of the skin. J Clin Oncol. 2011;29(25):3419–26.
26. Foote MC, McGrath M, Guminski A, Hughes BG, Meakin J, Thomson D, et al. Phase II study of single-agent panitumumab in patients with incurable cutaneous squamous cell carcinoma. Ann Oncol. 2014;25(10):2047–52.
27. Lewis CM, Glisson BS, Feng L, Wan F, Tang X, Wistuba II, et al. A phase II study of gefitinib for aggressive cutaneous squamous cell carcinoma of the head and neck. Clin Cancer Res. 2012;18(5):1435–46.
28. Ferrarotto R, Heymach JV, Glisson BS. MYB-fusions and other potential actionable targets in adenoid cystic carcinoma. Curr Opin Oncol. 2016;28(3):195–200.
29. Airoldi M, Pedani F, Succo G, Gabriele AM, Ragona R, Marchionatti S, et al. Phase II randomized trial comparing vinorelbine versus vinorelbine plus cisplatin in patients with recurrent salivary gland malignancies. Cancer. 2001;91(3):541–7.
30. Licitra L, Cavina R, Grandi C, Palma SD, Guzzo M, Demicheli R, et al. Cisplatin, doxorubicin and cyclophosphamide in advanced salivary gland carcinoma. A phase II trial of 22 patients. Ann Oncol. 1996;7(6):640–2.
31. Ferrarotto R, Mitani Y, Diao L, Guijarro I, Wang J, Zweidler-McKay P, et al. Activating NOTCH1 mutations define a distinct subgroup of patients with adenoid cystic carcinoma who have poor prognosis, propensity to bone and liver metastasis, and potential responsiveness to Notch1 inhibitors. J Clin Oncol Off J Am Soc Clin Oncol. 2017;35(3):352–60.
32. Grotz TE, Tarantola TI, Otley CC, Weaver AL, McGree ME, Jakub JW. Natural history of merkel cell carcinoma following locoregional recurrence. Ann Surg Oncol. 2012;19(8):2556–62.
33. Ouaz K, Robier A, Lescanne E, Bobillier C, Moriniere S, Bakhos D. Cancer of the external auditory canal. Eur Ann Otorhinolaryngol Head Neck Dis. 2013;130(4):175–82.
34. Mauzo SH, Ferrarotto R, Bell D, Torres-Cabala CA, Tetzlaff MT, Prieto VG, et al. Molecular characteristics and potential therapeutic targets in Merkel cell carcinoma. J Clin Pathol. 2016;69(5):382–90.
35. Tai PT, Yu E, Winquist E, Hammond A, Stitt L, Tonita J, et al. Chemotherapy in neuroendocrine/Merkel cell carcinoma of the skin: case series and review of 204 cases. J Clin Oncol Off J Am Soc Clin Oncol. 2000;18(12):2493–9.
36. Devaney KO, Ferlito A, Rinaldo A. Endolymphatic sac tumor (low-grade papillary adenocarcinoma) of the temporal bone. Acta Otolaryngol. 2003;123(9):1022–6.
37. Kawabata S, Hollander MC, Munasinghe JP, Brinster LR, Mercado-Matos JR, Li J, et al. Epidermal growth factor receptor as a novel molecular target for aggressive papillary tumors in the middle ear and temporal bone. Oncotarget. 2015;6(13):11357–68.
38. Sbeity S, Abella A, Arcand P, Quintal MC, Saliba I. Temporal bone rhabdomyosarcoma in children. Int J Pediatr Otorhinolaryngol. 2007;71(5):807–14.
39. Raney RB, Walterhouse DO, Meza JL, Andrassy RJ, Breneman JC, Crist WM, et al. Results of the Intergroup Rhabdomyosarcoma Study Group D9602 protocol, using vincristine and dactinomycin with or without cyclophosphamide and radiation therapy, for newly diagnosed patients with low-risk embryonal rhabdomyosarcoma: a report from the Soft Tissue Sarcoma Committee of the Children's Oncology Group. J Clin Oncol. 2011;29(10):1312–8.
40. Walterhouse DO, Pappo AS, Meza JL, Breneman JC, Hayes-Jordan AA, Parham DM, et al. Shorter-duration therapy using vincristine, dactinomycin, and lower-dose cyclophosphamide with or without radiotherapy for patients with newly diagnosed low-risk rhabdomyosarcoma: a report from the Soft Tissue Sarcoma Committee of the Children's Oncology Group. J Clin Oncol Off J Am Soc Clin Oncol. 2014;32(31):3547–52.
41. Malempati S, Hawkins DS. Rhabdomyosarcoma: review of the Children's Oncology Group (COG) Soft-Tissue Sarcoma Committee experience and rationale for current COG studies. Pediatr Blood Cancer. 2012;59(1):5–10.
42. Cascinelli N. Margin of resection in the management of primary melanoma. Semin Surg Oncol. 1998;14(4):272–5.
43. Mocellin S, Pasquali S, Rossi CR, Nitti D. Interferon alpha adjuvant therapy in patients with high-risk melanoma: a systematic review and meta-analysis. J Natl Cancer Inst. 2010;102(7):493–501.
44. Eggermont AM, Chiarion-Sileni V, Grob JJ, Dummer R, Wolchok JD, Schmidt H, et al. Adjuvant ipilimumab versus placebo after complete resection of high-risk stage III melanoma (EORTC 18071): a randomised, double-blind, phase 3 trial. Lancet Oncol. 2015;16(5):522–30.
45. Larkin J, Chiarion-Sileni V, Gonzalez R, Grob JJ, Cowey CL, Lao CD, et al. Combined nivolumab and ipilimumab or monotherapy in untreated melanoma. N Engl J Med. 2015;373(1):23–34.
46. Cureoglu S, Tulunay O, Ferlito A, Schachern PA, Paparella MM, Rinaldo A. Otologic manifestations of metastatic tumors to the temporal bone. Acta Otolaryngol. 2004;124(10):1117–23.
47. Postow MA, Callahan MK, Wolchok JD. Immune checkpoint blockade in cancer therapy. J Clin Oncol Off J Am Soc Clin Oncol. 2015;33(17):1974–82.
48. Ferris RL, Blumenschein G Jr, Fayette J, Guigay J, Colevas AD, Licitra L, et al. Nivolumab for recurrent squamous-cell carcinoma of the head and neck. N Engl J Med. 2016;375:1856–67.

49. Chow LQ, Haddad R, Gupta S, Mahipal A, Mehra R, Tahara M, et al. Antitumor activity of Pembrolizumab in biomarker-unselected patients with recurrent and/or metastatic head and neck squamous cell carcinoma: results from the phase Ib KEYNOTE-012 expansion cohort. J Clin Oncol. 2016;34(32):3838–45.
50. Kaufman HL, Russell J, Hamid O, Bhatia S, Terheyden P, D'Angelo SP, et al. Avelumab in patients with chemotherapy-refractory metastatic Merkel cell carcinoma: a multicentre, single-group, open-label, phase 2 trial. Lancet Oncol. 2016;17(10):1374–85.
51. Nghiem PT, Bhatia S, Lipson EJ, Kudchadkar RR, Miller NJ, Annamalai L, et al. PD-1 blockade with pembrolizumab in advanced Merkel-cell carcinoma. N Engl J Med. 2016;374(26):2542–52.

Temporal Bone Cancers and Quality of Life

32

John R. de Almeida

Introduction

Cancers involving the temporal bone and their treatment may be associated with a tremendous impact on health-related quality of life. Several critical structures course through the temporal bone and its proximity. Anatomic structures such as the pinna, vascular structures such as the internal carotid artery and jugular bulb, nervous structures such as the facial nerve, and sensorineural structures such as the cochlea and vestibular apparatus may be affected by diseases in this region. Injury to these structures may create facial disfigurement, cause hearing and vestibular impairment, cause pain, and cause chronic ear dysfunction, thereby affecting patients' physical, emotional, and social well-being.

The World Health Organization defines quality of life as an "individuals' perception of their position in life in the context of the culture and value systems in which they live and in relation to their goals, expectations, standards, and concerns. It is a broad ranging concept affected in a complex way by the person's physical health, psychological state, level of independence, social relationships, personal beliefs and their relationship to salient features of their environment" [1]. Quality of life is an important concept as it is patient-reported and helps clinicians advise patients on the morbidity of treatments and their expected impact on living. Often patient perceptions of their own quality of life following treatment do not necessarily correlate with the perceptions of their treating physicians [2, 3], thus reinforcing the importance of measuring and reporting this outcome.

Proper measurement of quality of life requires instruments that are both reliable and valid. These concepts are of paramount importance in the evaluation of the quality of life particularly because there is no gold standard way of measuring this concept. It can be measured both generically with generic quality of life instruments and specifically with disease-specific instruments. As one would not use a thermometer to measure blood pressure, or a sphygmomanometer to measure body temperature, similar application of the wrong disease-specific instrument would result in erroneous interpretation. Currently there is no validated disease-specific instrument to measure quality of life as it relates to patients with cancers of the temporal bone. However, a multitude of head and neck cancer-specific instruments, as well as symptom-specific instruments, exist to better quantify quality of life in these patients.

The main challenge in measuring quality of life in patients with cancers affecting the temporal bone is the amount of heterogeneity both in disease processes and in treatment approaches. For example, cancers of the parotid gland, external auditory canal, mastoid, nasopharynx, infratemporal fossa, and cutaneous malignancies subjacent to the temporal bone may affect patients' quality of life in different ways. Similarly, patients treated with parotidectomy and mastoidectomy for parotid gland malignancies may have a different impact on treatment compared to patients undergoing total temporal bone resection for an external auditory canal cancer. Further, the impact of adjuvant therapies such as radiotherapy and chemotherapy may also impact quality of life in various ways.

Given the rarity of cancers involving the temporal bone, the full impact of these cancers on quality of life is not well studied. Several factors including disease extent, histopathology, modalities of treatment, facial nerve function, impact on hearing and balance, and cosmetic impairment may all contribute to patients' health-related quality of life. Furthermore, several patient-specific factors may affect how they perceive their disease and their health, such as their value system, personal supports, cultural beliefs, and upbringing.

J. R. de Almeida, M.D., M.Sc.
Department of Otolaryngology — Head and Neck Surgery, University Health Network, Toronto, ON, Canada

Department of Otolaryngology — Head and Neck Surgery, Princess Margaret Cancer Centre, University of Toronto, Toronto, ON, Canada
e-mail: john.dealmeida@uhn.ca

P. W. Gidley, F. DeMonte (eds.), *Temporal Bone Cancer*, https://doi.org/10.1007/978-3-319-74539-8_32

Quality of Life Instruments

A number of measurement tools or instruments have been used to measure quality of life in patients with malignancies of the temporal bone. A summary of basic psychometric properties of quality of life instruments for temporal bone cancer is summarized in Table 32.1. In the absence of a truly disease-specific or site-specific quality of life measurement tool, however, generic instruments such as the 36-item Medical Outcomes Study Short Form Health Survey (SF-36) have been used [3–5]. This instrument was developed to measure quality of life over eight domains (physical functioning, role limitations due to physical health, role limitations due to emotional problems, energy/fatigue, emotional well-being, social functioning, pain, and general health) [3]. Although this instrument has been validated in several countries and in multiple languages, the challenge with applying it to tumors of the temporal bone is the inherent lack of content validity. That is to say that, on the surface, this instrument does not fully delve into components of quality of life affected by diseases in this anatomic area. For example, the impact of cancers of the temporal bone on hearing and communication is not addressed by the SF-36. Nevertheless, the SF-36 has been used in patients with diseases of the temporal bone. For example, in one study, this instrument was used to demonstrate a deterioration in quality of life in patients after surgery via a transpetrosal approach for petroclival meningiomas [5].

Disease-specific instruments may be used to overcome the inherent lack of content validity with generic instruments. For diseases affecting the temporal bone, a disease-specific instrument must address the components of quality of life affected by diseases of the temporal bone. The Glasgow Benefit Inventory (GBI) is a validated otolaryngologic-specific instrument composed of 18 items and 3 domains (social, physical, general) [6]. This instrument was originally validated in several populations undergoing otolaryngologic procedures such as middle ear surgery, cochlear implantation, middle ear surgery to eradicate ear infection, tonsillectomy, and rhinoplasty. Each item is scored on a Likert-type scale up to 5 with a score of 3 indicating no change, a score of 5 indicating maximum improvement, and a score of 1 indicating maximum detriment after surgery. The resultant score ranges from −100 to 100. The main limitation with the GBI is the lack of validation in patients with temporal bone cancers. As such, the full realm of quality of life impact from certain modalities of treatment such as radiation therapy is not covered by the GBI. Nevertheless, the GBI has been used to measure quality of life in patients undergoing surgery for external auditory canal cancers with lateral temporal bone resection [7]. In this study the GBI was used as a disease-specific instrument to demonstrate that reconstruction of the external auditory canal with a rolled-up skin graft combined with tympanoplasty may improve quality of life after lateral temporal bone resection in comparison to those not reconstructed.

Although not entirely disease-specific, a multitude of head and neck cancer-specific instruments have been developed that may be used to measure quality of life for temporal bone cancer. Eight such instruments used to measure quality of life in patients with head and neck cancer were summarized in a systematic review [8]. These instruments include the University of Washington Quality of Life (UWQOL) instrument [9], the European Organization for Research and Treatment of Cancer (EORTC) Head and Neck-35 (HN35) module [10], the Functional Assessment of Cancer Therapy-Head and Neck (FACT-HN) [11], the Head and Neck Radiotherapy

Table 32.1 Quality of life instruments for cancers of the temporal bone

Instrument	Number of domains	Number of items	Disease-specific items (i), domains (d)	Reliable	Valid	Content validity
Generic quality of life instruments						
SF-36	8	36	–	+	+	–
Disease-specific quality of life instruments						
GBI	3	18	Problems related to ear (i)	+	+	±
Head and neck cancer-specific quality of life instruments						
UWQOL	9	12	Appearance (i), chewing (i)	±	+	±
EORTC-HN35	7	35	Trismus (i)	+	+	–
FACT-HN	5	38	Appearance (i)	+	+	–
HNRQ	6	22	–	+	±	–
QL-H&N	3	29	–	±	±	–
QLQ	4	19	–	–	±	–
QOL-RTI/H&N	4	39	–	+	+	–
HNQOL	4	21	–	+	±	–
Anterior skull base-specific quality of life instruments						
ASB-QOL	6	35	Appearance (i)	+	+	–
SBI	11	41	Cognitive (d), neurologic (d), appearance (i)	+	+	–

Questionnaire (HNRQ) [12], the Quality of Life Instrument for Head and Neck Cancer (QL-H&N) [13], the Quality of Life Questionnaire for Advanced Head and Neck Cancer (QLQ) [14], the Quality of Life-Radiation Therapy Instrument Head and Neck Module (QOL-RTI/H&N) [15], and the University of Michigan Head and Neck Quality of Life (HNQOL) [16].

Each of these instruments has its own merits, and although they are germane to mucosal head and neck cancers, their relevance or validity in measuring quality of life of patients with cancers of the temporal bone has still not been established. The UWQOL contains two disease-specific items, one for appearance and one for chewing, both of which may be relevant to temporal bone disease processes [9]. This instrument is relatively short comprising 12 items and is relatively easy to complete. General quality of life topics such as impact on role functioning and emotional impact are not comprehensively covered in the UWQOL. The EORTC-HN35 is a well-validated instrument that serves as an additional module to the cancer-specific EORTC-QLQ30 instrument [10]. This instrument has seven domains (pain, swallowing, senses, speech, social eating, social contact, and sexuality), many of which have some relevance to temporal bone cancers but none of which is entirely disease-specific. One item related to jaw opening is pertinent to patients who have temporal bone diseases, but in general the instrument is well-suited to mucosal head and neck cancers. The FACT-HN also is specific to head and neck cancers [11]. The 11 disease-specific items contain 1 item related to appearances. In general, however, several disease-specific aspects are not assessed such as jaw dysfunction as well as hearing and communication. The HNRQ is a 22-item interviewer-administered instrument that is comprised of six dimensions (skin, throat, oral stomatitis, digestion, energy, psychosocial) [12]. In addition to lacking disease-specific items or dimensions relevant to temporal bone disease, this instrument focuses on the quality of life impairment experienced by patients undergoing radiotherapy and not surgery. The QL-H&N is a 29-item quality of life instrument with three domains (physical, social, psychological) [13]. Noticeably this instrument lacks several areas of content validity relevant to temporal bone cancers such as items relevant to appearance, hearing and communication, and jaw dysfunction. The QLQ is a 19-item questionnaire with four domains (physical, functional/mood, psychological, and attitude to treatment) [14]. This instrument has not had significant psychometric testing with no available data on reliability and minimal evidence of validity. The QOL-RTI/H&N is a 39-item instrument comprised of four domains (functional, emotional, family, general) [15]. Although the instrument has undergone psychometric evaluation, it has not been widely used and lacks content validity for temporal bone cancers. The HNQOL is a 21-item instrument divided into four domains (pain, emotion, communication, eating) [16]. Like the other head and neck cancer-specific instruments, items relevant to mucosal head and neck cancers are assessed. However, many general quality of life questions are missing.

Given the absence of a truly disease-specific or location-specific instrument for temporal bone cancers or diseases of the lateral skull base, investigators may consider using instruments designed for measuring quality of life in the anterior skull base. Currently two such instruments exist, the Skull Base Inventory (SBI) and the Anterior Skull Base (ASB) Quality of Life [17, 18]. The SBI is a 41-item instrument with 11 domains (5 physical subdomains and 6 nonphysical domains including cognitive, emotional, financial, family, social, spiritual). This instrument was validated for patients with diseases of the anterior and central skull base [19]. Although there are some domains and items that may have cross-relevance to patients with diseases of the lateral skull base (e.g., cognitive, neurological domains and appearance item), there are many deficiencies of this instrument as it relates to measuring quality of life. For example, the SBI does not cover hearing and communication. The Anterior Skull Base Quality of Life Questionnaire is a 35-item instrument with 6 domains (performance, physical function, vitality, pain, specific symptoms, impact on emotions). The specific symptoms relate to problems experienced with anterior skull base pathology such as nasal, visual, and appearance issues.

Symptom-Specific Instruments for Temporal Bone Cancers

Facial Paralysis and Disfigurement Instruments

Given the course of the facial nerve through the temporal bone and parotid gland, it is not uncommon for facial paralysis to result from either the disease process itself or from the management of the disease process. Paralysis of the face is associated with depression, lower self-reported attractiveness, lower mood, and lower quality of life [20]. Facial paralysis is perceived by society to decrease quality of life, and members of society generally place significant value on minimizing the ill effects of facial paralysis [21]. Interestingly, however, patients with facial paralysis generally perceive their disability to be less than observers [22].

A recent systematic review identified 28 questionnaires assessing facial paralysis. Three of these instruments were validated for measuring quality of life in facial paralysis patients, the Facial Clinimetric Evaluation Scale (FACE), the Facial Disability Index (FDI), and a questionnaire to study aberrant nerve generation (Borodic) [23]. Although there is no truly disease-specific instrument for lateral skull base surgery, measurement of the impact of temporal bone cancers should incorporate some measure of facial nerve dysfunction given the impact this has on patient quality of life. One of several instruments may be used to capture the impact of facial paralysis on patient quality of life.

Still other questionnaires have been used to measure appearance and quality of life related to appearance changes or facial disfigurement following head and neck cancer treatment. One systematic review identified the following instruments to measure appearance after head and neck cancer: the UWQOL, the EORTC-HN35, the Head and Neck Survey (H&NS), and the Derriford Appearance Scale (DAS) [24]. The UWQOL instrument has a single item for appearance, one for anxiety and one for mood. The EORTC-HN35 has 35 disease-specific items, 1 of which relates to appearance, 2 items relate to social contact with friends and family, 1 relates to going out in public, 1 relates to physical contact with friends and family, and 1 relates sexual libido. The Head and Neck Survey is comprised of 11 items, of which 4 are related to appearance (1 relates to appearance and work, 1 to appearance and social activity, 1 to appearance and self-esteem, and 1 to appearance and recreational activity) [25]. Each item has 5-point Likert scale. This instrument has good test-retest reliability (0.88) and internal consistency (0.89) and good convergent validity with other instruments. Intra-rater reliability and stability have not been tested for the H&NS. The Derriford Appearance Scale (DAS) has not been validated for use in patients with head and neck cancer but is a validated instrument for facial appearance [26, 27]. It aims to measure psychological distress and dysfunction related to patients with appearance issues. The 59-item DAS (DAS59) has six different factors including general self-consciousness about appearance, social self-consciousness about appearance, sexual and bodily self-consciousness about appearance, facial self-consciousness about appearance, and physical distress and dysfunction. The DAS59 has good internal consistency (0.74–0.98), good test-retest reliability (0.86), good stability (postoperative scores differ from preoperative), as well as good convergent validity with other instruments. Table 32.2 reviews the content and strengths of each of these instruments.

Hearing Loss Instruments

Patients with temporal bone cancers may develop hearing loss either due to their disease process or due to its management. Surgical resection of structures of the middle ear during a lateral temporal bone resection with subsequent free tissue reconstruction, for example, may leave patients with a maximal conductive hearing loss. Although the cochlea is often delineated as an organ at risk during radiotherapy planning, sensorineural hearing loss may result from irreversible damage to the cochlea. Lastly, many chemotherapeutic agents may be ototoxic, particularly platinum-based agents commonly used in the management of head and neck cancers.

Single-sided deafness is not uncommon in patients treated for cancers of the temporal bone because of the proximity to critical auditory structures. This may result in an inability to properly localize sounds as well as an impairment of speech

Table 32.2 Symptom-specific instruments for temporal bone cancer

Instrument	Number of items	Number of domains	Relevant domains	Reliable	Valid
Facial paralysis instruments					
FACE	15	6	Facial movement, facial comfort, oral function, eye comfort, lacrimal control, social function	+	+
FDI	10	3	Disability Social Emotional	+	+
Borodic	n/a	5	Quality of life, self-image, social interaction, impairment of peripheral vision, perception of appearance	–	±
Facial appearance instruments					
UWQOL	12	9	Appearance	+	+
EORTC-HN35	35	7	Appearance	+	+
H&NS	11	4	Appearance and work, appearance and social activity, appearance and self-esteem, appearance and recreational activity	+	+
Derriford Appearance Scale (59 item)	59	6	General self-consciousness, social self-consciousness, sexual and bodily self-consciousness, facial self-consciousness, physical distress and dysfunction	+	+
Hearing loss instruments					
APHAB	24	4	Ease of communication, reverberation, speech understanding in background noise, aversiveness of sounds	+	+
SSQ	49	3	Speech hearing items, spatial hearing items, qualities of hearing items	+	+
GHABP	n/a	n/a	Assessment of hearing in four environments	+	+
SHQ	24	3	Localization, speech in noise, speech in quite	+	+
HHIA	25	2	Emotional, social/situational	+	+

perception in background noise. Hearing assistive devices that reroute sounds to the unaffected ear may be used in certain circumstances to mitigate the effect on quality of life.

Several instruments have been developed to capture the quality of life impact associated with hearing loss. Many of these instruments have been used to quantify the benefit of hearing assistive devices but are useful in assessing hearing-related quality of life particularly as it relates to single-sided deafness [28]. Instruments used to measure the impact of hearing rehabilitation include the Abbreviated Profile of Hearing Aid Benefit (APHAB) [29]; the Speech, Spatial and Qualities of Hearing Scale (SSQ) [30]; the Glasgow Hearing Aid Benefit Profile (GHABP) [31]; the Spatial Hearing Questionnaire (SHQ) [32]; and the Hearing Handicap Inventory for Adults (HHIA) [33]. The APHAB consists of 24 items divided into 4 subscales (ease of communication, reverberation, speech understanding in background noise, aversiveness of sounds) [29]. It is relatively simple to complete and may aid in quantifying hearing loss-related quality of life. The SSQ contains 49 items divided over 3 subscales (speech hearing items, spatial hearing items, and qualities of hearing items) [30]. The instrument purports to assess hearing disability with attention to hearing speech in competing contexts, to assess spatial hearing, and to assess qualities of speech such as clarity, identifiability of speakers, and different sounds. The GHABP assesses hearing rehabilitation in four prespecified environments (listening to television, having conversation in quiet, having conversation in busy street, having conversation in a group) [31]. For each environment in which the respondent experiences disability, they are asked about their initial disability, handicap, hearing aid use, hearing aid benefit, residual disability, and hearing aid satisfaction. The SHQ is a 24-item instrument which is comprised of three domains demonstrated through factor analysis (localization, speech in noise, speech in quite) [32]. Lastly, the HHIA is a 25-item instrument with two subscales (emotional, social/situational) [33]. Scores on this instrument correlate with pure-tone averages as well as word recognition scores suggesting good validity.

As with facial paralysis, one of many instruments may be used to measure the impact of hearing loss on quality of life after treatment of temporal bone cancers. However, many of these instruments may be of limited usefulness in this population, as hearing rehabilitation is not always a therapeutic option.

Quality of Life

Quality of Life for Skull Base Cancers

Over the past several decades, there has been significant evolution in the management of head and neck cancers. Evolution in treatment philosophy has resulted in an emphasis on preserving quality of life. Because of the location of many of these cancers, the quality of life implications are tremendous. Moreover, many cancers are associated with an overall poor prognosis, and treating oncologists are faced with a delicate balance of quantity and quality of life.

Over the past two to three decades, an abundance of literature has emerged particularly as it related to anterior skull base malignancies. In comparison, there has been a relative dearth of studies assessing quality of life for temporal bone and lateral skull base malignancies. However, many of the findings are applicable to both populations albeit with site-specific variability.

Early studies evaluating quality of life for patients with anterior skull base malignancies demonstrated that many of them suffer even after surviving their cancers. One study showed that as many as 89% of long-term survivors have ongoing physical complaints, with unsightly physical appearance being the most common complaint [34]. In addition, almost two thirds of the same survivors were dissatisfied by their surgical treatment. Following treatment, Gil et al. reported that 26% of patients will experience a deterioration in their quality of life following surgery for a skull base tumor [35].

Several factors have been shown to be associated with worsening of quality of life in patients with skull base cancer. Malignancy, radiotherapy, age, comorbidities, larger tumors, and tumor recurrences have all been shown to adversely affect patients' quality of life [19, 35–37]. Despite evidence to suggest long-standing physical complaints after treatment, most studies of quality of life in patients with skull base cancers seem to demonstrate a similar temporal trend following treatment. Patients experience a temporary decline in their quality of life between 3 and 6 months after surgery with a subsequent return to baseline at roughly 1 year following treatment [35, 37–39].

Quality of Life for Temporal Bone Cancers

Cancers affecting the temporal bone can be broad-ranging, extending from primary external auditory canal carcinoma to parotid malignancies with temporal bone extension to cutaneous malignancies with temporal bone involvement to nasopharyngeal carcinomas. Histopathologies may similarly vary including squamous cell carcinomas, basal cell carcinomas, minor salivary gland malignancies, and nasopharyngeal carcinomas to name a few. While surgical treatment is an important modality for many cancers, other treatment modalities such as radiotherapy and chemotherapy may also have an impact on patients' quality of life.

Surgery

Surgical procedures of temporal bone and surrounding structures may vary from sleeve resection of the external auditory canal to total temporal bone resection. In some instances, a simple mastoidectomy with facial nerve skeletonization is required for malignancies of the parotid gland; and for tumors of the jugular foramen, Fisch-type procedures may be required. The quality of life implications for any of these surgeries depend on the approach used as well as the extent of surgery.

For patients with early external auditory canal squamous cell carcinomas treated with lateral temporal bone resection, one study demonstrated good hearing preservation (75%) and corresponding quality of life in patients with lateral temporal bone resection reconstructed with a rolled-up split thickness skin graft compared to those who did not have a skin graft [7]. The hearing preservation corresponded to significantly higher quality of life scores as measured using the Glasgow Benefit Inventory in this study reinforcing the impact of hearing loss on quality of life and the importance for measurement of hearing-related quality of life. Total temporal bone resection, on the other hand, may be associated with significant quality of life impairments. In one study of 13 survivors after temporal bone resection, the main factors affecting quality of life were pain, appearance, and anxiety [40]. Although 69% of the patients reported good quality of life, many patients were encumbered by pain issues, problems with their temporomandibular joint function, and changes in their appearance. Interestingly, in this study facial nerve function did not seem to affect quality of life.

Another study reported quality of life outcomes for patients who had either temporal bone resections or parotidectomy with adjuvant radiotherapy [41]. This study focused primarily on facial nerve function, disfigurement, and hearing loss. Several measurement tools were used to address appearance issues (UWQOL, EORTC-HN35), hearing-related quality of life (APHAB, GBI), and general quality of life (Auckland Quality of Life Questionnaire (AQLQ), the General Health Questionnaire (GHQ)). With respect to appearances, both pinna resection ($p = 0.03$) and flap reconstruction ($p = 0.04$) resulted in statistically lower appearance scores based on the UWQOL appearance item. Interestingly, a House-Brackmann facial nerve score of >3 did not correlate with poorer appearance scores on either the UWQOL or EORTC-HN35 appearance items. It is unclear whether this is related to surgical correction or reconstruction as opposed to patients' acceptance of their deformity in lieu of surviving their cancer. With respect to hearing and communication, patients with temporal bone resections were more likely to have problems with binaural hearing, which in turn affected their ability to communicate with ease. In addition, patients suffered from a variety of physical complaints including swallowing difficulty, difficulty with mouth opening, as well as difficulty eating. Physical symptoms, communication difficulties, and social disturbances were all associated with poor global quality of life.

Patients with hearing loss following management of temporal bone cancers surprisingly do not correlate strongly with poor overall QOL scores [41]. This is likely due to the ability of patients to cope with adversities and functional limitations following surviving their cancers. Hearing rehabilitations, where possible, may provide some functional restoration with potential to improve overall quality of life. Recent reports suggest that patients who sustain cochlear and auditory pathway damage with radiation doses in excess of 30 Gy may be amenable to hearing rehabilitation. Case reports and small case series suggest that cochlear implantation may be possible in patients having sustained radiation injury to the cochlea, suggesting that the retrocochlear pathways are relatively spared from radiation injury [42]. In one study, the authors compared the patients with profound deafness after radiotherapy for nasopharyngeal carcinoma with patients who were non-irradiated and found similar hearing benefit with the aid of cochlear implantation in radiated vs. non-irradiated ears using the APHAB [42–44]. Adunka et al. describe experience in cochlear implantation in a patient who underwent a labyrinth preserving temporal bone resection with free tissue reconstruction with the caveats that there is no cochlear fibrosis, chronic suppurative otitis media with cholesteatoma, or significantly impaired soft tissue and wound healing issues. Other hearing rehabilitations options include bone-anchored hearing aids (BAHAs) for those patients whose soft tissues and bone would tolerate such procedure [45].

Much like with hearing rehabilitation, facial reconstructive surgery for facial paralysis and disfigurement may have a perceived benefit on quality of life from a societal perspective [21]. Members of the general public perceive the quality of life associated with unilateral facial paralysis to be less than that associated with monocular blindness, and individuals would be willing to sacrifice years of living in exchange for reconstructive procedures to improve appearances [46]. These findings stress the importance of adequate and sound facial reanimation procedures to achieve symmetry at rest with the use of static and dynamic slings, neuromuscular tone with nerve grafting where possible, and soft tissue augmentation with free tissue reconstruction after surgical resection. Surprisingly, the perceived impairment of quality of life created by facial paralysis and disfigurement, however, is not reflected with actual quality of life losses in patients with facial paralysis [28]. This incongruence is likely due to quality of life patient adaptation after surviving cancer.

Radiotherapy

Lambert et al. reviewed the impact of radiotherapy for head and neck cancers on the temporal bone [47]. Radiotherapy may injure the cochlea causing sensorineural hearing loss, may alter middle ear function by damaging the Eustachian tube and middle ear, and may result in temporal bone osteoradionecrosis.

The cochlea is often delineated as an organ at risk during radiation planning but has been shown to be susceptible to injury with higher radiation doses. Doses of between 30 and 50 Gy may result in irreversible damage to the cochlea and permanent sensorineural hearing loss with pathological evidence of fibrosis of the cochlea [48–50], even with the advent of intensity-modulated radiotherapy (IMRT), as many as half (46%) of patients treated for nasopharyngeal carcinoma may develop hearing loss [51].

Damage to the middle ear after radiation for parotid or nasopharyngeal cancers may cause chronic serous otitis media, otorrhea, and/or conductive hearing loss. As many as 26% of patients with parotid cancers may suffer from middle ear dysfunction [52, 53]. Ongoing middle ear issues can impact the quality of life of these patients necessitating multiple doctor's visits as well as long-term topical and systemic therapies.

The treatment of nasopharyngeal carcinomas with definitive radiotherapy often has an impact on temporal bone structures because of the anatomic proximity. Using the UWQOL, one study evaluated the impact of treatment on quality of life for patients with NPC [54]. Overall patients rated themselves as having a "good" quality of life but noted problems with dry mouth, chewing, and ear problems. The authors concluded that conformal radiotherapy sparing both salivary glands and the temporal bone may help minimize morbidity and optimize quality of life outcomes for these patients.

Other Functional Limitations and Quality of Life

Although treatment of cancers involving the temporal bone may result in a number of functional sequelae, not all of these functional limitations are necessarily associated with a reduction or impairment in quality of life. It is, however, important to consider relevant functional limitations associated with treatment as these may often lead to an impact in quality of life. Temporal lobe necrosis, temporal bone osteoradionecrosis, and chronic suppurative otitis media are a few such sequelae of treatment with implications on quality of life. These sequelae of treatment and resulting functional deficits are difficult to quantify in the absence of validated measurement instruments, but they are nonetheless important considerations with respect to quality of life.

Temporal lobe necrosis is a rare complication of treatment, but the impact on quality of life may potentially be severe. This clinical entity may be associated with memory loss, headaches, vertigo, and neurological deficits such as sensory aphasia, cranial neuropathy, and epilepsy [55]. Many of these deficits may result in a functional and quality of life decline.

Temporal bone osteoradionecrosis may represent a chronic problem after radiotherapy for patients with temporal bone cancers. Sequestra of bone and exposure of bone particularly in the external canal are early signs of this chronic disease process. It may also be associated with fistula formation, malignant otitis externa, skull base osteomyelitis, meningitis, brain abscess, and even carotid artery aneurysms [47].

Chronic suppurative otitis media may afflict those with head and neck cancers affecting the temporal bone. Radiation-associated otitis media may occur in up to 26% of patients receiving radiotherapy for parotid cancers [52]. The etiology of this disease process seems primarily related to fibrosis of the Eustachian tube primarily in nasopharyngeal carcinomas. Regardless of the etiology, the long-standing otorrhea, associated hearing loss, and requirement of ventilation tubes can dramatically impact patient quality of life.

Future Research Efforts in Quality of Life

Future research efforts to delineate the impact of temporal bone disease and quality of life should be focused on development of a reliable and valid disease and site-specific instrument for measurement of quality of life. Use of a valid instrument may explore deficiencies in quality of life following treatment and help to counsel patients on potential impact of therapy. Such instruments must include items and domains related to general functioning, social well-being, emotional well-being, the impact of facial disfigurement and paralysis, the impact of unilateral or bilateral hearing loss, the impact of chronic ear dysfunction, as well as other physical and functional limitations (e.g., jaw dysfunction and cognitive impairment) (Fig. 32.1).

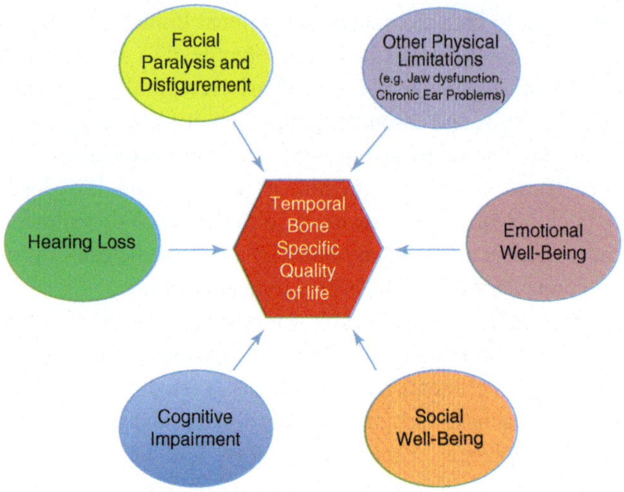

Fig. 32.1 Proposed dimension of quality of life for temporal bone cancers

References

1. World Health Organization (WHO). Rehabilitation after cardiovascular diseases, with special emphasis on developing countries: report of a WHO expert committee. WHO technical report series 831. Geneva: WHO; 1993.
2. Gil Z, Abergel A, Spektor S, Khafif A, Fliss DM. Patient, caregiver, and surgeon perceptions of quality of life following anterior skull base surgery. Arch Otolaryngol Head Neck Surg. 2004;131(11):1276–81.
3. Ware JE, Sherbourne CD. The MOS 36-item short-form health survey (SF-36). Med Care. 1992;30(6):473–83.
4. Lang DA, Neil-Dwyer G, Garfield J. Outcome after complex neurosurgery: the caregiver's burden is forgotten. J Neurosurg. 1999;91(3):359–63.
5. Neil-Dwyer G, Lang DA, Davis A. Outcome from complex neurosurgery: an evidence based approach. Acta Neurochir. 2000;142(4):367–71.
6. Robinson K, Gatehouse S, Browning GG. Measuring benefit in otorhinolaryngologic surgery and therapy. Ann Otol Rhinol Laryngol. 1996;105(6):415–22.
7. Morita S, Nakamura Y, Homma A, et al. Hearing preservation after lateral temporal bone resection for early-stage external auditory canal carcinoma. Audiol Neurootol. 2014;19(6):351–7.
8. Ringash J, Bezjak A. A structured review of quality of life instruments for head and neck cancer patients. Head Neck. 2001;23(3):201–13.
9. Hassan SJ, Weymuller EA. Assessment of quality of life in head and neck cancer patients. Head Neck. 1993;15:485–96.
10. Bjordal K, Kaasa S. Psychometric validation of the EORTC core quality of life questionnaire, 30-item version and a diagnosis-specific module for head and neck cancer patients. Acta Oncol. 1992;31:311–21.
11. Cella DF. F.A.C.I.T. manual, version 4. Evanston, NY: Centre on Outcomes, Research and Education, Evanston Northwestern Healthcare and Northwestern University; 1997.
12. Browman GP, Levine MN, Hodson ID, et al. The head and neck radiotherapy questionnaire: a morbidity/quality of life instrument for clinical trials of radiation therapy in locally advanced head and neck cancer. J Clin Oncol. 1993;11(5):863–72.
13. Morton RP, Witterick IJ. Rationale and development of a quality-of-life instrument for head-and -neck cancer patients. Am J Otolaryngol. 1995;16(5):284–93.
14. Rathmell AJ, Ash DV, Howes M, et al. Assessing quality of life in patients treated for advanced head and neck cancer. Clin Oncol. 1991;3:10–6.
15. Trotti A, Johnson DJ, Gwede C, et al. Development of a head and neck companion module for the Quality of Life-Radiation Therapy Instrument (QOL-RTI). Int J Radiat Oncol Biol Phys. 1998;4292:257–61.
16. Terrell JE, Nanavati KA, Esclamado RM, et al. Head and neck cancer-specific quality of life. Arch Otolaryngol Head Neck Surg. 1997;123:1125–32.
17. de Almeida JR, Vescan AD, Gullane PJ, et al. Development of a disease-specific quality of life questionnaire for anterior and central skull base pathology—the skull base inventory. Laryngoscope. 2012;122(9):1933–42.
18. Gil Z, Abergel A, Spektor S, et al. Development of a cancer-specific anterior skull base quality-of-life questionnaire. J Neurosurg. 2004;100(5):813–9.
19. Larjani S, Monteiro E, Witterick I, et al. Preliminary cross-sectional reliability and validity of the Skull Base Inventory (SBI) quality of life questionnaire. J Otolaryngol Head Neck Surg. 2016;45(1):45.
20. Nellis JC, Ishii M, Byrne PJ, Boahene KD, Dey JK, Ishii LE. Association among facial paralysis, depression, and quality of life in facial plastic surgery patients. JAMA Facial Plast Surg. 2016;19(3):190–6.
21. Su P, Ishii LE, Joseph A, et al. Societal value on surgery for facial reanimation. JAMA Facial Plast Surg. 2016;19(2):139–46.
22. Goines JB, Ishii LE, Dey JK, et al. Association of facial paralysis-related disability with patient and observer perceived quality of life. JAMA Facial Plast Surg. 2016;18(5):363–9.
23. Ho AL, Scott AM, Klassen AF, et al. Measuring quality of life and patient satisfaction in facial paralysis patients: a systematic review of patient reported outcome measures. Plast Reconstr Surg. 2012;130(1):91–9.
24. Djan R, Penington A. A systematic review of questionnaires to measure the impact of appearance on quality of life for head and neck cancer patients. J Plast Reconstr Aesthet Surg. 2013;66(5):647–59.
25. Gliklich RE, Goldsmith TA, Funk GF. Are head and neck specific quality of life measures necessary? Head Neck. 1997;19:474–80.
26. Klassen A, Jenkinson C, Fitzpatrick R, Goodacre T. Measuring quality of life in cosmetic surgery patients with a condition-specific instrument: the Derriford scale. Br J Plast Surg. 1998;51(5):380e4. [Epub 1998/10/15]
27. Harris D, Carr T, Moss T. Manual for Derriford appearance scale 59 (DAS59). Avon: Musketeer Press; 2004. p. 38.
28. Kitterick PT, Lucas L, Smith SN. Improving health related quality of life in single-sided deafness: a systematic review and meta-analysis. Audiol Neurootol. 2015;20(Suppl 1):79–86.
29. Cox RM, Alexander GC. The abbreviated profile of hearing aid benefit. Ear Hear. 1995;16:176–86.
30. Gatehouse S, Noble W. The speech, spatial and qualities of hearing scale (SSQ). Int J Audiol. 2004;43:85–9.
31. Gatehouse S. Glasgow hearing aid benefit profile: derivation and validation of a client-centered outcome measure for hearing-aid services. J Am Acad Audiol. 1999;10:80–103.
32. Tyler RS, Perreau AE, Ji H. Validation of the spatial hearing questionnaire. Ear Hear. 2009;30:466–74.
33. Newman CW, Weinstein BE, Jacobson GP, Hug GA. The hearing handicap inventory for adults: psychometric adequacy and audiometric correlates. Ear Hear. 1990;11:430–3.
34. Fukuda K, Saeki N, Mine S, et al. Evaluation of outcome and QOL in patients with craniofacial resection for malignant tumors involving the anterior skull base. Neurol Res. 2000;22(6):545–50.

35. Gil Z, Abergel A, Spektor S, et al. Quality of life following surgery for anterior skull base tumors. Arch Otolaryngol Head Neck Surg. 2003;129(12):1303–9.
36. Deckard NA, Harrow BR, Barnett SL, Batra PS. Comparative analysis of quality of life metrics after endoscopic surgery for sinonasal neoplasms. Am J Rhinol Allergy. 2015;29(2):151–5.
37. Castelnuovo P, Lepera D, Turri-Zanoni M, et al. Quality of life following endoscopic endonasal resection of anterior skull base cancers. J Neurosurg. 2013;119(6):1401–9.
38. McCoul ED, Anand VK, Schwartz TH. Improvements in site-specific quality of life 6 months after endoscopic anterior skull base surgery: a prospective study. J Neurosurg. 2012;117(3):498–506.
39. Abergel A, Fliss DM, Margalit N, Gil Z. A prospective evaluation of short-term health-related quality of life in patients undergoing anterior skull base surgery. Skull Base. 2010;20(1):27–33.
40. De Casso C, Kwhaja S, Davies S, et al. Effect of temporal bone resection on temporomandibular joint function: a quality of life study. Otolaryngol Head Neck Surg. 2010;142(1):85–9.
41. Kwok HCK, Morton RP, Chaplin JM, et al. Quality of life after parotid and temporal bone surgery for cancer. Laryngoscope. 2002;112:820–33.
42. Soh JM, D'Souza VD, Sarepaka GL, Ng WN, Ong CS, Low WK. Cochlear implant outcomes: a comparison between irradiated and non-irradiated ears. Clin Exp Otorhinolaryngol. 2012;5(Suppl 1):S93–8.
43. Chua DY, Tan HK. Successful rehabilitation with cochlear implant in post-irradiation induced hearing loss in nasopharyngeal carcinoma patient. Ann Acad Med Singap. 2007;36(1):74–7.
44. Adunka OF, Buchman CA. Cochlear implantation in the irradiated temporal bone. J Laryngol Otol. 2007;121(1):83–6.
45. Marzo SJ, Benscoter B, Leonetti JP. Contemporary options for lateral skull base reconstruction following tumor extirpation. Curr Opin Otolaryngol Head Neck Surg. 2011;19(5):330–4.
46. Sinno H, Thibaudeau S, Izadpanah A, Tahiri Y, Christodoulou G, Zuker R, Lin SJ. Utility outcome scores for unilateral facial paralysis. Ann Plast Surg. 2012;69(4):435–8.
47. Lambert EM, Gunn GB, Gidley PW. Effects of radiation on the temporal bone in patients with head and neck cancer. Head Neck. 2016;38(9):1428–35.
48. Oh YT, Kim CH, Choi JH, Kang SH, Chun M. Sensory neural hearing loss after concurrent cisplatin and radiation therapy for nasopharyngeal carcinoma. Radiother Oncol. 2004;72:79–82.
49. Pan CC, Eisbruch A, Lee JS, Snorrason RM, Ten Haken RK, Kileny PR. Prospective study of inner ear radiation dose and hearing loss in head-and neck cancer patients. Int J Radiat Oncol Biol Phys. 2005;61:1393–402.
50. van der Putten L, de Bree R, Plukker JT, et al. Permanent unilateral hearing loss after radiotherapy for parotid gland tumors. Head Neck. 2006;28:902–8.
51. Hsin CH, Chen TH, Young YH, Liu WS. Comparison of otologic complications between intensity-modulated and two-dimensional radiotherapies in nasopharyngeal carcinoma patients. Otolaryngol Head Neck Surg. 2010;143:662–8.
52. Hsu MM, Young YH, Lin KL. Eustachian tube function of patients with nasopharyngeal carcinoma. Ann Otol Rhinol Laryngol. 1995;104:453–5.
53. Young YH, Hsieh T. Eustachian tube dysfunction in patients with nasopha-ryngeal carcinoma, pre- and post-irradiation. Eur Arch Otorhinolaryngol. 1992;249:206–8.
54. Talmi YP, Horowitz Z, Bedrin L, et al. Quality of life of nasopharyngeal carcinoma patients. Cancer. 2002;94(4):1012–7.
55. Mou YG, Sai K, Wang ZN, Zhang XH, Lu YC, Wei DN, Yang QY, Chen ZP. Surgical management of radiation induced temporal lobe necrosis patients with nasopharyngeal carcinoma: report of 14 cases. Head Neck. 2011;33(10):1493–500.

Index

P. W. Gidley, F. DeMonte (eds.), *Temporal Bone Cancer*, https://doi.org/10.1007/978-3-319-74539-8

N

U

V

W

X

The manufacturer's authorised representative in the EU is Springer Nature Customer Service Centre GmbH, Europaplatz 3, 69115 Heidelberg, Germany. If you have any concerns regarding our products, please contact ProductSafety@springernature.com

Printed and bound by CPI Group (UK) Ltd, Croydon, CR0 4YY
30/09/2026
02225479-0001